*Education, Ethics and Empathy*

# API Medicine
# A-Clinical Compendium 2025

*Education, Ethics and Empathy*

# API Medicine A-Clinical Compendium 2025


***Editors***

**Jyotirmoy Pal** MD(General Medicine) FRCP FICP FACP WHO Fellow
Professor
Department of General Medicine
University College of Medicine and Sagore Dutta Medical College
Kamarhati, West Bengal, India
Former Dean, Indian College of Physicians (ICP)
President-Elect, Association of Physicians (API)

**Nandini Chatterjee** MD FRCP(London, Glasgow) FICP
Professor
Department of Medicine
Institute of Postgraduate Medical Education and Research (IPGMER)
Kolkata, West Bengal, India
API Scientific Convener
Ex-Editor, Journal of the Indian Medical Association (JIMA)
Editor, Bengal Physician Journal



JAYPEE

**JAYPEE BROTHERS MEDICAL PUBLISHERS**

*The Health Sciences Publisher*

**New Delhi | London**

JAYPEE Jaypee Brothers Medical Publishers (P) Ltd

**Headquarters**
EMCA House
23/23-B, Ansari Road, Daryaganj
New Delhi 110 002, India
Landline: +91-11-23272143, +91-11-23272703
+91-11-23282021, +91-11-23245672
E-mail: jaypee@jaypeebrothers.com

**Corporate Office**
Jaypee Brothers Medical Publishers (P) Ltd.
4838/24, Ansari Road, Daryaganj
New Delhi 110 002, India
Phone: +91-11-43574357
Fax: +91-11-43574314
E-mail: jaypee@jaypeebrothers.com

**Overseas Office**
JP Medical Ltd.
83, Victoria Street, London
SW1H 0HW (UK)
Phone: +44-20 3170 8910
Fax: +44(0)20 3008 6180
E-mail: info@jpmedpub.com

Website: www.jaypeebrothers.com
Website: www.jaypeedigital.com



**Inquiries for bulk sales may be solicited at:** jaypee@jaypeebrothers.com

*API Medicine: A-Clinical Compendium 2025* / ***Jyotirmoy Pal, Nandini Chatterjee***

*First Edition*: **2025**

ISBN: 978-93-6616-804-3

*Printed in India*

## DISCLAIMER

# EDITORIAL BOARD

# Contributors

**Abha Gupta** MBBS MD
Professor of Medicine
LLRM Medical College
Meerut, Uttar Pradesh, India

**Abhay Kumar** MBBS MS(General Surgery) MCh(Cardiothoracic and Vascular Surgery)
Cardiothoracic and Vascular Surgeon
Aakash Healthcare Super Speciality Hospital
Dwarka, New Delhi, India

**Abhay Sahoo** MBBS MD(General Medicine) DM(Endocrinology and Metabolism) FACE(Fellowship in American College of Endocrinology)
Senior Consultant
Department of Endocrinology and Metabolism
Apollo Hospitals
Bhubaneswar, Odisha, India

**Abhishek Dixit** DM(Neurology)
Associate Consultant
Department of Neurology
BLK-Max Super Speciality Hospital
MAX Healthcare
Rajendra Place, New Delhi, India

**Abhishek Shrivastava** MBBS MD(General Medicine) DM(Endocrinology) DEM(Endocrinology)
Endocrinologist
Medical College Colony
Jabalpur, Madhya Pradesh, India

**Abhishek Singhai** MBBS MD(General Medicine)
Associate Professor
General Medicine
AIIMS, Bhopal
Bhopal, Madhya Pradesh, India

**Abhranil Dhar** MBBS MD(General Medicine) DM(Endocrinology)
Junior Resident
Department of Endocrinology
IPGME&R
Kolkata, West Bengal, India

**Akash Pawar** MBBS MD(General Medicine)
Assistant Professor
General Medicine
AIIMS, Bhopal
Bhopal, Madhya Pradesh, India

**Akhilesh Kumar Singh** MD(Medicine)
Professor
Department of Medicine
SN Medical College
Agra, Uttar Pradesh, India

**Amandeep Kaur** MBBS MD(Medicine)
Associate Professor
AIIMS, Bathinda
Bathinda, Punjab, India

**Anand Dev** MBBS MD(General Medicine)
General Physician
Anand Kumar Clinic
Patna, Bihar, India

**Anand Kate** MBBS MD(Cardiology)
Cardiologist
Ameya General Hospital
Nagpur, Maharashtra, India

**Aneesha G** MBBS MD(General Medicine) DNB(Obstetrics and Gynecology) MNAMS MSc(Clinical Embrology)
Consultant
NOVA IVF Fertility Center
Gurugram, Haryana, India

**Anirban Paul** MBBS MS(Orthopedics)
Orthopedic Surgeon
New Town Nursing Home
Kolkata, West Bengal, India

**Anismita Basu** MBBS MD(General Medicine)
Junior Resident
Calcutta National Medical
Kolkata, West Bengal, India

**Anupama YJ** MBBS MD(General Medicine) DNB(Nephrology)
Consultant Nephrologist
Nanjappa Hospital
Shivamogga, Karnataka, India

**Aradhya Sekhar Bagchi** MBBS MD(Internal Medicine)
Senior Resident (Neurology)
NIMHANS
Bengaluru, Karnataka, India

**AR Balamurugan** MD(General Medicine) MBBS Diploma in Tuberculosis and Chest Diseases(DTCD) Internal Medicine
Pulmonologist
Swasam Speciality Clinic
Chennai, Tamil Nadu, India

**Arghya Chattopadhyay** MBBS MD(General Medicine) DM(Clinical Immunology and Rheumatology)
Consultant Rheumatology
Fortis Anandapur
Kolkata, West Bengal, India

**Arjun Tandon** MBBS Senior Resident DM(Interventional Cardiology)
Department of Interventional Cardiology
IMS-BHU
Varanasi, Uttar Pradesh, India

**Arunangshu Banerjee** MD(Medicine) DM(Nephrology)
Nephrologist, Astha Medical Center
Bardhaman, West Bengal, India

**Arup Kumar Kundu** MD FRCP FICP MNAS
Ex-Professor of Medicine and In-Charge, Division of Rheumatology
Department of Medicine
RG Kar Medical College
Kolkata, West Bengal, India

**Ashutosh Chaturvedi** MBBS MS(Neurosurgery) MCh(Neurosurgery)
Neurosurgeon, Galaxy Hospital
Varanasi, Uttar Pradesh, India

**Ashwini C** MBBS MDRD EDiR
Consultant
Manipal Hospitals Radiology Group
Bengaluru, Karnataka, India

**Asish Kumar Basu** MBBS DT&H Dip(Cardiology) MD(Medicine) DM(Endocrine)
Endocrinologist and Diabetologist
Apollo Clinic
Kolkata, West Bengal, India

**Atanu Chandra** MD(Medicine) DNB(Medicine) MRCP(UK)
Assistant Professor
Department of Internal Medicine
Bankura Sammilani Medical College
Bankura, West Bengal, India

**Atul Mehrotra** MBBS MD(General Medicine) Diploma in Tuberculosis and Chest Diseases(DTCD)
Consultant Physician
Mehrotra Family Clinic
Lucknow, Uttar Pradesh, India

**Azifa Taj Nazer** MBBS PG Resident(General Medicine)
Post Graduate Trainee
Department of General Medicine
All India Institute of Medical Sciences, Kalyani
Kalyani, West Bengal, India

**Balachandra R** MBBS MS(General Surgery) Diploma(Diabetology)
Diabetologist
Lakshmana Multispeciality Hospital
Madurai, Tamil Nadu, India

**Bhagirath B Solanki** MBBS MD(Psychiatry)
Professor and Head
Department of Medicine
BJ Medical College and Civil Hospital
Ahmedabad, Gujarat, India
Life member of IMA, APG, API, CSI, RSSDI

**Bharatsing D Rathod** MBBS MD(General Medicine)
Associate Professor
All India Institute of Medical Sciences, Nagpur
Nagpur, Maharashtra India

**Bhaskar Ghosh** MBBS MD(General Medicine) DNB(Neurology) MNAMS DM
Neurologist
BR Singh Hospital and Center for Medical Education and Research
Eastern Railway
Kolkata, West Bengal, India

**Bhupen Barman** MD(General Medicine)
Professor
Department of General Medicine
All India Institute of Medical Sciences, Guwahati
Guwahati, Assam, India

**Biva Bhakat** MBBS MD(General Medicine)
Consultant, Private Clinic
Kolkata, West Bengal, India

**Boudhayan Das Munshi** MBBS DNB(General Medicine) Fellowship in Diabetology(JIPMER) MNAMS
Associate Professor General Medicine
All India Institute of Medical Sciences, Kalyani
Kalyani, West Bengal, India

**Chiranjita Phukan** MBBS MD(Medicine)
Associate Professor of Medicine
Gauhati Medical College
Guwahati, Assam, India

**Debaditya Chatterjee** MBBS MD(General Medicine)
General Physician
Apollo Medical Center
Kolkata, West Bengal, India

**Debaleena Mukherjee** MBBS MD(General Medicine) DM(Neurology)
Senior Resident
Department of Neurology
Institute of Post Graduate Medical Education and Research and Seth Sukhlal Karnani Memorial Hospital
Kolkata, West Bengal, India

**Debalina Sarkar** MBBS MD DM(Endocrinology)
Clinical Tutor
Department of Endocrinology
Medical College
Kolkata, West Bengal, India

**Deepak Kumar** MBBS MD(Anesthesiology)
Assistant Professor (Emergency Medicine)
AIIMS, Patna
Patna, Bihar, India

**Deepanjan Bhattacharya** MBBS MD(Pediatrics) DM(Cardiology)
Assistant Professor
Department of Cardiology
All India Institute of Medical Sciences, Kalyani
Kalyani, West Bengal, India

**Deepthi Vemula** MD MBBS(Internal Medicine)
Professor
Department of General Medicine
KIIT University
Bhubaneswar, Odisha, India

**Deepu Peter** MBBS MD(General Medicine)
Assistant Professor
Department of Pulmonary Medicine
Command Hospital (NC)
Udhampur, Jammu and Kashmir, India

**Dipanjan Bandyopadhyay** MBBS MD FIACM
Senior Consultant
Department of Internal Medicine
Thalamus Institute of Medical Sciences
Siliguri, West Bengal, India

**Dipesh Kumar Dhoot** DM(Nephrology) MD(General Medicine) MBBS
Nephrologist/Renal Specialist
Mission Hospital
Durgapur, West Bengal, India

**Gouranga Santra** MBBS MD(General Medicine) FICP FIACM
Professor and Head
Department of Medicine
Deben Mahata Govt Medical College
Purulia, West Bengal, India

**Gwenette A War** MBBS MD(General Medicine)
Assistant Professor
Department of General Medicine
All India Institute of Medical Sciences, Guwahati
Guwahati, Assam, India

**Harshita Vaddi** MBBS
Senior Resident
All India Institute of Medical Sciences, Bibinagar
Bibinagar, Telangana, India

**Jaydeep Majumdar** MBBS DNB FVRS
Consultant in Susrut Eye Foundation and Research Center
Kolkata, West Bengal, India

**Jayeeta Bhowmick** MBBS (MC Cal) (Gold Medalist) MD(IPGMER Cal) (Gold Medalist) DM(Gastroenterology) MRCP(SCE Gastro and Hepato, UK)
Assistant Professor and Acting Head
Department of Gastroenterology
AIIMS, Kalyani
Kalyani, West Bengal, India

**Joydeep Mukherjee** MBBS MD DM(Neurology)
Neurologist
Department of Neurology
NIMHANS
Bengaluru, Karnataka, India

**Jyoti Jha** MBBS MD(General Medicine)
General Physician
Khushi Medical Center
Najafgarh, New Delhi, India

**Kanchan Kiran Kujur** MBBS MD(General Medicine)
Assistant Professor
AIIMS, Deoghar
Deoghar West Bengal, India

**Kaushik Basu** MBBS MD(General Medicine) DM(Rheumatology)
Rheumatologist
HealthETC
Kolkata, West Bengal, India

**Kaushik Biswas** MBBS MD(General Medicine) DM(Endocrinology)
Senior Consultant
Medica Superspecialty Hospital
Kolkata, West Bengal, India

**Kausik Bhar** MBBS MD(General Medicine)
General Physician
Department of Internal Medicine
The West Bengal University of Health Sciences
Kolkata, West Bengal, India

**Keshao Nagpure** MBBS MD(General Medicine)
Assistant Professor
All India Institute of Medical Sciences, Raipur
Raipur, Chhattisgarh, India

**Khemeswar Agasti** MBBS MD(General Medicine)
General Practitioner
Department of General Medicine
SCB Medical College
Cuttack, Odisha, India

**Kirandeep Kour** MD DM(Endocrinology)
Assistant Professor
Department of General Medicine
AIIMS, Jammu
Jammu and Kashmir, India

**Kiran Vadapalli** MBBS MD(General Medicine) DM(Critical Care Medicine) DNB(CCM)
Assistant Professor
AMCU, Rangaraya Medical College and Government Hospital
Kakinada, Andhra Pradesh, India

**Kripasindhu Gantait** MBBS MD(Medicine) DSc FICP FIACM FIAMS
Professor and Head
Jhargram Government Medical College
Jhargram, West Bengal, India

**Krishna Padarabinda Tripathy** MBBS MD(General Medicine)
Professor
KIIT University
Bhubaneswar, Odisha, India

**Kutty Sharada Vinod** MBBS DM(Pulmonary Critical Care and Sleep Medicine) MD(Medicine) European Diploma in Adult Respiratory Medicine (Switzerland) MRCP SCE(Respiratory Medicine)
Associate Professor
Department of Internal Medicine
AIIMS, Mangalagiri
Mangalagiri, Andhra Pradesh, India

**Madhuchanda Kar** MBBS MD(General Medicine) PhD
Oncologist
Department of Oncology
Peerless Hospital
Kolkata, West Bengal, India

**Mahesh Ravikumar Jansari** MBBS MD(Pulmonology)
Associate Professor
Department of Pulmonary Medicine
AIIMS, Kalyani
Kalyani, West Bengal, India

**Mainak Mukhopadhyay** MBBS MD(General Medicine) DM(Cardiology) FESC
Cardiologist
Department of Cardiology
Manipal Hospitals
Broadway, Kolkata, West Bengal, India

**Manish Khandare** MBBS MD(Dermatology, Venereology and Leprology)
Assistant Professor
Department of Dermatology, STD and Leprosy
AIIMS, Bhopal
Bhopal, Madhya Pradesh, India

**Man Mohan Mehndiratta**
MD(Medicine) DNB(Medicine) DM(Neurology) FAAN FANA FAMS MNAMS FRCP FICP FIAN
Principal-Director
Department of Neurology
BLK-Max Super Speciality Hospital, MAX Healthcare
Rajendra Place, New Delhi, India

**Manuj Kumar Sarkar** MBBS MD(Internal Medicine)
Associate Professor
Department of General Medicine
All India Institute of Medical Sciences, Deoghar
Deoghar, Jharkhand, India

**Md Jamil** MBBS MD(General Medicine)
Associate Professor
Department of General Medicine
AIIMS, Guwahati
Guwahati, Assam, India

**Mohd Asif** MBBS MD(General Medicine)
Assistant Professor
All India Institute of Medical Sciences, Mangalagiri
Mangalagiri, Andhra Pradesh, India

**Monica Gupta** MBBS(AIIMS) MD(AIIMS) DNB MAMS FIMSA FIACM
Professor
Government Medical College and Hospital
Chandigarh, India

**Mrinal Kanti Roy** MBBS MD(General Medicine) DM(Neurology)
Neurologist
Lifeline Medicity
Kalyani, West Bengal, India

**Mudalsha Ravina** MBBS DNB(Nuclear Medicine)
Associate Professor
AIIMS, Raipur
Raipur Chhattisgarh, India

**Mugundhan Krishnan** MBBS MD(General Medicine) DM(Neurology)
Professor and Head
Department of Neurology
Government Kilpauk Medical College
Chennai, Tamil Nadu, India

**Nandini Chatterjee** MD FRCP(London, Glasgow) FICP
Professor
Department of Medicine
Institute of Postgraduate Medical Education and Research (IPGMER)
Kolkata, West Bengal, India
API Scientific Convener
Ex-Editor, Journal of the Indian Medical Association (JIMA)
Editor, Bengal Physician Journal

**Naresh Kumar Midha** MBBS MD(General Medicine)
Associate Professor
AIIMS, Jodhpur
Jodhpur, Rajasthan, India

**Narmada Prasad Patel** MBBS MD(General Medicine)
Associate Professor of Medicine
LN Medical College
Bhopal, Madhya Pradesh, India

**Nazneen Nahar Begam** MBBS(Gold Medalist) MD(Tropical Medicine) DM(Infectious Diseases)
Consultant
Department of Infectious Diseases
Sarvodaya Hospital
Faridabad, Haryana, India

**Neeradi Charan** MBBS MD(General Medicine)
Assistant Professor
Department of General Medicine
All India Institute of Medical Sciences, Bibinagar
Bibinagar, Telangana, India

**Neeraj Kapoor** MBBS MD(General Medicine)
Assistant Professor
Shri Ram Murti Smarak Institute of Medical Sciences
Bareilly, Uttar Pradesh, India

**Niladri Das** MBBS MD(Internal Medicine) DM(Endocrinology)
Endocrinologist
Private Clinic
West Bengal, India

**Niket Verma** MBBS MD(Medicine)
Assistant Professor
Department of Medicine
AIIMS, Bathinda
Bathinda, Punjab, India

**Nishant Tomar** MD(Pediatrics) DrNB Student(Neurology)
Department of Neurology
BLK-Max Super Speciality Hospital, MAX Healthcare
Rajendra Place, New Delhi, India

**Nishi Kant** MBBS MD(General Medicine) DM(Endocrinology)
Diabetologist
Rockland Hospital
New Delhi, India

**Nongmaithem Bikash Singh** MBBS
Junior Resident
AIIMS, Delhi
New Delhi, India

**Onkar Awadhiya** MBBS MD(General Medicine)
Assistant Professor
Department of General Medicine
All India Institute of Medical Sciences, Nagpur
Nagpur, Maharashtra, India

**Pankaj Singhania** MBBS MD(General Medicine) DM(Endocrinology)
Endocrinologist
Arogyam Health Care
Purulia, West Bengal, India

**Paramita Bhattacharya** BPT MPT(Neurology)
Physiotherapist, Apollo Hospital
Chennai, Tamil Nadu, India

**Parthajit Das** MBBS MD FRCP(London) FRCP(Edinburgh) MRCP(Rheumatology) MSC(Sports Medicine)
Rheumatologist, Asian Institute of Immunology and Rheumatology
Kolkata, West Bengal, India

**Partha Sarkar** MBBS MD FICP
Professor and Head
Department of General Medicine
Tamralipto Govt Medical College and Hospital
Tamluk, West Bengal, India

**Pavithra Ravi** MBBS
Resident Doctor
SRM Medical College Hospital and Research Center
Chennai, Tamil Nadu, India

**Piyush Kumar Gupta** MBBS MD(Community Medicine)
Senior Resident
AIIMS, Rishikesh
Rishikesh, Uttarakhand, India

**Plawan Mazumdar** MBBS MD(Internal Medicine)
General Physician
Arogya Bongaigaon
Bongaigaon, Assam, India

**Pooja Baradia** MBBS MD(Medicine)
PG Resident
LN Medical College and JK Hospital
Bhopal, Madhya Pradesh, India

**Poulami Das** MBBS MD(General Medicine)
Cardiologist, Private Clinic
Bhandup West, Mumbai, Maharashtra, India

**Pradeep K Maheshwari** MBBS MD(General Medicine)
Additional Professor
Department of Pediatrics
All India Institute of Medical Sciences, Patna
Patna, Bihar, India

**Pranita** MD(General Medicine)
Associate Professor
Department of General Medicine
AIIMS, Raipur
Raipur, Chhattisgarh, India

**Prashant G Badole** MBBS
Senior Resident
All India Institute of Medical Sciences, Raipur
Raipur, Chhattisgarh, India

**Pratap Sharma** MBBS MD PhD
Professor, Department of Pediatric
AIIMS, Delhi
New Delhi, India

**Preeti Singh Dhoat** MBBS MD(General Medicine)
Professor and Head
Department of General Medicine
AIIMS, Bathinda
Bathinda, Punjab, India

**Priyanka B** MBBS MS(Ophthalmology) PMCH FMRF
Associate Professor
Department of Ophthalmology
AIIMS, Bhopal
Bhopal, Madhya Pradesh, India

**Priyank Rastogi** MBBS MD(General Medicine)
General Physician
Hindu Rao Hospital
New Delhi, India

**Puranjoy Chakrabarty** MBBS MD(General Medicine) DM(Nephrology)
Nephrologist/Renal Specialist
Samaritan Clinic Private Limited
Kolkata, West Bengal, India

**Rahul K Adhikary** MBBS MD
General Medicine Specialist
Private Clinic
Darjeeling, West Bengal, India

**Rajashree Khot** MBBS MD DNB Diploma for Management in Diabetes
Associate Professor
All India Institute of Medical Sciences, Nagpur
Nagpur, Maharashtra, India

**Rajat Kanti Goswami** MBBS MD(General Medicine) DM(Endocrinology)
Senior Consultant Physician (Diabetic and Internal Medicine)
Inner Health Diagnostic Center
Kolkata, West Bengal, India

**Raj Datta** MBBS BCS(Health) FCPS(Medicine) MD(Gastroenterology)
Gastroenterologist
Popular Diagnostic Center
Dhaka, Bangladesh

**Rajesh Bhawani** MBBS MD(General Medicine)
Associate Professor
Shri Lal Bahadur Shastri Government Medical College
Mandi, Himachal Pradesh, India

**Rajesh Kumar** MBBS MD(Anatomy)
Assistant Professor
Department of Anatomy
AIIMS, Patna
Patna, Bihar, India

**Rakesh Kumar** MBBS MD(General Medicine)
Associate Professor at Centre for Community Medicine, All India Institute of Medical Sciences
New Delhi, India

**Rakhi Sanyal** MBBS MD(Pharmacology)
General Physician
Manipal Hospital Broadway (AMRI Hospitals)
Kolkata, West Bengal, India

**Rana Bhattacharjee** MBBS MD(General Medicine) MRCP DM(Endocrinology) FACE
Endocrinologist
Department of Endocrinology
Institute of Post-Graduate Medical Education and Research and Seth Sukhlal Karnani Memorial Hospital
Kolkata, West Bengal, India

**Ravikant** MBBS MD(General Medicine) DM(Endocrinology)
Endocrinologist
Diabetes and Endocrine Clinic
Kolkata, West Bengal, India

**Ritasman Baisya** MBBS MD(General Medicine) DM(Rheumatology)
Assistant Professor
Department of Rheumatology and Clinical Immunology
AIIMS, Kalyani
Kalyani, West Bengal, India

**Ritu** MBBS MD(General Medicine)
Assistant Professor
AIIMS, Jammu
Jammu and Kashmir, India

**Ruhani Ahuja**
JR 3rd Year of Medicine
SN Medical College
Agra, Uttar Pradesh, India

**Rohini Rokkam** MBBS MD(General Medicine)
Assistant Professor
Department of General Medicine
AIIMS, Raipur
Raipur, Chhattisgarh, India

**Rohit Raina** MBBS MD(General Medicine)
Assistant Professor
Department of Medicine
AIIMS, Bathinda
Bathinda, Punjab, India

**Rohit Singh** MBBS MS(General Surgery)
General Surgeon
Proctologist
Sushruta Anorectal Institute
New Delhi, India

**Ruthra Kumaran** MBBS MD(General Medicine)
Associate Professor
AIIMS, Jammu
Jammu, Jammu and Kashmir, India

**Rupak Chatterjee** MBBS MD(Tropical Medicine)
General Physician/Internal Medicine Specialist
Woda Diagnostics LLP
Kolkata, West Bengal, India

**Sabu Augustine** MBBS MD(Internal Medicine)
Associate Professor, Head In-Charge
Department of General Medicine
All India Institute of Medical Sciences, Madurai
Madurai, Tamil Nadu, India

**Sagar Khadanga** MBBS MD(General Medicine)
Associate Professor
Department of General Medicine
AIIMS, Bhopal
Bhopal, Madhya Pradesh, India

**Sagar Sangole** MBBS Currently Pursuing MD(General Medicine)
Senior Resident
Department of Internal Medicine
All India Institute of Medical Sciences, Nagpur
Nagpur, Maharashtra, India

**Saikat Datta** MBBS MD(General Medicine)
Consultant Physician, Private Clinic
Siliguri, West Bengal, India

**Saikat Ghosh** MBBS MS(Orthopedics)
Assistant Professor
Department of Neuromedicine
North Bengal Medical College and Hospital
Siliguri, West Bengal, India

**Saikat Mondal** MBBS MD(General Medicine)
Assistant Professor
AIIMS, Kalyani
Kalyani, West Bengal, India

**Sakthivadivel V** MBBS MD(General Medicine)
Additional Professor
All India Institute of Medical Sciences
Bibinagar, Telangana, India

**Sambit Das** MBBS MD(Internal Medicine) DM(Endocrinology)
Consultant Endocrinologist and Diabetologist
Apollo Hospitals
Bhubaneswar, Odisha, India

**Sandeep Thareja** MBBS MD(General Medicine) DM(Gastroenterology)
General Officer
Army Research and Referral Hospital
New Delhi, India

**Sandipta Ray** MBBS Diploma in Child Health(DCH) MD(Pediatrics) DM(Cardiology)
Cardiologist
Manipal Hospitals
Kolkata, West Bengal, India

**Sangram S Biradar** MD FICP FACP(USA) FRCP(Glasgow and Ireland ) FACC(USA) FCSI FEAC
Consulting Doctor
SB Medical Center
Gulbarga, Karnataka, India

**Sanjay Bandyopadhyay** MBBS MD(General Medicine) DM(Gastroenterology) DNB(General Medicine)
Senior Consultant
Woodland Hospital
Kolkata, West Bengal, India

**Sanjay Tandon** MBBS MD(Cardiology)
Consultant
Tandon's Clinic
Lucknow, Uttar Pradesh, India

**Santosh Kumar Nayan** MBBS MD(General Medicine)
Senior Consultant
Indira Gandhi Institute of Medical Sciences
Sheikhpura, Patna, Bihar, India

**S Anita Nambiar** MBBS MD(General Medicine)
Senior Consultant
Department of Internal Medicine
Lakeshore Hospital and Research Center
Kochi, Kerala, India

**Santosh Kumar Swain** MBBS MS(ENT) DNB(ENT) MNAMS MBA
Professor
All India Institute of Medical Sciences, Bhubaneswar
Bhubaneswar, Odisha, India

**Sarabmeet Singh Lehl** MBBS MD(Medicine)
Professor
Government Medical College
Chandigarh, India

**Satyendra Khichar** MD(General Medicine)
Professor
Department of Medicine
All India Institute of Medical Sciences, Jodhpur
Jodhpur, Rajasthan, India

**Sayan Kar** MBBS
Senior Resident
Department of General Medicine
AIIMS, Kalyani
Kalyani, West Bengal, India

**Shafat Iqbal Bhati** MBBS MD(Internal Medcine)
Assistant Professor
Faculty of Medicine
Aligarh Muslim University
Aligarh, Uttar Pradesh, India

**Shambo Samrat Samajdar** MBBS MD DM(Clinical Pharmacology) Post Graduate Diploma in Clinical Endocrinology and Diabetes(RCP-UK) Fellowship in Respiratory and Critical Care(WBUHS)
Consultant Physician
Department of General Medicine
HealthETC
Kolkata, West Bengal, India

**Shounak Basak** MBBS DNB(General Medicine)
Senior Resident
AIIMS, Kalyani
Kalyani, West Bengal, India

**Shrikant Mukewar** MBBS MD(Medicine) DM(Gastroenterology)
Director and Senior Gastroenterologist
Midas Hospital
Nagpur, Maharashtra, India

**Shrivarthan R** MBBS MD(General Medicine) DM(Neurology)
Consultant
Department of Neurology
MGM Healthcare Pvt Ltd
Chennai, Tamil Nadu, India

**Siddharth Singh** MBBS MD(General Medicine)
Junior Resident
JN Medical College
Belagavi, Karnataka, India

**Silima Subhasnigdha Tarenia** MBBS MS(General Medicine) DM(Endocrinology)
Consulting Physician
Medica Superspecialty Hospital
Kolkata, West Bengal, India

**Sirshendu Pal** MBBS
Junior Resident Doctor
Department of Community Medicine
AIIMS, New Delhi
New Delhi, india

**Smita Gupta** MBBS DNB(General Medicine)
Professor and Head
Shri Ram Murti Smarak Institute of Medical Sciences
Bareilly, Uttar Pradesh, India

**Snehansu Shekhar Samanta** MBBS MD(General Medicine)
Assistant Professor
Calcutta National Medical College and Hospital, Beniapukur
Kolkata, West Bengal, India

**Soumya Bhowmik** MBBS MD DNB(Internal Medicine) DM & DrNB(Neurology)
Assistant Professor
Department of Neurology
AIIMS, Kalyani
Kalyani, West Bengal, India

**Sreemanta Madhab Baruah** MBBS MD(General Medicine)
Diabetologist, Medicine Specialist
Dr Damani's Nursing Home
Dibrugarh, Assam, India

**Sreesha S** MBBS MD(General Medicine)
General Practitioner
Private Clinic
Vatakara, Kerala, India

**Srikant Behera** MBBS MD(General Medicine)
Assistant Professor
Department of General Medicine
AIIMS, Bhubaneswar
Bhubaneswar, Odisha, India

**S Sreenivas** MBBS MD(General Medicine)
General Physician
Sreenivas Clinic
Dondaparthy, Visakhapatnam, India

**Subhendu Jana** MBBS MD(General Medicine)
PGT
IPGMER SSKM Hospital
Kolkata, West Bengal, India

**Sudeshna Guha Thakurta Ghosh** MBBS MD(General Medicine)
Assistant Professor
Midnapore Medical College and Hospital
Midnapore, West Bengal, India

**Sukdev Manna** MBBS MD(General Medicine) DM(Clinical Immunology and Rheumatology)
Assistant Professor
Department of Rheumatology and Clinical Immunology
AIIMS, Kalyani
Kalyani, West Bengal, India

**Sumit Chatterjee** (Medicine Specialist) MBBS(Hon) MD(Medicine) Gold Medalist
Assistant Professor
JNM Medical College
Aligarh, Uttar Pradesh, India

**Sumit Chakrabarti** MBBS MD(Endocrine) MD(General Medicine)
Endocrinologist
North Bengal Medical College
Thiknikata, West Bengal, India

**Sunita Kumbhalkar** MBBS MD(General Medicine)
Professor
Department of General Medicine
AIIMS, Nagpur
Nagpur, Maharashtra, India

**Surbhi Dogra** MBBS MD(Pediatrics) Fellowship in Pediatric Gastroenterology and Hepatology
Pediatric Gastroenterologist
Apollo Hospitals
Gandhinagar, Ahmedabad, India

**Sushil Kumar** MBBS MD(General Medicine)
Assistant Professor
Department of General Medicine
AIIMS, Deoghar
Deoghar, Jharkhand, India

**Swarnadip Hazra** MBBS MD(General Medicine)
General Medicine Specialist
Private Clinic
Darjeeling, West Bengal, India

**Tapas Bandyopadhyay** DNB(General Medicine) MD(Internal Medicine)
Senior Consultant and Post Graduate Faculty, Medica Superspecialty Hospital
Kolkata, West Bengal, India

**Taranpreet Kour** MBBS MD(General Medicine)
Assistant Professor
Department of General Medicine
AIIMS, Jammu
Jammu and Kashmir, India

**Uddalak Chakraborty** MBBS MD(General Medicine) DM(Neurology)
Neurologist, VDC Clinic
Kolkata, West Bengal, India

**U Meenakshisundaram** MBBS MD(Internal Medicine) DM(Neurology)
Director and Senior Consultant
MGM Healthcare Pvt Ltd
Chennai, Tamil Nadu, India

**Upoma Saha** MBBS
Senior Resident
Department of General Medicine
Calcutta National Medical College and Hospital
Kolkata, West Bengal, India

**Uppara Kadiyala Rakesh** MBBS MD(General Medicine)
Assistant Professor
All India Institute of Medical Sciences, Mangalagiri
Mangalagiri, Andhra Pradesh, India

**Vahini Golla** MBBS MD(General Medicine) CCEBDM
Assistant Professor
Department of General Medicine
All India Institute of Medical Sciences, Bibinagar
Bibinagar, Telangana, India

**Vijay Karthik Bhogaraju** MBBS MD DM(Rheumatology) MRCP(Rheumatology)
Senior Resident
All India Institute of Medical Sciences, Rishikesh
Rishikesh, Uttarakhand, India

**Col Vikas Marwah** MBBS MD(Respiratory Medicine) MRCP SCE(Respiratory Medicine)
Senior Advisor and Head
Department of Respiratory Medicine
Army Hospital Research and Referral
New Delhi, India

**Vishakha Jain** MD(Medicine) PGDGM(Geriatric Medicine)
Additional Professor and Head
All India Institute of Medical Sciences Bibinagar
Bibinagar, Telangana, India

**Vishal Agarwal** MBBS MD(General Medicine) DM(Endocrinology)
General Physician
SB Aggarwal Clinic
New Delhi, India

**Visvesvaran Salitteeswaran** MBBS MD(General Medicine)
Assistant Professor
Department of General Medicine
Saveetha Medical College
Chennai, Tamil Nadu, India

**Vivek Paul Chowdhury** MBBS MD(General Medicine)
General Physician
Private Clinic
Siliguri, West Bengal, India

**Yasmee Khan** MBBS MD(General Medicine)
Associate Professor
Department of General Medicine
AIIMS, Bhopal
Bhopal, Madhya Pradesh, India

# Preface

It is with pleasure and pride, we present the "*API Medicine: A-Clinical Compendium 2025*". This novel publication of the Association of Physicians of India (API) is being published for the first time as a fourth volume along with Update and Progress in Medicine at APICON 2025. It endeavors to rejuvenate interest in clinical medicine, an art more than science that is on its way to oblivion.

It covers a wide range of relevant clinical topics that will assist not only in postgraduate examinations but also day-to-day decision making.

There is an ocean of information on the internet these days, and it is too vast and deep for even the most avid reader to fully encompass. The topics dealt with are chosen to help our students and practitioners to approach clinical problems analytically with suitable algorithms and diagrams.

The differential diagnosis has been discussed with gradual exclusion by clinical clues, which give the reader a thrilling experience and flavor of clinical analysis.

We thank the entire editorial team for their commendable effort in producing this comprehensive treatise for internists and hope it will be useful in daily practice.

On behalf of the Editorial Board, We extend heartfelt gratitude to the dedicated team at Jaypee Brothers Medical Publishers for their tireless efforts in ensuring the timely compilation of this book. Special thanks to Shri Jitendar P Vij (Group Chairman), Mr Ankit Vij (Managing Director), Mr MS Mani (Group President), Ms Chetna Malhotra (Senior Director—Professional Publishing, Marketing, and Business Development), Ms Pooja Bhandari [Director—Production (Books and Journals)], Mr Sabyasachi Hazra (Associate Director—Publishing), Mrs Nedup Bhutia Pillai (Assistant Manager, Print Publishing), Ms Bhavana Sharma (Project Manager), and the entire team for their invaluable support in making this volume a seamless accomplishment.

**Jyotirmoy Pal**
**Nandini Chatterjee**

# Contents

## SECTION 10: NEUROLOGY

## SECTION 11: ONCOLOGY



## SECTION 12: PULMONOLOGY



## SECTION 13: RHEUMATOLOGY

## SECTION 14: DERMATOLOGY



## SECTION 15: HEPATOLOGY



## SECTION 16: INTERNAL MEDICINE

CHAPTER 1

# An Approach to a Case of Recurrent DVTs in a 25-year-old Lady

*Monica Gupta, Sarabmeet Singh Lehl*

**CASE VIGNETTE**

A 25-year-old, unmarried lady working in a MNC presents with painful swelling in the right leg for 8–10 days. She has been a regular middle distance runner, but now finds it difficult to cope and therefore visits her general physician. The GP finds that the right leg is swollen up to the upper thigh, slightly tender, and has a circumference 3 cm more than the left limb. Her vitals are within normal range. The 12-lead electrocardiogram (ECG) is normal. On further questioning, there is no recent injury, hospitalization, surgery, long-distance travel in a flight or bus, rheumatologic problems or, medication intake like OCP. Family history did not suggest hematologic or autoimmune diseases. She confirms that about 2 years ago, she had similar swelling in the same leg, and as per her records, it was classified as a "provoked" DVT of the calf veins related to musculoskeletal injury in the right knee for which she was advised ambulation using a knee brace. She was prescribed Warfarin anticoagulation for 3 weeks. Then she was lost to follow-up. The GP finds the clinical probability Wells score for DVT as >2 (high).

## PROVISIONAL DIAGNOSIS

- *Classification of the first DVT event*:
  - *Unprovoked versus provoked*: The first DVT cannot be clearly classified as either fully provoked or unprovoked.
  - *Risk factors*: No typical major risk factors (e.g., surgery >30 min, trauma, or prolonged immobility). No minor transient risk factors like short-duration surgery or travel. Persistent factors (e.g., obesity, autoimmune disorders) should be considered.
  - *Learning point*: Traditional classification of DVT as provoked or unprovoked is no longer recommended by the European Society of Cardiology. Minor transient factors may carry a higher recurrence risk than some major factors.
- *Well's clinical prediction rule for DVT*:
  - *Score calculation*: Based on available information, the patient's score is 1 point (from knee brace use), placing her in the low to moderate likelihood category.
  - *Learning point*: Other conditions mimicking DVT (e.g., Baker's cyst rupture, meniscal tear, and cellulitis) must be ruled out, especially in athletes.
  - *Risk of recurrence*: Patients with persistent major risk factors (e.g., cancer) have a higher recurrence risk (20.7%) compared to noncancer cases (6.8%). Annual recurrence risk after stopping anticoagulation in unidentified risk factor cases is approximately 7.9%.
- *Diagnosis when Well's criteria are not met*:
  - *D-dimer testing*: A D-dimer test should be performed if suspicion is high despite a low Well's score. A result > 500 ng/mL indicates a high probability of DVT.
  - *Learning point*: D-dimer is reliable for outpatient diagnosis but less useful in hospitalized or postoperative patients due to potential false elevation.

## DIFFERENTIAL DIAGNOSIS

- *Primary DVT versus recurrent DVT:*
  - Primary DVT: First occurrence, often requiring risk factor identification (provoked vs. unprovoked).
  - Recurrent DVT: Consider prior history of DVT and ongoing symptoms or risk factors (e.g., persistent thrombophilia, residual DVT on imaging).
- *Provoked DVT*:
  - Transient risk factors: Recent surgery, trauma, prolonged immobility, hormonal therapy, pregnancy.
  - Persistent risk factors: Active cancer, autoimmune disorders, obesity, and nephrotic syndrome.
- *Unprovoked DVT*: No identifiable risk factor, requiring investigation for underlying conditions (e.g., occult malignancy, inherited thrombophilia).
- *Thrombophilia-related DVT*:
  - Inherited: Factor V Leiden, prothrombin gene mutation.
  - Acquired: Antiphospholipid syndrome (APS), especially in young, premenopausal women without other risk factors.
- *Mimickers of DVT:*
  - Musculoskeletal causes: Baker's cyst rupture, meniscal tear, muscle strain, or tendon injury.
  - Infectious/Inflammatory: Cellulitis, venous insufficiency, or post-thrombotic syndrome.

- *Pulmonary embolism (PE)*: Consider in cases of proximal DVT or if symptoms include shortness of breath, chest pain, or hypoxemia.

## CLINICAL APPROACH

- *Pretest probability assessment*: Assess symptoms (swelling, redness, tenderness) and history (prior DVT, risk factors like oral contraceptives, COVID-19, family history).
  - Evaluate signs of limb-threatening ischemia (cyanosis, reduced pulses) and systemic signs (tachycardia, hypoxia, elevated JVP).
  - Explore risk factors: Hereditary thrombophilia, autoimmune diseases, malignancy, immobility, surgery, pregnancy, hormonal therapy.
- *Wells clinical prediction rule*: A score >2 indicates high probability; imaging with compression ultrasound (CUS) is recommended.
- *Compression ultrasound (CUS) diagnosis*: New noncompressible segment—indicates new DVT.
  - Ipsilateral recurrent DVT: Requires comparison with previous CUS; ≥4 mm thrombus diameter increase suggests recurrence.
  - Contralateral DVT: CUS sensitivity: 90% (proximal) and 60% (distal), specificity: ~100%.
- *Algorithm for nondiagnostic CUS*: Repeat CUS in 5–7 days if high/moderate suspicion.
  - Use D-dimer if CUS is inconclusive.
  - Consider venography or repeated CUS at 2–7 days for persistent doubts.
- *Role of D-dimer testing*: Helps exclude DVT in low-probability cases with high negative predictive value.
  - Elevated D-dimer in high clinical suspicion may support diagnosis, but prolonged elevation post-DVT reduces specificity.
- *Distinction between proximal and distal DVT*:
  - Proximal DVT: Involves popliteal, femoral, or iliac veins; higher PE risk.
  - Distal DVT: Involves peroneal, tibial veins; risk of progression to proximal DVT.
- *Laboratory investigations*:
  - Routine tests: CBC, peripheral smear, liver/renal function, ESR, coagulation profile.
  - Specific clues: Elevated hematocrit (myeloproliferative), prolonged aPTT (lupus anticoagulant), schistocytes (DIC/TTP-HUS).
- *Evaluation for thrombophilia/hypercoagulability*: Inherited thrombophilia—factor V Leiden, prothrombin G20210A, protein C/S, antithrombin deficiency.
  - Acquired conditions: APS, myeloproliferative disorders (JAK2), PNH.
  - Testing is indicated for young (<45 years) patients with unprovoked recurrent DVT or family history of VTE.
- *Timing of thrombophilia testing*: Perform after an anticoagulation-free period—
  - Warfarin: At least 5 days.
  - DOACs: 2–3 days.
  - Aim for a minimum 2-week gap when feasible.
- *Impact on management*:
  - Thrombophilia testing guides long-term anticoagulation decisions and may help in primary prevention for at-risk relatives.

**TABLE 1: Testing for thrombophilia in different settings.**

| Thrombophilic factor that can be tested | Acute thrombosis | Heparin therapy | Warfarin therapy | DOAC* |
|---|---|---|---|---|
| Factor V Leiden | Yes | Yes | Yes | Yes |
| Prothrombin G20210A | Yes | Yes | Yes | Yes |
| Antiphospholipid antibodies | Yes | Yes | Yes | Yes |
| Lupus anticoagulant§ | Yes | No | Avoid | No |
| Protein C deficiency | Yes | Yes | No | No |
| Protein S deficiency | Avoid | Yes | No | No |
| Antithrombin deficiency | Avoid | No | Yes | No |

*Direct oral anticoagulants

§LAC antibody

  - Avoid routine testing to prevent anxiety and unnecessary healthcare costs.
  - Ideally these tests should be performed after an anticoagulation-free period of at least two weeks, when feasible. However, a minimum of 5 days for warfarin-free period or 2–3 days for DOAC-free period is reasonable. **Table 1** summarizes the clinical setting and the drugs that may interfere with the results.
- As per the revised Sapporo criteria, our patient meets the diagnostic criteria for APS. She has two events of venous thrombosis and the three types of aPL are positive (these will be repeated at 12 weeks). A substantial number (44%) of triple-positive APS patients develop recurrent VTE over 10-year, even after adequate anticoagulation. These patients have a 10-fold higher risk of first VTE and two- to sixfold higher risk of recurrent VTE than general population.
- For most patients with acute proximal DVT (e.g., popliteal, femoral, or iliac vein DVT), anticoagulation is mandatory to decrease VTE recurrence, provided the risk of bleeding is not high. Considering the intermediate risk of PE in our patient, and a diagnosis of APS, she needs to be started urgently on anticoagulation.

## PATHOPHYSIOLOGY

### Antiphospholipid Antibody Syndrome (APS) and Risk of Recurrent VTE

- *Mechanism*: APS is an autoimmune disorder characterized by the presence of antiphospholipid antibodies (aPL) which include lupus anticoagulant, anticardiolipin antibodies, and anti-β2-glycoprotein I antibodies. These antibodies promote a hypercoagulable state by interfering with endothelial function, platelet activation, and coagulation pathways.
- *Risk of recurrent VTE*: Triple-positive APS patients have a 10-fold higher risk of first VTE and a two- to sixfold increased risk of recurrence compared to the general population, even with anticoagulation. This is due to persistent activation of coagulation and impaired fibrinolysis.

### Pathophysiology of PE in APS (Fig. 1)

- *Thrombus formation*: In APS, abnormal thrombi form due to endothelial damage, platelet aggregation, and overactivation

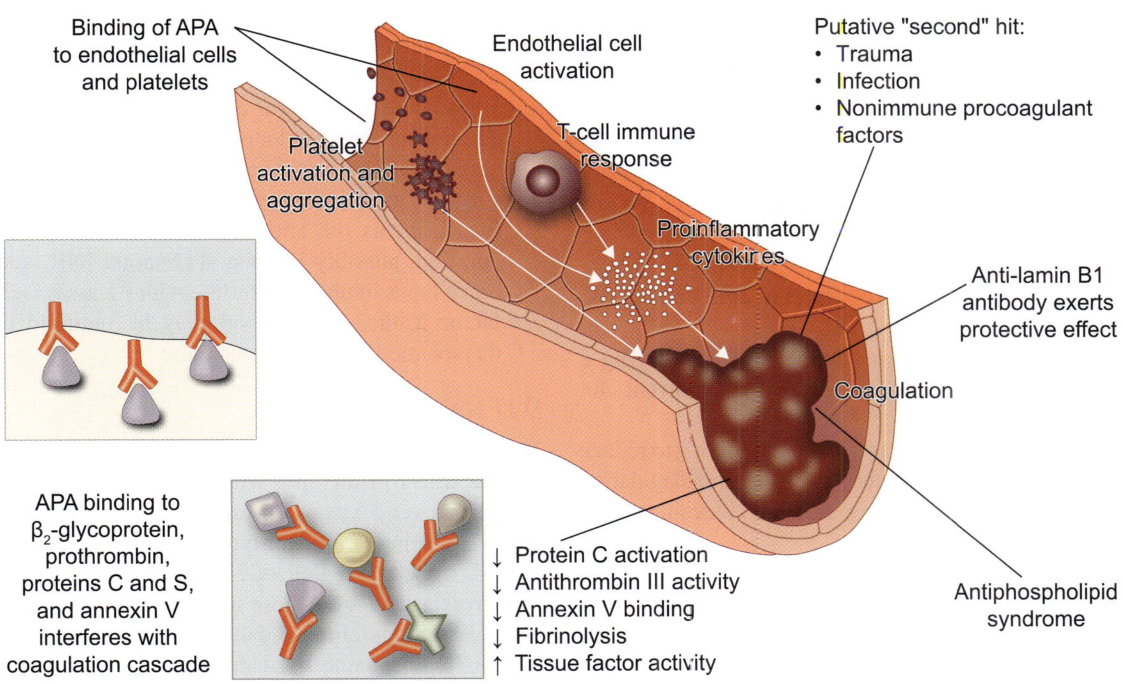


**FIG. 1:** Pathogenic mechanisms in antiphospholipid syndrome.
*Source*: Hanly JG. Antiphospholipid syndrome: an overview. CMAJ. 2003;168(13):1675-82.

of coagulation factors. These thrombi can embolize from deep veins to the pulmonary arteries, leading to PE.

- *Clinical risk estimation (modified Wells score)*: PE risk is evaluated using a scoring system based on factors like prior VTE, heart rate >100 beats/min, immobilization, and clinical signs of DVT. A score of 2–6 indicates intermediate PE risk, which aligns with our patient's profile.

## Indications for Anticoagulation

- *Acute proximal DVT*: Anticoagulation is essential in proximal DVT (popliteal, femoral, iliac veins) to prevent thrombus extension and PE, unless contraindicated due to high bleeding risk.
- *APS and PE risk*: Given APS and intermediate PE risk, anticoagulation is critical to reduce morbidity and mortality. It works by inhibiting thrombin generation and platelet aggregation, thus preventing clot propagation and embolization.

**TABLE 2: Anticoagulant drugs.**

| Drug | Dosage |
|---|---|
| Unfractionated heparin (UFH) | 80 units/kg IV bolus, then continuous IV infusion @18 units/kg/h (minimum 5 days) |
| LMWH (Enoxaparin) | 1 mg/kg SC BD (minimum 5 days) |
| Fondaparinux | 5–10 mg SC OD (minimum 5 days) |
| Warfarin | Initiate at a dose of 2–5 mg orally OD following LMWH or UFH and overlap until desired INR, maintenance dose is generally between 2–10 mg OD |
| Apixaban | 10 mg BD for 1 week, then 5 mg BD, reduce dose to 2.5 mg BD after 6 months |
| Rivaroxaban | 15 mg BD for 3 weeks, then 20 mg OD |
| Dabigatran | 150 mg BD |
| Edoxaban | 60 g OD |

# TREATMENT AND PREVENTION

- For recurrent DVT, initial treatment involves prompt anticoagulation with either unfractionated heparin (UFH), low-molecular-weight heparin (LMWH), or fondaparinux for at least 5 days. From day 2, oral anticoagulants like warfarin (target INR 2.0–3.0), dabigatran, or edoxaban can be added, requiring a 5-day UFH/LMWH bridge. Rivaroxaban and apixaban can be used as monotherapy without a heparin bridge.
- EULAR recommends warfarin (VKA) as the first-line anticoagulant for triple-positive APS, targeting an INR of 2–3 for VTE and 3–4 for arterial thrombosis. DOACs, particularly rivaroxaban, are not advised due to their higher risk of arterial thrombosis, especially stroke, in triple-positive APS patients. However, in single or double aPL-positive cases, DOACs may be considered individually, with dabigatran showing some favorable evidence over other DOACs.
- Warfarin initially reduces protein C and S levels faster than factors II and X, creating a temporary procoagulant state. To prevent this, overlapping warfarin with another anticoagulant, such as heparin, is recommended during the initial phase of therapy.

Please refer to **Table 2** for the dosages of the various anticoagulant drugs.

Predicting bleeding risk in patients with VTE is challenging, as available scoring models are not reliable for clinical use. The long-term risk of major bleeding during anticoagulation ranges from 1 to 6.5% annually, which is 2–3 times higher than the risk of death from recurrent VTE. However, this risk may not apply to patients who have previously tolerated anticoagulation well (like in this case). The ACCP recommends assessing bleeding risk based on factors such as advanced age, liver or kidney disease, cancer, alcohol abuse, thrombocytopenia, antiplatelet therapy, poor anticoagulant control, recent surgery, and prior bleeding or stroke.

## Anticoagulant Timeline

Since patients with APS require lifelong anticoagulation, 3 phases can be identified.

- *Anticoagulation therapy begins* immediately following a DVT diagnosis, typically lasting 7–21 days, to prevent clot propagation.
- The *primary treatment phase* lasts 3 months, aiming to reduce the risk of VTE recurrence. After this phase, anticoagulation may be stopped if the recurrence risk is low, bleeding risk is high, or if the patient prefers.
- For patients with unprovoked VTE, *extended anticoagulation* is recommended beyond 3 months to prevent further VTE episodes.
- In some cases, *indefinite anticoagulation* may be necessary if the recurrence risk remains high, reducing recurrence by 80–90%. Please refer to **Table 3** for the optimal duration of anticoagulation.

**TABLE 3: Optimal duration of anticoagulation in various settings.**

| Type of VTE | % risk of recurrence at 1 year | Optimal duration of treatment |
|---|---|---|
| Isolated distal DVT | 0.5 | 3 months |
| Proximal DVT with major transient risk factors (provoked) | 1 | 3 months |
| Proximal DVT with minor transient risk factors (provoked) | 3–8 | 3 months |
| DVT in pregnancy/estrogen use (provoked) | 3–8 | 3 months |
| Proximal DVT with no major transient risk factors (unprovoked) | 3–8 | 3 months |
| Proximal recurrent DVT with major transient risk factors (provoked) | 3–8 | 3 months-indefinite |
| Proximal recurrent DVT with no major transient risk factors (unprovoked) | 8–10 | Indefinite |
| Pulmonary embolism (unprovoked) | >10 | Indefinite |
| VTE associated with active cancer | 20 | Indefinite or till cancer active |
| VTE associated with APS | 8–10 | Indefinite |

- The patient was administered anticoagulation with LMWH subcutaneous injection, 60 mg/12 h for one week. The patient evolved uneventfully during hospital stay and an overlap of 5 days with a VKA was done to achieve stable INR of 2–3. The patient agreed to long-term oral warfarin after explaining hervarious facts about her condition.
- Current guidelines recommend a VKA-based regimen (warfarin) as the anticoagulation of choice for a longer duration, possibly lifelong. The target INR is kept at 2–3. Since lupus inhibitors interfere with PT assays, chromogenic factor X therapeutic level may be required to ascertain therapeutic INR in these patients.

## DVT Re-occurrence

Thrombotic APS is associated with a high risk of recurrent VTE despite warfarin therapy, with recurrence rates ranging from 3 to 24% over 5 years. Ensuring treatment adherence, regular INR monitoring, and identifying potential drug interactions are crucial. If the target INR of 2–3 is insufficient, adding LMWH or increasing the VKA dose to achieve an INR of 3–4 may be necessary. Some clinicians also consider adding aspirin while maintaining the same VKA dose. Fondaparinux can be used as an alternative for patients who are allergic to LMWH or have suspected HIT.

The patient has now completed 3 months of warfarin therapy and is fully compliant. The involved leg has normalized, and she is able to run two miles daily. A repeat test for APS at 12 weeks confirms the diagnosis. Given her health insurance and willingness to afford newer medications, options for safer treatments may be considered, taking into account her APS diagnosis and previous history of VTE.

- Given that APS is a multisystem disease, the patient should undergo assessments for potential involvement of the cardiac valves, nervous system, kidneys, and hematological system, particularly checking for thrombocytopenia. General advice on reducing cardiovascular and thrombotic risk factors should be provided. For any upcoming surgeries or procedures, it's important to minimize interruption of anticoagulation and encourage early ambulation. A repeat CUS should be performed to establish a new baseline for future DVT comparisons. Additionally, the patient should be evaluated for post-thrombotic syndrome, which is more likely to develop in cases of ipsilateral recurrent DVT.
- The patient should be informed about the increased risk of developing another thrombosis, preeclampsia, miscarriage, or intrauterine growth restriction. She should be advised against pregnancy while on warfarin due to its teratogenic risks. If she plans to conceive, she will need to switch to LMWH throughout the pregnancy. Additionally, low-dose aspirin may be prescribed in the preconception period. After delivery, she can continue LMWH for 6–8 weeks or return to warfarin. Both LMWH and warfarin are safe to use while breastfeeding.

## Points to Ponder

- *Complexity of recurrent DVT*: Recurrent deep vein thrombosis (DVT) in young patients without clear risk factors, especially in the same leg, presents significant diagnostic and treatment challenges.
- *Treatment approach*: Initial management of acute recurrent DVT mirrors that of the first episode, emphasizing prompt and effective anticoagulation.
- *Risk of recurrence*: Patients with a second DVT are at high risk for future episodes, necessitating consideration of *lifelong anticoagulation* to prevent further occurrences.
- *Anticoagulant selection*: Direct oral anticoagulants (DOACs) are preferred for their convenience, efficacy, and safety, though *vitamin K antagonists (VKAs)* and *heparins* may be more suitable in specific cases.
- *Need for evidence-based guidelines*: Continued research and development of robust, evidence-based guidelines are essential to improve long-term outcomes for patients with recurrent DVT.

## MULTIPLE CHOICE QUESTIONS

1. **What is the most likely diagnosis for this 25-year-old female with a painful, swollen leg and history of a previous DVT?**
   A. Deep vein thrombosis (DVT)
   B. Peripheral artery disease
   C. Cellulitis
   D. Acute myocardial infarction
2. **What is the first diagnostic step in this patient's management, given the clinical suspicion of DVT and a Wells score of >2?**
   A. Immediate surgery
   B. Compression ultrasonography (CUS)
   C. CT pulmonary angiogram
   D. D-dimer test
3. **Given this patient's previous history of a "provoked" DVT, what should be considered next in terms of risk assessment for recurrence?**
   A. Evaluate for underlying thrombophilia
   B. Start aspirin for primary prevention
   C. Begin long-term anticoagulation therapy
   D. Discontinue all anticoagulants
4. **What is the most appropriate anticoagulation therapy for a young female with a history of recurrent DVT, considering this is a second episode of thrombosis?**
   A. Aspirin alone
   B. Vitamin K antagonist (Warfarin) with a target INR of 2–3
   C. No anticoagulation needed
   D. Direct oral anticoagulants (DOACs) like apixaban
5. **What is the recommended approach for managing this patient if she wishes to conceive in the future, considering her history of DVT and the use of warfarin?**
   A. Continue warfarin throughout pregnancy
   B. Discontinue anticoagulation during pregnancy
   C. Switch to low molecular weight heparin (LMWH) during pregnancy
   D. Use a combination of warfarin and aspirin

### Answers

1. (A); 2. (B); 3. (A); 4. (B); 5. (C)

## SUGGESTED READINGS


1. Stevens SM, Woller SC, Kreuziger LB, et al. Antithrombotic Therapy for VTE Disease: Second Update of the CHEST Guideline and Expert Panel Report. Chest. 2021;160:e545-608.
2. Mazzolai L, Ageno W, Alatri A, et al. Second consensus document on diagnosisand management of acute deep vein thrombosis: updated document elaboratedby the ESC Working Group on aorta and peripheral vascular diseases and the ESC Working Group on pulmonary circulation and right ventricular function. Eur J Prev Cardiol. 2022;29:1248-63.
3. Ortel TL, Neumann I, Ageno W, et al. American Society of Hematology 2020 guidelines for management of venous thromboembolism: treatment of deepvein thrombosis and pulmonary embolism. Blood Adv. 2020;4:4693-738.
4. Konstantinides SV, Meyer G, Becattini C, et al. 2019 ESC Guidelines for the diagnosis and management of acute pulmonary embolism developed in collaborationwith the European Respiratory Society (ERS). Eur Heart J. 2020;41:543-603.
5. McCormack T, Harrisingh MC, Horner D, et al. Venous thromboembolism inadults: summary of updated NICE guidance on diagnosis, management, andthrombophilia testing. BMJ. 2020; 369:m1565.
6. Mwansa H, Zghouzi M, Barnes GD. Unprovoked Venous Thromboembolism: The Search for the Cause. Med Clin North Am. 2023;107:861-82.
7. Kyrle PA. How I treat recurrent deep-vein thrombosis. Blood. 2016;127:696-702.
8. Tumian NR, Hunt BJ. Clinical Management of Thrombotic Antiphospholipid Syndrome. J Clin Med. 2022;11:735.
9. Miyakis S, Lockshin MD, Atsumi T, et al. International consensus statement on an update of the classification criteria for definite antiphospholipid syndrome (APS). J Thromb Haemost. 2006;4:295-306.
10. McKean SC, Ross JJ, Dressler DD, Scheurer DB (Eds). Principles and Practice of Hospital Medicine, 2nd edition. McGraw-Hill Education; 2017.

CHAPTER
2

# An Approach to a Case of Tuberculosis of Pericardium

*Sakthivadivel V, Neeradi Charan*

**CASE VIGNETTE**

A 35-year-old male presents with a 3 weeks history of dyspnea, chest pain, and low-grade fever. He reports recent weight loss, night sweats, and fatigue. His chest pain is a dull ache, worsening when lying down and relieved when sitting forward. Examination reveals a heart rate of 120 beats/min, BP of 95/65 mm Hg, respiratory rate of 22 breaths/min, temperature of 37.8°C, raised jugular venous pressure (JVP), and muffled heart sounds. Chest imaging shows cardiomegaly, and electrocardiogram (ECG) reveals low-voltage QRS complexes. Echocardiogram confirms a huge pericardial effusion with strands and early right atrial and ventricular diastolic collapse. Pericardiocentesis yields straw-colored fluid with high protein, lymphocyte predominance, and elevated ADA; Gram-stain and culture is negative for infection. Xpert MTB, AFB stain, and culture are negative for *Mycobacterium tuberculosis*.

## PROVISIONAL DIAGNOSIS

Tuberculous pericardial effusion with possible cardiac tamponade.

## DIFFERENTIAL DIAGNOSIS

- *Infective causes*:
  - *Viral:* Common cause of acute pericarditis**.** Echovirus and coxsackievirus are most common causes among viruses. Other viruses like adenovirus, Epstein–Barr virus, CMV, influenza, mumps, varicella, HIV, hepatitis B, and SARS-CoV-2 also cause pericarditis
  - *Bacteria*: *Staphylococcus, Streptococcus, Haemophilus,* and *Pneumococcus* commonly causes pericardial involvement. *Rickettsia, Chlamydia, Borrelia, Mycoplasma, Treponema, Ureaplasma, Nocardia, Tropheryma* also can cause pericarditis.
  - *Fungal*: *Histoplasma, Aspergillus, Blastomyces, Coccidioides,* and *Candida*
  - *Parasitic: Echinococcus, Entamoeba, Toxoplasma*
- *Inflammatory causes*: Autoimmune diseases like SLE, RA, Sjögren's syndrome.
- *Metabolic causes*: Uremia, hypothyroidism, dialysis associated, ovarian hyperstimulation syndrome, IgG4 disease, inflammatory bowel disease.
- *Neoplastic causes*: Cancer of lung, breast, esophagus, melanoma and lymphoma
- *Trauma*: Hemopericardium may result from blunt trauma, penetrating injuries, and iatrogenic damage to the myocardium aorta, or coronary arteries.
- Radiation
- *Drugs and toxins*: Hydralazine, doxorubucine, cyclophosphamide, phenytoin, and isoniazid

## IDIOPATHIC CLINICAL APPROACH

- *TB pericardium* **(Fig. 1)**: It contributes to 60–80% of acute pericarditis and 75% of constrictive pericarditis in high-risk areas.
- *Clinically presents in three forms*: Pericardial effusion, constrictive pericarditis, and a combination of effusion with constriction:
  - Tuberculous pericardial effusion (TBPE) presents with a diverse range of clinical symptoms and have to be contemplated in the differential diagnosis of pericarditis, especially in cases that do not resolve spontaneously
  - Usually presents insidiously with systemic symptoms as fever, sweats at night, exhaustion, and loss of weight. Other common symptoms include chest pain, cough, and dyspnea.

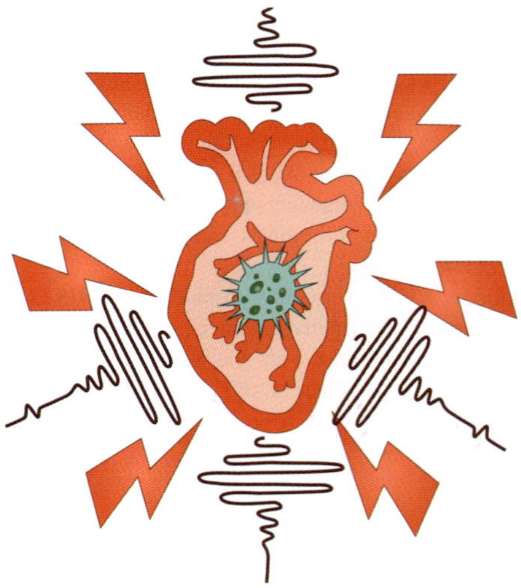

**FIG. 1:** TB in pericardium.

- Acute TB pericarditis rarely causes severe pain.
- Right hypochondriac discomfort may be present due to liver congestion.
- In pericardial effusion without tamponade, cardiovascular examination may not yield any findings.
- JVP is distinctly high, with discernible *x* descent and nonexistent descent with retained respiratory variation in tamponade.
- The cardiac impulse may be difficult to feel and the heart sounds may be attenuated if the effusion is substantial. In percussion, cardiac dullness can extend to the right of the sternum. Friction rub may be heard.
- *Beck's triad*: Hypotension, inaudible heart sounds, and elevated JVP is a key indicator of severe tamponade. Paradoxical pulse is classically present in tamponade.
- *Respiratory system*: Tubular breath sounds may be audible in the left axilla or base due to bronchial compression by large effusion (Ewart's sign).
- The wide variation in symptoms is due to how quickly pericardial fluid builds up. Rapid accumulation of 100–150 mL of pericardial fluid can result in tamponade. In contrast, slow accumulation can accommodate up to 1–2 L of fluid before tamponade occurs.
- *Constrictive pericarditis:* It's a consequence of untreated TBPE. Presents with Symptoms of fluid overload and/or diminished cardiac output. Kussmaul sign (absence of inspiratory diminution of JVP), discernible Y descent and pericardial knock (rare) are seen.
- *Effusive constrictive pericarditis:* Pulsus paradoxus, lack of kussmaul sign, less significant Y descent and pericardial knock.
- About 90% of patients have cardiomegaly, 30% of patients have signs of active TB, 40–60% have pleural effusion on a chest radiograph. Pericardial calcification suggests constriction.
- *ECG:* Nonspecific ST-T wave changes, PR-segment depression, and ST-segment elevation appear in about 9–11% of cases of TB pericarditis. A significant pericardial effusion is suggested by low voltage complexes (QRS amplitude <5 mm in limb leads and <10 mm in precordial leads). Electrical alternans, an indicator of tamponade, is rare.
- *Echocardiography:*
  - Fluid with fibrinous strands are typical but not unique to a TBPE.
  - Small pericardial effusions initially appear over the posterobasal left ventricle and expand anteriorly, laterally, and around the left atrium as fluid increases.
  - *Cardiac tamponade*: Right ventricle collapse in early diastole, right atrial collapse in late diastole, marked variation in size of RV and LV, and inspiratory shift of interventricular septum.
  - *Constrictive pericarditis*: Moderate biatrial dilatation, septal shudder, and inspiratory shift of interventricular septum.
- *Chest CT and/or MRI:* Lymphadenopathy, pericardial thickening, and pericardial effusion. Mediastinal and tracheobronchial (with hilar sparing) lymph node involvement is characteristic; it is >10 mm and has hypodense centers and matting.
- While TSTs and IGRAs are helpful in identifying TB infection, they are unable to differentiate between latent and active TB disease. Hence, their role is limited.
- Diagnosis confirmation requires pericardial fluid analysis TBPE are usually exudative in nature with high protein content, raised cell count with lymphocytic preponderance. Fluid smear microscopy and culture for MTB have very low sensitivity. Adenosine deaminase (ADA) level above 40 U/L in a lymphocyte-predominant effusion strongly suggests TB in high prevalence settings. One study found that a pericardial lymphocyte/neutrophil ratio of ≥1.0 had a high sensitivity, and specificity for diagnosing tuberculous pericardial effusion.
- Xpert MTB/RIF and IFN-$\gamma$ testing on pericardial fluid has moderate sensitivity and high specificity for diagnosing TBPE. While not recommended by the INDEX guidelines, it can still be useful for diagnosing TBPE.
- Finding tubercle bacilli in a pericardial fluid smear or culture, as well as recognizing tubercle bacilli or caseating granulomas on pericardial histological examination, confirms the diagnosis of tuberculous pericardial effusion.
- *Viral:* Acute onset and follows self-limiting course. It's associated with viral prodrome.
- *Bacteria:* Usually cause purulent pericardial effusion. Often fatal if not treated early. Extra pericardial infection is important component in clinical picture.
- *Inflammatory causes*: Clinically silent. Usually associated with other serositis.
- *Neoplastic causes*: Primary tumors rarely cause pericardial effusion. Malignancy must be considered in any case of rapidly accumulating and recurrent pericardial effusion or cardiac tamponade at presentation.
- *Radiation:* The patient may experience acute pericarditis with or without effusion shortly after radiation therapy. Pericardial effusion with or without tamponade, and constrictive pericarditis are all common forms of late-onset pericardial illness.

## PATHOPHYSIOLOGY

- TB bacilli can enter the pericardium by retrograde lymphatic spread from nearby lymph nodes, bloodstream transfer from a primary infection, rarely direct contiguous spread from neighbouring infected structures.
- The immune response to the TB bacilli is responsible for the clinical manifestations. Bacillus protein antigens cause delayed hypersensitivity, activating lymphocytes to generate lymphokines, which in turn stimulate macrophages and promote the development of granulomas.
- Two primary mechanisms coerce the presentation of pericarditis:
  i. Accumulation of fluid in the pericardium, compress the cardiac chambers during the entire cardiac cycle, thereby hampering the contraction and relaxation.
  ii. Pericardial thickening with minimal or no effusion, leading to impaired cardiac filling during diastole (constriction).
- Tuberculous pericarditis (TBP) progresses through four pathological phases, each associated with distinct clinical manifestations:
  - *Phase 1: Fibrinous exudation*—Marked by preliminary polymorphonuclear leukocytosis, an excess of

mycobacteria, and the early development of granulomas featuring loosely organized macrophages and T-cells. This is the least common phase.

- *Phase 2: Serosanguineous effusion*—The exudate primarily consists of lymphocytes, accompanied by monocytes and foam cells, and tubercle bacilli present in low concentrations. This is the most common phase, where patients often present with heart failure symptoms due to large pericardial effusion, with or without tamponade.
- *Phase 3: Absorption and granuloma formation*—The effusion is absorbed, leading to granulomatous caseation and pericardial thickening caused by fibrin, collagen, and fibrosis. Patients show signs of constrictive pericarditis, though echocardiography reveals thick fibrinous fluid encircling the heart.
- *Phase 4*: *Constrictive scarring*—The fibrosing pericardium squeezes around the heart and as well as calcify, forming a fibrocalcific shell that limits diastolic filling, ensuing in the classic syndrome of constrictive pericarditis. The diagnosis is proved by echocardiography when there is no remaining pericardial fluid.

## TREATMENT AND PREVENTION

- *Hemodynamic stabilization*: Urgent pericardiocentesis if signs of tamponade are present
- *Specific antituberculous therapy*:
  - In areas with a high incidence of tuberculosis, pericardial effusion is generally regarded as tuberculosis until an alternative etiology is clearly identified. Additionally, treatment is often initiated before a bacteriological diagnosis is confirmed.
  - ATT significantly improves survival in tuberculous pericarditis. It has been shown to reduce mortality from 80–90% in the preantibiotic era to 8–17% in HIV-negative patients and 17–34% in HIV-positive individuals. A 6-month weight-based ATT regimen includes HRZE for 2 months, followed by HRE for 4 months is used to treat TBPE.
- *Adjunctive steroid therapy*:
  - The INDEX guidelines recommend corticosteroids for all patients with TB pericarditis and pericardial effusion as a conditional recommendation. Prednisolone can be administered at a dose of 1 mg/kg for 4 weeks, followed by 0.5 mg/kg for 4 weeks, then tapering over next 4 weeks.
  - Corticosteroids may hasten clinical improvement, prevent development of constriction, and reduce the need for pericardiectomy.
- *Surgical management*:
  - Even with prompt treatment, 30–60% of patients develop constrictive pericarditis for which surgical pericardiectomy is the treatment of choice.

### Points to Ponder

- *Forms of TBPE:* Pericardial effusion, constrictive pericarditis, or a combination of both.
- *Cardiac tamponade:* Suggested by Beck's triad (hypotension, muffled heart sounds, elevated jugular venous pressure).
- *Fluid accumulation*: The speed of fluid accumulation is more critical than the volume for tamponade development.
- *Diagnostic features*: Exudative effusion with lymphocytic predominance and elevated ADA levels.
- *Confirmation:* Tubercle bacilli in pericardial fluid smear or culture, or caseating granulomas on histology.
- Treatment: Early initiation of antitubercular therapy (ATT) improves survival.
- *Steroids:* May accelerate clinical improvement, prevent constriction, and reduce the need for pericardiectomy.

## MULTIPLE CHOICE QUESTIONS

**1. Which of the following viruses commonly causes acute pericarditis?**
A. ECHO virus
B. Hepatitis B virus
C. Epstein–Barr virus
D. Cytomegalovirus

**2. What is the most common complication of untreated TB pericardial effusion?**
A. Constrictive pericarditis
B. Pleural effusion
C. Cardiac arrhythmia
D. Pulmonary embolism

**3. In suspected TBPE, pericardial fluid analysis shows?**
A. High protein, low ADA
B. Low protein, low ADA
C. High protein, high ADA
D. Low protein, high ADA

**4. Which clinical feature would most likely suggest cardiac tamponade?**
A. Sharp chest pain worsening with inspiration
B. Pulsus paradoxus
C. Persistent low-grade fever
D. Cough and night sweats

**5. Which finding on echocardiography is most concerning for tamponade?**
A. Large pericardial effusion
B. Collapsed right atrium during diastole
C. Normal ventricular wall motion
D. Echogenic pericardium

### Answers

1. (A); 2. (A); 3. (C); 4. (B); 5. (B)

## SUGGESTED READINGS


1. Index-TB-Guidelines.pdf [Internet]. [cited 2024 Nov 5]. Available from: https://tbcindia.mohfw.gov.in/wp-content/uploads/2023/05/5585665076Index-TB-Guidelines.pdf
2. Mayosi BM, Burgess LJ, Doubell AF. Tuberculous Pericarditis. Circulation. 2005;112(23):3608-16.
3. Willner DA, Goyal A, Grigorova Y, et al. Pericardial Effusion. In: StatPearls [Internet]. Treasure Island (FL): StatPearls Publishing; 2024 [cited 2024 Nov 14]. Available from: http://www.ncbi.nlm.nih.gov/books/NBK431089/.
4. Chau E, Sarkarati M, Spellberg B. Adenosine Deaminase Diagnostic Testing in Pericardial Fluid. JAMA. 2019;322(2):163.
5. Reuter H, Burgess L, van Vuuren W, et al. Diagnosing tuberculous pericarditis. QJM. 2006;99:827.
6. Yu G, Zhong F, Shen Y, et al. Diagnostic accuracy of the Xpert MTB/RIF assay for tuberculous pericarditis: A systematic review and meta-analysis. PLoS ONE. 2021;16(9):e0257220.
7. Mori S, Bertamino M, Guerisoli L, et al. Pericardial effusion in oncological patients: current knowledge and principles of management. Cardiooncology. 2024;10(1):8.
8. Evans DJ. The use of adjunctive corticosteroids in the treatment of pericardial, pleural and meningeal tuberculosis: Do they improve outcome? Respiratory Medicine. 2008;102(6):793-800.

CHAPTER 3

# An Approach to a Case of Heart Failure with Preserved Ejection Fraction

*Deepanjan Bhattacharya*

## CASE VIGNETTE

A 34-year-old lady presented with progressive dyspnea on exertion and bipedal edema for the past 3 months, without any history of orthopnea, paroxysmal nocturnal dyspnea, palpitations, angina, or syncope, nor there was any family history of cardiac illness.

Examination showed pulse rate of 96 beats/min, regular and normal volume with no radio-radial or radio-femoral delay. Blood pressure was 96/74 mm Hg in the right upper limb and 108/76 mm Hg in the left lower limb. Pitting bipedal edema was present.

Jugular venous pressure was elevated 8 cm above clavicle, with prominent *v* wave and *y* descent. There was no cardiomegaly. Auscultation showed normal S1 and normally split S2 with loud pulmonary component and audible LV-S3. Systemic examination was otherwise unremarkable.

A 12-lead electrocardiogram showed sinus rhythm with first-degree atrioventricular block, low amplitude QRS in limb leads, and QS pattern in $V_1$-$V_3$ (Pseudoinfarct pattern). Chest X-ray showed no cardiomegaly with Grade I pulmonary venous hypertension.

Transthoracic echocardiogram showed concentric left ventricular hypertrophy with speckling bright myocardium and good biventricular function. There was grade III diastolic dysfunction, mild pulmonary arterial hypertension (pulmonary artery systolic pressure = 42 mm Hg) and with mild pericardial effusion. Global longitudinal strain was markedly reduced with apical sparing (cherry on top appearance). NT-proBNP was also elevated (2,420 pg/mL).

Cardiac magnetic resonance imaging showed good biventricular systolic function with impairment of diastolic function and elevated native T1 value (1,200 ms). Postcontrast imaging showed delayed enhancement of the subendocardium predominantly at mid and basal segments of interventricular septum, along with reversal of myocardial suppression on TI scout images. Coronary angiogram was normal.

Myocardial biopsy showed revealed interstitial eosinophilic deposits that were positive for Congo Red stain with apple-green birefringence on polarization, suggestive of amyloidosis.

Considering the possibility of myeloma-related amyloidosis, serum protein electrophoresis was done, which was negative for "M band." Immunoglobulin profile was normal; however, free kappa chains were markedly elevated (1,530 mg/L). Bone marrow biopsy showed clusters of CD138 positive plasma cells with kappa light chain restriction

## PROVISIONAL DIAGNOSIS

Provisional diagnosis of the case was heart failure with preserved ejection fraction (HFpEF). On workup, the diagnosis was infiltrative cardiomyopathy due to AL amyloidosis secondary to plasma cell myeloma.

## DIFFERENTIAL DIAGNOSIS

Other causes of HFpEF include ATTR amyloidosis, hemochromatosis, sarcoidosis, hypertrophic cardiomyopathy, coronary artery disease and secondary to hypertension and aging.

## CLINICAL APPROACH

Heart failure (HF) is a complex clinical syndrome characterized by inefficient myocardial performance, resulting in compromised blood supply to the body, due to impairment of ventricular filling or ejection of blood to the systemic circulation.

Based on echocardiogram, HF is classified into:
- Heart failure with reduced ejection fraction (HFrEF): Patients with an LVEF ≤40%
- Heart failure with improved ejection fraction (HFimpEF): Patients with a previous LVEF ≤40% and a subsequent measurement of LVEF >40%
- Heart Failure with mildly reduced ejection fraction (HFmrEF): Patients with an LVEF 41–49%
- Heart failure with preserved ejection fraction (HFpEF): Patients with an LVEF ≥50%

For diagnosis of HFpEF, HFA-PEFF and $H_2$FPEF scoring systems are used **(Table 1)**.

**TABLE 1: HFA-PEFF and $H_2FPEF$ scoring systems.**

| HFA-PEFF score | $H_2FPEF$ score |
|---|---|
| **Major criteria (2 points each)**<br>• Septal e′ <7 cm/s or lateral e′ <10 cm/s or E/e′ >15 or TR velocity >2.8 m/sec<br>• LAVI >34 mL/m² or LVMI >149 (male) or >122 (female) g/m² and RWT >0.42 g<br>• NT-proBNP >220 pg/mL or BNP >80 pg/mL (in sinus rhythm)<br>• NT-proBNP >660 pg/mL or BNP >240 pg/mL(in atrial fibrillation)<br>**Minor criteria (1 point each)**<br>• E/e′ 9–14 or GLS <16%<br>• LAVI 29–34 mL/m² or LVMI >115 (male) or >95 (female) g/m² or RWT >0.42 g or LV wall thickness >12 mm<br>• NT-proBNP 125–220 pg/mL or BNP 35–80 pg/mL (in sinus rhythm)<br>• NT-proBNP 365–660 pg/mL or BNP 105–240 pg/mL (in atrial fibrillation)<br>2–4 points → Diastolic stress echocardiogram or invasive cardiac catheterization ≥5 → HFpEF | • Heavy (BMI >30 kg/m²) – 2<br>• Hypertensive (≥2 antihypertensive drugs) – 1<br>• Atrial fibrillation (paroxysmal/persistent) – 3<br>• Pulmonary hypertension (PASP >35 mm Hg) – 1<br>• Elderly (Age >60 years) – 1<br>• Filling pressure (E/e′ > 9) – 1<br>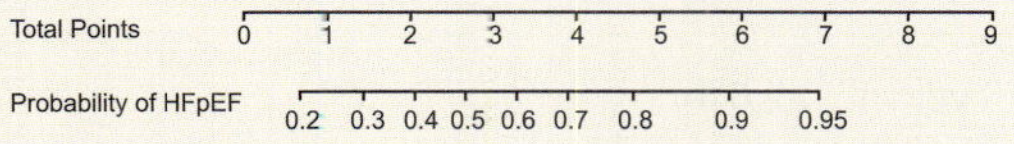 |

On clinical examination, patients can have features of left heart failure (orthopnea, paroxysmal nocturnal dyspnea, pulmonary edema) or congestive cardiac failure (bipedal edema, elevated JVP). Cardiomegaly is characteristically absent.

On auscultation, S1 is usually normal (can be variable if patient is in atrial fibrillation) with a loud P2 (in cases with pulmonary hypertension) and prominent LV S3.

Electrocardiogram is usually unremarkable except for occasional findings of left atrial enlargement (P mitrale), left ventricular hypertrophy or atrial fibrillation. Echocardiogram shows a preserved LVEF (≥50%) with varying degrees of diastolic dysfunction, pulmonary hypertension and a distended inferior vena cava.

Further workup includes cardiac MRI for LGE pattern, and workup for amyloidosis including 99mTc-pyrophosphate scan and serum free light chain assay.

## PATHOPHYSIOLOGY

In HFpEF, there is significant remodelling of the left ventricle resulting in incomplete myocardial relaxation, increased ventricular stiffness with subsequent decreased ventricular distensibility. There can be additional infiltration as seen in amyloidosis or sarcoidosis. Contributory factors include advanced age, hypertension, diabetes mellitus, renal dysfunction, coronary artery disease and obesity.

This results in a shift in the Frank–Starling mechanism initially during exercise and eventually at rest, and elevated left ventricular filling pressures.

Physiologic reserve is also markedly decreased leading to diminished exercise capacity. Peripheral oxygen extraction during exercise is also impaired, along with reduced total arterial compliance during submaximal and peak exercise. The exact etiology of this impairment is unclear but may be due to intrinsic deficiencies in the function of skeletal muscle, vascular endothelium, or mitochondria.

## TREATMENT AND PREVENTION

Lifestyle changes and risk factor modification are important parts of therapy, which include weight reduction, low salt diet, control of hypertension and diabetes mellitus.

Diuretics have been shown to reduce mortality and heart failure hospitalization (HFH) in the optimize HF study. The TOPCAT trial also demonstrated reduction of HFH by aldosterone antagonists.

Use of ARNI is controversial, as the PARAGON HF trial did not show any reduction in mortality or HFH.

Sodium-glucose cotransporter-2 (SGLT-2) inhibitors (dapagliflozin and empagliflozin) are considered the mainstay of therapy. Both the DELIVER and EMPEROR PRESERVED trials showed significant reduction in cardiovascular mortality, HFH, decline in renal function and improvement in quality of life.

Atrial fibrillation mandates need for anticoagulation irrespective of $CHA_2DS_2VASc$ score, while beta-blockers and non-DHP calcium channel blockers are used for control of heart rate.

CardioMEMS is a wireless device placed in the pulmonary artery which monitors changes in pulmonary artery pressure. It helps to titrate therapy on the basis of pulmonary capillary wedge pressure. In the CHAMPION trial, it was associated with significant reduction of HFH.

Coronary revascularization is indicated only in patients with significant coronary artery obstruction.

In patients with AL amyloid, treatment of underlying plasma cell neoplasia is required. In patients with ATTR amyloidosis, treatment modalities include.

- Inhibitors of TTR gene expression – Patisiran, Inotersen, Revusiran
- Tetramer stabilizer – Tafamidis, Diflunisal

## Points to Ponder

- Normal left ventricular ejection fraction does not rule out heart failure.
- Diastolic function testing and strain imaging are useful tools.
- In suspected cardiac amyloidosis, cardiac MRI, Tc99m pyrophosphate scan and serum free light chain assay are an essential part of workup.
- ATTR amyloidosis requires targeted therapy against TTR.
- SGLT-2 inhibitors are the only medications with proven mortality benefit in HFpEF.

## MULTIPLE CHOICE QUESTIONS

**1. All are markers of elevated left atrial filling pressures except:**

A. E/e' >15
B. TR velocity >2.8 m/s
C. LA volume indexed>34 mL/m$^2$
D. None of the above

**2. All are treatment modalities for ATTR amyloidosis?**

A. Patisiran
B. Inotersen
C. Tafamidis
D. All of the above

**3. Which of these medicines have shown clinical benefit in HFpEF?**

A. Dapagliflozin
B. Bisoprolol
C. Vericiguat
D. Carvedilol

**4. Which type of cardiac amyloidosis has worst prognosis?**

A. AL
B. ATTR (senile)
C. AA
D. ATTR (wild)

**5. Which of the following is an intervention for HFpEF?**

A. Cardiac resynchronisation therapy
B. CardioMEMs
C. Coronary sinus reducer
D. Enhanced External Counterpulsation

### Answers

1. (D); 2. (D); 3. (A); 4. (A); 5. (B)

## SUGGESTED READINGS


1. Heidenreich PA, Bozkurt B, Aguilar D, et al. 2022 AHA/ACC/HFSA Guideline for the Management of Heart Failure: A Report of the American College of Cardiology/American Heart Association Joint Committee on Clinical Practice Guidelines. J Am Coll Cardiol. 2022;79(17):e263-e421
2. Reddy YNV, Kaye DM, Handoko ML, et al. Diagnosis of Heart Failure With Preserved Ejection Fraction Among Patients With Unexplained Dyspnea. JAMA Cardiol. 2022;7(9):891-99.
3. McDonagh TA, Metra M, Adamo M, et al. ESC Scientific Document Group. 2023 Focused Update of the 2021 ESC Guidelines for the diagnosis and treatment of acute and chronic heart failure. Eur Heart J. 2023 ;44(37):3627-39. Erratum in: Eur Heart J. 2024;45(1):53.
4. O'Connor CM, Abraham WT, Albert NM, et al. Predictors of mortality after discharge in patients hospitalized with heart failure: an analysis from the Organized Program to Initiate Lifesaving Treatment in Hospitalized Patients with Heart Failure (OPTIMIZE-HF). Am Heart J. 2008;156(4):662-73.
5. Pitt B, Pfeffer MA, Assmann SF, et al; TOPCAT Investigators. Spironolactone for heart failure with preserved ejection fraction. N Engl J Med. 2014;370(15):1383-92.
6. Chandra A, Vaduganathan M, Lewis EF, et al; PARAGON-HF Investigators. Health-Related Quality of Life in Heart Failure With Preserved Ejection Fraction: The PARAGON-HF Trial. JACC Heart Fail. 2019;7(10):862-74.
7. Solomon SD, McMurray JJV, Claggett B, et al; DELIVER Trial Committees and Investigators. Dapagliflozin in Heart Failure with Mildly Reduced or Preserved Ejection Fraction. N Engl J Med. 2022;387(12):1089-98.
8. Anker SD, Butler J, Filippatos G, et al; EMPEROR-Preserved Trial Investigators. Empagliflozin in Heart Failure with a Preserved Ejection Fraction. N Engl J Med. 2021;385(16):1451-61.
9. Adamson PB, Abraham WT, Aaron M, et al. CHAMPION trial rationale and design: the long-term safety and clinical efficacy of a wireless pulmonary artery pressure monitoring system. J Card Fail. 2011;17(1):3-10.

CHAPTER

4

# An Approach to a Case of Cardiac Manifestations of Connective Tissue Disease

*Sunita Kumbhalkar, Keshao Nagpure*

## CASE VIGNETTE

In December 2022, a 56-year-old female patient presented with a 1-month history of tingling and numbness in both the lower and upper limbs, followed by distal symmetrical weakness starting in the lower limbs and later involving the upper limbs. The patient also reported large ulcers on both distal lower limbs and blackish discoloration of the fingers and toes for 1 month. **Figure 1A** she did not report any cardiorespiratory symptoms at presentation. Additionally, she had a 4-year history of pain and swelling in the small joints of the hands and feet, accompanied by morning stiffness, for which she had intermittently taken alternative medications. The patient was a known case of diabetes mellitus and hypothyroidism and was on regular treatment.

Initial investigations revealed microcytic hypochromic anemia (hemoglobin –6.9 g/dL), neutrophilic leukocytosis (total count –16,006/mm$^3$), elevated ESR (46 mm/h) and CRP (>90 mg/L) levels. Rheumatoid factor and anti-CCP antibodies were positive, while ANA was negative. ANA immunoblot, p-ANCA, and c-ANCA were also negative. Her HbA1c - 9.27%, and TSH was 7.43 µIU/mL. Kidney and liver function tests were within normal limit. An arterial Doppler study of the upper limbs was normal. A nerve conduction study indicated axonal sensory-motor neuropathy. A skin biopsy suggestive of ulceration and thrombosis of small and medium size vessels with degeneration of collagen consistent with rheumatoid vasculitis. **(Figs. 1B and C)**. Fundus examination and urinary albumin excretion were normal.

The 12-lead ECG was within normal limits; however, the 2D echocardiogram revealed mild global left ventricular (LV) hypokinesia, an LVEF of 50%, thickened mitral and aortic valves, and grade 1 diastolic dysfunction, with no evidence of clots, vegetations, or pulmonary embolism.

The patient was treated with pulse steroid therapy, followed by oral steroids, methotrexate and hydroxychloroquine, and two doses of Rituximab (1 g each, administered 2 weeks apart), antiplatelets, statins, ACE inhibitors and beta-blockers. Blood sugar levels were strictly managed using insulin and oral hypoglycemic agents. The patient responded well to treatment, showing rapid healing of leg ulcers, nonprogression of digital gangrene, and improved neurological function over the following 6 months. However, she was lost to follow-up for 1 year.

In February 2024, she presented with shortness of breath and sudden blackening of the left hand. On examination, the left hand was swollen with blackish discoloration, extending to the wrist and lower third of the forearm. There was an ulcer with black slough on the right lower limb, tenderness, and blisters. The left brachial pulse was present, but the radial pulse was not palpable. A venous Doppler of the left upper limb showed complete lumen-occluding echogenic material in the axillary, brachial, ulnar, cephalic, basilic, and median cubital veins, suggestive of thrombosis. An arterial Doppler of the left upper limb

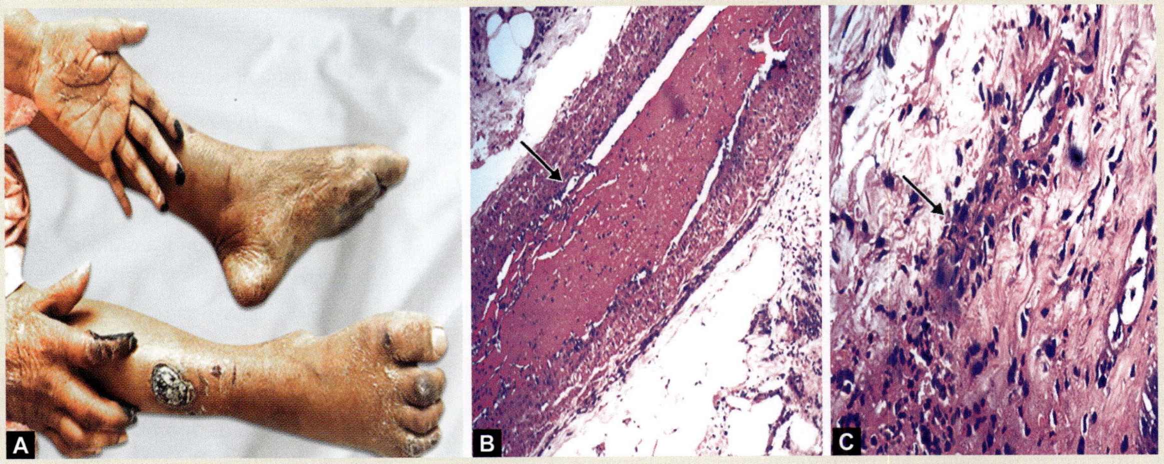


**FIGS. 1A TO C:** (A) Showing digital gangrene and ulcer. (B) (Low power) and (C) (high power) – skin biopsy showing vasculitis.

revealed atherosclerotic changes in the radial and ulnar arteries as vessel wall calcification. The axillary, brachial, radial, and ulnar arteries demonstrated normal colour flow, patency, velocity, and triphasic waveforms. No abnormal narrowing or thrombus was seen. CRP elevated at 90 mg/L, ESR was 42 (mm/h), and antiphospholipid antibodies were negative. The DAS28-CRP score was 4.25, indicating moderate disease severity. 2D echocardiogram revealed worsening global LV hypokinesia, LVEF of 25–30%, moderate mitral and tricuspid regurgitation, mild pulmonary artery hypertension, TAPSE of 15 mm, and a collapsing IVC, with no vegetations, clots, or pulmonary embolism was noted. Cardiac angiography was planned, however refused by relatives. Due to poor LV function, Rituximab was not given, and the patient was treated with cyclophosphamide injections, along with steroids, DMARDs, and treatment for heart failure and anticoagulation. The patient received six doses of cyclophosphamide, additional immunosuppressive therapy, antiplatelets with statins, anticoagulation, and comprehensive heart failure management.

## PROVISIONAL DIAGNOSIS

Rheumatoid arthritis with systemic rheumatoid vasculitis presenting as peripheral neuropathy, digital gangrene and vasculitis ulcers with venous thrombosis with heart failure with reduced ejection fraction.

## DIFFERENTIAL DIAGNOSIS

Refer to **Table 1**.

## CLINICAL APPROACH

Patients with connective tissue diseases (CTDs) may present with valvular, myocardial, pericardial inflammation, coronary artery disease, vasculitis, myocardial fibrosis, heart failure, as well as pulmonary arterial hypertension. Cardiovascular diseases (CVD) are leading cause morbidity and mortality in patients with connective tissue diseases. Therefore, all the patients with CTDs are clinically evaluated for CVD. CVD in CTD may be asymptomatic or characterized by subtle, usually atypical symptoms (Patients with RA are less likely to report chest pain than those without RA). Detailed history taking includes traditional risk factors for CVD including smoking, hypertension, diabetes mellitus, hyperlipidemia, and obesity. The nontraditional risk factors associated with CVD in CTDs include severity of the disease, more extra-articular manifestation at presentation, corticosteroids, NSAIDs, immunosuppressants and the low socioeconomic status. The increased risk of CAD results from both traditional risk factors and factors unique to these CTDs.

Physical examination includes detailed head to toe examination to look for articular and extra-articular manifestations of CTDs. This includes examination of all joints, peripheral pulses, dermatological examination for rash typical for particular CTD, nail changes, vasculitis manifestations, signs of heart failure and comprehensive examination of cardiovascular system. Disease activity of CTDs has been assessed as per disease activity indices.

The standard initial tests for cardiac evaluation in CTDs are a 12-lead ECG and exercise ECG, though the latter is often not feasible in CTD patients. Transthoracic echocardiography (TTE) is the primary tool for diagnosing certain cardiac issues in CTDs, while stress echocardiography, combining TTE with stress (physical, pharmacological), is a highly effective, cost-efficient method for diagnosing coronary artery disease. Stress myocardial perfusion scintigraphy (MPS) is another valuable noninvasive tool for coronary disease diagnosis. More recently, cardiovascular magnetic resonance (CMR) has emerged as the gold standard for evaluating heart structure and function, myocardial inflammation, and coronary abnormalities, including aneurysms. CMR has proven particularly useful in assessing

**TABLE 1: Cardiovascular manifestations of connective tissue diseases.**

| Connective tissue disease | Cardiovascular disease |
|---|---|
| Rheumatoid arthritis 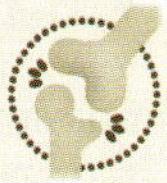 | • Accelerated atherosclerosis<br>• Coronary artery disease (CAD)<br>• Congestive heart failure<br>• Cardiomyopathy<br>• Peripheral arterial disease (PAD)<br>• Pericarditis<br>• Myocarditis and endocarditis<br>• Pulmonary hypertension<br>• Rheumatoid nodule/granuloma<br>• Secondary cardiac amyloidosis<br>• Mitral valve insufficiency, aortic valve insufficiency<br>• Conduction abnormalities<br>• Rheumatoid vasculitis |
| Systemic lupus erythematosus 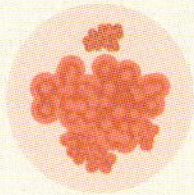 | • Pericarditis, pericardial effusion<br>• Lupus myocarditis-cardiomyopathy<br>• Heart failure<br>• Coronary artery disease<br>• Endocarditis (Libman–Sacks endocarditis)<br>• Congenital heart blocks |
| Systemic sclerosis | • Myocardial fibrosis-cardiomyopathy<br>• Pulmonary hypertension<br>• Conduction defects |
| Ankylosing spondylitis 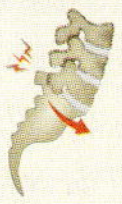 | • Coronary artery disease<br>• Conduction defects<br>• Aortic valve insufficiency<br>• Left ventricular dysfunction |
| Psoriatic arthritis | • Conduction defects<br>• CAD<br>• Peripheral arterial disease |
| Inflammatory myopathies | • Myocarditis<br>• CAD |
| Systemic vasculitis 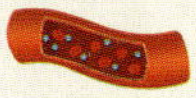 | • CAD<br>• PAD<br>• Myocardium, pericardium, endocardium, and conduction system involvements |
| Antiphospholipid syndrome 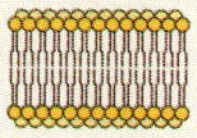 | • CAD<br>• PAD<br>• Valvular heart disease – mitral and aortic valve stenosis/insufficiency<br>• Deep venous thrombosis, pulmonary embolism<br>• Nonbacterial thrombotic endocarditis |

cardiac involvement in rheumatic diseases like vasculitis, SLE, rheumatoid arthritis, and scleroderma, making it an important tool for rheumatologists.

## PATHOPHYSIOLOGY

Cardiovascular diseases in connective tissue diseases are due to various pathophysiologic processes **(Fig. 2)**, such as myocardial and vascular inflammation, accelerated atherosclerosis, myocardial ischemia due to micro- or macrovascular disease, abnormal coronary vasoreactivity and/or myocardial fibrosis. The underlying mechanisms vary across different CTDs but are generally linked to autoimmune dysregulation and chronic inflammation. Immune complex deposits in the heart can trigger autoimmune responses and activate the complement system. Persistent inflammation leads to oxidative stress, which, along with increased fibroblast activity, contributes to myocardial fibrosis. Chronic inflammation also causes monocyte accumulation, upregulates adhesion molecules, releases proinflammatory cytokines, and promotes the breakdown of vascular matrix, all of which contribute to endothelial dysfunction and early coronary atherosclerosis.

## TREATMENT AND PREVENTION

Cardiovascular disease in connective tissue diseases varies in frequency and requires individualized treatment based on disease type and severity. Treatment typically involves immunosuppressive or immunomodulatory therapies, especially during active disease phases, tailored to disease activity, organ involvement, and comorbidities. Life-threatening complications like myocarditis and vasculitis are treated with pulse methylprednisolone, followed by oral steroids and intensive immunosuppression (cyclophosphamide or Rituximab). Steroid doses should be minimized, with a taper attempted in remission or low disease activity.

In primary antiphospholipid syndrome (APS) or APS associated with CTDs and thrombosis, Warfarin is the preferred treatment. Rivaroxaban should be avoided due to recurrent thrombosis risk. Low-dose aspirin with hydroxychloroquine is recommended for thrombosis prevention in antiphospholipid antibody-positive SLE patients.

*CTD medications can influence CVD risk and severity*:

- Corticosteroids should be cautiously, for shortest period of time in lowest possible dosage, if long-term steroids required, steroid sparing strategy with long-term immunosuppressive agents to be considered.
- NSAIDs should be used cautiously, especially in patients with existing CVD or risk factors. Selective COX-2 inhibitors should be avoided, with naproxen preferred when necessary.
- Conventional DMARDs (Methotrexate, hydroxychloroquine, sulfasalazine) reduce cardiovascular risk, while leflunomide and cyclosporine can induce hypertension and should be avoided in high-risk patients.
- TNF blockers reduce CVD risk in rheumatoid arthritis, but Infliximab and Rituximab should be avoided in severe heart failure.

Preventing CVD in CTD patients involves controlling both traditional and nontraditional risk factors. This includes managing dyslipidemia, diabetes, hypertension, and obesity, following lifestyle changes like a healthy diet, regular exercise, and smoking cessation. Blood pressure and blood sugar should be monitored regularly, especially in patients on NSAIDs, cyclosporine, or corticosteroids. Early diagnosis and optimal disease management can significantly reduce CVD risk in CTD patients.

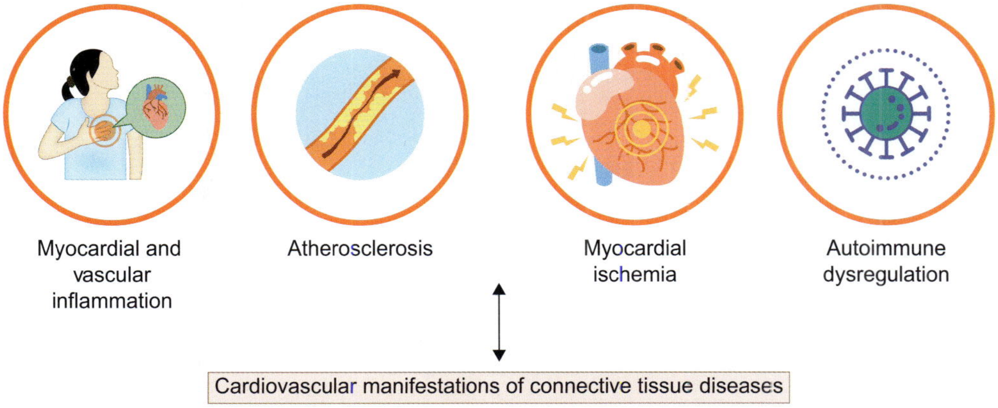


**FIG. 2:** Cardiovascular diseases in connective tissue disorders result from a variety of pathophysiological mechanisms.

### Points to Ponder

- Connective tissue disorders are important risk factor for cardiovascular diseases.
- Cardiovascular disease may be initial manifestation or late features of poorly controlled, long standing connective tissue disease.
- CVD in connective tissue diseases arises from inflammation, accelerated atherosclerosis, myocardial ischemia, and myocardial fibrosis and vasculitis.
- Cardiovascular disease in CTD can range from mild pericarditis to severe life threatening myocarditis and systemic vasculitis.
- Early recognition of clinical features, identifying risk factors, and implementing preventive measures to manage and reduce the impact of CVD in these patients.
- Timely treatment of underlying CTD and treat to target strategy lower the rate of cardiovascular disease in CTDs.
- Treatment options varies from simple anti-inflammatory drugs for mild disease to aggressive immunosuppression for severe life-threatening CVDs.

## MULTIPLE CHOICE QUESTIONS

**1. What is the most frequent cardiac manifestation of systemic lupus erythematosus?**
a. Myocarditis
b. Pericarditis
c. Libman–Sacks endocarditis
d. Coronary artery disease

**2. Drug of choice for deep venous thrombosis in patient with antiphospholipid syndrome is:**
A. Rivaroxaban
B. Apixaban
C. Warfarin
D. Fondaparinux

**3. Which of the following is most common valvular abnormality in patients with rheumatoid arthritis?**
A. Mitral regurgitation
B. Mitral stenosis
C. Aortic stenosis
D. Aortic regurgitation

**4. Which of the following is appropriate treatment for myocarditis in 50-year-old female patient with SLE ?**
A. Methotrexate and pulse methylprednisolone
B. Cyclophosphamide and pulse methylprednisolone
C. Hydroxychloroquine and pulse methylprednisolone
D. Only pulse methylprednisolone

**5. Which of the following drug should be avoided in patient with hypertension and increased cardiovascular risk in patients with connective tissue disease?**
A. Methotrexate
B. Sulfasalazine
C. Hydroxychloroquine
D. Leflunomide

### Answers

1. (B); 2. (C); 3. (A); 4. (B); 5. (D)

## SUGGESTED READINGS

1. Ali RA, Hussein H, Almoallim H. Cardiovascular Diseases and Rheumatology. In Skills in Rheumatology, Singapore: Springer, 2021.
2. Pan SY, Tian HM, Zhu Y, et al. Cardiac Damage in Autoimmune Diseases: Target Organ Involvement That Cannot Be Ignored. Frontiers in Immunology. 2022;13: 1056400.
3. Mavrogeni S. Assessment of Cardiovascular Involvement in Connective Tissue Disease: Let's Open Pandora's Box. Mediterr J Rheumatol. 2016;27(3):91-3.
4. Hedar AM, Stradner MH, Roessler A, et al. Autoimmune Rheumatic Diseases and Vascular Function: The Concept of Autoimmune Atherosclerosis. J Clin Med. 2021;10(19):4427.
5. Drosos GC, Thomas K, Boumpas D, et al. EULAR Recommendations for Cardiovascular Risk Management in Rheumatic and Musculoskeletal Diseases, Including Systemic Lupus Erythematosus and Antiphospholipid Syndrome. Annals of the Rheumatic Diseases. 2022;81(6):768-79.

CHAPTER 5

# An Approach to a Case of Ejection Systolic Murmur at the Base of Heart

*Mainak Mukhopadhyay, Sandipta Ray*

**CASE VIGNETTE**

A 63-year-old hypertensive gentleman with regular history of smoking, attended OPD with complaint of effort angina and dyspnea on exertion over last 6 months. He had a recent history of transient loss of consciousness (TLOC) with spontaneous complete recovery while running to catch a bus. His past medical history or family history was noncontributory. He was on tablet telmisartan 40 mg once daily for hypertension. On clinical examination, he was afebrile and without any pallor or clubbing or cyanosis, pulse rate was 78 beats/min, regular, slow rising and delayed peaking with carotid thrill bilaterally, sans any radio-radial or radio-femoral delay. BP was 130/80 mm Hg in both upper limbs. There was no pedal edema and JVP was not raised. On cardiovascular examination, there was no cardiomegaly but sustained apical impulse and thrill in right upper parasternal area. On auscultation, $S_1$ was normal with soft $A_2$ (aortic component of $S_2$) and grade 4 harsh ejection systolic murmur (ESM) in right upper parasternal area radiating toward the carotids best heard with the diaphragm of the stethoscope while patient in sitting and leaning forward position. The intensity of murmur reduced on standing and on strain phase of Valsalva and remain unchanged on squatting or leg raising or handgrip. There was bilateral normal breath sound and other system examination including fundoscopy was noncontributory.

## PROVISIONAL DIAGNOSIS

The patient was clinically diagnosed to be functional NYHA class II due to symptomatic severe valvular aortic stenosis of degenerative etiology; in sinus rhythm without any feature of infective endocarditis.

## DIFFERENTIAL DIAGNOSIS

Common differential diagnosis of ESM at the base of heart are:

- *Aortic stenosis (AS)*: Harsh ESM of AS is best heard in the right upper parasternal area in sitting posture with the diaphragm of the stethoscope. The murmur radiates toward the carotids. With severity, the duration of murmur increases with delayed peaking and is often associated with thrill. Grade 4 murmur is usually associated with >50 mm Hg pressure gradient, whereas delayed peaking is often associated with 75 mm Hg above gradient. Severe AS is associated with a delayed aortic component of second heart sound ($A_2$) and paradoxical splitting **(Fig. 1)**. Paradoxical split is usually associated with a gradient of > 100 mm Hg or LV systolic pressure >160 mm Hg. AS can be valvular, subvalvular or supravalvular. Valvular AS is having valvular click, supravalvular AS is often characterized by differential limb BP, and subvalvular AS is often associated with aortic regurgitation (AR). Often, degenerative AS murmur is quite conspicuous in the apical area; it is called the Gallavardin effect and may mimic mitral regurgitation (MR) murmur.
- *Pulmonary stenosis (PS)*: ESM of PS is best heard in a left upper parasternal area with radiation toward the back. Valvular PS murmur is often associated with valvular click. Although the PS murmur increases with inspiration, the click decreases with inspiration. With progressive severity, the click tends toward the first heart sound and finally merges with $S_1$. In such a situation, the intensity of $S_1$ will vary with respiration.
- *Hypertrophic obstructive cardiomyopathy (HOCM)*: ESM of HOCM is best heard in the mid precordium, and the murmur increases on standing from squatting and in the Valsalva strain phase. HOCM is often associated with MR.
- *High output flow status*: Sometimes, even with a normal valve, owing to high flow status [e.g., anemia, thyrotoxicosis, fever,

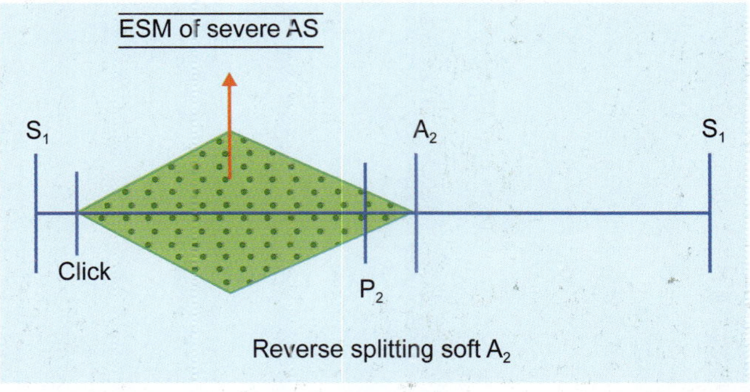


**FIG. 1:** Ejection systolic murmur (ESM) of severe valvular aortic stenosis (AS).

ventricular septal defect (VSD), patent ductus arteriosus (PDA), and atrial septal defect], outflow tract ESM may be audible. But hardly the intensity ever crosses beyond grade 3, and they are never associated with any ejection click.

- *Chronic mitral regurgitation due to posterior mitral leaflet flail/prolapse*: The holosystolic-murmur radiates to the base of the heart when it is due to the posterior leaflet prolapse or flail. In that case, it may be confused with the long ESM of severe AS and is often impossible to differentiate clinically. In the subsequent normal beat of ventricular premature contraction (VPC), the murmur of AS increases in intensity, whereas the murmur of MR remains the same.

## DIAGNOSIS

Resting ECG showed left ventricular hypertrophy (LVH) and resting echo Doppler study **(Figs. 2 and 3)** showed the mean gradient across thickened and restricted and calcified aortic valve is 62 mm Hg with LVH and good LV systolic function but grade 3 diastolic function with elevated filling pressure with LA borderline dilated.

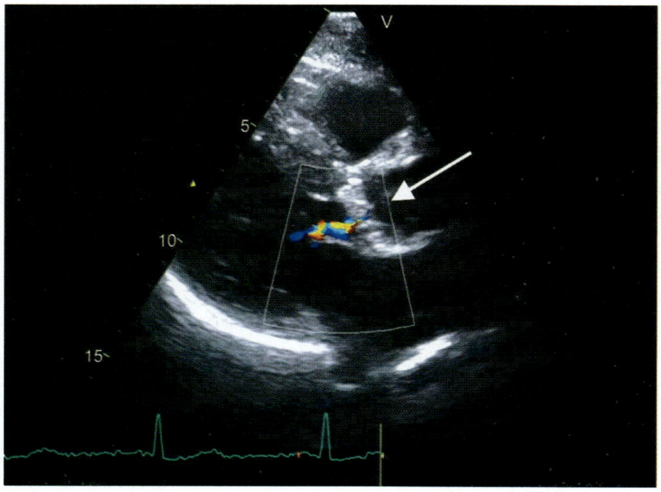


**FIG. 2:** Parasternal long axis (PLAX) view in echo Doppler showing calcified and thickened aortic valve leaflets.

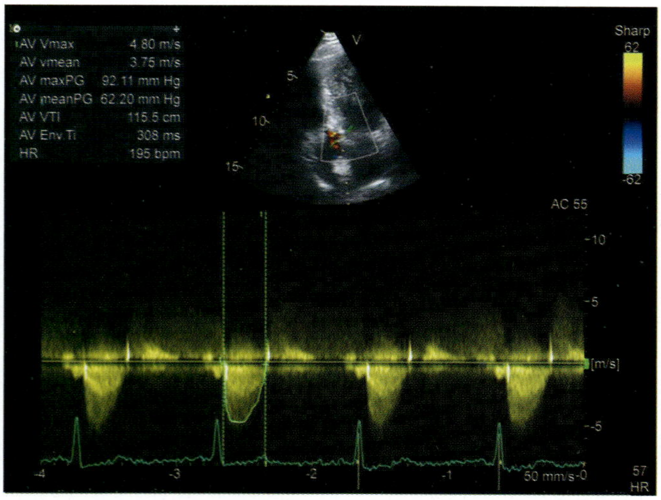


**FIG. 3:** Apical five-chamber view in echo Doppler showing severe gradient across calcified and thickened aortic valve leaflets.

## PATHOPHYSIOLOGY

In AS, the aortic valve becomes narrowed, restricting blood flow from the left ventricle into the aorta and onward to the rest of the body.

Common causes:

- *Age-related degenerative changes*: The most common cause in older adults, where the valve thickens and calcifies.
- *Congenital valve defects*: Some individuals are born with a bicuspid aortic valve, which is more prone to stenosis.
- *Rheumatic heart disease*: Although less common in developed countries, this is still common in developing countries, and it is often associated with mitral valve disease.

Aortic stenosis causes a cascade of hemodynamic changes, beginning with increased left ventricular pressure and hypertrophy, followed by reduced stroke volume, increased atrial pressure, and eventually left heart failure. If untreated, it can lead to severe complications, including heart failure and sudden cardiac death.

Important pathophysiological features of aortic stenosis are:

- Pressure gradient across aortic valve
- Increased left ventricular pressure (both systolic and end diastolic)
- LVH and fibrosis
- Aortic mean pressure is decreased
- Decreased stroke volume
- Prolonged LV ejection period
- Increased left atrial pressure
- Decreased coronary perfusion

## CLINICAL APPROACH

Symptoms of severe aortic stenosis are:

- *Angina*—due to reduced coronary blood flow (for prolonged ejection period, diastolic period gets shortened) or may be due to associated coronary artery disease.
- *Syncope*—may be at rest (arrhythmia related) or during activities (reduced forward flow).
- *Dyspnea* from heart failure or pulmonary congestion—predominantly due to diastolic failure followed by systolic failure.
- *Fatigue*

Without treatment, severe aortic stenosis has a poor prognosis. The typical survival is only 2–3 years after the onset of symptoms (e.g., chest pain, syncope, or heart failure). Valve replacement significantly improves survival and quality of life, particularly if done before the onset of irreversible heart damage.

## TREATMENT AND PREVENTION

Symptomatic severe AS must undergo surgical replacement of aortic valve otherwise mortality risk increases significantly. Medical management has got a limited role in severe AS. For patients with feature of failure may get benefitted with diuretics. For our patient cardiothoracic and vascular surgery (CTVS) consultation was done. Patient underwent preprocedural coronary angiography showing minor coronary artery disease and subsequent surgical aortic valve replacement (SAVR) was done with bioprosthetic aortic valve uneventfully. Patient received aspirin plus Warfarin with target INR 2.5 for initial 6 months post SAVR, subsequently on Aspirin alone only with satisfactory postoperative follow-up recovery. For patients who are having very high SAVR risk, now a days they undergo transcatheter aortic valve replacement (TAVR).

## Points to Ponder

- *Effort-related symptoms*: The combination of effort angina, dyspnea on exertion, and a history of TLOC suggests possible aortic stenosis as a cause of obstructive cardiac pathology.
- *Examination findings*: Slow-rising pulse with delayed carotid upstroke ("pulsus parvus et tardus") and a right parasternal thrill are classic signs of severe aortic stenosis.
- *Characteristic murmur*: The harsh ejection systolic murmur radiating to the carotids, reducing with standing or Valsalva, is diagnostic of valvular aortic stenosis.
- *Normal blood pressure and absence of cyanosis*: These findings rule out severe left ventricular dysfunction or systemic vascular compromise at this stage.
- *Red flags*: Transient loss of consciousness during exertion in a patient with aortic stenosis suggests significant left ventricular outflow obstruction, warranting urgent evaluation and possible intervention.

## MULTIPLE CHOICE QUESTIONS

1. **The commonest congenital anomaly of aortic valve is bicuspid aortic valve.**
   A. True
   B. False
2. **Pulsus parvus et tardus is characterized by rapid rise.**
   A. True
   B. False
3. **Severe valvular AS is having mean transvalvular pressure gradient > 40 mm Hg.**
   A. True
   B. False
4. **The commonest cause of severe aortic stenosis in elderly is rheumatic.**
   A. True
   B. False
5. **Symptomatic severe aortic stenosis can be treated with medical management only.**
   A. True
   B. False

### Answers

1. (A); 2. (B); 3. (A); 4. (B); 5. (B)

## SUGGESTED READINGS


1. Libby P, Bonow RO, Mann DL, et al. Braunwald's Heart Disease, Single Volume: A Textbook of Cardiovascular Medicine. Elsevier; 2021.
2. Fuster V, Narula J, Vaishnava P, et al. Fuster and Hurst's The Heart, 15th edition. McGraw Hill Professional; 2022.
3. Loscalzo J, Fauci AS, Kasper DL, et al. Harrison's Principles of Internal Medicine, Twenty-First Edition (Vol. 1 & Vol. 2). McGraw Hill Professional; 2022.
4. Bundrick JB, Litin SC. Clinical pearls in general internal medicine. Mayo Clinic Proceedings [Internet]. 2010;86(1):70-4.
5. Jose VJ. Cardiology: Clinical methods. JP Medical Ltd; 2017.

CHAPTER
6

# An Approach to a Case of Digital Gangrene and Its Management

*Vivek Paul Chowdhury, Poulami Das, Partha Sarkar*

### CASE VIGNETTE

A 62-year-old male with history of poorly controlled type 2 diabetes mellitus and smoking presents with painful, dusky discoloration of his left second toe, progressing over the last 10 days. He reports an intense cold sensation and episodes of throbbing pain in the affected digit, which worsens upon exposure to cold. Physical examination revealed cyanotic, mottled skin on distal phalanx, absent dorsalis pedis pulse and delayed capillary refill time **(Fig. 1)**.

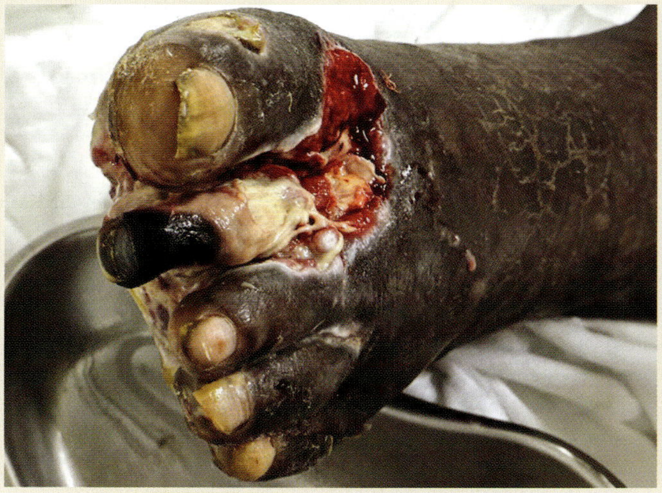

**FIG. 1:** Cyanotic, painful, and dusky discoloration of patient's toe.

## PROVISIONAL DIAGNOSIS

Peripheral artery disease due to uncontrolled type 2 diabetes mellitus.

## DIFFERENTIAL DIAGNOSIS

The patient's presentation suggests an ischemic process leading to digital gangrene.

The differentials include:

- *Vasospastic disorders*: Raynaud's phenomenon, especially precipitating in the presence of cold or stress.
- *Vasculitis*: Potential causes include polyarteritis nodosa, cryoglobulinemia, granulomatosis with polyangiitis, and thromboangiitis obliterans.
- *Connective tissue disease*: SLE, APLA, systemic sclerosis, Sjögren's disease and MCTD.
- *Infective causes*: Bacterial endocarditis, scrub typhus causing pan-digital gangrene.
- *Arterial embolism or thrombosis*: Secondary to atrial fibrillation or vascular plaque rupture.
- *Other causes*: Hypercoagulable states like polycythemia and thrombocytopenia, intra-arterial injection of drugs like pentazocine and promethazine.

## CLINICAL APPROACH

### Signs and Symptoms

Digital gangrene often begins with coldness and discoloration, progressing to cyanosis, pallor and pain. Patient may report with numbness, tingling or throbbing pain, especially if vasospasm or embolism is involved.

- *Ischemic phase*: Presents with pain, cold intolerance and pallor.

- *Progression to gangrene*: Cyanosis and subsequent necrosis of affected areas, potentially leading to tissue loss, if left untreated.

### History and Physical Examination

A thorough history is essential to uncover comorbidities (e.g., diabetes, smoking), medication use (e.g., beta-blockers) and family history of vascular or autoimmune diseases. Physical examination should assess pulses, capillary refill time and skin temperature. Evaluate for any ulcers, dry gangrene in the hands or feet.

### Classification of Digital Gangrene

- *Dry gangrene*: Commonly seen in chronic ischemia or vasculitis with a demarcated area of tissue loss.
- *Wet gangrene*: Often associated with infection, inflammation and rapid tissue necrosis, commonly leading to sepsis if untreated.
- *Gas gangrene*: Typically follows trauma or infection with *Clostridium* species, though rare in isolated digital gangrene cases.

### Diagnostic Evaluation

Diagnosis requires a multimodal approach with laboratory and imaging studies:

- *Laboratory tests*: Assess blood glucose, HbA1c, inflammatory markers (ESR, CRP), coagulation profile and autoantibody screen (ANA, antiphospholipid antibodies) if systemic disease is suspected.
- *Imaging*:
  - *Doppler ultrasound*: Identifies blood flow abnormalities in peripheral vessels.
  - *Angiography*: Digital subtraction angiography (DSA) or CT angiography provides a detailed view of vascular occlusions or stenoses.
  - *MRI or MR angiography:* For soft tissue and vascular anatomy in cases where conventional angiography is inconclusive.

## PATHOPHYSIOLOGY

Digital gangrene arises from a critical reduction in blood flow to the affected digit, leading to ischemia and tissue necrosis. Underlying mechanisms include:

- *Atherosclerosis and diabetes*: Chronic endothelial damage, vascular occlusions and microvascular complications lead to impaired circulation.
- *Vasospasm*: Raynaud's phenomenon or sympathetic nervous system overactivity can cause episodic reduction in blood flow which may result in tissue necrosis over time.
- *Inflammation and autoimmune processes:* In vasculitis or connective tissue diseases, inflammation damages the vessel wall, leading to occlusion and ischemia.

## TREATMENT AND PREVENTION

Early recognition and management are vital to prevent irreversible tissue loss. Management strategies include:

- *Medical management*:
  - *Vasodilators:* Calcium channel blockers (e.g., nifedipine) and phosphodiesterase inhibitors (e.g., sildenafil) can help increase blood flow in cases with vasospasm.
  - *Antiplatelet agents:* Low dose aspirin or clopidogrel to prevent thrombosis in high-risk patients.
  - *Anticoagulants:* In cases of arterial embolism or thrombosis anticoagulants like heparin or warfarin is indicated.
  - *Glycemic control:* Strict control of blood glucose levels is essential in diabetic patients to reduce further vascular damage.
  - *Analgesics:* Pain management with NSAIDs or opioids if necessary for severe pain.
- *Surgical management*:
  - *Revascularization procedures:* Angioplasty or arterial bypass may be considered in patients with accessible occlusive disease.
  - *Sympathectomy:* For refractory cases with significant vasospasm, sympathetic nerve interruption can improve blood flow.
  - *Debridement or amputation:* For non-viable tissues, surgical debridement or amputation may be necessary to prevent infection.
  - *Skin grafting:* If reconstruction is needed, healthy tissue from another area of the body is used to cover the missing or damaged area.
- *Adjuctive therapy*:
  - *Hyperbaric oxygen therapy (HBOT):* HBOT may improve oxygenation and promote wound healing in chronic cases.
  - *Wound care:* Regular cleaning, debridement and application of topical agents (e.g., silver sulfadiazine) to prevent infection.

### Points to Ponder

- ❑ *Importance of early recognition:* Digital gangrene is a potentially life-altering condition that requires prompt recognition and aggressive, multifaceted management approach. Identifying the underlying etiology, optimizing medical management and considering surgical intervention are key to prevent tissue loss and improve patient's outcome.
- ❑ *Diabetic patients*: Often present with neuropathy of insidious onset and may lack the typical pain response seen in ischemic events.
- ❑ *Cold weather and vasospasm*: Exposure to cold temperatures can precipitate vasospasm and worsen the gangrene.
- ❑ *Smoking cessation*: Smoking is a critical risk factor and cessation can significantly reduce progression risk.
- ❑ *Long-term monitoring*: Patients with underlying systemic disease like lupus or diabetes should undergo routine follow-up to monitor vascular health.

## MULTIPLE CHOICE QUESTIONS

**1. What type of gangrene is likely to occur due to poor circulation in an area of the body?**
- A. Wet gangrene
- B. Dry gangrene
- C. Gas gangrene
- D. Viral gangrene

**2. Which statement accurately describes wet gangrene?**
- A. Can be due to infection and always produces gas
- B. Can be due to infection and typically does not produce gas
- C. Leads to little or no damage to infected tissues
- D. Amputation is the only treatment modality

**3. A 30-year-old woman who is allergic to penicillin is diagnosed with gas gangrene. What is the best treatment for her?**
- A. Ampicillin (2 g IV q4h) + Vancomycin (1 g IV q12h)
- B. Metronidazole (500 mg IV q6h)
- C. Ciprofloxacin (400 mg IV q6–8h) + Clindamycin (600–900 mg IV q6–8h)
- D. Cefoxitin (2 g IV q6h) + Clindamycin (600–900 mg IV q6–8h)

**4. A 34-year-old male patient with history of smoking 1 packet of cigarettes every day presents with exertional pain and darkening of skin of the fingers in both upper limbs. On examination radial and ulnar pulses are feeble. Angiography of his upper extremity shows smooth tapering segmental lesions in the distal arterial vessels. Which treatment has the highest chance of success?**
- A. Cilostazol
- B. Heparin and surgical methods
- C. High dose steroids
- D. Smoking cessation

**5. Which one of the following drug should be avoided in a 38-year-old woman with complaints of bluish discoloration and pain in her fingertips?**
- A. Prazosin
- B. Clonidine
- C. Diltiazem
- D. Isradipine

### Answers

1. (B); 2. (B); 3. (D); 4. (D); 5. (B)

## SUGGESTED READINGS

1. Diormandy JA, Rutherford RB. Management of peripheral arterial disease (PAD). J Vasc Surg. 2000;31(1):1-296.
2. Soyoye DO, Abiodun OO, Ikem RT, et al. Diabetes and peripheral arterial disease: A review. World J Diabetes. 2021;15(6):827-38.
3. Powell JT, Varty K. Arterial occlusive diseases of the extremities. Harrison's Principles of internal medicine, 20th edition, McGraw Hill; 2016.
4. Thompson MM, Nasim A. Revascularization Techniques in Limb Ischemia. Vasc Endovascular Surg. 2021;52(4):12-8.
5. Zelman S. Diabetic foot and digital gangrene. Int J Diabetes Dev Coun. 2019;39(3):232-9.
6. Mills JL, Conte MS, Armstrong DG, et al. The Society for Vascular Surgery Lower Extremity Threatened Limb Classification System: Risk Stratification based on wound, ischemia and foot infection (WIFI). J Vasc Surg. 2014;59(1):220-34.
7. Norgren L, Hiatt WR, Dormandy JA, et al. Inter Society Consensus for the management of Peripheral Arterial Disease (TASC II). Eur J Vasc Endovasc Surg. 2007;33(Suppl 1):S1-S75.
8. Hinchliffe RJ, Forsythe RO, Apelqvist J, et al. Guidelines on the diagnosis and management of peripheral arterial disease. Surgical perspective. Eur J Vasc Endovasc Surg. 2020;60(3):364-73.

CHAPTER

7

# An Approach to a Case of Reporting an ECG

*Partha Sarkar, Snehansu Shekhar Samanta*

**CASE VIGNETTE**

A 66-year-old female presents with altered mental status and agitation. Systematic ECG analysis using the checklist reveals features such as sinus rhythm, a normal cardiac axis, and no significant deviations in P waves, PR interval, or QRS complex. A detailed evaluation of the ST and T wave segments confirms no acute ischemic changes. Practice in such cases reinforces the critical role of a systematic approach and highlights how ECG can provide valuable diagnostic insights at the bedside.

## PROVISIONAL DIAGNOSIS

Anticholinergic toxicity due to promethazine overdose in the context of polypharmacy and chronic alcohol use.

## DIFFERENTIAL DIAGNOSIS

- Delirium tremens (alcohol withdrawal)
- Serotonin syndrome (venlafaxine)
- Neuroleptic malignant syndrome
- Sepsis with systemic inflammatory response syndrome (SIRS)
- Stroke or intracranial pathology

## CLINICAL APPROACH

- *History*: Detailed medication use, timing, and dosages; alcohol use pattern.
- *Examination*: Look for anticholinergic signs (e.g., dry skin, dilated pupils, tachycardia).
- *Toxidrome identification*: Match clinical signs to anticholinergic features.
- *Investigations*: ECG for cardiac arrhythmias, serum electrolytes, liver/kidney function tests, and toxicology screen.

## PATHOPHYSIOLOGY

Anticholinergic toxicity results from competitive inhibition of muscarinic acetylcholine receptors, disrupting parasympathetic nervous system signaling. This leads to symptoms such as tachycardia, hypertension, and altered mental status. Central nervous system effects stem from impaired cholinergic transmission, while peripheral effects include dry mucosa, mydriasis, and urinary retention.

## MANAGEMENT AND PREVENTION

- *Supportive care*: Airway, breathing, and circulation (ABC) stabilization.

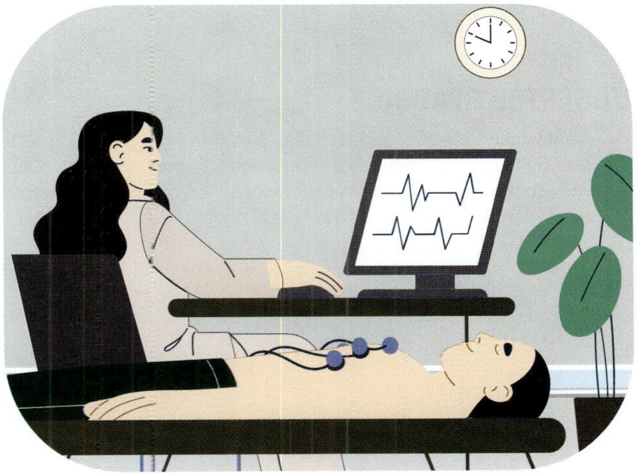

**FIG. 1:** Continuous ECG monitoring.

- *Decontamination*: Activated charcoal if within ingestion window.
- *Antidote*: Administer physostigmine under close monitoring in severe cases.
- *Symptom control*: Benzodiazepines for agitation; IV fluids for hydration; cooling measures for hyperthermia.
- *Monitoring*: Continuous ECG and vitals for arrhythmias or hemodynamic instability **(Fig. 1)**.

## PREVENTION

- Educate patients on proper dosing of medications and risks of polypharmacy.
- Screen high-risk individuals for misuse of over-the-counter drugs.
- Close monitoring of elderly patients on anticholinergic drugs.
- Avoid prescribing anticholinergics to individuals with a history of substance abuse.

## Points to Ponder

- A checklist is essential to avoid errors of omission.
- It is cheap, available and offers valuable information at the bedside.
- Daily practice using a checklist is the way to improve one's ability to read an ECG.
- This should be supplemented by reading of relevant text.

## MULTIPLE CHOICE QUESTIONS

**1. The most common cause of a LAA in the ECG is:**
A. IHD
B. Mitral stenosis
C. Cardiomyopathy
D. Hypertensive heart disease

**2. Bazett's formula is used for:**
A. Calculation of the QTc
B. Calculation of the heart rate
C. Detection of LVH
D. Detection of RVH

**3. True about the U wave:**
A. It is always abnormal
B. It is discordant with the T wave
C. It is a feature of hyperkalemia
D. It is caused by repolarization of the Purkinje fibers

**4. The T wave is normally negative in lead aVR and in:**
A. Lead V1
B. Lead V6
C. Lead aVF
D. Lead I

**5. The J point is the:**
A. The end of the T wave
B. The junction between QRS complex and the ST segment
C. The starting point of the QRS complex
D. The highest point of the QRS complex

### Answers

1. (A); 2. (A); 3. (D); 4. (A); 5. (B)

## SUGGESTED READINGS

1. Goldberger AL, Goldberger ZD, Shvilkin A. Clinical Electrocardiography: A Simplified Approach, Expert Consult: Online and Print,8: Clinical Electrocardiography: A Simplified Approach. Elsevier Health Sciences; 2012.
2. Wagner GS, Strauss DG. Marriott's practical electrocardiography 13e. Lippincott Williams & Wilkins; 2021.
3. Mattu A. ECGs for the Emergency physician 1. John Wiley & Sons; 2013.
4. An Introduction to Electrocardiography, 8th edition by Leo Schamroth.

# CHAPTER 8

# An Approach to a Case of Absent Peripheral Pulses

***Bhupen Barman, Gwenette A War, Ashwini C***

## CASE VIGNETTE

A 45-year-old female with no known comorbidities presented with intermittent episodes of abdominal pain, sudden in onset and dull in character, with no radiation. She reported no associated symptoms such as fever, loose stools, or rectal bleeding. On general physical examination, there was a notable radio-radial delay. Blood pressure measurements across all four limbs revealed a significant discrepancy, and oxygen saturation was 97% on room air. Auscultation detected bruits over both carotid and renal arteries. The systemic examination was otherwise unremarkable. Laboratory investigations showed elevated inflammatory markers, including C-reactive protein (CRP) and erythrocyte sedimentation rate (ESR). MRI angiography of the aorta and its branches confirmed the diagnosis of Takayasu arteritis **(Fig. 1)**.

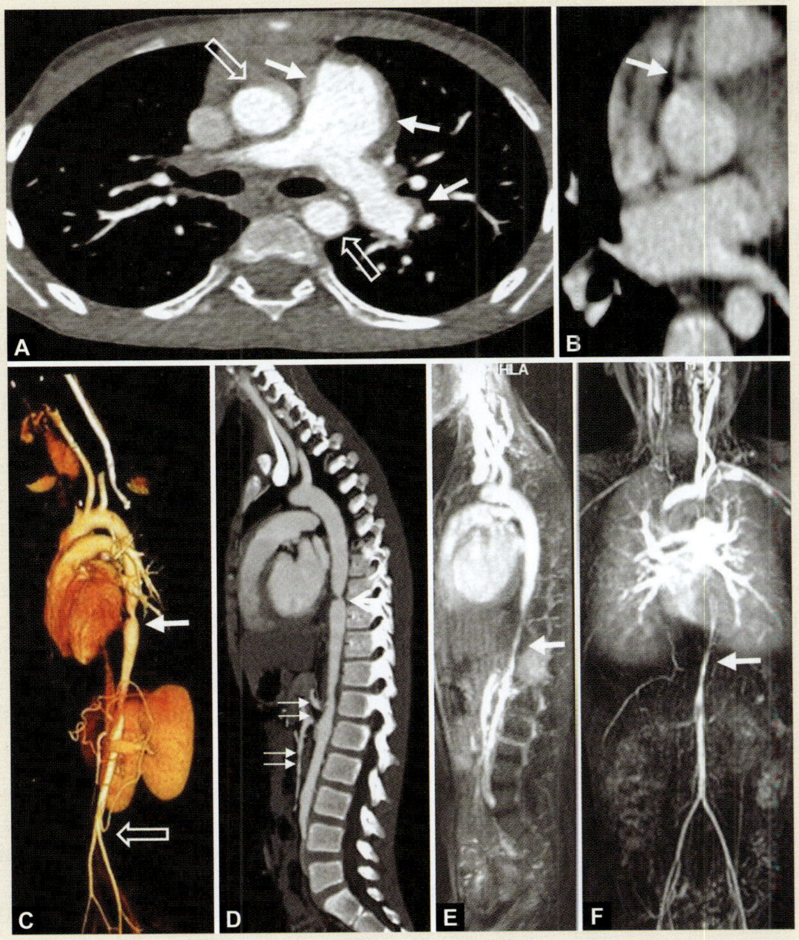

**FIGS. 1A TO F:** CTA and MRA images show TA type V, C (+), P (+) disease. Axial CTA image (A) showing diffuse wall thickening of PA and its main branches, ascending and descending thoracic aorta. Axial CT image (B) shows focal RCA stenosis. Sagittal CTA, VRT and MPR images (C and D) shows showing diffuse aortic wall thickening with focal stenosis of descending aorta, diffuse wall thickening of supra and infrarenal abdominal aorta with stenosis of celiac trunk and SMA with large IMA collateral. MRA with oblique sagittal and coronal reconstructions images (E and F) on follow-up shows progression of stenosis.

## PROVISIONAL DIAGNOSIS

*Vasculitis*: Takayasu arteritis.

## DIFFERENTIAL DIAGNOSES

- Tubercular aortitis
- Syphilitic aortitis
- Fibromuscular dysplasia
- Coarctation of aorta
- Thoracic outlet syndrome

### Clinical Approach

Approaching a patient with absent peripheral pulses demands meticulous clinical reasoning, as it encompasses a wide spectrum of etiologies with variable presentations, locations, and severities. This variability underscores the importance of a thorough, integrated history and physical examination, enabling the identification of systemic and localized manifestations. Proper evaluation not only aids in diagnosis but also provides an opportunity to address the patient's condition holistically, potentially impacting their health from head to toe.

### History

- The clinical manifestation of absent peripheral pulse mainly includes claudication in the involved limb. This is typically described as cramps, fatigue or pain in the involved limb which improves upon rest **(Table 2)**.
- Involvement of the common carotid arteries leads to visual manifestations, syncope and stroke.
- Abdominal pain, vomiting and nausea are the common features of involvement of abdominal aorta, celiac and superior mesenteric artery.
- Young onset hypertension can be a presenting symptom if renal artery is involved.
- <10% manifest as chest pain and myocardial infarction which are the leading cause of mortality.

### Examination

*Inspection*: The involved limb might show:

- Shiny skin
- Absent hair
- Pallor
- Edema
- Thickened nails
- *Blood pressure difference*: The normal blood pressure difference between both upper limbs is < 10 mm Hg, and between the upper and lower limbs, it is < 20 mm Hg

*Palpation*:

- *Pulse*: Feeble or absent peripheral pulses
- Cold extremities
- Edema

*Auscultation*:

- *Bruits:* Heard over the stenosed vessel **(Table 1)**

Fundoscopy to screen for vasculitis.

### Clinical Significance

Refer to **Table 2**.

**TABLE 1: Sites for auscultation of bruit.**

| Artery involved | Site of bruit |
|---|---|
| Internal/External carotid artery | Anterior neck |
| Subclavian artery | Supraclavicular |
| Axillary artery | Infraclavicular |
| Thoracic aorta | Left interscapular |
| Abdominal aorta | Epigastrium |
| Celiac | Epigastrium |
| Renal | Upper abdominal quadrants, lumbar |
| Aorto-iliac bifurcation | Umbilicus |
| Common femoral | Inguinal |
| Superficial femoral | Femoral triangle |
| Popliteal | Popliteal fossa |

**TABLE 2: Causes of absent peripheral pulse.**

| | |
|---|---|
| Congenital causes | • Coarctation of aorta<br>• Anomalous peripheral artery |
| Intrinsic disease of the artery | • Atherosclerosis<br>• Fibromuscular dysplasia<br>• Thromboangiitis obliterans<br>• Vasculitis (Takayasu arteritis)<br>• Atheroembolism |
| Vasospastic disorders | • Raynaud's phenomenon |
| Extrinsic compression | • Thoracic outlet syndrome<br>• Neoplasms<br>• Trauma |

## PATHOPHYSIOLOGY

Takayasu arteritis is a vasculitis disorder affecting medium and large vessels, characterized by panarteritis that leads to vessel wall inflammation and subsequent stenosis. Microscopically, the affected vessels exhibit intimal fibrosis, degeneration of the internal elastic lamina, and medial scarring. These changes result in narrowing of the vessels, impairing blood flow and causing a range of clinical manifestations depending on the arteries involved. The aorta and its branches are predominantly affected, with the subclavian artery commonly leading to arm claudication and Raynaud's phenomenon. Involvement of the common carotid artery can result in visual disturbances, syncope, and transient ischemic attacks, while renal artery involvement often manifests as hypertension and, in severe cases, renal failure.

The classification criteria for Takayasu arteritis are shown in **Figure 2**.

Takayasu arteritis can also be classified radiologically as follows:

- *Type I*: Involvement of the aortic branches (brachiocephalic trunk, carotid and subclavian artery)
- *Type II*:
  - *Type IIa*: Involvement of the aorta at its ascending portion and or at the aortic arch.
  - *Type IIb*: Involvement of the descending thoracic aorta with or without ascending thoracic branches

## 2022 AMERICAN COLLEGE OF RHEUMATOLOGY/EULAR CLASSIFICATION CRITERIA FOR TAKAYASU ARTERITIS

### ABSOLUTE REQUIREMENTS

- Age 60 years at the time of diagnosis
- Evidence of vasculitis on imaging[a]

### ADDITIONAL CLINICAL CRITERIA

| | |
|---|---|
| Female sex | +1 |
| Angina or ischemic cardiac pain | +2 |
| Arm or leg claudication | +2 |
| Vascular bruit[b] | +2 |
| Reduced pulse in upper extremity[c] | +2 |
| Carotid artery abnormality[d] | +2 |
| Systolic blood pressure difference in arm 20 mm Hg | +1 |

### ADDITIONAL IMAGING CRITERIA

| | |
|---|---|
| Number of affected arterial territories (select one)[e] | |
| • One artery territory | +1 |
| • Two arterial territories | +2 |
| • Three or more arterial territories | +3 |
| Symmetric involvement of paired arteries[f] | +1 |
| Abdominal aorta involvement with renal or mesenteric involvement[g] | +3 |
| Sum the score of 10 items, if present. A score of ≥5 points is needed for the classificat on of Takayasu arteritis. | |

[a]Evidence of vasculitis in the aorta and branch arteries must be confirmed by vascular imaging (e.g., computed tomography, catheter based, magnetic resonance angiography, ultrasound, positron emission tomography).

[b]Bruit detected by auscultation of a large artery including the aorta, carotid, subclavian, axillary, brachial, renal or iliofemoral arteries.

[c]Reduction or absence of pulse by physical examination of the axillary, brachial or radial arteries.

[d]Reduction or absence of pulse of the carotid artery or tenderness of the carotid artery.

[e]Number of arterial territories with lumlnal change (stenosis, occlusion or aneurysm) detected by angiography or ultrasonography from the following nine territories: Thoracic aorta, abdominal aorta, mesenteric, left or right carotid, lelt or right subclavian, or renal arteries.

[f]Bilateral luminal damage (stenosls, occlusion or aneurysm) detected by angiography or ultrasonography in any of the following paired vascular territories: Carotid, subclavian or renal arteries.

[g]Luminal damage (stenosis, occlusion or aneurysm) detected by angiography or ultrasonography involving the abdominal aorta and either the renal or mesenteric arteries.

**FIG. 2:** 2022 American College of Rheumatology/EULAR classification criteria for Takayasu arteritis.

- *Type III*: Involvement of the thoracic and abdominal aorta distal to the arch and its main branches.
- *Type IV*: Involvement of the abdominal aorta and renal branches
- *Type V*: Generalized involvement of all aortic segments.

Additionally, involvement of the coronary and pulmonary arteries should be indicated as C (+) or P (+), respectively.

The outcome measures in disease activity assessment of Takayasu arteritis are assessed by the "presence of constitutional symptoms, new-bruits, acute phase reactants (APR) or new angiographic features" as used in a study from the National Institute of Health (NIH), or by the Indian Takayasu's Arteritis Score (ITAS) scoring. ITAS score is a useful clinical tool to measure the severity of disease during patient monitoring. Persistently high ITAS score despite therapy suggests poor control of the disease. This score is to be used only if abnormality is present and new within the past 3 months and ascribed to current active vasculitis. Each of the below listed condition is given a score of +1.

- *Systemic*: Malaise/weight loss of >2 kg, myalgia, arthralgia or arthritis, headache
- *Abdominal*: Severe abdominal pain
- *Genitourinary*: Recent history of spontaneous abortion
- *Renal*: SBP >140 mm Hg, DBP >90 mm Hg
- *Neurological*: Stroke, seizures, syncope, vertigo/dizziness
- *Cardiovascular*: Bruits, pulse inequality, new onset loss of pulses, claudication, carotidynia, aortic incompetence, myocardial infarct/angina, cardiomyopathy/cardiac failure

A score of ≥2 points is suggestive of active disease.

## TREATMENT AND PREVENTION

Glucocorticoids are the mainstay of treatment for remission induction in TAK. Details of treatment algorithm has been given as flowchart adopted from 2018 Update of the EULAR recommendations for the management of large vessel vasculitis **(Flowchart 1)**.

Takayasu arteritis diagnosis requires clinical evaluation confirmed by imaging. Localized disease may benefit from lower initial glucocorticoid doses (25–30 mg/day). csDMARDs such as methotrexate, mycophenolate mofetil, leflunomide, azathioprine, or cyclophosphamide are used based on tolerance and disease severity. The treatment goal is sustained remission with normalized acute-phase reactants and glucocorticoid tapering without relapse. Relapses are classified as *major* (ischemia or progressive aortic inflammation) or *minor* (active disease without severe complications). Off-label biologics like tocilizumab and TNF inhibitors may be used in refractory cases, with switching considered for intolerance.

## CONCLUSION

Takayasu arteritis is a chronic large-vessel vasculitis affecting young females, causing arterial stenosis, occlusion, or aneurysms. Symptoms depend on the vessels involved, with hallmark features including absent pulses, claudication, and bruits. Diagnosis relies on elevated inflammatory markers and imaging, such as MRI angiography. Treatment centers on glucocorticoids, with immunosuppressants or biologics for refractory cases. Regular disease monitoring using ITAS or NIH criteria ensures effective management and better outcomes.

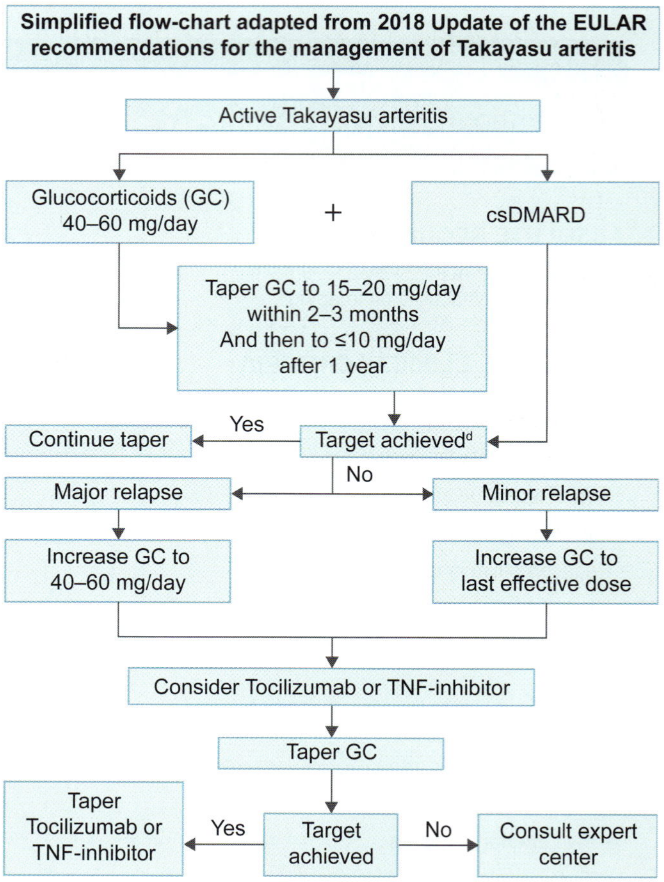


**FLOWCHART 1:** Simplified flowchart showing treatment of Takayasu arteritis.

### Points to Ponder

- Absence of peripheral pulses with systemic symptoms like hypertension or abdominal pain should prompt consideration of Takayasu arteritis to avoid delayed diagnosis.
- MRI angiography is the gold standard for diagnosing vascular involvement and monitoring disease progression in Takayasu arteritis.
- Tools like ITAS or NIH criteria help assess disease activity, guiding treatment adjustments and preventing complications.
- Glucocorticoid-sparing strategies using immunosuppressants or biologics are crucial in managing relapsing or refractory cases while minimizing long-term steroid side effects.

## MULTIPLE CHOICE QUESTIONS

**1. The most common artery involved in Takayasu arteritis is?**

A. Common carotid artery
B. Renal artery
C. Subclavian artery
D. Aortic arch

**2. Amongst the below listed conditions, which connective tissue disorder has the strongest association with Raynaud's phenomenon?**

A. Dermatomyositis
B. Systemic sclerosis
C. Systemic lupus erythematosus
D. Rheumatoid arthritis

**3. All of the following drugs can be used in the treatment of Raynaud's phenomenon, except:**

A. Diltiazem
B. Nifedipine
C. Prazosin
D. Clonidine

**4. All of the following drugs can be used in the treatment of aortic dissection, except:**

A. Esmolol
B. Labetalol
C. Hydralazine
D. Verapamil

**5. The most common pathophysiology associated with ascending aortic aneurysm is:**
   A. Atherosclerosis
   B. Vasculitis
   C. Medial degeneration
   D. Syphilis

## Answers

1. (C); 2. (B); 3. (D); 4. (C); 5. (C)

## SUGGESTED READINGS


1. Wennberg PW. Approach to the patient with peripheral arterial disease. Circulation. 2013;128(20):2241-50.
2. Seyahi E. Takayasu arteritis: an update. Curr Opin Rheumatol. 2017;29(1):51-6.
3. Grayson PC, Ponte C, Suppiah R, et al; DCVAS Study Group. 2022 American College of Rheumatology/EULAR classification criteria for Takayasu arteritis. Ann Rheum Dis. 2022;81(12):1654-60.
4. Zhu FP, Luo S, Wang ZJ, et al. Takayasu arteritis: imaging spectrum at multidetector CT angiography. Br J Radiol. 2012;85(1020):e1282-92.
5. Kerr GS, Hallahan CW, Giordano J, et al. Takayasu arteritis. Ann Intern Med. 1994;120(11):919-29.
6. Misra R, Danda D, Rajappa SM, et al, Indian Rheumatology Vasculitis (IRAVAS) group. Development and initial validation of the Indian Takayasu Clinical Activity Score (ITAS2010). Rheumatology (Oxford). 2013;52(10):1795-801.
7. Hellmich B, Agueda A, Monti S, et al. 2018 Update of the EULAR recommendations for the management of large vessel vasculitis. Ann Rheum Dis. 2020;79(1):19-30.

CHAPTER 9

# An Approach to a Case of Hemorrhagic Stroke in a Patient with Chronic Atrial Fibrillation

*Uddalak Chakraborty*

## CASE VIGNETTE

A 58-year-old hypertensive male patient with a prior history of cardioembolic stroke presented with a new-onset right hemiparesis. Brain imaging revealed a left gangliocapsular bleed with minimal mass effect **(Fig. 1)**. He was diagnosed to have non-valvular atrial fibrillation (NVAF) and was initiated on nicoumalone 2 mg during his prior stroke. His blood parameters revealed an International normalized ratio (INR) of 1.8.

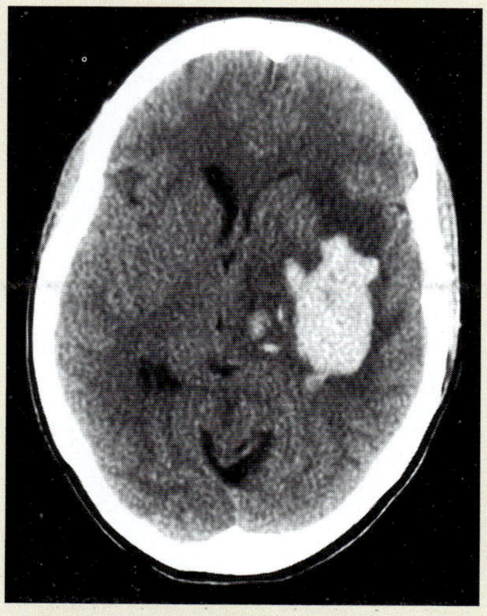

**FIG.1:** NCCT brain shows left gangliocapsular bleed with minimal mass effect.

## THERAPEUTIC DILEMMA

In the above-mentioned case, the patient was on anticoagulation and had suffered a hemorrhagic stroke. Anticoagulation therapy in these scenarios serves as a double-edged sword; continuing anticoagulation will promote hematoma expansion, hence worsening the outcome of a hemorrhagic stroke whereas withholding anticoagulation may promote recurrent thromboembolic vascular events. In order to mitigate this therapeutic dilemma, we need to formulate our treatment strategies which tends to balance the risk of hematoma expansion against the risk of thromboembolic stroke.

## DIFFERENTIAL DIAGNOSIS

The treatment strategies can be divided based on patients with chronic atrial fibrillation who are anticoagulation naïve or not on any anticoagulation and patients who are receiving anticoagulation therapy. However, every patient needs to be individualized and personalized risk/benefit analysis is to be done. The therapeutic inertia and further management have been highlighted in **Table 1**.

**TABLE 1: Therapeutic challenges and way forward in hemorrhagic stroke in a patient with chronic atrial fibrillation.**

| Therapeutic challenges | Measures |
|---|---|
| Risk of hematoma expansion | Stop anticoagulation |
| Iatrogenic coagulopathy | Reversal of anticoagulation |
| Surgical intervention if required | Perioperative management of atrial fibrillation |
| Prophylaxis for AF | When to initiate anticoagulation |
| Risk analysis of thromboembolic events | Use conventional scores and judgement |

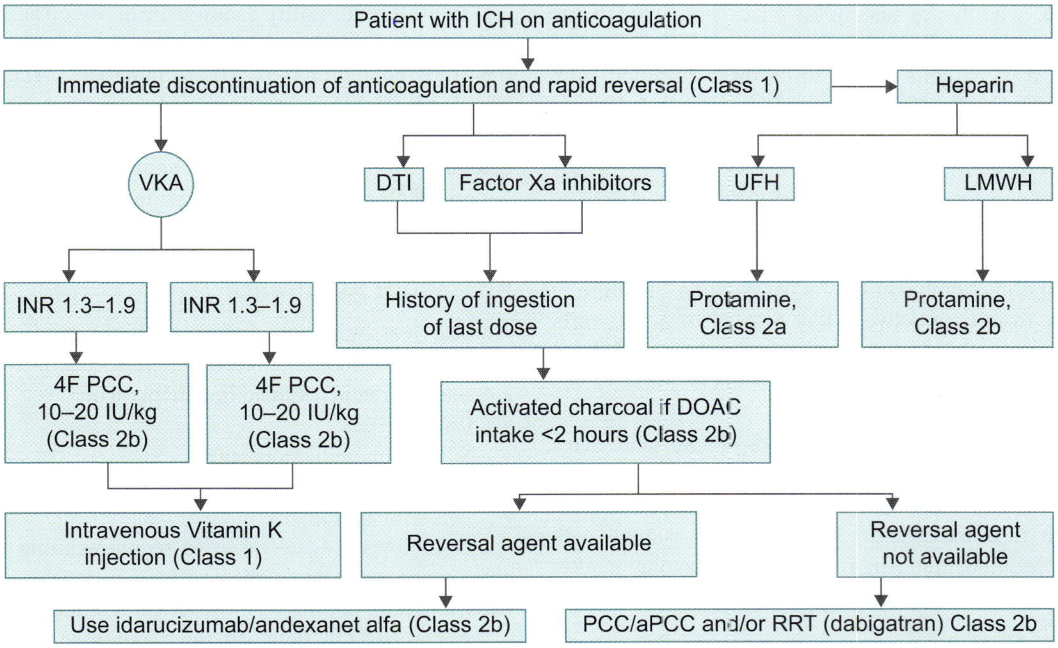


**FLOWCHART 1:** Anticoagulation reversal in hemorrhagic stroke.

(aPCC: activated prothrombin complex concentrate; DOAC: direct oral anticoagulant; DTI: direct thrombin inhibitors; ICH: intracerebral hemorrhage; INR: international normalized ratio; LMWH: low molecular weight heparin; PCC: prothrombin complex concentrate; RRT: renal replacement therapy; UFH: unfractionated heparin; VKA: vitamin K antagonists)

Withdrawal of anticoagulant and reversal of the same **(Flowchart 1)** is the mainstay of initial management to prevent hematoma expansion in hemorrhagic stroke which has a direct impact on morbidity and mortality.

## CLINICAL APPROACH

The primary challenge is managing anticoagulation in the setting of hemorrhagic stroke. Initial steps involve stopping anticoagulation to prevent further hematoma expansion and considering reversal agents if necessary. Surgical interventions, such as hematoma evacuation, may be needed depending on the severity and location of the bleed.

The case involves a hypertensive patient with chronic atrial fibrillation (AF) on anticoagulation therapy. Hemorrhagic stroke in this context often results from anticoagulation-induced bleeding complications, which create a therapeutic dilemma: balancing the prevention of thromboembolic events with the risk of worsening hemorrhage.

*Evidence-based notes*:

- Reversal of anticoagulation in presence of left ventricular assist device/mechanical valves was not associated with immediate left ventricular assist device (LVAD)/valve thrombosis if the patient is optimally anticoagulated.
- Higher rate of hematoma expansion has been observed in patients receiving fresh frozen plasma (FFP) compared to PCC for anticoagulation reversal (INCH trial).
- The efficacy of hemostatic measures like recombinant factor VIIa and TXA to limit hematoma expansion in spontaneous intracerebral hemorrhage is not well established.

## TREATMENT AND PREVENTION

- *Initial management*: Cease anticoagulation and use reversal agents to control bleeding. Consider surgical options for significant bleeds.
- *Anticoagulation resumption*: Based on risk factors like thromboembolism and the type of AF, resumption timing is tailored—usually between 6 days to several weeks.
- *Alternatives for high-risk patients*: In patients who cannot tolerate long-term anticoagulation, options like left atrial appendage closure or catheter ablation are recommended.

### Hemorrhagic Stroke Requiring Surgical Intervention: Specific Considerations in Chronic AF

Surgical modalities like decompressive craniectomy, hematoma evacuation, external ventricular drainage have been considered as life-saving measures capable enough to reduce mortality and limit functional disability in hemorrhagic strokes especially in infratentorial bleeds. Any emergency intervention should be performed at the earliest preferably within 48 hours of ictus to provide a good outcome. If a patient is on anticoagulation, adequate reversal should be arranged simultaneously which should not defer any emergency intervention. In patients with atrial fibrillation, perioperative management should focus more on rate control compared to rhythm control, bridging with UFH compared to LMWH.

### Resuming Anticoagulation after Hemorrhagic Stroke

The million-dollar questions you encounter once you stabilize and manage the hemorrhagic stroke is when to resume anticoagulation, whether to resume at all or not, what if the patient bleeds again. In absence of any universal consensus, individualization of patients serves to be the best guide from case-to-case scenario. The physician needs to focus on the type of AF (valvular/nonvalvular), risk of thromboembolic events, risk of recurrent bleeding.

- *High risk of thromboembolism:* This group encompassing patients with mechanical heart valves, LVAD, left atrial clot warrants early resumption of anticoagulation to prevent thromboembolic complications. As per existing literature, it is advisable to initiate between day 6 to 14 of event; early initiation warranted for mechanical mitral valves (4–7 days) compared to delayed initiation for mechanical aortic valves (7–14 days).
- *Low risk of thromboembolism:* $CHA_2DS_2$-VASc score helps in assessing the risk of vascular events in patients with nvAF. Anticoagulation is recommended in patients with $CHA_2DS_2$-VASc score ≥2 in males and ≥3 in females. In patients with low risk of thromboembolism, resuming anticoagulation after 7–8 weeks after ICH may be optimal after risk benefit analysis.

## Patients with Contraindication to Long-/Short-term Anticoagulation

Data from PROTECT-AF and PREVAIL trial have endorsed the use of the WATCHMAN device for closure of left atrial appendage in patients with contraindication to long-term anticoagulation. Although the rates of ischemic events with left atrial appendage closure (LAAC) did not demonstrate noninferiority compared to warfarin, rates of recurrent bleeds and hemorrhagic stroke were considerably lower. In patients with LAAC, dual antiplatelets for 6 months followed by single antiplatelets tend to confer lower bleeding risk and hemorrhagic stroke compared to anticoagulation.

## Patients with Amyloid Angiopathy

Amyloid angiopathy has increasingly been recognized these days as an important etiology of ICH, especially lobar bleeds. The transient focal neurological episodes (TFNE) tend to mimic transient ischemic attacks and once these patients are initiated on antiplatelets, they tend to bleed. The patients are usually diagnosed based on the modified Boston 2.0 criteria.

There is a markedly increased risk of recurrence of hemorrhage in patients with prior lobar bleeds compared to non-lobar ICH. European guidelines recommend against initiation or resumption of anticoagulation in patients with prior lobar bleeds, definite or probable cerebral amyloid angiopathy (CAA). LAAC/catheter ablation has been suggested as a modality in these patients.

## Oral Anticoagulation and Risk of ICH

The risk of recurrent hemorrhagic stroke in patients with AF, treated with oral anticoagulation who survived a previous ICH range from 1.3 to 7.4%. A 10-fold increased risk of ICH has been reported in patients on oral anticoagulation with a 30- to 90-day mortality ranging from 40–60%. Moreover, the annual rate of ICH in patients receiving VKA ranges from 0.3–0.6% compared to 0.1–0.2% in patients receiving NOACs. The HAS-BLED score designed to predict risk of bleed in patients on anticoagulation is limited by risk stratification and categorization, lack of external validation, no consideration of genetic factors, specific medications, etiologies like amyloid angiopathy.

## Risk of ICH Recurrence

Among various risk factors which predict chances of recurrent bleeding, meticulous monitoring is warranted once anticoagulation is resumed in patients with:

- Lobar bleeds
- Subarachnoid hemorrhage
- Pre-existing cerebral microbleeds
- Amyloid angiopathy

Guidelines tend to differ in recommending resumption of anticoagulation in hemorrhagic stroke; European guidelines favor early initiation compared to American guidelines **(Table 2)**.

A comparison between the recommendations have been listed in **Table 3**.

**TABLE 2: Resumption of anticoagulation based on categories of patients as per European guidelines.**

| Type of bleed | OAC resumption |
|---|---|
| Lobar bleed | • If CAA suspected and microbleeds >5, OAC may be avoided<br>• If microbleeds <5, OAC should be resumed between 4 to 8 weeks after risk/benefit analysis |
| Non-lobar bleeds | OAC should be resumed between 4 to 8 weeks after risk/benefit analysis |
| Patients with mechanical valves | OAC should be resumed not earlier than 6 days, however resumption after 13 days is considerably safe |

(CAA: cerebral amyloid angiopathy; OAC: oral anticoagulation)

**TABLE 3: Comparison of several guidelines on resumption of anticoagulation.**

| Guideline | Recommendation for OAC resumption |
|---|---|
| ACC expert committee | 4 weeks waiting for DOAC |
| CHEST guidelines | • 48 hours to 4 weeks based on risk/benefit analysis<br>• DOAC preferred<br>• LAAC for high risk of recurrent bleeding |
| ESC | 2–4 weeks for re-initiation |
| EHRA | 4–8 weeks waiting |

(ACC: American College of Cardiology; CHEST: American College of Chest Physicians; DOAC: direct oral anticoagulant; EHRA: European Heart Rhythm Association; ESC: European Stroke Congress; LAAC: left atrial appendage closure)

## Points to Ponder

- Hemorrhagic stroke in chronic atrial fibrillation warrants a multidisciplinary assessment including cardiologists, neurologists, and neurosurgeons to decide upon the management.
- Personalized risk estimation, balance between risk of hematoma expansion and thromboembolic risk, estimation of recurrence risk helps in optimal management of these subgroup of patients.
- Hematoma expansion should be prevented by prompt withdrawal of anticoagulation and reversal of the same in order to prevent morbidity and mortality in hemorrhagic stroke.
- Anticoagulation may be initiated earlier in cases with high risk of thromboembolism to prevent vascular events.
- In patients with contraindications to long-term anticoagulation, left atrial appendage closure/catheter ablation may be considered as alternate modalities.

## MULTIPLE CHOICE QUESTIONS

**1. Which of the following is the reversal agent for dabigatran related bleeding?**

A. Andexanet alfa
B. Protamine
C. Idarucizumab
D. Ticagrelor

**2. Which of the following is a Class 1 recommendation for anticoagulation reversal in patients receiving Vitamin K antagonists?**

A. PCC
B. FFP
C. RRT
D. Injection vitamin K

**3. Which of the following has the highest risk of thromboembolic events among the following if not anticoagulated optimally?**

A. $CHA_2DS_2$-VASc score 1
B. Mechanical heart valve
C. Lone AF
D. Triple vessel disease

**4. Which of the following scores are used to predict bleeding risk after initiating anticoagulation?**

A. HAS-BLED
B. HEMORRHAGES
C. ATRIA
D. All of the above

**5. Which of the following modalities are used to prevent thromboembolic events in patients with contraindication to long-term anticoagulation?**

A. Left atrial appendage closure
B. Intra-aortic balloon pump
C. SA node ablation
D. Automated defibrillator implantation

### Answers

1. (C); 2. (D); 3. (B); 4. (D); 5 (A)

## SUGGESTED READINGS

1. Greenberg SM, Ziai WC, Cordonnier C, et al.; American Heart Association/American Stroke Association. 2022 Guideline for the Management of Patients With Spontaneous Intracerebral Hemorrhage: A Guideline From the American Heart Association/American Stroke Association. Stroke. 2022;53(7):e282-e361.
2. Kuramatsu JB, Sembill JA, Gerner ST, et al. Management of therapeutic anticoagulation in patients with intracerebral haemorrhage and mechanical heart valves. Eur Heart J. 2018;39(19):1709-23
3. Chao TF, Liu CJ, Lin YJ, et al. Oral Anticoagulation in Very Elderly Patients With Atrial Fibrillation: A Nationwide Cohort Study. Circulation. 2018;138(1):37-47.
4. Viles-Gonzalez JF, Kar S, Douglas P, et al. The clinical impact of incomplete left atrial appendage closure with the Watchman Device in patients with atrial fibrillation: a PROTECT AF (Percutaneous Closure of the Left Atrial Appendage Versus Warfarin Therapy for Prevention of Stroke in Patients With Atrial Fibrillation) substudy. J Am Coll Cardiol. 2012;59(10):923-9

CHAPTER 10

# A Case-based Discussion on Hypogonadism

*Pankaj Singhania, Debalina Sarkar, Abhranil Dhar, Rana Bhattacharjee, Asish Kumar Basu*

**CASE VIGNETTE**

A 17-year-old female presented with complaint of failure to gain height along with poor development of secondary sexual characteristics and failure to attain menarche. Her birth history was uneventful. Her height was 134 cm (–4,94 SDS, HA: 10 years), target height SDS (–0.53 SDS), she weighed 33 kg (–2.48 SDS, WA: 12 years). Her bone age was 11–12 years and body segment ratio were 1.06. Head to toe inspection revealed presence of high arched palate, low set ears, low posterior hairline, multiple pigmented nevi, short webbed neck, shield chest and short 4th metacarpals. Carrying angle was: right 21° and left 18°. Her sexual maturity was prepubertal. Investigations revealed serum FSH 154 mIU/mL, LH 38 mIU/mLl, estradiol <20 pg/mL. USG lower abdomen revealed hypoplastic uterus and streak ovaries. Her karyotype showed 45,XO. The case was provisionally diagnosed as Turner syndrome.

## PROVISIONAL DIAGNOSIS

Based on the clinical presentation and investigations, the provisional diagnosis is *Turner syndrome*. This is a chromosomal disorder characterized by a complete or partial absence of one X chromosome, often leading to short stature, delayed puberty, and a range of physical abnormalities.

- Short stature, below the expected target height, short webbed neck, shield chest.
- Poor development of secondary sexual characteristics, prepubertal sexual maturity, and failure to attain menarche.
- Elevated FSH (154 mIU/mL) and LH (38 mIU/mL) suggesting primary ovarian insufficiency.
- Estradiol < 20 pg/mL indicating low estrogen levels.
- Ultrasound (USG) showing hypoplastic uterus and streak ovaries.
- Karyotype 45,XO

## DIFFERENTIAL DIAGNOSIS

### Noonan Syndrome

- *Distinguishing features:* Short stature, webbed neck, and shield chest can resemble Turner syndrome, but Noonan syndrome is autosomal dominant and can occur in both sexes.
- *Investigative clues:* Normal karyotype (46,XX), heart defects (like pulmonary stenosis), and normal or mildly elevated FSH and LH

### Müllerian Agenesis (Mayer–Rokitansky–Küster–Hauser Syndrome)

- *Distinguishing features:* Primary amenorrhea with normal secondary sexual characteristics development, absent or underdeveloped uterus, and normal ovarian function.
- *Investigative clues:* Normal karyotype (46,XX), normal hormone levels (FSH, LH), absence of uterus or only a rudimentary one on imaging

### Androgen Insensitivity Syndrome (AIS)

- *Distinguishing features:* Individuals with AIS are phenotypically female with male (46,XY) karyotype, presenting with primary amenorrhea, normal breast development, and absent or sparse pubic hair.
- *Investigative clues:* Male karyotype (46,XY), normal or elevated LH, low or absent FSH, and high testosterone levels.

## CLINICAL APPROACH

Symptoms and presenting features of hypogonadism vary depending on age, sex, and severity **(Fig. 1 and Flowchart 1)**.

- *Neonatal period*:
  - Cryptorchidism/Micropenis in an otherwise normally sexually differentiated male suggests hypogonadotropic hypogonadism.
  - Lymphedema, webbed neck may give clue for Turner syndrome.
  - Eunuchoid body habitus suggests central cause.
- *Adolescence*:
  - Failure of onset of puberty
  - Amenorrhea, absent breast development (in females)
  - Inadequate testicular growth (in males)
  - Absent/Decreased sense of smell
  - Inadequate growth spurt
  - No/less erections and shaving (in males)
  - Turner stigmata—increased carrying angle, webbed and short neck, high arched palate, short 4th metacarpals
  - Verbal learning disability/ADHD/autism (in Klinefelter syndrome)

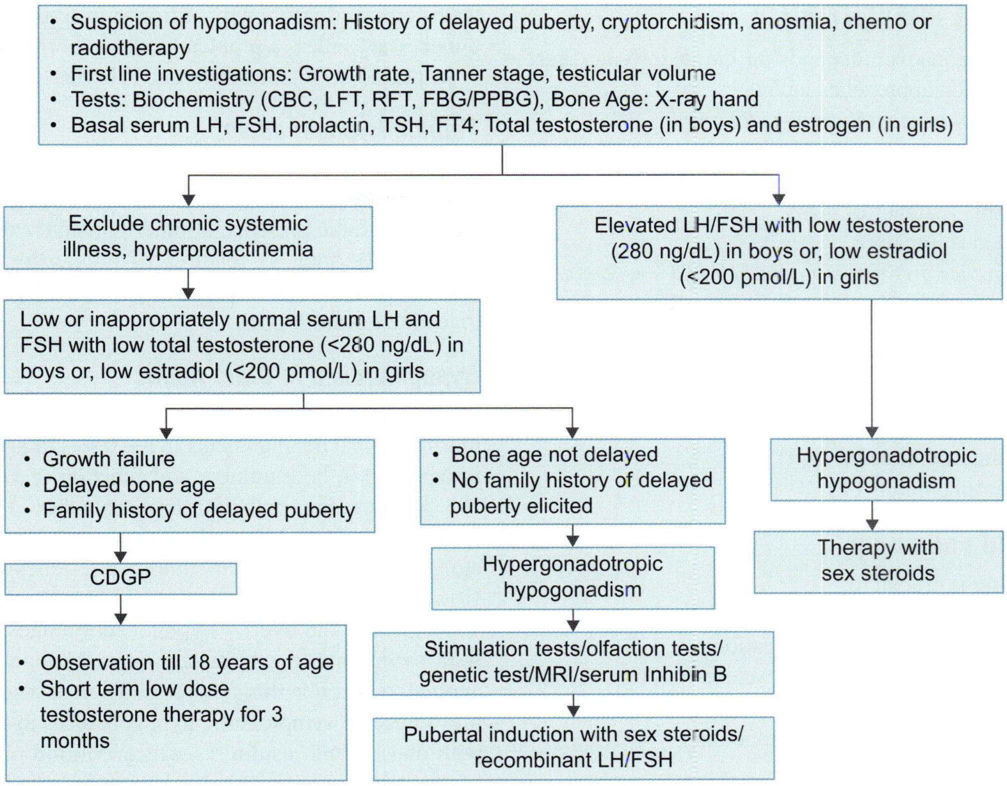


**FLOWCHART 1:** Clinical approach to hypogonadism.

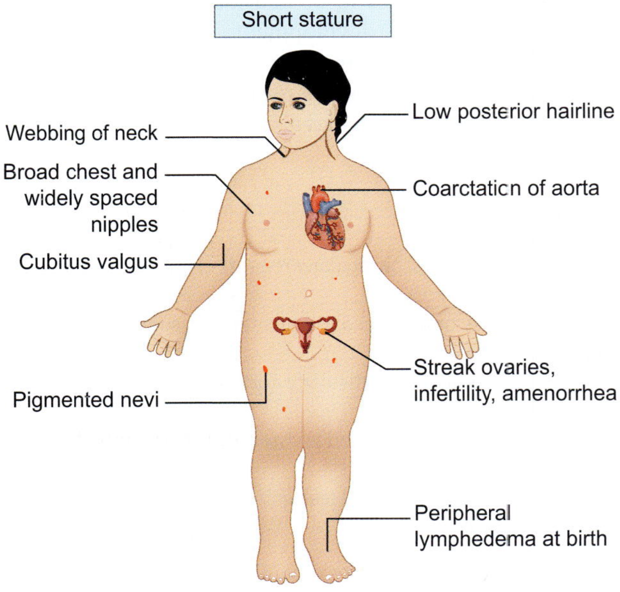


**FIG. 1:** Characteristic features of a girl with Turner syndrome.
*Courtesy*: Image by Lecturio.

- *Adulthood*:
  - Erectile dysfunction (in men)
  - Fatigue
  - Osteoporosis
  - Infertility
  - Decreased muscle mass and strength
  - Decreased bone density
  - Hair loss or thinning
  - Gynecomastia (in men)
  - Hot flashes and vaginal dryness

*Physical examination may reveal*:
- Arm span > height
- Minimal axillary and pubic hair
- Reduced body hair distribution
- Genital abnormalities (e.g., micropenis and undescended testicles)
- Decreased muscle mass

## DIAGNOSTIC EVALUATION

- Hormone level assessments:
  - Testosterone (total)—low in all forms of hypogonadism, free testosterone if total testosterone borderline or, any abnormality in SHBG suspected (steroid use, nephrotic syndrome)
  - Luteinizing hormone (LH)—low in hypo hypo, high in hyper hypo
  - Follicle-stimulating hormone (FSH)—low in hypo hypo, high in hyper hypo
  - Prolactin
  - Thyroid function test
  - Estrogen (in women)—low in all forms of hypogonadism
- *Imaging studies*:
  - Hypothalamic–pituitary magnetic resonance imaging (MRI)
  - Testicular ultrasound (in men)
  - Ovarian ultrasound (in women)
- Semen analysis (in men):

**Genetic testing (in suspected genetic disorders)**

## TREATMENT AND PREVENTION

Treatment for hypogonadism depends on the underlying cause, age, and sex. Common approaches include:

- *Testosterone replacement therapy (TRT)*:
  - Oral
  - Injectable
  - Transdermal (patches or gels)
  - Subcutaneous implants
- *Gonadotropin therapy (recombinant LH/ hCG, recombinant FSH/ hMG):* Used for secondary hypogonadism, especially to achieve fertility.
- *Hormone replacement therapy (HRT) in women*: Used to treat estrogen deficiency
- *Fertility treatments (in men and women):*
  - Intrauterine insemination (IUI)
  - In vitro fertilization (IVF)

### Monitoring and Follow-up

Regular monitoring is crucial to:

- Adjust treatment as needed
- Monitor for side effects and complications
- *Check hormone levels*: Monitor midcycle testosterone in male.
- Assess bone density and muscle mass
- Evaluate fertility and reproductive function

### Hypogonadism in Men versus Women

#### *In Men*

Initial laboratory testing should include 2 early morning (8 AM to 10 AM) serum testosterone measurements. Two total testosterone levels <280 ng/dL are generally considered sufficient to diagnose biochemical hypogonadism. Only patients with symptoms associated with clinical hypogonadism should be treated for low testosterone. Measurement of free testosterone levels is generally unnecessary unless a problem with sex hormone-binding protein is suspected or, total testosterone is borderline.

#### *Female Hypogonadism*

Hypergonadotropic hypogonadism mimics premature ovarian insufficiency. The diagnosis of female hypogonadism becomes trickier with the presence of other potential causes of prolonged amenorrhea, such as features of polycystic ovary syndrome (PCOS). Features of hyperandrogenism, insulin resistance may give clue toward PCOS.

#### *Hypogonadism in Older Adults*

Age-related progressive testicular dysfunction is underpinned by morphological derangements in the testes of aged men including a reduction in both number and function of Leydig cells, germ cell degeneration, reduction in the number of Sertoli cells and areas of fibrosis. Although testosterone levels decrease with aging, real and universal "andropause" does not exist in men. However, in a small minority of elderly men (>70 year of age), T declines to the overtly hypogonadal range, and if associated with symptoms, the term late-onset hypogonadism has been applied to describe this syndrome. There is also there is growing prevalence of symptomatic hypogonadism in middle-aged men with obesity and insulin resistance. Morbid obesity (BMI >40) has been linked to hypothalamic hypogonadism.

#### *Hypogonadism in Children and Adolescents*

Pubertal induction needs to be considered for future fertility prospect as well as development of secondary sexual characteristics. Optimization of height also needs to be considered. Psychosocial issues regarding non development of secondary sexual characteristics also needs to be addressed.

### Points to Ponder

- ❑ *Early diagnosis*: Early identification of Turner syndrome can improve management outcomes, particularly regarding growth, puberty induction, and cardiac care.
- ❑ *Growth and puberty*: The significant growth delay (height SDS –4.94) and absence of secondary sexual characteristics suggest the need for growth hormone therapy and estrogen replacement to induce puberty.
- ❑ *Cardiovascular concerns*: Turner syndrome patients are at risk for cardiovascular abnormalities, particularly aortic coarctation and bicuspid aortic valve. Regular echocardiography is recommended.
- ❑ *Fertility implications*: Streak ovaries typically lead to infertility, but ovarian tissue cryopreservation and assisted reproductive technologies offer potential options for family planning.
- ❑ *Psychosocial support*: Given the challenges related to physical development, infertility, and potential learning difficulties, comprehensive psychosocial support is essential to improve the patient's quality of life.

## MULTIPLE CHOICE QUESTIONS

1. **What is the most likely diagnosis for the 17-year-old female above with the described clinical features?**
   A. Klinefelter syndrome
   B. Turner syndrome
   C. Premature ovarian insufficiency
   D. Hypopituitarism

2. **The patient's karyotype shows 45,XO. Which of the following is a common feature of Turner syndrome?**
   A. Long limbs and tall stature
   B. Webbed neck and low set ears
   C. High levels of estradiol
   D. Enlarged uterus with normal ovaries

**3. In the above given case, the serum levels of FSH and LH are significantly elevated while estradiol is low. This suggests what in the patient:**

A. Hypothalamic dysfunction
B. Primary ovarian insufficiency
C. Normal pubertal development
D. Hyperprolactinemia

**4. The patient's bone age is 11–12 years despite being 17 years old. This suggests:**

A. Delayed puberty
B. Accelerated bone growth
C. Normal pubertal progression
D. Early menarche

**5. Which of the following is typically seen on ultrasound in patients with Turner syndrome?**

A. Enlarged uterus with normal ovaries
B. Hypoplastic uterus and streak ovaries
C. Polycystic ovaries
D. Normal uterus and ovaries

## Answers

1. (B); 2. (B); 3. (B); 4 (A); 5. (B)

## SUGGESTED READINGS


1. Melmed S, Auchus RJ, Goldfine AB, et al. Williams Textbook of Endocrinology E-Book. Elsevier Health Sciences; 2024.
2. Robertson RP. DeGroot's Endocrinology, E-Book: Basic Science and Clinical Practice. Elsevier Health Sciences; 2022.
3. Simoni M, Huhtaniemi IT. Endocrinology of the testis and male reproduction. Springer; 2017.
4. Winters SJ, Huhtaniemi IT. Male hypogonadism: Basic, Clinical and Therapeutic Principles. Humana Press; 2017.
5. Gravholt CH, Andersen NH, Christin-Maitre S, et al. Clinical practice guidelines for the care of girls and women with Turner syndrome. European Journal of Eur J Endocrinol. 2024;190(6):G53–151.

CHAPTER 11

# An Approach to a Case of Discrepant Thyroid Function Tests

***Anand Kate***

**CASE VIGNETTE**

A 25-year-old man, referred with the diagnosis of TSHoma, who had Duchenne muscular dystrophy (DMD) of childhood onset. Biochemical evaluation for low bone density showed discrepant TFTs, confirmed on different assay platforms. Although TPOAb and TgAb were negative, thyroid ultrasonography showed heterogeneous echotexture with pseudonodules. The TRH test showed a normal increase of the TSH after TRH stimulation, and MRI scan showed a 3 mm left-sided pituitary lesion. Sequencing of THRB and ALB did not identify any pathogenic variants. With T3 administration being contraindicated due to DMD, a LAR-SMS trial (20 mg/day) was undertaken, with normalization of FT4 and FT3.

Twelve months later FT4 became elevated again, while FT3 levels were within the normal range. LAR-SMS dosage was increased up to 30 mg/28 days without improvement.

Thyroid function was rechecked using a two-step assay platform and found to be normal [FT4 14.8 pmol/L, RR 10–20, Total T4 (TT4) 118.9 nmol/L, RR 69.0–141.0 nmol/L].

Thyroxine binding globulin (TBG) levels were low (13 µg/mL RR 14–31).

## PROVISIONAL DIAGNOSIS: BIOTIN ASSAY INTERFERENCE

- *Assay interference*:
  - Assay interference in thyroid function testing has been estimated as occurring in up to 1% of all tests performed.
  - Given the widespread testing of thyroid function in clinical practice, assay interference is an important consideration.
  - The issue of assay interference arises because there are several different methods used to measure thyroid stimulating hormone (TSH), total and free thyroxine (T4), and total and free triiodothyronine (T3), including radioimmunoassay, immunometric assay, and tandem mass spectrometry.
  - Differences in sensitivity, specificity, and standardization can result in significant variability between these methods.
- *Interference in TFT by antibodies*:
  - The gold standard free T4 assay is one that uses the equilibrium dialysis method although this is not widely available.
  - The FT4 assay platforms in routine use are not always robust and can be affected by serum antibodies.
  - The commonest cause of a falsely high TSH is assay interference from human anti-murine antibodies (HAMA) or thyroid hormone autoantibodies (THAAbs).
  - Rheumatoid factor (RF) is an antibody directed against human IgG and is often present in people with autoimmune disease—particularly rheumatoid arthritis.
  - RF can also interfere with TFT assays and should be considered if the clinical picture is suggestive.
  - Other antibodies such as anti-streptavidin and anti-ruthenium antibodies can also cause assay interference
- *Biotin interferes with TFT*: Biotin is used with increasing frequency as a health supplement for healthy skin, hair and nails. Biotin can interfere with certain TFT assays. Ylli D et al. conducted a prospective study of possible biotin interference in thyroid-related laboratory assays, with a comparison of different commonly used assay platforms. They reported a daily dose of Biotin 10 mg was shown to interfere with specific assays for TSH, FT4, TT3, and Tg. Physicians must be aware of the potential risk of erroneous test results in subjects taking biotin supplements.

## DIFFERENTIAL DIAGNOSIS

Clinical history with detailed questioning leads to clarity whether patient is on supplements.

Thyroid function tests: Discordant scenarios—

- Differential diagnosis of normal TSH **(Table 1)**
- Differential diagnosis of low TSH **(Table 2)**
- Differential diagnosis of high TSH **(Table 3)**

Algorithmic free T4 based approach to interpret thyroid function tests **(Flowchart 1)**.

### Diagnosis: Biotin Assay Interference

Thyroxine binding globulin (TBG) levels were low due to corticosteroid treatment.

**TABLE 1: Differential diagnosis of normal TSH.**

| Disorder | FT4 | FT3 | Thyroid status |
|---|---|---|---|
| Resistance to thyroid hormone beta | High | High | Euthyroid/ Hyperthyroid |
| Resistance to thyroid hormone alpha | Lower or lower half of normal range | High or upper half of normal range | Hyperthyroid |
| MCT8 deficiency | Low or lower half of normal range | High or upper half of normal range | Cerebral hypothyroidism with peripheral hyperthyroidism |

**TABLE 2: Differential diagnosis of low TSH.**

| Disorder | FT4 | FT3 | Thyroid status |
|---|---|---|---|
| Graves' disease | High | High | Hyperthyroid |
| Neonatal thyrotoxicosis | High | High | Hyperthyroid |
| Hashitoxicosis | High | High | Hyperthyroid |
| Euthyroid sick syndrome | Low/ Normal | Low | Euthyroid |
| Biotin interference | High | High | Euthyroid |
| Central hypothyroidism | Low | Normal/ Low | hypothyroid |

He was also taking biotin as a supportive therapy for DMD, which might have caused interference with avidin/streptavidin-based assay methods.

Discordant TFT is a diagnostic challenge:
- While interpretation of thyroid function testing is usually straightforward, accurate interpretation becomes significantly more challenging when the parameters do not behave as would be expected in normal negative feedback.
- In such cases, uncertainty regarding further investigation and management arises.
- An important abnormal pattern encountered in clinical practice is that of high normal or raised free thyroxine (FT4) with inappropriately nonsuppressed or elevated TSH.

Rule out assay interference before considering rare diagnoses:
- In a patient who is clinically euthyroid with elevated FT4 and an inappropriately normal or raised TSH, the most likely cause is assay interference.

**TABLE 3: Differential diagnosis of high TSH.**

| Disorder | FT4 | FT3 | Thyroid status |
|---|---|---|---|
| Congenital/Acquired hypothyroidism | Low/ Normal | Normal | Hypothyroid/ Euthyroid |
| Subclinical hypothyroidism | Normal | Normal | Euthyroid |
| TSHOma | High | High | Hyperthyroid |

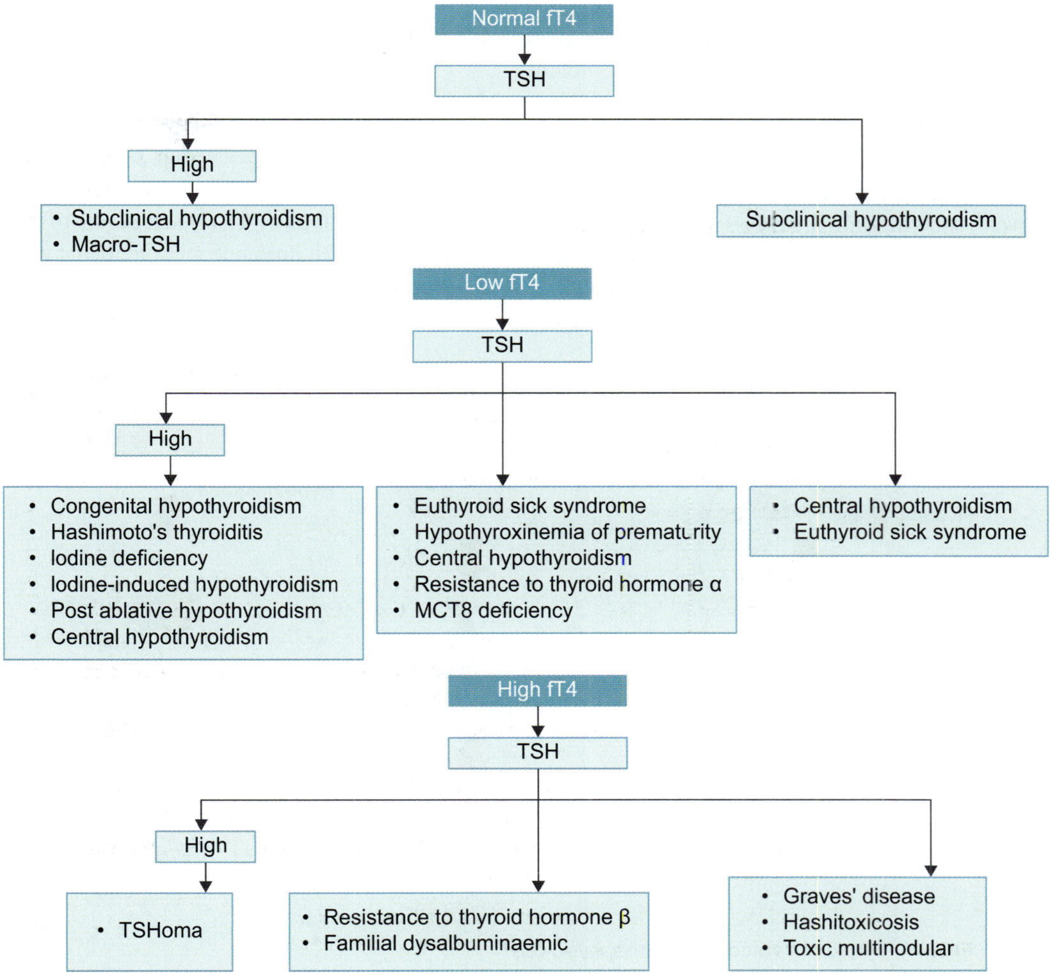


**FLOWCHART 1:** Differential diagnosis for normal free T4.

- Interference should firstly be excluded before considering rarer conditions such as resistance to thyroid hormone and TSH-secreting pituitary adenoma (TSHoma).
- Repeat thyroid function tests should be sent to another laboratory using a different assay to unmask assay interference if this is suspected.
- Focused drug history and family history of thyroid function abnormalities should be specifically sought in these patients.

Differentiate between RTH and TSHoma:
- When assay interference has been excluded, consideration should be given to resistance to thyroid hormone (RTH) and TSHoma.
- Biochemical, dynamic testing, and imaging can be used to differentiate between the two conditions.
- An algorithmic approach to investigation ensure that a diagnosis is reached in this clinical conundrum.

## CLINICAL APPROACH

- *Diagnosis confirmation*: A comprehensive evaluation is essential due to the complexity of the case, including the history of Duchenne muscular dystrophy (DMD) and suspected TSHoma. Discrepant thyroid function tests (TFTs) and imaging findings suggest the need for careful diagnostic assessment. Differentiating true TSHoma from other causes of abnormal TFTs, such as thyroid hormone resistance or assay interference, is crucial.
- *Imaging and hormonal assessment*: The 3 mm pituitary lesion observed on MRI raises suspicion for a TSHoma, but a normal TSH response to the TRH stimulation test suggests otherwise. Further imaging, if necessary, should include follow-up MRIs and pituitary function tests to assess lesion stability and potential growth.
- *Trial of treatment*: The trial of long-acting somatostatin (LAR-SMS) aimed to suppress TSH secretion and normalize thyroid hormone levels, showing initial success with FT4 and FT3 normalization. The re-elevation of FT4 after 12 months may indicate partial resistance or the need for dose adjustment.
- *Thyroid function re-evaluation*: Given the inconsistent TFT results, a repeat assessment using a reliable two-step assay platform revealed normal thyroid hormone levels. This highlights the importance of using accurate assays to confirm thyroid status, avoiding misinterpretation due to assay discrepancies.
- *Management of low TBG*: The low TBG levels should be taken into account, as they may affect total thyroid hormone measurements. Regular monitoring of free T4 (FT4) and total T4 (TT4), along with TBG levels, is essential to ensure accurate evaluation and guide ongoing management.

This approach emphasizes the need for accurate diagnostics, tailored therapeutic trials, and careful monitoring in complex endocrine cases.

## PATHOPHYSIOLOGY (FIGS. 1 AND 2)

Discrepant thyroid function tests (TFTs) occur when laboratory results do not align with the clinical picture, often due to factors affecting hormone levels or assay accuracy. Common causes include:
- *Thyroid hormone resistance*: Mutations in the thyroid hormone receptor (THRB) can lead to tissue insensitivity, resulting in elevated thyroid hormones with normal or high TSH levels.
- *Pituitary disorders*: TSH-secreting pituitary adenomas (TSHomas) or nontumorous pituitary dysfunction can cause inappropriate TSH secretion despite abnormal thyroid hormone levels.
- *Assay interference*: Autoantibodies, heterophile antibodies, or abnormal proteins can interfere with immunoassays, leading to falsely elevated or suppressed results.
- *Thyroid binding protein abnormalities*: Changes in thyroid-binding globulin (TBG), albumin, or transthyretin levels can alter total hormone measurements without affecting free hormone levels.

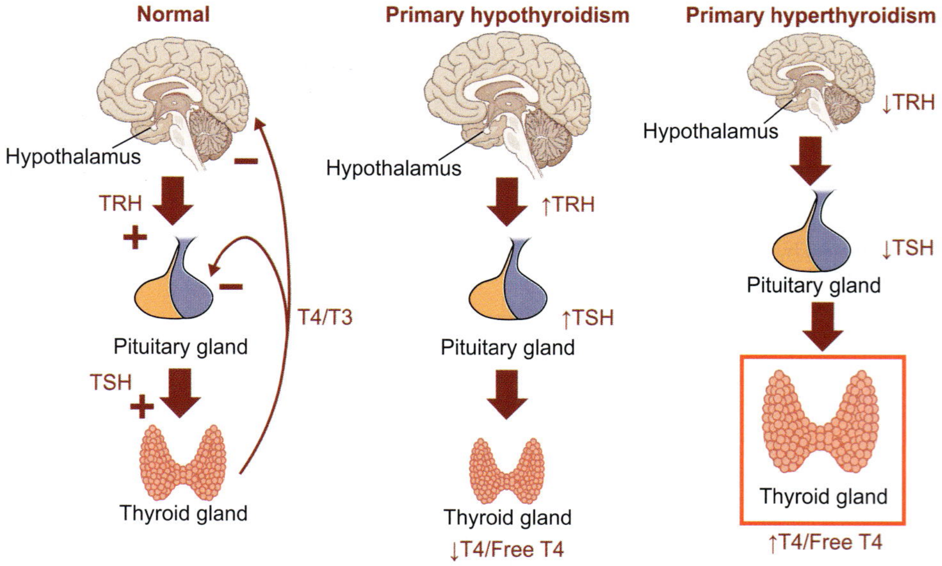


**FIG. 1:** Thyroid physiology and pathophysiology.
Source: Kurian M, Kapoor N. Interpretation of thyroid function tests. 2018.

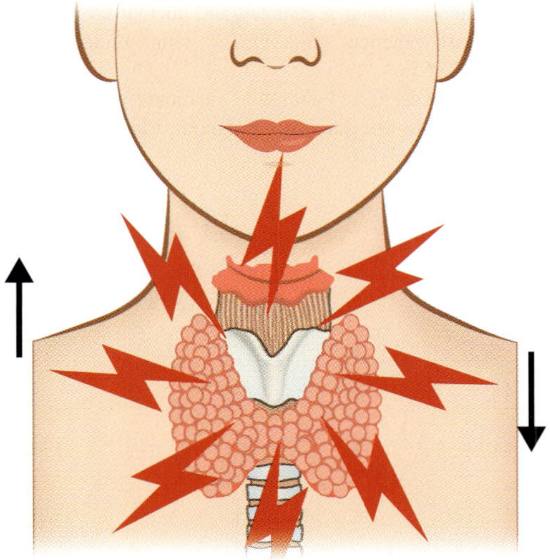

**FIG. 2:** The image depicting a visual representation of thyroid dysfunction.

- *Nonthyroidal illness*: Acute or chronic illnesses can impact thyroid function tests, causing alterations in hormone levels due to changes in hormone metabolism or binding.

## TREATMENT AND PREVENTION

- *Somatostatin analog therapy*: Initial treatment with LAR-SMS at 20 mg/day, which helped normalize thyroid hormone levels (FT4 and FT3). However, due to a later increase in FT4, the dose was increased to 30 mg/28 days without sufficient improvement.
- *Monitoring and adjustment*: Continuous monitoring of thyroid function tests using a reliable assay platform is crucial, as discrepancies in hormone levels were noted initially and needed accurate reassessment.
- *Avoidance of T3 therapy*: Direct T3 administration was contraindicated due to the patient's Duchenne muscular dystrophy, requiring careful management with other therapeutic options.
- *Regular thyroid function tests*: Periodic evaluation of thyroid hormones (FT4, FT3, and TSH) using accurate and consistent testing methods to avoid misinterpretation of lab results.
- *MRI follow-up*: Routine imaging to monitor the pituitary lesion for any changes, given the presence of a small left-sided pituitary abnormality.
- *Bone health monitoring*: Due to the patient's history of low bone density, ensure ongoing assessment and management of bone health, including calcium and vitamin D supplementation if needed.
- *Multidisciplinary care*: Collaboration with endocrinology, neurology, and other specialists to tailor management, especially given the complexity of DMD and potential contraindications for typical treatments.
- *Monitoring of thyroxine binding globulin*: Given the low TBG levels, consider evaluating factors that could affect thyroid hormone levels and ensure that thyroid function is interpreted in light of TBG status.

### Points to Ponder

- *Assay accuracy*: Use reliable and consistent assay platforms to avoid discrepancies in thyroid function tests.
- *DMD considerations*: In patients with Duchenne muscular dystrophy, contraindications for certain treatments like T3 must be carefully considered.
- *Pituitary monitoring*: Small pituitary lesions, even if asymptomatic, require periodic imaging follow-up for changes.
- *Somatostatin analog efficacy*: Dosage adjustments may be necessary if initial somatostatin analog therapy fails to maintain thyroid hormone levels.
- *TBG impact*: Low thyroxine binding globulin (TBG) levels can influence thyroid hormone interpretation and management decisions.

## MULTIPLE CHOICE QUESTIONS

**1. What was the primary reason T3 administration was contraindicated in this patient?**
   A. Elevated TSH levels
   B. Presence of a pituitary lesion
   C. Duchenne muscular dystrophy (DMD)
   D. Low bone density

**2. What imaging finding was identified in this patient with TSHoma?**
   A. Thyroid nodules
   B. Enlarged pituitary gland
   C. 3 mm left-sided pituitary lesion
   D. Bilateral adrenal enlargement

**3. Which therapy was initially used to manage this patient's TSHoma?**
   A. Levothyroxine
   B. Radioactive iodine
   C. T3 administration
   D. Long-acting release somatostatin (LAR-SMS)

**4. Why the thyroid function was reassessed using a two-step assay platform?**
   A. To check for pituitary hormone levels
   B. Due to discrepancies in initial thyroid function tests
   C. To confirm the presence of TPO antibodies
   D. To evaluate calcium levels

**5. What abnormal finding was noted regarding thyroxine binding globulin (TBG) in this patient?**
   A. Elevated TBG levels
   B. Normal TBG levels
   C. Low TBG levels
   D. Unmeasurable TBG levels

### Answers

1. (C); 2. (C); 3. (D); 4. (B); 5. (C)

## SUGGESTED READINGS


1. Ross DS, Burch HB, Cooper DS, et al. 2016 American Thyroid Association guidelines for diagnosis and management of hyperthyroidism and other causes of thyrotoxicosis. Thyroid. 2016;26(10):1343-1421.
2. Spencer CA, LoPresti JS. Influence of TSH and thyroid hormone assays on the diagnosis and management of subclinical thyroid dysfunction. Front Endocrinol (Lausanne). 2018;9:173.
3. De Groot LJ, Abalovich M, Alexander EK, et al. Management of thyroid dysfunction during pregnancy and postpartum: an Endocrine Society clinical practice guideline. J Clin Endocrinol Metab. 2012;97(8):2543-65.
4. Demers LM, Spencer CA. Laboratory medicine practice guidelines: laboratory support for the diagnosis and monitoring of thyroid disease. Thyroid. 2003;13(1):3-126.

CHAPTER

12

# An Approach to a Case of Exercise Planning in Type 2 Diabetes Mellitus: Overcoming Barriers

*Plawan Mazumdar*

**CASE VIGNETTE**

A 45-year-old female Mrs Bimala (name changed) suffering from type 2 diabetes in the last 4 years having a BMI of 28. She is a housewife and leads a sedentary life-style. She is on metformin 1 g twice daily and her current HbA1c is 7.5%. She does not have any comorbidities.

## PROVISIONAL DIAGNOSIS

Type 2 diabetes mellitus with suboptimal glycemic control (HbA1c 7.5%) in a 45-year-old sedentary female with obesity (BMI 28).

## DIFFERENTIAL DIAGNOSIS

- *Hypertension*: Obesity and sedentary lifestyle increase the risk of elevated blood pressure.
- *Dyslipidemia*: Type 2 diabetes and obesity are risk factors for abnormal lipid profiles.
- *Nonalcoholic fatty liver disease (NAFLD)*: Common in type 2 diabetes and obesity, often asymptomatic.
- *Diabetic nephropathy*: Long-standing diabetes can lead to kidney damage; monitor kidney function.
- *Vitamin D deficiency*: Common in obesity and can worsen insulin resistance.

## CLINICAL APPROACH

### Analysis of Sedentary Behavior of Mrs Bimala

#### *Barriers*

After detailed discussion and analysis with Mrs Bimala, we identified two barriers. Firstly, the lack of knowledge about the benefits of PA and lack of idea about the type and amount of activity suitable for her and secondly, other priorities (like household works, children's care) are more important for her, leaving little time for her own PA.

#### *Motivators*

While interacting with her we also found that she liked socializing and she had the sense that physical activity with others generates social bonding.

#### *Creating the Habit of PA*

**Pick the Cue, Choose a Reward, Execute the Routine**

On analyzing her daily routine, we found that on week days. She accompany her son in the morning to the school bus stop. While returning from there she takes a different longer route, walks leisurely and on the way spend some time in the local park socializing with her neighbors. We identified accompanying her son to the bus stop as the cue, taking the different route to reach the park as the behavior and socializing with neighbors at the park as the reward. We suggested to her that while coming back from bus stand rather than walking leisurely if she does brisk walking or jogging then she will reach the park early and that behavior will generate more time for socializing. She immediately agreed to the idea. Then we informed her about the various health benefit of aerobic exercise and suggested that while returning, walk briskly (5.6 km/h) to the park which will take around 10–15 minutes, four times a week and jogging (9.6 km/h) once a week. Thus, a habit of physical activity was created.

#### *Clearance for PA*

Pre-exercise medical clearance is not necessary for asymptomatic individual undergoing treatment for diabetes who wish to begin low or moderate intensity PA. So, Mrs Bimala does not need any clearance for her structured physical activity.

### Advice and Calculation of Volume of Aerobic Physical Activity

#### *Recommendations*

Refer to **Figure 1**.

#### *Calculations for Mrs Bimala*

Brisk walking (5.6 km/h) on level ground is a 3.8 MET activity. Jogging (9.6 km/h) on level ground is a 10 MET activity. So,

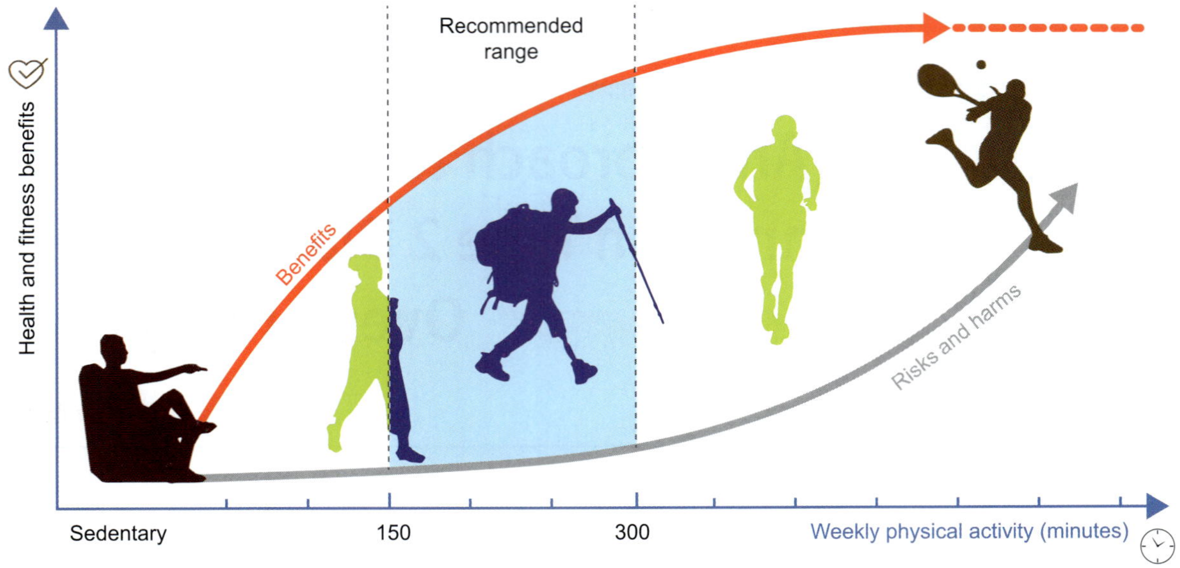


**FIG. 1:** WHO guidelines on physical activity and sedentary behavior (2020).

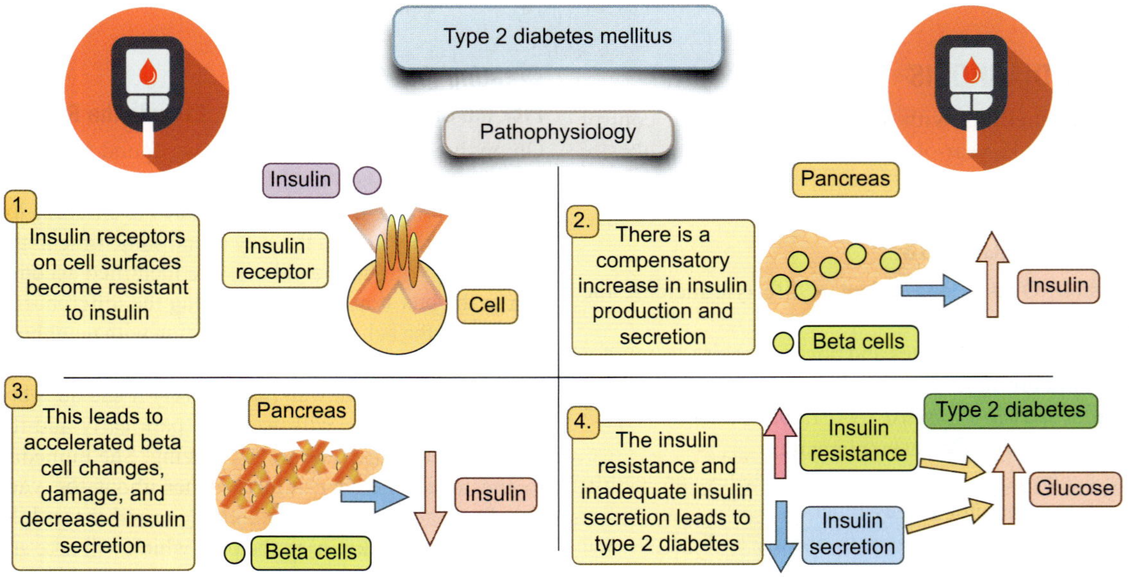


**FIG. 2:** Pathophysiology of T2DM.

*Source*: EZmed. Type 2 diabetes mellitus: Symptoms, diet, medication, treatment, risk factors, definition-EZMeD [Internet]. EZmed. 2023. Available from: https://www.ezmedlearning.com/blog/type-2-diabetes-mellitus-symptoms-medications.

at start we recommended 15 minutes of brisk walking 4 days/week (which was later increased to 30 minutes) and 10 minutes of jogging 1 day/week.

$(30 \times 3.8 \times 4)/60$ plus $(10 \times 10 \times 1)/60 = 9.3$ MET- h/week

So, this is the individualized aerobic exercise plan for Mrs Bimala fulfilling the minimum required energy expenditure per week.

## PATHOPHYSIOLOGY (FIG. 2)

- *Insulin resistance:* In type 2 diabetes, insulin resistance occurs due to impaired function of insulin receptors in muscle, fat, and liver cells, leading to elevated blood glucose levels.
- *Beta-cell dysfunction:* Over time, the pancreas loses its ability to produce adequate insulin in response to elevated blood glucose levels.
- *Obesity:* Mrs Bimala's BMI of 28 indicates obesity, which exacerbates insulin resistance, as excess adipose tissue, especially visceral fat, releases inflammatory cytokines and fatty acids that impair insulin signaling.
- *Sedentary lifestyle:* Physical inactivity worsens insulin resistance and contributes to poor glycemic control.
- *Metformin:* This oral medication helps lower blood glucose by decreasing hepatic glucose production and improving insulin sensitivity. However, her HbA1c of 7.5% indicates suboptimal control, suggesting the need for further interventions in lifestyle or medication management.

## TREATMENT AND PREVENTION

### Resistance, Flexibility, and Balance Advice

- We recommended 2–3 weekly sessions of resistance training targeting all major muscle groups on nonconsecutive days (Physical Activity Guidelines Advisory Committee, 2008).
- To mitigate the effects of sedentary behavior, she was advised to break prolonged sitting with brief standing bouts (<5 min), light walking every 20–30 minutes, and 15 minutes of walking after meals.
- We recommended 2–3 yoga sessions per week to improve flexibility, muscular strength, and balance.

### Execution of the Plan

Checklist before starting the aerobic exercise plan **(Table 1)**.

**TABLE 1: Exercise plan for Mrs Bimala.**

| | |
|---|---|
| **Exercise plan (Turner et al., 2019) for Mrs Bimala** | |
| *For starting exercise* | |
| Glucose trend monitoring before exercise | Not required (required if on Insulin/Sulphonylureas) |
| Do not exercise if feeling unwell or history of level 3 hypoglycemia within 24 hours | |
| Glucose level 99–270 mg/dL | **OK to exercise** (may need one serve carb, if exercise is more than 60 minutes and on Insulin/Sulphonylureas) |
| Glucose level 72–98 mg/dL | **Exercise with caution.** Monitor trend. May need additional carbohydrate if duration of exercise is > 60 minutes (if on insulin or sulphonylureas then, need to take one or two servs of fast acting carb, start exercise only if sugar is >98 mg/dL). Need one serv of slow act carb if exercise duration > 30 minutes |
| Glucose level below 72 mg/dL | **Do not exercise** |
| Glucose level above 270 mg/dL | **Exercise with caution,** if feeling well. Monitor trend /adequate hydration |
| *During exercise* | |
| Glucose below 98 mg/dL | Continue exercise with caution. Need fast acting carbohydrate if next meal is not due in 30 minutes. One, two and four servs per hour for mild, moderate and vigorous exercise respectively |
| Glucose below 72 mg/dL | STOP exercise. Treat hypoglycemia accordingly. After glucose increases above 72 mg/dL, need to take one serv slow acting carbohydrate if next meal is not due in 30 minutes. Only to resume exercise if glucose is above 98 mg/dL |
| Glucose rises above pre-exercise level | Exercise with caution. This may be due to missed medication or effect of food consumed within 90 minutes. Prepare for fall in glucose later |
| **After exercise** (if on insulin or sulphonylurea) | |
| • Need monitoring for post exercise hypoglycemia if there is an increase in the intensity and duration of exercise or starting a new exercise<br>• If there is post exercise hypoglycemia, then after treatment of the event need to check glucose every 2 hours till 6 hours post exercise<br>• If exercise is being done in the afternoon, then need to monitor for nocturnal hypoglycemia<br>• If there is nighttime hypoglycemia, then glucose should be checked at bedtime, 2 AM and after awaking<br>• If glucose is < 126 mg/dL before bed, then extra carb should be taken<br>• Adjustment of Insulin dose with post exercise meal, or additional carbohydrates following exercise may be required | |

### Points to Ponder

- *Lifestyle modification*: Emphasize the need for increased physical activity and reduced sedentary behavior to improve insulin sensitivity.
- *Weight management*: Focus on weight reduction strategies to lower BMI and enhance glycemic control.
- *Glycemic control optimization*: HbA1c of 7.5% suggests room for improvement; consider dietary adjustments or therapy intensification.
- *Long-term complications*: Address preventive measures for diabetes-related complications despite the absence of current comorbidities.
- *Patient education*: Reinforce the importance of regular monitoring and adherence to lifestyle changes alongside medication.

## MULTIPLE CHOICE QUESTIONS

1. **What is the recommended initial management strategy for a 45-year-old female with type 2 diabetes mellitus, suboptimal glycemic control (HbA1c 7.5%), obesity (BMI 28), and a sedentary lifestyle?**
   - A. Increase the dose of metformin
   - B. Add insulin therapy
   - C. Initiate lifestyle modifications with emphasis on diet and physical activity
   - D. Switch to a different oral hypoglycemic agent
2. **What is the target HbA1c level for most adults with type 2 diabetes, according to current guidelines?**
   - A. <6%
   - B. <7%
   - C. <8%
   - D. <9%
3. **Given Mrs Bimala's BMI of 28, what is the recommended goal for weight loss to improve her type 2 diabetes management?**
   - A. 10–15% of her total body weight
   - B. 2–5% of her total body weight
   - C. 5–10% of her total body weight
   - D. No weight loss is necessary
4. **Which of the following is a potential complication for a patient with type 2 diabetes and suboptimal glycemic control?**
   - A. Hypoglycemia
   - B. Diabetic retinopathy
   - C. Hyperkalemia
   - D. Osteoporosis
5. **For a sedentary patient with type 2 diabetes, what is the recommended amount of physical activity per week to help manage blood glucose levels and improve overall health?**
   - A. 30 minutes of moderate-intensity exercise once a week
   - B. 150 minutes of moderate-intensity aerobic exercise per week
   - C. 60 minutes of high-intensity exercise per week
   - D. 30 minutes of low intensity walking daily

### Answers

1. (C); 2. (B); 3. (C); 4. (B); 5. (B)

## SUGGESTED READINGS

1. Myers J, Kokkinos P, Arena R, et al. The impact of moving more, physical activity, and cardiorespiratory fitness: Why we should strive to measure and improve fitness. Prog Cardiovasc Dis. 2021;64:77-82.
2. Committee Physical Activity Guidelines Advisory (2018). Physical Activity Guidelines Advisory Committee Scientific Report. Washington, DC: US. Department of Health and Human Services.
3. Turner G, Quigg S, Davoren P, et al. Resources to Guide Exercise Specialists Managing Adults with Diabetes. Sports Medicine – Open. 5, Article number: 20; 2019.
4. Committee Physical Activity Guidelines Advisory. Physical Activity Guidelines Advisory Committee Scientific Report. Washington, DC: US Department of Health and Human Services; 2018.
5. Lear SA, Hu W, Rangarajan S, et al. The effect of PA on mortality and cardiovascular disease in 130000 people from 17 high-income, middle-income, and low-income countries: the PURE study. Lancet. 2017;390:2643-54.
6. MacIntosh BR, Murias JM, Keir DA, et al. What is Moderate to Vigorous Exercise Intensity? Front Physiol. 2021;12:682233.
7. Myers J, Kokkinos P, Arena R, et al. The impact of moving more, physical activity, and cardiorespiratory fitness: Why we should strive to measure and improve fitness. Prog Cardiovasc Dis. 2021;64:77-82.
8. WHO guideline on physical activity and sedentary behaviour (2020). Geneva: World Health Organization; 2020. Licence: CC BY-NC-SA 3.0 IGO. ISBN 978-92-4-001512-8 (electronic version) ISBN 978-92-4-001513-5 (print edition).

CHAPTER 13

# A Case-based Approach to Type 2 Diabetes Mellitus

*Nishi Kant, Jyoti Jha*

**CASE VIGNETTE**

A 50-year-old woman with a history of type 2 diabetes mellitus (T2DM) and acute coronary syndrome (ACS) presented for follow-up care. At the time of diagnosis, her HbA1c was 8.8%, which improved to 7.8% with initial metformin therapy. Despite these improvements, her obesity (BMI 32.1 kg/m$^2$) and dyslipidemia (LDL 66 mg/dL, HDL 34 mg/dL, TG 185 mg/dL) posed significant cardiovascular risks.

To achieve tighter glycemic control and address her cardiovascular profile, an SGLT2 inhibitor was initiated. This choice was based on its benefits, including HbA1c reduction, weight loss, and cardioprotection. Patient education emphasized dietary modifications, weight management, and the importance of adhering to treatment protocols. Follow-ups were scheduled to monitor clinical outcomes and ensure the safety and efficacy of the therapy. This case highlights the importance of personalized treatment strategies that integrate glycemic control with cardiovascular risk management in patients with T2DM.

## PROVISIONAL DIAGNOSIS

Type 2 diabetes mellitus (T2DM) with a history of acute coronary syndrome (ACS) and obesity.

## DIFFERENTIAL DIAGNOSIS

- Dyslipidemia-related metabolic syndrome
- Nonalcoholic fatty liver disease (NAFLD)
- Hypertensive cardiovascular disease

## CLINICAL APPROACH

- Comprehensive evaluation of glycemic status (HbA1c, fasting glucose)
- Lipid panel and blood pressure assessment
- Screening for microvascular complications (e.g., retinopathy, nephropathy)
- Cardiovascular risk stratification

## PATHOPHYSIOLOGY (FIG. 1)

Type 2 diabetes mellitus results from insulin resistance and relative insulin deficiency, leading to hyperglycemia and metabolic dysfunction. Chronic hyperglycemia exacerbates endothelial damage, increases oxidative stress, and accelerates atherosclerosis, heightening cardiovascular risk.

## TREATMENT AND PREVENTION

### Treatment

- Initiate SGLT2 inhibitors for glycemic control and cardioprotection.
- Continue metformin therapy.
- Lifestyle modifications, including dietary counseling and weight loss interventions.
- Statins for dyslipidemia management.
- Antiplatelet therapy if indicated for cardiovascular protection.

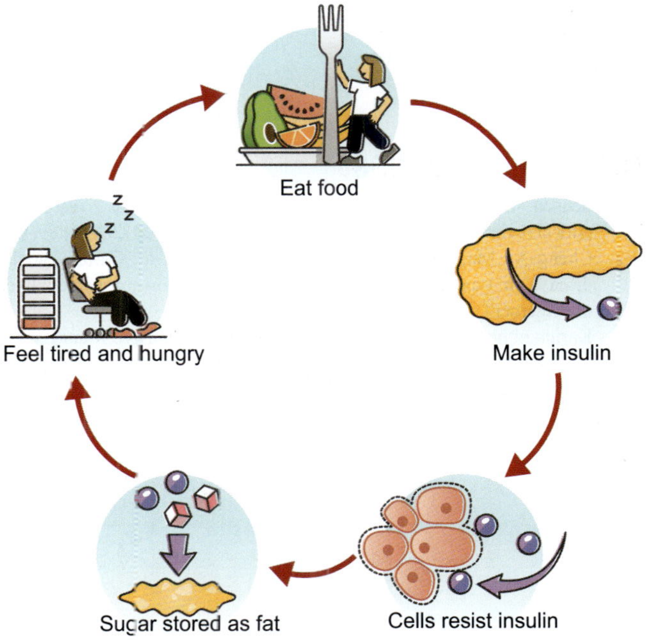


**FIG. 1:** Insulin resistance.

## Prevention

- Regular physical activity and balanced diet to prevent metabolic deterioration.
- Routine monitoring of glycemic and cardiovascular parameters.
- Patient education on lifestyle modifications and medication adherence.
- Early screening for diabetes-related complications to ensure timely intervention.

## Points to Ponder

- *Tailored therapy*: Selecting treatment strategies that align with individual patient profiles, such as using SGLT2 inhibitors for patients with T2DM and cardiovascular risks, ensures optimal outcomes.
- *Glycemic and cardiovascular goals*: Achieving HbA1c targets (≤7%) and addressing comorbid conditions like dyslipidemia and hypertension are crucial in comprehensive T2DM management.
- *Risk-benefit analysis*: Balancing efficacy and safety is vital, especially in elderly patients with multiple comorbidities, to avoid adverse effects like hypoglycemia.
- *Early detection*: Monitoring markers such as microalbuminuria helps in identifying complications like diabetic nephropathy early, allowing timely intervention.
- *Multifactorial approach*: Combining lifestyle modifications, pharmacotherapy, and patient education enhances glycemic control and mitigates long-term complications of T2DM.

## MULTIPLE CHOICE QUESTIONS

**1. Which class of drugs provides both glycemic control and cardioprotection in patients with T2DM and cardiovascular disease?**
A. DPP-4 inhibitors
B. SGLT2 inhibitors
C. GLP-1 receptor agonists
D. Sulfonylureas

**2. What is the recommended HbA1c target for most patients with T2DM and cardiovascular comorbidities?**
A. ≤6.5%
B. ≤7%
C. ≤7.5%
D. ≤8%

**3. Which of the following metabolic abnormalities is not commonly associated with T2DM?**
A. Hyperglycemia
B. Dyslipidemia
C. Hypernatremia
D. Insulin resistance

**4. Which pharmacological agent is preferred for weight management in T2DM patients?**
A. Insulin
B. SGLT2 inhibitors
C. TZDs
D. DPP-4 inhibitors

**5. What is a key clinical marker for early detection of diabetic nephropathy in T2DM patients?**
A. Elevated LDL cholesterol
B. Increased HbA1c
C. Microalbuminuria
D. Retinopathy

### Answers

1. (B); 2. (B); 3. (C); 4. (B); 5. (C)

## SUGGESTED READINGS

1. Scheen AJ. DPP-4 inhibitors in the management of type 2 diabetes: a critical review of head-to-head trials. Diabetes Metab. 2012;38(2):89-101.
2. Cheng-Xu Ma, Xiao-Ni Ma, Cong-Hui Guan, et al. Cardiovascular disease in type 2 diabetes mellitus: progress toward personalized management. Cardiovasc Diabetol. 2022;21(1):74.
3. Karunarathna I, P Jayathilaka, Pradeep. Comprehensive Management of Type 2 Diabetes Mellitus: From Prevention to Novel Therapeutic Approaches. Endocrinol Res Pract. 2024;16(3):153-72.
4. Zinman B, Wanner C, Lachin JM, et al. Empagliflozin, cardiovascular outcomes, and mortality in type 2 diabetes. N Engl J Med. 2015;373(22):2117-28.
5. Nathan DM, Genuth S, Lachin J, et al. Intensive diabetes treatment and cardiovascular outcomes in type 2 diabetes. N Engl J Med. 2005;353(24):2643-53.
6. American Diabetes Association. Standards of Medical Care in Diabetes – 2024. Diabetes Care. 2024;47(Suppl. 1):S1-S148.

CHAPTER 14

# An Approach to a Case of Galactorrhea in a 20-year-old Woman

*Sambit Das, Vishal Agarwal*

## CASE VIGNETTE

A 20-year-old girl was referred to endocrinological consultation for galactorrhea for past 2 months and oligomenorrhea for past 6 months. Pelvic ultrasounds performed by a gynecologists, multifollicular ovaries with no features suggestive of polycystic ovarian disease and routine laboratory workup revealed normal levels of serum androgens, testosterone and androstenedione, however, serum prolactin levels were high (up to 252 µg/L; normal range, 5–25 µg/L). There was no history of intake of oral contraceptives or any gastric motility drug like domperidone in the recent past. The patient had history of intermittent headache. Owing to high suspicion of pituitary adenoma, a magnetic resonance imaging (MRI) of the pituitary was performed which revealed a microadenoma of size 6 mm × 7 mm × 9 mm diameter. With this clinical background, along with laboratory finding of hyperprolactinemia and MRI revealing a microadenoma, the diagnosis of prolactinoma was made, and cabergoline therapy was started at the dose of 0.5 mg/week with gradual up-titration of the dose until normalization of prolactin levels. The clinical course was indolent with responsiveness to cabergoline with complete normalization of prolactin level over 16 months, and an 80% shrinkage in pituitary tumor size, associated with full recovery of the clinical syndrome. The cabergoline therapy was gradually withdrawn over next 2 years.

## PROVISIONAL DIAGNOSIS

Prolactinoma (pituitary microadenoma) with hyperprolactinemia.

## DIFFERENTIAL DIAGNOSIS

- *Hypothyroidism:* It can cause secondary hyperprolactinemia due to increased TRH drive, though thyroid function tests were normal.
- *Polycystic ovarian syndrome (PCOS):* Oligomenorrhea and galactorrhea, but pelvic ultrasound did not support PCOS.
- *Medications-induced hyperprolactinemia:* Exclusion of drugs like antipsychotics or domperidone, which can elevate prolactin levels.
- *Pituitary stalk effect:* Lesions affecting the pituitary stalk can lead to hyperprolactinemia, but MRI showed a microadenoma, not a stalk lesion.
- *Chest wall injury or herpes zoster:* It can cause hyperprolactinemia, but no history of chest trauma or relevant conditions.

## CLINICAL APPROACH

Galactorrhea must be distinguished from pathological nipple discharge associated with breast tumors. Tumor-related discharge typically originates from a single duct, is bloody or serosanguineous, and is often accompanied by a palpable breast lump. In contrast, galactorrhea presents as bilateral, multiductal, milky discharge, which may vary in color from yellow to green or brown. When the diagnosis is uncertain, Sudan IV staining can confirm the presence of milk in the discharge.

### History and Clinical Examination

- *Medication and pregnancy history:* Assess for medications and pregnancy to rule out drug-induced or pregnancy-related galactorrhea.
- *Symptom review:* Consider symptoms like loss of libido, oligomenorrhea/amenorrhea, erectile dysfunction, and gynecomastia.
- *Mass effect symptoms:* Look for signs of sellar or suprasellar mass, such as headaches or visual field defects.
- *Physical examination:* Diagnose galactorrhea by examining the patient in a sitting position, leaning forward, and gently massaging the areolae from all quadrants toward the nipple.
- *Prolactin testing timing:* Avoid prolactin areolae measurement shortly after breast examination to prevent transient prolactin elevation.

### Laboratory Evaluation and Imaging

- *Prolactin measurement:* A single serum prolactin test is usually sufficient; avoid nipple stimulation or vigorous exercise 30 minutes before.
- *Hook effect:* In macroprolactinomas (≥10 mm), falsely low prolactin levels may occur due to the "Hook effect" in immunoassays; a 1:100 serum dilution can prevent this.

- *Macroprolactin interference:* Macroprolactins, large isoforms with low biological activity, may cause asymptomatic hyperprolactinemia; polyethylene glycol screening is recommended.
- *Secondary causes:* Check thyroid-stimulating hormone (TSH) and creatinine to rule out secondary hyperprolactinemia.
- *Imaging and further tests:* Gadolinium-enhanced MRI (or CT if contraindicated) is essential for pituitary evaluation. Perform visual field testing for macroadenomas and assess pituitary hormones. BMD testing (DEXA) is advised for patients with secondary hypogonadism at risk of osteoporosis.

## PATHOPHYSIOLOGY (FIG. 1)

Hyperprolactinemia usually leads to symptomatology pertaining to galactorrhea-amenorrhea complex. However, in patients with galactorrhea and normal menses, the prolactin levels are usually normal. The following are the common causes of galactorrhea encountered in clinical practice:

- *Physiological galactorrhea*: In neonates, transplacental estrogen transfer can cause temporary galactorrhea, known as "witch's milk." Physiological prolactin increases can also occur during pregnancy, breastfeeding, strenuous exercise and stress, etc.
- *Disorder involving hypothalamus and pituitary*: Pituitary stalk compression from dorsally extending suprasellar or sellar mass lesions can cause hyperprolactinemia and galactorrhea, a phenomenon known as the "stalk effect". These lesions impair dopamine transport from the hypothalamus to the anterior pituitary, reducing dopamine's inhibitory effect on lactotroph cells. Such lesions include large non-prolactin-secreting pituitary adenomas, parasellar masses, or granulomatous infiltration of the hypothalamus. Serum prolactin levels in these cases are rarely above 200 μg/L. Prolactinomas, the most common pituitary adenomas, are classified as microadenomas (<10 mm) or macroadenomas (≥10 mm). Prolactin levels above 250 μg/L typically indicate a prolactinoma, while levels exceeding 500 μg/L suggest a macroprolactinoma.
    - *Thyroid disorders*: Hypothyroidism increases thyrotropin-releasing hormone (TRH) drive, which directly stimulates pituitary lactotrophs, leading to hyperprolactinemia. Therefore, thyroid function tests should be conducted in all patients presenting with galactorrhea-amenorrhea complex symptoms.
- *Chronic kidney disease:* In chronic kidney disease, decreased clearance of prolactin leads to hyperprolactinemia. Correction of hyperprolactinemia and galactorrhea typically occurs within days after renal transplantation.
- *Drug induced:* Drug-induced hyperprolactinemia is a common cause in clinical practice, often due to antipsychotics, gastrointestinal promotility agents, and verapamil. Medications like domperidone and antipsychotics block dopamine D2 receptors on pituitary lactotrophs, disrupting the inhibitory effect of hypothalamic dopamine on prolactin secretion.
- *Hyperestrogenemia:* Estrogen directly stimulates lactotroph proliferation and prolactin secretion, and indirectly increases prolactin by inhibiting hypothalamic dopamine neurons. High estrogen levels during pregnancy cause lactotroph hyperplasia and may promote the growth of pre-existing prolactinomas. Oral contraceptives containing estrogens can also contribute to hyperprolactinemia.
- *Chest wall lesions:* Injury to chest wall, herpes zoster, burns, can lead to hyperprolactinemia. Afferent signal from chest wall is relayed through the spinal cord to hypothalamus, leading to reduction of dopamine signaling, thereby inducing hyperprolactinemia.
- *Idiopathic galactorrhea:* Occasionally, in few cases, no apparent cause of hyperprolactinemia is identified; and this is termed as idiopathic galactorrhea.

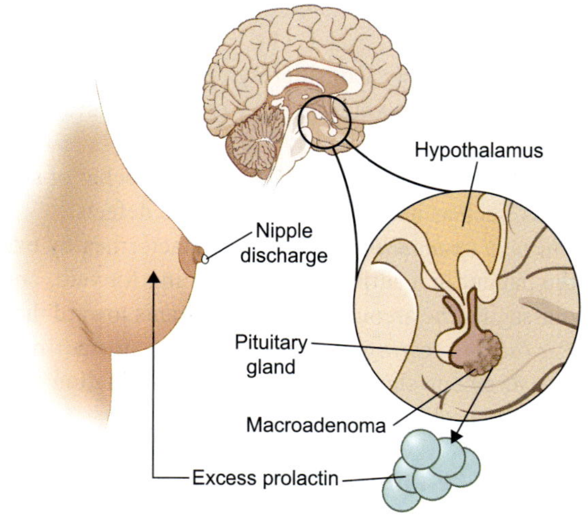


**FIG. 1:** Depicting pathophysiology of galactorrhea.
*Source*: Cleveland Clinic; 2022.

## TREATMENT AND PREVENTION

After exclusion of an underlying breast pathology, treatment is usually indicated for bothersome galactorrhea. The management involves reassurance and treatment of the underlying condition.

Discontinuation of the causative medication in drug-induced hyperprolactinemia usually suffices in such cases. If continuation of the drug is warranted depending on patient's clinical profile as in cases of antipsychotics use, switching to other class of dug with lower or no potential to cause hyperprolactinemia is warranted.

Medical therapy is the treatment of choice for symptomatic prolactinomas. Dopamine agonists are effective in normalising prolactin levels and reducing tumor size. Both cabergoline and bromocriptine are efficacious for management of hyperprolactinemia due to prolactinomas, however, cabergoline is more effective and better tolerated than bromocriptine with lesser side effects. Asymptomatic microprolactinoma does not warrant treatment. Surgery or radiation therapy is rarely needed for prolactinomas.

## Points to Ponder

- Hyperprolactinemia is common in clinical practice.
- Careful history regarding drug intake is of utmost importance while evaluating a case of hyperprolactinemia.
- Assay interferences due to "hook effect" and "macroprolactin" should be taken into account while interpreting serum prolactin reports.
- *Dopamine agonists*: Cabergoline and bromocriptine are the mainstay of treatment of hyperprolactinemia.

## MULTIPLE CHOICE QUESTIONS

1. **What is the most likely diagnosis in this 20-year-old female with galactorrhea, oligomenorrhea, and elevated serum prolactin levels?**
   A. Hypothyroidism
   B. Polycystic ovary syndrome (PCOS)
   C. Prolactinoma
   D. Pituitary stalk effect
2. **What imaging finding was consistent with the diagnosis of prolactinoma in this patient?**
   A. Large pituitary adenoma
   B. Pituitary microadenoma (6 mm × 7 mm × 9 mm)
   C. Cystic lesion in the ovaries
   D. Enlargement of the thyroid gland
3. **Which of the following treatments was initiated for the diagnosis of prolactinoma in this case?**
   A. Levothyroxine
   B. Cabergoline therapy
   C. Oral contraceptive pills
   D. Insulin therapy
4. **Which of the following conditions is most likely to cause secondary hyperprolactinemia in a patient with normal thyroid function?**
   A. Prolactinoma
   B. Pituitary stalk effect
   C. Hypothyroidism
   D. Polycystic ovary syndrome (PCOS)
5. **What was the outcome after treatment with cabergoline in this patient?**
   A. No improvement in prolactin levels
   B. Complete normalization of prolactin levels and tumor shrinkage
   C. Development of ovarian cysts
   D. Worsening of galactorrhea

### Answers

1. (C); 2. (B); 3. (B); 4. (B); 5. (B)

## SUGGESTED READINGS


1. Atluri S, Sarathi V, Goel A, et al. Etiological profile of galactorrhoea. Indian J Endocrinol Metab. 2018;22(4):489-93.
2. Barbieri RL. Breast [Internet]. Yen & Jaffe's Reproductive Endocrinology: Physiology, Pathophysiology, and Clinical Management: 8th edition. Elsevier Inc; 2019. 248-255.e3 p. Available from: https://doi.org/10.1016/B978-0-323-47912-7.00010-X
3. Huang W, Molitch ME. Evaluation and management of. Am Fam Physician. 2012;85(11):1073-80.
4. Aliberti L, Gagliardi I, Dorizzi RM, et al. Hypeprolactinemia: still an insidious diagnosis. Endocrine [Internet]. 2021;72(3):928-31.
5. Stojkovic M, Radmanovic B, Jovanovic M, et al. Risperidone Induced Hyperprolactinemia: From Basic to Clinical Studies. Front Psychiatry. 2022;13(May):1-9.
6. Auriemma RS, Pirchio R, Pivonello C, et al. Approach to the Patient with Prolactinoma. J Clin Endocrinol Metab [Internet]. 2023;108(9):2400-23.
7. Junqueira DR, Bennett D, Huh SY, et al. Clinical Presentations of Drug-induced Hyperprolactinaemia: A Literature Review. Pharmaceut Med [Internet]. 2023;37(2):153-66.
8. Glezer A, Garmes HM, Kasuki L, et al. Diagnosis of hyperprolactinemia in women: A Position Statement from the Brazilian Federation of Gynecology and Obstetrics Associations (Febrasgo) and the Brazilian Society of Endocrinology and Metabolism (SBEM). Arch Endocrinol Metab. 2024;68:1-9.
9. Fachi MM, de Deus Bueno L, de Oliveira DC, et al. Efficacy and safety in the treatment of hyperprolactinemia: A systematic review and network meta-analysis. J Clin Pharm Ther. 2021;46(6):1549-56.

CHAPTER
15

# A Case-based Approach to Gynecomastia

*Abhay Kumar Sahoo*

## CASE VIGNETTE

A 17-year-old male **(Fig. 1)** was referred from general surgery to our endocrine clinic with bilateral breast enlargement, gradually progressing over the past 1 to 2 years. He reported tenderness but without any nipple discharge, pruritus, or skin changes. He denied any systemic symptoms like recent weight loss, fever, night sweats, or changes in appetite, and had an unremarkable medical history. There was no history of chest trauma. He had not been on any medications and categorically denied the use of anabolic steroids, recreational drugs, or over-the-counter supplements. He reported normal pubertal development and denied any issues with libido or erectile function. There was no family history of breast cancer, endocrine disorders, or similar conditions. Physical examination revealed gynecomastia, more pronounced on the left side. The breast tissue was firm and glandular, subareolar, tender, and mobile, without skin changes or cervical/axillary lymphadenopathy, with a disk diameter of 3 cm bilaterally. Sexual maturity rating (SMR) was B3, A1, P4, and testicular volume 20 mL bilaterally (without masses or tenderness), consistent with tanner stage 4. His vitals were normal and anthropometric parameters were height: 170 cm, weight: 85 kg, BMI: 29.4 kg/m$^2$ (overweight), arm span: 172 cm, upper to lower segment ratio: 0.9. Hormonal profile revealed serum total testosterone: 350 ng/dL (300–1,000), serum estradiol: 45 pg/mL (<20 in males), LH: 5 IU/L (1.24–7.8), FSH: 4 IU/L (1.5–12.4 IU/L), prolactin: 10 ng/mL (2–18). Other biochemistry was ALT: 22 U/L (7–56), AST: 18 U/L (10–40), total bilirubin: 0.8 mg/dL (0.1–1.2), serum creatinine: 0.9 mg/dL (0.7–1.3), TSH: 1.8 μIU/mL (0.4–4.0), FT4: 1.2 ng/dL (0.8–1.7), FT3: 3.2 pg/mL (2.3–4.2), beta-hCG: <1 IU/L (<2), alpha-fetoprotein (AFP): 2 ng/mL (<10). Breast ultrasound revealed bilateral subareolar hypoechoic nodules consistent with glandular tissue without any suspicious masses or calcifications. Radiological workup was previously done by the surgeon, in which testicular ultrasound showed normal echotexture of both testes with no focal lesions or masses. Chest X-ray showed normal cardiac and mediastinal silhouettes, clear lung fields, and no evidence of gynecomastia-related thoracic pathology.

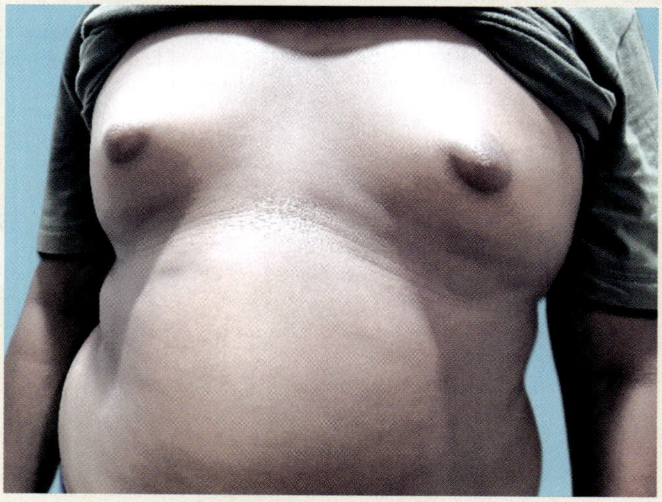

**FIG. 1:** A 17-year-old male with gynecomastia.

## PROVISIONAL DIAGNOSIS

Diagnosis of pubertal gynecomastia was made, parents were reassured, diet/lifestyle modifications were advised for weight loss, and tamoxifen trial was started, with an advice of regular follow-up.

## DIFFERENTIAL DIAGNOSES

- *Physiological gynecomastia*: Commonest cause of gynecomastia. Typically occurring during puberty, this benign condition arises due to transient hormonal fluctuations, primarily an imbalance between estrogen and androgen levels. This condition is self-limiting, generally resolving within six months to two years without intervention.
- *Pathological gynecomastia*:
  - o *Endocrine disorders*:
    - Hyperthyroidism: Excessive thyroid hormone levels can increase sex hormone-binding globulin (SHBG), leading to a relative increase in estrogen.
    - Hypogonadism: Both hypergonadotropic and hypogonadotropic hypogonadism can cause gynecomastia. Conditions like Klinefelter syndrome (47,XXY karyotype) result in decreased androgen production and a relative increase in estrogen activity.
    - Adrenal tumors: These can secrete estrogen or estrogen precursors, disrupting the androgen-estrogen balance.
  - o *Systemic diseases*:
    - Chronic liver disease: Impaired hepatic metabolism of estrogens can lead to increased circulating estrogen levels.
    - Chronic kidney disease: Impaired renal clearance of prolactin and alterations in sex hormone metabolism can contribute to gynecomastia.
  - o *Neoplasms*:
    - Testicular tumors: Germ cell tumors (e.g., seminomas) may secrete beta-hCG, which stimulates estrogen production.
    - Adrenal tumors: Adenomas or carcinomas that secrete estrogen or androgen precursors.
    - Pituitary adenomas: Prolactinomas or tumors secreting gonadotropins can alter the hormonal milieu.
  - o *Drug-induced gynecomastia*:
    - Medications like antiandrogens (e.g., spironolactone), anabolic steroids, certain antipsychotics (e.g., risperidone), and antiulcer drugs (e.g., cimetidine) can interfere with estrogen metabolism or androgen action.
  - o *Genetic conditions*:
    - Androgen insensitivity syndrome: Mutations in the androgen receptor gene lead to a partial or complete inability to respond to androgens, resulting in a higher ratio of estrogenic activity.
- *Pseudogynecomastia*: Characterized by adipose tissue accumulation in the breast region without glandular proliferation, often associated with obesity. Differentiation from true gynecomastia is achieved through clinical examination and imaging modalities such as ultrasonography.

## CLINICAL APPROACH

- *Detailed history*: Comprehensive history focusing on the onset, duration, and progression of breast enlargement. Inquire about systemic symptoms, past medical history, drug usage, family history of endocrine or breast disorders, and lifestyle factors including substance use.
- *Physical examination*:
  - o Thorough breast examination to evaluate tissue characteristics (firmness, tenderness, disk diameter) and distinguish between glandular and adipose tissue.
  - o Assessment of secondary sexual characteristics and genital examination to determine testicular volume using an orchidometer and detect signs of hypogonadism.
  - o Anthropometric measurements including BMI, arm span, and upper to lower segment ratio.
- *Laboratory investigations*:
  - o *Hormonal profile:* Quantification of serum testosterone, estradiol, luteinizing hormone (LH), follicle-stimulating hormone (FSH), and prolactin to evaluate endocrine function and identify hormonal imbalances.
  - o *Liver and renal function tests:* Assessment of hepatic and renal function to rule out systemic causes of gynecomastia.
  - o *Thyroid function tests:* Measurement of thyroid-stimulating hormone (TSH) and free thyroid hormones to exclude thyroid dysfunction (primary or secondary).
  - o *Tumor markers:* Measurement of beta-hCG and alpha-fetoprotein (AFP) to screen for neoplastic etiologies, particularly testicular and germ cell tumors.
- *Imaging studies*:
  - o *Breast ultrasound:* To differentiate glandular from fatty tissue and detect any suspicious masses or architectural distortions indicative of malignancy.
  - o *Testicular ultrasound:* To exclude testicular tumors or other abnormalities.
  - o *Chest X-ray:* To rule out thoracic pathology and assess for mediastinal masses that might secrete hormones.

## PATHOPHYSIOLOGY

Gynecomastia occurs when there is an imbalance between estrogen and testosterone levels, leading to increased estrogenic activity in the breast tissue. This results in the proliferation of glandular tissue, causing breast enlargement. It can be triggered by physiological changes (puberty, aging), certain medications (e.g., antiandrogens, spironolactone), or underlying conditions (e.g., liver disease, hypogonadism) that alter hormone levels.

## TREATMENT AND PREVENTION

- *Reassurance and monitoring:* Most cases of physiological gynecomastia resolve spontaneously. Patients should be reassured of the benign nature of the condition and monitored periodically to assess for resolution or progression.

- *Addressing underlying causes:* Discontinuation or substitution of causative medications should be considered. Management of underlying systemic or endocrine disorders should be initiated to address the root cause of gynecomastia.
- *Medical management:*
  - *Selective estrogen receptor modulators (SERMs):* Tamoxifen (10–20 mg daily) or raloxifene (60 mg daily) can be effective in reducing breast size and alleviating tenderness in persistent gynecomastia.
  - *Aromatase inhibitors:* Anastrozole may be used in cases with elevated estrogen levels, although their efficacy is less established compared to SERMs.
  - *Androgens:* Testosterone replacement therapy is indicated in cases of hypogonadism to normalize androgen levels and counteract estrogen effects.
- *Surgical management:* Indicated for long-standing gynecomastia, significant psychological distress, or when medical treatment is ineffective. Surgical options include liposuction and subcutaneous mastectomy, tailored to the severity and tissue composition of the gynecomastia.

### Points to Ponder

- *Accurate diagnosis is the key:* Differentiating physiological from pathological gynecomastia is critical to avoid unnecessary investigations and interventions. A thorough clinical and laboratory evaluation is essential.
- *Role of endocrinologist:* The involvement of endocrinologists, apart from surgeons, can optimize diagnosis and management, particularly in complex or persistent cases of gynecomastia.
- *Patient education:* Educating patients and their families about the natural course of gynecomastia, potential causes, and treatment options is crucial for ensuring adherence to management plans and setting realistic expectations for outcomes.
- *Psychosocial impact:* Gynecomastia can lead to significant psychosocial distress, particularly in adolescent males, affecting self-esteem and social interactions. Holistic care should be offered addressing all domains, including psychological aspects.

## MULTIPLE CHOICE QUESTIONS

1. **What is the most likely diagnosis for the 17-year-old male with bilateral breast enlargement, firm glandular tissue, and normal pubertal development?**
   A. Gynecomastia
   B. Breast cancer
   C. Hormonal imbalance due to thyroid dysfunction
   D. Testicular tumor
2. **Which of the following findings is consistent with the diagnosis of gynecomastia in this patient?**
   A. Nipple discharge and skin changes
   B. Firm, glandular, tender, mobile breast tissue without skin changes
   C. Abnormal testicular volume and tenderness
   D. Positive family history of breast cancer
3. **The hormonal profile of this patient reveals an elevated level of which hormone that may contribute to gynecomastia?**
   A. Total testosterone
   B. Estradiol
   C. Prolactin
   D. LH
4. **Given the normal testicular ultrasound and absence of systemic symptoms, what is the most appropriate next step in management for this patient?**
   A. Start hormonal therapy with antiestrogens
   B. Perform genetic testing for Klinefelter syndrome
   C. Observe with regular follow-up and monitor breast changes
   D. Refer for breast biopsy
5. **Which of the following is an expected finding in this patient's sexual maturity rating (SMR)?**
   A. SMR B5, A5, P5
   B. SMR B3, A1, P4
   C. SMR B2, A2, P3
   D. SMR B4, A3, P4

### Answers

1. (A); 2. (B); 3. (B); 4. (C); 5. (B)

## SUGGESTED READINGS


1. Shirwaikar A, Shirwaikar A. Gynaecomastia: A Review of Pathophysiology and Management. J Clin Endocr. 2019;102(4):213-21.
2. Cohen SA, Speiser PW. Gynecomastia in Endocrine Disorders: Mechanisms and Management. Endocrinol Metab Clin North Am. 2018;47(2):235-46.
3. Sato T, Hirose T. Estrogen-related Mechanisms in Gynaecomastia: Insights from Hormonal Imbalance. J Reprod Med. 2020;44(5):509-15.
4. Rajasekaran M, Balamurugan A. The Role of Surgery in Severe Gynaecomastia. Plast Reconstr Surg. 2021;147(1):37-45.
5. Mazzola J, Fitzgerald B. Diagnosis and Treatment of Gynaecomastia: A Comprehensive Review. Surg Clin North Am. 2017;97(3):675-88.
6. Araujo AB, Wittert GA. Androgen Deficiency and its Role in Gynaecomastia in Older Men. J Androl. 2019;40(3):223-30.
7. Brown MD, Pearson J. Endocrine Causes of Gynaecomastia: A Diagnostic Approach. Clin Endocrinol. 2018;89(2):206-12.
8. Sener S, Ozdiler E. Hormonal Imbalance in Gynaecomastia: Pathogenesis and Management Approaches. J Clin Med. 2020;9(6):1657.

CHAPTER 16

# An Approach to the Case of Pituitary Apoplexy

*Sumit Chakrabarti*

**CASE VIGNETTE**

A 39-year-old homemaker from a remote village in West Bengal presents with anorexia, fatigue, and asthenia for the last 3–4 years. She is pale, with no history of overt blood loss, fever, or jaundice. She received a blood transfusion during her last childbirth 6 years ago, followed by lactation failure and delayed, scanty menstruation. She has been amenorrheic for the past couple of years and has no history of headaches or visual disturbances. On examination, she has mild pallor, normal vitals, no edema, and mild splenomegaly.

Laboratory tests show Hb 7.5 g% with microcytic hypochromic cells, mild hyponatremia (Na 128), and normal WBC and platelet counts. Her cortisol level is low at 2.9 mcg/dL, with low ACTH (10.9 pg/mL). TSH, total T4, prolactin, LH, and FSH are within range. MRI reveals a partial empty sella with normal posterior pituitary bright spots. The patient's symptoms, including reduced axillary and pubic hair, suggest a possible pituitary dysfunction.

## PROVISIONAL DIAGNOSIS

A diagnosis of Sheehan's syndrome subsequent to pituitary apoplexy, likely due to peripartum hemorrhage, leading to empty sella was made.

## DIFFERENTIAL DIAGNOSIS

- *Cerebrovascular accident*: Intracerebral or subarachnoid hemorrhage
- Acute encephalitis syndrome
- Lymphocytic hypophysitis
- Acute adrenal insufficiency
- Complicated migraine

## CLINICAL APPROACH

Diagnosis of pituitary apoplexy can be challenging due to nonspecific symptoms, requiring a high index of suspicion. Apoplexy occurs from hemorrhage or infarction of the pituitary gland, often within an adenoma when its growth exceeds the blood supply. Postpartum hemorrhage, especially in pregnancy when the pituitary enlarges, can lead to apoplexy, resulting in Sheehan's syndrome, but significant hemorrhage may not always be apparent.

Typical symptoms include severe headache, vomiting, visual disturbances, and loss of consciousness, though not all are present. Risk factors for pituitary apoplexy include systemic hypertension, diabetes, major surgery, head injury, coagulopathy, and conditions such as dengue, snake bites, and sickle cell anemia. The pituitary gland's rich vascular supply makes anterior pituitary hormone deficiency the primary feature after vascular damage, while posterior pituitary is usually spared or transiently affected, leading to temporary diabetes insipidus.

Growth hormone deficiency presents with nonspecific signs such as wrinkling of skin and subtle personality changes. Cortisol deficiency is more acute and manifests with hypotension, poor appetite, weight loss, hyponatremia, hyperkalemia, and hypoglycemia. Low ACTH in pituitary apoplexy contrasts with Addison's disease, where high ACTH causes skin pigmentation. Reduced DHEAS from low ACTH can lead to loss of axillary and pubic hair, a key diagnostic clue.

Thyroid hormone deficiency results in secondary hypothyroidism with nonspecific symptoms such as fatigue, constipation, and dry skin. Loss of lactotroph cells can cause lactation failure, particularly in postpartum women, pointing to Sheehan's syndrome. In women, gonadotroph loss leads to secondary hypogonadism, causing menstrual irregularities, amenorrhea, and menopausal symptoms. In men, secondary hypogonadism manifests as low testosterone, reduced libido, and erectile dysfunction.

## PATHOPHYSIOLOGY

The patient's symptoms suggest pituitary dysfunction, likely due to partial pituitary insufficiency following postpartum hemorrhage, which may have led to Sheehan's syndrome (pituitary apoplexy). The hypopituitarism seen in this case is characterized by low cortisol and ACTH levels, indicating adrenal insufficiency. This can occur due to damage to the corticotroph cells in the anterior pituitary. Additionally, the patient's low LH and FSH levels suggest secondary hypogonadism, which is common in pituitary disorders. The presence of partial empty sella on MRI further supports the diagnosis of pituitary insufficiency, where damage to the pituitary gland reduces its size and function.

## TREATMENT AND PREVENTION

Management principles include initial supportive measures to maintain homeostasis, followed by pituitary hormone replacement as needed. Surgical intervention, such as transsphenoidal decompression, may be considered in cases with visual deficits or prolonged unconsciousness.

For patients with hypotension or hypovolemic shock, rapid infusion of isotonic saline is crucial, and blood transfusion may be necessary in cases of blood loss or postpartum hemorrhage. Investigations, including routine lab tests, hormonal evaluation, and pituitary imaging (CT or MRI), should be completed promptly.

Cortisol replacement is the first priority, starting with hydrocortisone IV (100 mg stat, followed by 50–100 mg thrice daily). After stabilization, oral hydrocortisone (25–30 mg/day) or prednisolone (5–10 mg/day) can be used. Thyroid replacement with L-thyroxine (1.6–1.8 mcg/kg/day) is initiated if secondary hypothyroidism is present, but cortisol replacement should be prioritized if both adrenal and thyroid axes are deficient.

Monitoring involves serum free or total T4 levels, keeping them within the mid-normal range, as TSH measurement can be misleading. In women, combined oral contraceptive pills (COCPs) are used to manage secondary hypogonadism and reestablish menstruation. For men, testosterone replacement is recommended, with monitoring of hemoglobin and prostate-specific antigen (PSA). DHEAS can be used to address loss of libido.

### Points to Ponder

- Pituitary apoplexy has become rarer in the present era, a good history and detailed examination in an appropriate setting may provide clue to the clinician.
- Baseline investigation and neuroimaging are to be done first.
- Endocrine evaluation, especially cortisol status is to be evaluated at the earliest.
- Cortisol replacement is lifesaving, should be started on strong clinical suspicion after sending baseline blood samples, if deferred for lab reports for confirmation, may prove to be fatal. Cortisol replacement should be started first, L-thyroxine to be started simultaneously or after cortisol is initiated.
- A conservative approach is commonly preferred. Transsphenoidal decompression of pituitary may be opted where vision is threatened and/or prolonged unconsciousness is observed.

## MULTIPLE CHOICE QUESTIONS

**1. What is the most likely diagnosis in a patient presenting with anorexia, fatigue, and amenorrhea following postpartum hemorrhage?**

A. Hyperthyroidism
B. Sheehan's syndrome
C. Polycystic ovary syndrome
D. Cushing's disease

**2. Which of the following findings is most indicative of secondary hypogonadism in a patient with pituitary insufficiency?**

A. High levels of LH and FSH
B. Low levels of LH and FSH
C. Elevated testosterone levels
D. Increased estradiol levels

**3. What is the most likely cause of the patient's low cortisol and ACTH levels?**

A. Primary adrenal insufficiency
B. Pituitary dysfunction
C. Excessive cortisol secretion
D. Hypothalamic disorder

**4. Which imaging finding is consistent with pituitary insufficiency in this patient?**

A. Brain metastasis
B. Partial empty sella
C. Brain hemorrhage
D. Pituitary adenoma

**5. Which of the following is the most appropriate next step in management for a patient with suspected Sheehan's syndrome?**

A. Initiate thyroid hormone replacement
B. Start cortisol replacement therapy
C. Prescribe oral contraceptives
D. Administer insulin therapy

### Answers

1. (B); 2. (B); 3. (B); 4. (B); 5. (B)

## SUGGESTED READINGS


1. Sheehan HL. Postpartum necrosis of the anterior pituitary. J Pathol Bacteriol. 1937;45(1):189-214.
2. Grossman A, Besser GM. Hypopituitarism and its causes. The Lancet. 2009;374(9697):1447-55.
3. Al-Huniti N, Dabeer S. Sheehan's syndrome: A review of the clinical features, diagnosis, and management. Endocrine Practice. 2014;20(4):376-83.
4. Gurnell M, Ezzat S. Pituitary apoplexy: Clinical features and management. Clinical Endocrinology. 2002;57(1):129-33.
5. Fleseriu M, Findling JW. Management of pituitary apoplexy: Challenges and advances. Endocrine Reviews. 2013;34(5):1-18.
6. Ghosh A, Maheshwari A. Pituitary hormone deficiencies following Sheehan's syndrome: A systematic review of diagnosis and management. JCEM. 2018;103(11):4042-50.

CHAPTER 17

# An Approach to a Case of Late-onset Hypogonadism

*Abhishek Shrivastava*

**CASE VIGNETTE**

Mr X was a 52-year-old male nonsmoker with a medical history of hypertension and type 2 diabetes. He had no prior history of hypogonadism or other endocrine disorders. Mr X reported a significant decrease in sexual desire over the past year, indicating decreased libido. He had also experienced difficulty achieving and maintaining erections sufficient for sexual intercourse, indicative of erectile dysfunction. Additionally, Mr X complained of persistent tiredness and lack of energy despite adequate sleep, suggesting fatigue. He had emotions of sadness, irritability, and diminished interest in daily activities, which were symptoms of depression. Despite regular physical activity, he had noticed a reduction in muscle strength and mass.

## PROVISIONAL DIAGNOSIS

Late-onset hypogonadism.

## DIAGNOSTIC DIAGNOSIS

### Laboratory Tests

Mr X's serum total testosterone level is 250 ng/dL, which was low (normal range: 300–1,000 ng/dL). His free testosterone level is 4 pg/mL, also low (normal range: 9–30 pg/mL). LH ("luteinizing hormone") and FSH ("follicle-stimulating hormone") levels were within normal ranges at 4.0 IU/L and 5.5 IU/L, respectively. His prolactin level was 10 ng/mL (normal range: 4–15 ng/mL).

## CLINICAL APPROACH

On general physical examination, Mr X appears well-nourished and in no acute distress. His vital parameters were: blood pressure—140/85 mm Hg, heart rate—78 beats/min, and his BMI—28. Specific signs include mild bilateral enlargement of breast tissue, indicative of gynecomastia, and a slight reduction in bilateral testicular volume, suggestive of testicular atrophy.

### Imaging Studies

A testicular ultrasound showed normal size and echotexture, with no masses or lesions detected. An MRI of the pituitary gland revealed normal findings, with no adenomas or abnormalities present.

### Additional Evaluations

A bone mineral density (DEXA) scan revealed a T-score of –1.5, indicating osteopenia. Given his existing hypertension and diabetes, Mr X's cardiovascular risk assessment indicates an elevated risk.

## TREATMENT AND PREVENTION

### Lifestyle Modifications

Mr X was advised to adopt lifestyle modifications to improve his overall health and manage his symptoms. To meet his nutritional demands, he was started on diet full of fruits, vegetables, and lean proteins. Regular physical activity was recommended, focusing on both aerobic and resistance training to enhance muscle mass and overall fitness. Aiming for a gradual reduction in BMI to below 25 is crucial for better health outcomes, particularly in managing his diabetes and hypertension.

### Pharmacological Treatment

Mr X was initiated on testosterone replacement therapy (TRT) to address his symptomatic testosterone deficiency. The chosen type of TRT was testosterone gel, applied daily as per the prescribed dosage. Indications for TRT include his low serum and free testosterone levels combined with his presenting symptoms. There were no contraindications present in his case. Regular monitoring and follow-up were essential, with evaluations of testosterone levels, hematocrit, and prostate-specific antigen (PSA) conducted every 3 months to ensure efficacy and safety of the treatment.

The case of Mr X illustrate the clinical presentation and management of late-onset hypogonadism (LOH) in older males. Imaging studies did not reveal any abnormalities **(Table 1)**.

## PATHOPHYSIOLOGY

Testosterone deficiency is due to impaired hypothalamic–pituitary–gonadal (HPG) axis function. In conditions like type 2 diabetes and hypertension, chronic inflammation, oxidative stress, and vascular dysfunction can disrupt gonadotropin release (LH/FSH), leading to reduced testosterone synthesis by the testes. Low testosterone levels contribute to decreased libido, erectile dysfunction, fatigue, muscle loss, and mood disturbances, creating a multifactorial impact on his physical and psychological health.

**TABLE 1: Patients with late-onset hypogonadism.**

| Feature | MR X |
|---|---|
| Age | 52 years |
| History of smoking | No |
| Medical history | Hypertension, type 2 diabetes |
| History of hypogonadism | No |
| Decreased libido | Yes |
| Erectile dysfunction | Yes |
| Fatigue | Yes |
| Depression/Emotional symptoms | Sadness, irritability, loss of interest |
| Decreased muscle strength | Yes |
| Physical examination findings | Well-nourished, BP—140/85 mm Hg, HR—78 bpm, BMI—28, mild bilateral gynecomastia, slight testicular atrophy |
| Serum total testosterone level | 250 ng/dL |
| Free testosterone level | 4 pg/mL |
| Additional evaluations | DEXA T-score: –1.5 (osteopenia), elevated cardiovascular risk |
| Treatment | Lifestyle modifications, TRT with testosterone gel |

## Points to Ponder

- The patient's symptoms may suggest late-onset hypogonadism linked to chronic conditions like diabetes and hypertension.
- Testosterone replacement therapy could address both physical and psychological manifestations.
- Studies indicate that LOH is a common condition affecting 2–5% of men over 40, with prevalence increasing with age.
- The EMAS (European Male Aging Study) found that approximately 30% of men aged 70 and above exhibit testosterone deficiency.
- The HIM (Hypogonadism in Males) study highlighted the prevalence of low testosterone in men with chronic conditions like diabetes and COPD, corroborating the findings in these cases.

## MULTIPLE CHOICE QUESTIONS

1. **Which of the following symptoms in Mr X is most indicative of testosterone deficiency?**
   A. Persistent tiredness and fatigue
   B. Difficulty maintaining erections
   C. Decreased libido
   D. Reduction in muscle strength and mass
2. **What is the most likely contributing factor to Mr X's erectile dysfunction given his medical history?**
   A. Hypogonadism
   B. Hypertension and diabetes
   C. Lack of physical activity
   D. Nonsmoking status
3. **Which diagnostic test is most appropriate to evaluate suspected testosterone deficiency in Mr X?**
   A. Fasting blood glucose
   B. Serum testosterone levels
   C. Complete blood count (CBC)
   D. Electrocardiogram (ECG)
4. **What is the first-line treatment for testosterone deficiency in a patient like Mr X with persistent symptoms and confirmed low testosterone levels?**
   A. Antidepressants
   B. Phosphodiesterase-5 inhibitors
   C. Testosterone replacement therapy
   D. Psychotherapy
5. **Which lifestyle modification would most likely benefit Mr X in managing his symptoms?**
   A. Smoking cessation
   B. Increased physical activity
   C. Low-sodium diet
   D. High-carbohydrate diet

### Answers

1. (C); 2. (B); 3. (B); 4. (C); 5. (B)

## SUGGESTED READINGS


1. Banov D, Biundo B, Ip K, et al. Testosterone Therapy for Late-Onset Hypogonadism: A Clinical, Biological, and Analytical Approach Using Compounded Testosterone 0.5-20% Topical Gels. Pharmaceutics. 2024;16(5):621.
2. Harman SM, Metter EJ, Tobin JD, et al. Longitudinal effects of aging on serum total and free testosterone levels in healthy men. Baltimore Longitudinal Study of Aging. J Clin Endocrinol Metab. 2001;86(2):724-31.
3. Lee DM, O'Neill TW, Pye SR, et al.; EMAS study group. The European Male Ageing Study (EMAS): design, methods and recruitment. Int J Androl. 2009;32(1):11-24.
4. Mulligan T, Frick MF, Zuraw QC, et al. Prevalence of hypogonadism in males aged at least 45 years: the HIM study. Int J Clin Pract. 2006;60(7):762-9.
5. Park JY, Seok JH, Cho KS, et al. Association of salivary testosterone levels during the post-awakening period with age and symptoms suggestive of late-onset hypogonadism in men. Ann Med. 2024;56(1):2356667.

CHAPTER

18

# An Approach to a Case of Nondiabetic Hypoglycemia

*Boudhayan Das Munshi, Azifa Taj Nazer, Shounak Basak, Saikat Mondal, Mahesh Ravikumar Jansari, Jayeeta Bhowmick*

## CASE VIGNETTE

A 55-year-old lady presented to the emergency department with complaints of recurrent episodes of giddiness, anxiety, palpitations and sweating. Capillary blood glucose (CBG) was found to be 47 mg/dL. She suffered from primary hypertension for the last five years for which she received telmisartan and amlodipine and primary hypothyroidism for last three years for which she received L-thyroxine 25 mcg once daily. Her vitals were found to be stable on admission. However, she continued to have recurrence of symptoms every few hours since admission and CBG was always found to show a value < 60 mg/dL. She was worked up extensively. Complete blood count, renal function tests, liver function tests, thyroid profile, fasting lipid profile were within normal limits. Triple serology was nonreactive. 8 AM serum cortisol, ACTH was normal. During one such episode of hypoglycemia when CBG was 37 mg/dL, blood for paired serum insulin and C-peptide was collected and analyzed.

Serum Insulin (330 µ IU/L) and fasting C-peptide (13.30 ng/mL) were found to be elevated. Polyethylene glycol (PEG) precipitation test was performed with another critical sample of blood when capillary blood glucose was 55 mg/dL. The **Table 1** shows a significant reduction in both insulin and C-peptide levels after PEG treatment, indicating decreased endogenous insulin secretion for a case with a CBG of 55 mg/dL.

Insulin autoantibodies was elevated [>3,000 µU/mL (N = 2.70 –24.80 µU/mL)].

Contrast enhanced CT scan of the abdomen revealed no pancreatic abnormality.

Sulphonylurea screen was negative. Beta-hydroxybutyrate could not be done.

She was initially treated with dextrose infusion followed by oral glucose. Subsequently after the initial reports of serum insulin and C-peptide she was started on uncooked cornstarch and diazoxide. The frequency of hypoglycemic episodes reduced. She was discharged after 2 weeks. On follow-up she had very few instances of hypoglycemia for which the diazoxide dose was increased and her hypoglycemic symptoms subsided with no recorded capillary blood glucose below 70 mg/dL.

**TABLE 1: Endogenous insulin secretion.**

| Parameter (for CBG = 55 mg/dL) | Pre-PEG | Post-PEG |
|---|---|---|
| Insulin (mIU/L) | 260.04 | 10.43 |
| C-peptide (ng/mL) | 11.22 | 3.18 |

## PROVISIONAL DIAGNOSIS

### Nondiabetic Hypoglycemia – Insulin Autoimmune Syndrome – Type 1 (Hirata's Disease)

This lady satisfied Whipple's criteria for hypoglycemia:

- Symptoms consistent with hypoglycemia.
- Low plasma glucose concentration.
- Relief of symptoms with correction of hypoglycemia.

During the episode of hypoglycemia, the critical sample plasma glucose was low with elevated fasting insulin and C-peptide. Beta-hydroxybutyrate was not done. Hormonal evaluation was unremarkable and noncontributory. Sulphonyl urea screen was negative. Abdominal imaging did not pick up any abnormality. Although an insulinoma could be missed during routine abdominal imaging however nuclear medicine imaging of the pancreas is expensive and is not routinely available. So, it's a preferable to proceed with polyethylene glycol (PEG) precipitation and assessment of insulin autoantibodies. Post-PEG precipitation decrease in insulin measured from the supernatant was suggestive of the insulin autoantibody syndrome. Elevated insulin autoantibodies was confirmed the diagnosis of insulin autoimmune syndrome.

## DIFFERENTIAL DIAGNOSIS

- *Artifactual hypoglycemia (without symptoms)*:
  - Reticulocytosis (polycythemia, sickle cell anemia)
  - Leucocytosis (leukemia)
  - Thrombocytosis
- *Fasting hypoglycemia (>5 hours from the last meal)*: The **Table 2** below compares different causes of hypoglycemia based on hormonal and metabolic responses.

TABLE 2: Different causes of hypoglycemia based on hormonal and metabolic responses.

| High insulin, low beta hydroxy butyrate, high glucagon response | Low insulin, high beta hydroxy butyrate, low glucagon response |
|---|---|
| Insulinoma | Ketotic hypoglycemia |
| Autoimmune syndrome (antibodies to insulin or the insulin receptor) | Prolonged exercise |
| Factitial due to exogenous insulin | Alcohol induced |
| Factitial due to insulin secretagogues | Glycogen storage diseases |
| Induced by nondiabetic medications | Isolated GH or cortisol deficiency |
| Noninsulinoma pancreatogenous hypoglycemia syndrome | |

- *Postprandial hypoglycemia (within 5 hours from the last meal)*:
    - Postbariatric surgery
    - Nesidioblastosis
    - Hereditary fructose intolerance
- *Associated with other disorder*:
    - Critical illness (liver failure, congestive heart failure, sepsis, renal failure)
    - Malnutrition
    - Adrenal insufficiency
    - Nonislet cell tumors

## Insulin Autoantibody Syndrome

- It is a cause of nondiabetic hypoglycemia. It is an uncommon cause of nondiabetic hypoglycemia characterized by high concentrations of insulin autoantibodies.
- It is of two types: (i) Hirata's disease (insulin autoantibody syndrome); and (ii) Anti-insulin receptor antibodies (Type B insulin resistance).
- The prognosis usually good with self-remission reported in majority of patients.
- Details of pathogenesis noted under pathophysiology section.

## Type B Insulin Resistance

- It occurs predominantly in middle-aged women of the Black race with obesity, hyperandrogenism and acanthosis nigricans.
- It is caused by anti-insulin receptor antibodies.
- The autoantibodies are partial agonists for the insulin receptor.

## Insulinoma

- Insulinomas are neuroendocrine insulin producing tumors.
- Extremely rare (1–4 new cases per million people/year).
- 4% are associated with multiple endocrine neoplasia type 1 (MEN-1)
- <10% are malignant.
- 10% are multiple.
- Slightly more common in females.
- Present usually in the fifth decade of life.
- Hypoglycemia—fasting/postexercise/postprandial.
- Biochemical testing—72 hours fasting test
- Diagnosis is made by hyperinsulinemic hypoglycemia, negative screening for oral hypoglycemic agents, negative insulin autoantibody testing.
- Imaging—transabdominal and endoscopic ultrasonography, CT scan abdomen, MRI abdomen.
- Negative imaging does not rule out the diagnosis.
- Selective arterial calcium stimulation with hepatic venous sampling—it is done if noninvasive imaging does not rule out the diagnosis. A $\geq$ 2-fold increase in insulin concentrations from baseline localizes the site of an insulinoma with a >90% sensitivity.

## Addison's Disease

- Primary adrenal insufficiency characterized by glucocorticoid deficiency with or without mineralocorticoid deficiency.
- In the western countries, autoimmune damage to the adrenal cortex by 21-hydroxylase antibodies.
- Hypoglycemia is rare in such scenarios. It is due to cortisol deficiency that interferes with counter-regulatory response during times of stress.
- The diagnosis is to be considered in a hypoglycemic patient with hyperpigmentation, hyponatremia, hyperkalemia and acidosis.

## Critical Illness-associated Hypoglycemia

- Occurs in sepsis, acute liver failure, congestive cardiac failure, end stage renal disease.
- It occurs due to impaired gluconeogenesis, increased peripheral glucose utilization and depletion of hepatic glycogen stores.

## Nonislet Cell Tumors

- Rare mesenchymal or epithelial tumors that can be benign or malignant.
- Clinically apparent and large usually (>10 cm)
- Hypoglycemia results from increased production of incompletely processed IGF-2.
- IGF-2 structurally mimics insulin. High levels can bind to insulin receptor and mimic the action of insulin.
- Serum insulin and C-peptide are, however, not elevated during the episode of hypoglycemia.

## Drugs Causing Hypoglycemia

- Drugs stimulating insulin secretion—quinolones, nonsteroidal anti-inflammatory drugs, antipsychotics, alpha- and beta-blockers.
- Transient hypoglycemia induced by cytolytic insulin release—pentamidine

## Ketotic Hypoglycemia

- It occurs during fasting/starvation/alcohol intake.
- Increase in plasma ketones occur during attempts at weight loss by prolonged adherence to ketogenic diet severely restricts carbohydrate intake to 20–50 g/day.
- Reduction in hepatic glucose production by hyperketonemia, which outweighs the diminished glucose utilization.

## Nesidioblastosis

- Postprandial hypoglycemia.
- Beta-cell hypertrophy, islet cell hyperplasia, increase in beta-cell mass.

- It should be considered as a diagnosis in a patient of hypoglycemia with a negative 72 hours fast, positive mixed meal test, no history of GI surgery and negative imaging for insulinoma.
- Selective arterial calcium stimulation will show diffuse insulin secretion.

## CLINICAL APPROACH

History taking, clinical examination, laboratory workup and imaging studies form the pillars for diagnosis of the causes of nondiabetic hypoglycemia.

1. Whipple's triad is used for confirmation of possible hypoglycemia:
   a. Symptoms of hypoglycemia
   b. Documented low blood glucose ( < 55 mg/dL)
   c. Improvement of symptoms of hypoglycemia on correction of low blood glucose.
2. At the very outset, it should be determined whether the patient has any end organ failure or hormonal contributory causes for hypoglycemia. If not, then it should be ascertained from history and laboratory follow-up whether the hypoglycemia is fasting or postprandial in nature. Fasting hypoglycemia occurs > 5 hours after the last meal intake while postprandial hypoglycemia occurs within 5 hours of intake of the last meal.

Factitial hypoglycemia is more likely to be found in (i) healthcare workers who are aware of adverse effects of drugs (ii) relatives of people living with diabetes mellitus in the same household (iii) those with mental illness, e.g., major depression.

The algorithm for nondiabetic hypoglycemia is explained below in **Flowchart 1**.

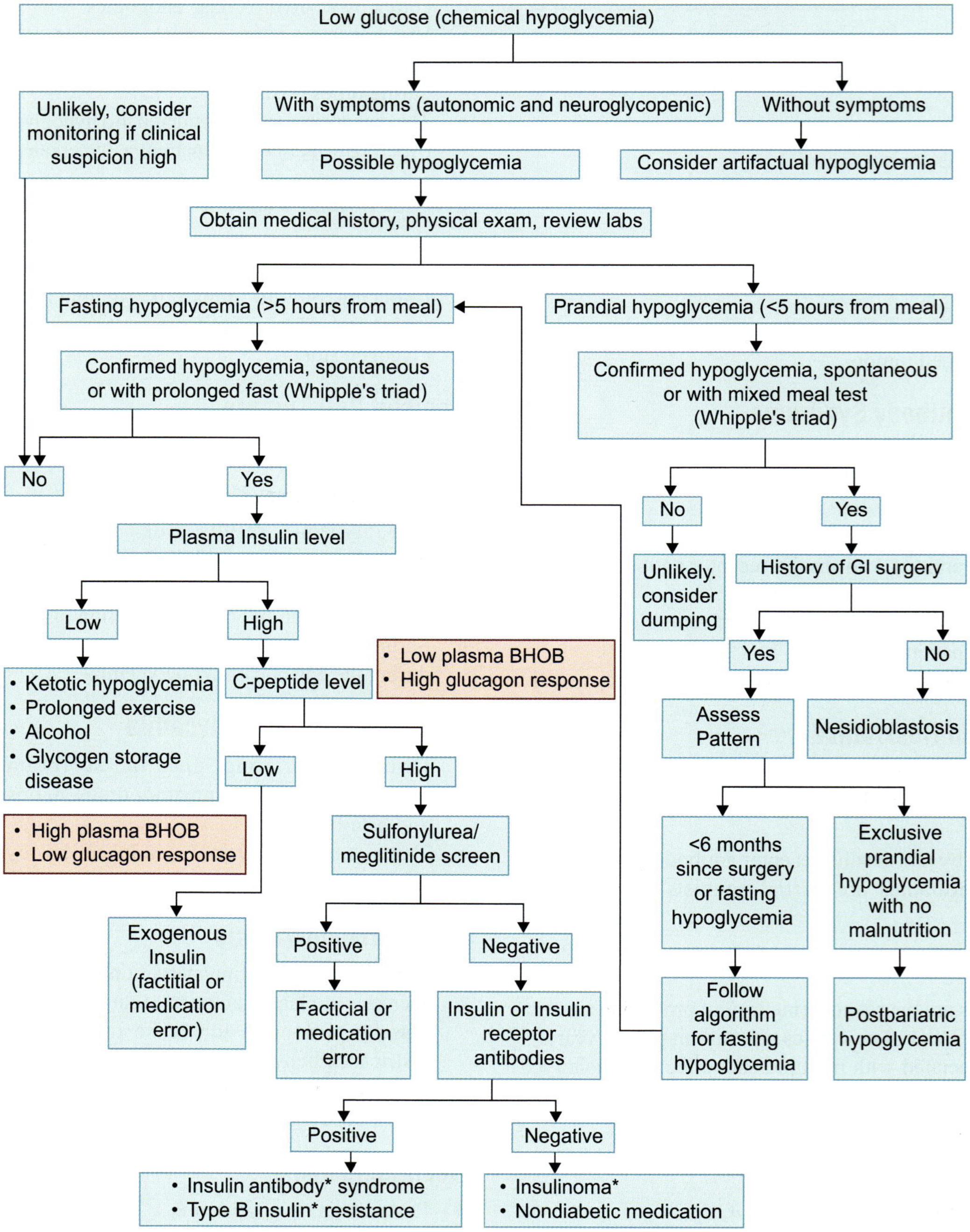


*May also present as prandial hypoglycemia.

**FLOWCHART 1:** Diagnostic algorithm for nondiabetic hypoglycemia.

**BOX 1: Laboratory parameter.**

- Serum insulin
- Serum C-peptide
- Plasma beta hydroxybutyrate
- Insulin autoantibodies
- Hormonal evaluation: TSH, free T4, T3, 8 AM serum cortisol, ACTH

Polyethylene glycol (PEG) precipitation test of insulin

The algorithm mentions the testing of several laboratory parameters. Some of them are listed in the below **Box 1**.

### Polyethylene Glycol Precipitation

The procedure for PEG precipitation involves the following steps:

1. Mix 20 µL of patient serum with an equal volume of 25% PEG 6,000 solution in 40 µM phosphate buffer.
2. Vortex the mixture for 10 seconds
3. Let the mixture stand in crushed ice for 5 minutes
4. Centrifuge the sample at 10,000 g for 2 minutes
5. Use the supernatant for an insulin assay

Following PEG precipitation, insulin assay in the supernatant if found to be decreased would be suggestive of the presence of insulin autoantibodies.

## PATHOPHYSIOLOGY

### Insulin Autoimmune Syndrome

Autoimmune syndromes are of two major types:

1. *Hirata's disease*: Antibodies directed against insulin.
2. *Flier's disease*: Antibodies directed against insulin receptor. It is also referred to as Type B insulin resistance.

Insulin autoantibodies (IAAs) are predominantly immunoglobulins (Ig) directed against endogenously released insulin in response to nutrient ingestion with a high binding capacity but low affinity to insulin. Patients may manifest hyperglycemia in the early absorptive phase of meal or oral glucose intake, when exogenous glucose appearance into circulation is maximal, followed by hypoglycemia in a few hours during the late prandial condition or postabsorptive state. Hypoglycemia is caused by the binding and release of insulin from the antigen-antibody complex independently of changes in glucose concentrations. So biochemically insulin and C-peptide are both elevated at the time of hypoglycemia. Insulin antibodies against exogenous insulin do not cause hypoglycemia as they are low binding and high affinity.

It may be associated with:

- Autoimmune (SLE, rheumatoid arthritis), hematological diseases (multiple myeloma, monoclonal gammopathy of undetermined significance)
- *Triggering factors*:
  - Medications: Drugs with sulfhydryl containing groups —methimazole, captopril, propylthiouracil, penicillin G.
  - Viral infections: Measles, mumps, rubella, varicella zoster, Coxsackie B, hepatitis C

## TREATMENT AND PREVENTION

### Insulin Autoimmune Syndrome

Prognosis of IAS is very good with self-remission in majority of the cases.

Treatment includes:

- *Dietary modification*:
  - Small frequent low carbohydrate meals
  - Uncooked cornstarch
- *Medications to decrease insulin secretion*:
  - Diazoxide
  - Somatostatin analogues like octreotide
- *Immunosuppressants*:
  - High dose corticosteroids
  - Azathioprine
  - Rituximab
- *Plasmapheresis*:
  - Treatment of associated hematological or immunological causes.
  - Avoidance of precipitating factors may help in prevention of IAS.

### Insulinoma

- Surgical enucleation of the tumor—open surgery preferred over laparoscopic.
- Pancreatectomy—distal or central depending on the location of the tumor. Indications includes:
  - Large tumor
  - Concern for malignancy or metastasis
- Inoperable causes are managed by medical management.
  - Drugs—diazoxide, streptozocin, verapamil, phenytoin, corticosteroids.
- *Nonsurgical*:
  - CT guided radiofrequency ablation
  - USG guided ablation with ethanol
  - Peptide receptor radionuclide therapy
- Robotic radiosurgery

### Addison's Disease

- Intravascular volume replacement
- Hydrocortisone—intravenous
- Identification and management of the precipitating cause—infection, hemorrhage.

### Nonislet Cell Tumors

- Surgery
- Chemotherapy
- Radiotherapy
- Medical therapy with glucocorticoids, GH or octreotide.

### Nesidioblastosis

- Low carbohydrate frequent meals
- Drugs—diazoxide, acarbose, verapamil, octreotide
- Refractory—partial pancreatectomy for severe neuroglycopenic symptoms

## Points to Ponder

- *Whipple's triad*: (a) Symptoms of hypoglycemia, (b) Documented low blood glucose (< 55 mg/dL), (c) Improvement of symptoms of hypoglycemia on correction of low blood glucose
- *Nondiabetic hypoglycemia*: Two broad types—(a) Fasting hypoglycemia (beyond 5 hours of meal intake), (b) Postprandial hypoglycemia (within 5 hours of meal intake).
- Insulin autoimmune syndrome (IAS, Hirata's disease) is an uncommon etiology in a patient with nondiabetic hypoglycemia.
- IAS is characterized by spontaneous hypoglycemia with high circulating insulin levels and positive anti insulin antibodies.
- IAS is known to resolve spontaneously in majority of the patients.

## MULTIPLE CHOICE QUESTIONS

**1. A 25-year-old male patient presented with symptoms of giddiness, confusion and sweating. Plasma glucose was recorded to be 50 mg/dL. The symptoms were relieved by the administration of glucose. Name this triad.**

A. Whipple's triad
B. Beck's triad
C. Virchow's triad
D. Sandblom triad

**2. A 35-year-old male patient presented to the emergency department with recurrent episodes of hypoglycemia. CT scan abdomen done showed the presence a tumor in the pancreas of size 1.5 × 1.5 cm. Which of the following fits into criteria for the diagnosis of hypoglycemia based on the above findings?**

A. Serum insulin < 6 μU/mL
B. C-peptide <0.6 ng/mL
C. Proinsulin to insulin ratio >0.2
D. Beta-hydroxybutyrate levels > 0.2 mmol/L

**3. A 30-year-old female with history of tuberculosis presented with giddiness. She has hyperpigmentation over the knuckles, oral mucosa, palmar creases, nipples and axilla. She had a BP = 80/50 mm Hg and heart rate = 100 beats/min. Investigations showed serum sodium = 129 mEq/L, capillary blood glucose = 54 mg/dL. What investigation could be ordered for diagnosis of the cause of hypoglycemia in this patient?**

A. Serum TSH, free T4
B. 8 AM serum cortisol, ACTH
C. MRI brain
D. Urine spot sodium

**4. A 42-year-old lady without diabetes presented to the OPD with recurrent episodes of hypoglycemia after having multiple arguments with her family members. Her parents have diabetes for which they were taking metformin and glimepiride. There was no other relevant significant contributory history. Investigations revealed hyperinsulinemic hypoglycemia. Nuclear imaging of the pancreas was noncontributory. Insulin autoantibodies were negative. What could be the possible diagnosis?**

A. Insulinoma
B. Insulin autoantibody syndrome
C. Surreptitious sulphonylurea intake
D. Malignancy

**5. A 30-year-old school teacher was diagnosed with hyperinsulinemic hypoglycemia. Which of the following is not a recommended therapeutic option?**

A. Diazoxide
B. Verapamil
C. Corticosteroids
D. Thiazide diuretics

### Answers

1. (A); 2. (C); 3. (B); 4. (C); 5. (D)

## SUGGESTED READINGS

1. Registration - Endotext [Internet]. Endotext. 2022 [cited 2024 Nov 2]. Available from: https://www.endotext.org/chapter/non-diabetic-hypoglycemia/
2. Galván R, Fernández-Riejos P, Martinez P, et al. Complete laboratory diagnosis of Insulin Autoimmune Syndrome. Pract Lab Med. 2023:36: e00320.
3. Reis MZR, Fernandes VO, Fontenele EGP, et al. Insulin autoimmune syndrome in an occidental woman: a case report and literature review. Arch Endocrinol Metab. 2018;62(5):566-70.
4. Kumar V, Gala D, Rafi I, et al. Autoimmune Hypoglycemia With Anti-Insulin Autoantibodies in an Eighty-One-Year-Old Woman Without Apparent Risk Factors. AACE Clin Case Rep. 2023;9(5):146-8.
5. Abeyagunawardena I, Madurapperuma C, Thuvarakan P, et al. Uncommon triggers of insulin autoimmune syndrome: a case report. J Med Case Rep. 2024;18(1):292.
6. Alrashidi E, Alessa T. Insulin Autoimmune Syndrome in a 25-Year-Old, Previously Healthy Kuwaiti Man. Case Rep Endocrinol. 2019: 2019:8919457.

CHAPTER

19

# An Approach to a Case of Diabetic Ketoacidosis

*Gouranga Santra*

**CASE VIGNETTE**

Mr X, a 35-year-old male was suffering from type 1 diabetes mellitus (T1DM) for last 20 years. He was on regular insulin therapy. Two days before admission in hospital, he began experiencing nausea, vomiting, and acute crampy pain in abdomen. His supine blood pressure (BP) was 90/50 mm Hg; and standing BP was 60/30 mm Hg. Pulse was 106 beats/min. Respiratory rate (RR) was 25 breaths/min. Oral temperature was 98.4°F. On systemic examination no neurodeficits were found. Chest was normal. Cardiovascular system revealed muffled heart sounds. Abdomen was soft and nontender. Liver and spleen were not palpable.

## DIFFERENTIAL DIAGNOSIS

Possible causes of acute presentation of the patient were acute surgical disorder (like pancreatitis); acute gastritis; sepsis; or diabetic ketoacidosis (DKA).

## LABORATORY REPORT

Lab reports revealed, serum $Na^+$ 138 mEq/L; $K^+$ 4.9 mEq/L; $HCO_3^-$ 8 mEq/L; $Cl^-$ 100 mEq/L; urea 30 mg/dL; creatinine 1.4 mg/dL; and sugar (random) 389 mg/dL. Total leukocyte count was 10,500/mm$^3$ (neutrophil 70%, lymphocyte 27%, eosinophil 2%, monocyte 1%). Hemoglobin was 14 g/dL. Hematocrit was 42%. Liver function test was normal but serum albumin was 3.5 g/dL. Serum amylase and lipase levels were normal.

## DISCUSSION

Very low serum $HCO_3^-$ (8 mEq/L) level suggested a significant acid-base disorder. So, in addition to evaluating abdominal pain, exploring the acid-base disorder was essential.

**What is next step?**

ABG analysis was done. Report showed: pH of 7.15; $HCO_3^-$ = 8 mEq/L; $PaCO_2$ = 20 mm Hg; and $PaO_2$ of 80 mm Hg. Report was suggestive of metabolic acidosis.

**Was it high anion gap metabolic acidosis (HAGMA) or normal anion gap metabolic acidosis (NAGMA)?**

Metabolic acidosis is due to production of acid (i.e., ketoacids, lactic acid), or lose of $HCO_3^-$ in urine or stool (i.e., diarrhea, renal tubular acidosis). Production of acid (e.g., in ketoacidosis) accumulates unmeasured anions resulting in high anion gap (AG). Processes that lose $HCO_3^-$ do not generate unmeasured anions and AG remains normal.

$$\text{Anion gap} = Na^+ - (HCO_3^- + Cl^-). \text{ Normal AG is } 10 \pm 2 \text{ mmol/L.}$$

Albumin is negatively charged, so low albumin is associated with a lower AG. Normal AG is 2.5 mEq/L lower, for every 1 g/dL drop in serum albumin (below 4.5 g/dL).

*Our patient's AG was*: $Na^+ - (HCO_3^- + Cl^-) = 138 - (8 + 100) =$ 30 mEq/L. So, it was HAGMA.

### Differential Diagnosis

*Differential diagnosis of HAGMA*: DKA; starvation ketoacidosis; ketoacidosis due to alcohol; Uremia from chronic kidney disease; lactic acidosis (from hypoxemia or shock), and toxins.

**Are all informations available to narrow the D/D of the patient's HAGMA?**

The patient denied any history of alcohol consumption or toxin ingestion. Serum lactate level was 1 mEq/L (normal = 0.5–1.5 mEq/L). Serum creatine was 1.4 mg/dL. Serum ketones came high (+++). High blood sugar and ketones, and history of T1DM suggested a diagnosis of DKA. High sugar and profound acidosis (pH of 7.15) were against starvation ketoacidosis. Absence of a significant alcohol history went against alcoholic ketoacidosis. Normal lactate level ruled out lactic acidosis. Uremic acidosis was also unlikely with a serum creatinine level of 1.4 mg/dL. So, diagnosis was narrowed down as HAGMA due to DKA.

**Had he isolated DKA or a mixed disorder?**

*Delta-delta gap*: Delta-delta gap is assessed to determine a mixed metabolic disorder. In delta-delta gap rise in AG above normal is compared with fall in $HCO_3^-$ below normal.

$$\Delta AG = \text{Pt's AG} - \text{normal AG}. \ \Delta HCO_3^- = 24 - \text{Pt's } HCO_3^-.$$

In simple AG acidosis, deltas are similar [extra anions (i.e., ketones) neutralize $HCO_3^-$ in equal proportions].

In HAGMA + NAGMA, fall in $HCO_3^-$ is greater than rise in AG.

In HAGMA + metabolic alkalosis, fall in $HCO_3^-$ due to HAGMA is antagonized by concurrent metabolic alkalosis. Here, fall in $HCO_3^-$ is lesser than increase in AG.

HAGMA + NAGMA has $\Delta AG/\Delta HCO_3^-$ ratio < 1.

HAGMA + metabolic alkalosis has $\Delta AG/\Delta HCO_3^-$ ratio > 2. (Probable if > 1).

In our patient serum albumin was 3.5 mg/dL. So, corrected normal AG = 10–2.5 = 7.5 mEq/L.

So, Δ AG was = 30–7.5 = 22.5 mEq/L. Δ $HCO_3^-$ was = 24–8 = 16 mEq/L.

So, reduction of bicarbonate ($\Delta HCO_3^-$) was lesser than elevation of anions (ΔAG), and $\Delta AG/\Delta HCO_3^-$ ratio was> 1.

So, the patient had possible concurrent metabolic alkalosis. As he had h/o recurrent vomiting, vomiting induced metabolic alkalosis was likely.

**Is there any associated respiratory acid-base disorder?**

In metabolic acidosis respiratory system hyperventilates to lower $PaCO_2$ and create respiratory alkalosis that returns pH closer to normal. Compensation greater or lesser than expected suggests an additional acid-base abnormality **(Table 1)**. Our patient's RR was elevated to 25 beats/min.

Pt's $HCO_3^-$ was 8 mEq/L (Normal = 24).

Expected $PaCO_2$ after compensation in metabolic acidosis, $PaCO_2 = 1.5 \times HCO_3^- + 8 \pm 2$ (Winter's formula). Here it was $1.5 \times 8 + 8 \pm 2 = 20 \pm 2$ mm Hg

Actual $PaCO_2$ (20 mm Hg) was similar suggesting that respiratory compensation was appropriate.

So, it was a case of HAGMA with vomiting induced concurrent metabolic alkalosis but with appropriate respiratory compensation.

**Is the diagnosis complete?**

Common cause of death in DKA is underlying precipitant. It must be identified.

The patient reported no h/o fever, cough, diarrhea, and focal neurodeficit. Urine revealed pus cell 3–4/HPF. Chest X-ray and ultrasonography of abdomen were normal. Serum lipase was normal. Patient confirmed that he was taking insulin regularly and properly.

**What would be the next test?**

12-lead ECG was done. It revealed inferior wall acute myocardial infarction (AMI). Trop T kit test was positive. So, AMI was the precipitant of DKA.

**TABLE 1: Expected compensation in acid-base disorders.**

| Acid-base abnormality | Primary change | Compensation |
|---|---|---|
| Metabolic acidosis | ↓ $HCO_3^-$ | ↓ $PaCO_2$ |
| Metabolic alkalosis | ↑ $HCO_3^-$ | ↑ $PaCO_2$ |
| Respiratory acidosis | ↑ $PaCO_2$ | ↑ $HCO_3^-$ |
| Respiratory alkalosis | ↓ $PaCO_2$ | ↓ $HCO_3^-$ |

## Final Diagnosis

A case of HAGMA due to DKA in T1DM along with vomiting induced metabolic alkalosis and a precipitating cause of DKA being inferior wall AMI.

## Treatment and Prevention

Fluid resuscitation was done with intravenous (IV) normal saline (NS) 1 L bolus, and subsequently with NS, half NS, and 5% Dextrose (when sugar came down < 250 mg/dL) with close monitoring forheart failure. IV insulin was given with dose titration until ketoacidosis was resolved. Potassium chloride (KCl) was given in each bottle of NS. No bicarbonate was given. AMI was treated with aspirin, low molecular weight heparin and β blocker. Cardiac catheterization done later revealed triple vessel disease. After stabilization, he underwent coronary artery bypass grafting and did well.

## Important Points for DKA Management

- *Fluid resuscitation*: To reduce risk of hyperchloremic acidosis, switch NS to 0.45% NaCl after volume is restored to correct free water deficit.
- *IV insulin*: Continue IV insulin until resolution of DKA. Criteria of resolution include random blood sugar <200 mg/dL and two of the following: serum $HCO_3^- \geq 15$ mEq/L, venous blood pH > 7.3 and AG ≤ 12 mEq/L. Start subcutaneous insulin 1–2 hours before stopping IV insulin to prevent insulin-free window to prevent rebound ketoacidosis.
- *Potassium supplement*: Insulin shifts $K^+$ back intracellular. Fluid resuscitation and correction of acidosis further lower serum potassium. Potassium needs supplementation throughout DKA management if $K^+$ is < 5– 5.2 mEq/L. Insulin should be started only if $K^+$ is > 3.3 mEq/L and hypokalemia should be corrected first.
- *Bicarbonate therapy*: It is recommended only in extreme acidosis when pH is <7.00. No bolus should be given. Only 50 mEq $NaHCO_3$ in 200 mL NS should be given IV slowly. Hypokalemia is a risk of bicarbonate therapy when urine output is restored. β-hydroxybutyric, acetoacetate and lactate are metabolizable and are potential bicarbonate.

# PATHOPHYSIOLOGY

*DKA pathogenesis*: Both insulin deficiency and glucagon excess are necessary for DKA to develop. Decreased ratio of insulin and glucagon (I:G) causes increased gluconeogenesis, glycogenolysis and ketone body formation. Ketosis results from marked increase in free fatty acid release from adipocyte, with a resulting shift toward ketone body synthesis in liver which ultimately leads to DKA. Precipitating factors aggravate imbalance of the ratio, and aggravate hyperglycaemia; and associated nausea and vomiting add to hypovolemia.

*Euglycemic DKA*: DKA can occur when diabetics are treated with SGLT-2 inhibitors. Patients have near normal glucose levels (mean 265 mg/dL) due to glucosuria, despite having insulin deficits. Mechanisms include: (1) Decreased insulin release (due to lower glucose levels); (2) Direct stimulation of glucagon release; and (3) Ketogenic effects of SGLT-2i.

Pharmacological effect of SGLTi persists 10–14 days after withdrawal of the drug. Relapse of DKA may occur during this time. To reduce risk of euglycemic DKA, avoid SGLT-2i in T1DM, in latent autoimmune diabetes of adult, and with concurrent insulin therapy in type 2 diabetes mellitus (T2DM).

*Hyperglycemic hyperosmolar state (HHS)*: For managing DKA, differentiating it from HHS is important. HHS is common in elderly individual and is seen in T2DM. Several weeks of polyurea, weight loss, decreased oral intake and mental confusion are associated with HHS. HHS causes profound dehydration, hypotension, and tachycardia. It is marked by absence of nausea, vomiting, pain abdomen and Kussmaul breathing. HHS has higher mortality than DKA.

Pathogenesis includes relative insulin deficiency and inadequate fluid intake. Insulin deficiency leads to glycogenolysis, gluconeogenesis, and impaired glucose utilization in skeletal muscle. Precipitating factors include cerebrovascular accident, AMI, sepsis, pneumonia, debilitating condition with water deprivation.

It is associated with marked hyperglycemia (800–1,000 mg/dL), serum osmolality >350 mOsm/L (Normal = 285–295 mOsm/kg $H_2O$) and profound fluid deficit (more in HHS 6–10 L vs. 5–6 L in DKA). Patients often have prerenal azotemia. In HHS acidosis and ketonemia are absent or mild. A small anion gap acidosis may occur due to increased lactic acid. Mild ketonemia may be due to starvation.

*Formula for calculation of serum osmolality*:

$$\text{Serum osmolality} = 2\,(Na^+) + 2\,(K^+) + \text{glucose (mg/L)}/18 + \text{BUN (mg/dL)}/2.8$$

*Diabetic Striatopathy (DS)*: Few patients with HHS may present with DS. DS is seen in HSS but not in DKA. CT scan of brain in DS is normal initially, but later it demonstrates hyperdensity in striatal region. Possible mechanism is hyper-viscosity leading to regional BBB disruption and metabolic damage. In HHS brain metabolism is shifted toward an anaerobic pathway in Krebs cycle causing depletion in GABA. This leads to attenuated inhibition of striatum resulting in hyperkinetic movements. Conversely, GABA can be readily resynthesized from acetoacetate in a ketotic milieu in DKA. DS is associated with female preponderance due to augmented sensitivity of dopaminergic receptors in postmenopausal period.

## Points to Ponder

- DKA should always be in differential diagnosis of acute abdomen in diabetic patients.
- Precipitating factors of DKA like AMI, sepsis., etc should be searched thoroughly.
- Potassium supplementation is essential in DKA except when serum $K^+$ is > 5–5.2 mEq/L.
- IV bicarbonate should be given only in severe acidosis with pH < 7.
- DKA may relapse with premature withdrawal of IV insulin, and subcutaneous insulin should have 1–2 hour overlap because of short half-life of IV insulin.

## MULTIPLE CHOICE QUESTIONS

**1. Euglycemic DKA is seen with:**
A. Metformin
B. Sulfonylurea
C. DPP-4 inhibitors
D. SGLT-2 inhibitors

**2. Diabetic striatopathy is seen with:**
A. DKA
B. HHS
C DKA with hyponatremia
D. DKA after recovery

**3. Insulin with potassium should be started in DKA:**
A. Irrespective of potassium level
B. Potassium level > 5 mEq/L
C. Potassium level < 5 mEq/L
D. Only with ECG changes of hypokalemia

**4. Bicarbonate infusion in DKA:**
A. Given with pH< 7.2
B. Given when pH is <7
C. It leads to hyperkalemia
D. Dose is 50 mEq slow IV TDS

**5. IV insulin in DKA should be continued until:**
A. pH returns to 7.4
B. AG returns to < 20 mEq/L
C. Subcutaneous insulin overlapped for 1–2 hours,
D. Serum $HCO_3^-$ is > 24 mEq/L

### Answers

1. (D); 2. (B); 3. (C); 4. (B); 5. (C)

## SUGGESTED READINGS

1. Lizzo JM, Goyal A, Gupta V. Adult Diabetic Ketoacidosis. 2023 Jul 10. In: StatPearls [Internet]. Treasure Island (FL): StatPearls Publishing; 2024.
2. Healy AM, Faherty M, Khan Z, et al. Diabetic ketoacidosis diagnosis in a hospital setting. J Osteopath Med. 2023;123(10):499-503.

CHAPTER

20

# An Approach to a Case of Sexual Dysfunction in DM

*Ravikant, Aneesha G, Balachandra R*

**CASE VIGNETTE**

A 49 years old male patient, married 15 years back, presented to diabetic clinic with complaints of inability to maintain erection during sexual intercourse for last 4 months. He is a diabetic since 10 years on basal bolus regimen of insulin for last 1 year and chronic smoker for last 22 years. Patient has no history of trauma previously or any previous hospitalization. His father has history of coronary artery disease and type 2 diabetes. On general examination patient had BMI of 28, obese habitus and acanthosis nigricans. His genital exam was normal with no loss of secondary sexual characteristics. All of his peripheral pulses were palpable. Rest of systemic exam was normal.

What is your provisional diagnosis and how would you investigate and treat this patient further?

## PROVISIONAL DIAGNOSIS

A middle aged man presenting with above mentioned complaints with associated comorbidities of obesity, diabetes, and significant history of smoking a provisional diagnosis of erectile dysfunction (ED) is to be considered.

## DIFFERENTIAL DIAGNOSIS

Drug induced causes of erectile dysfunction **Table 1**.

## CLINICAL APPROACH

An algorithm based clinical approach will help in timely diagnosis and guide for appropriate treatment in cases of sexual dysfunction in diabetes. The psychological and social factors influence the patient from expressing his concerns, as a clinicians, active search for cases of sexual dysfunction in diabetes patients is necessary. As in any case, history taking is first and most important step for diagnosis.

*History*: Detailed history taking with particle attention to age, comorbidities, addiction history, diabetes history, sexual history, drug history, family history, social history has to be considered.

*Age and comorbidities*: Sexual dysfunction incidence increases with age primarily driven by comorbid conditions like smoking, heart disease, hypertension, dyslipidemia and diabetes.

*Diabetes history*: Duration, level glycemic control, complications of diabetes, treatment compliance, type of diabetes are to be considered while taking history. Men with diabetes mellitus are at increased risk of erectile dysfunction. The prevalence of severe ED in men with diabetes mellitus is estimated to be 21.6%. In one of the study, prevalence of ED in type 1 and type 2 diabetes mellitus was 26% and 37% respectively. Compared to general population, people with diabetes are at 3.5 times risk for ED.

*Sexual history*: Onset of symptom and its severity, performance anxiety, problems with sexual partner, domestic violence should be enquired in sexual history.

*Drug history*: Drugs associated with erectile dysfunction has to be ruled out before considering organic causes for the same.

Below table mentions the few of the drugs associated with erectile dysfunction in men with diabetes mellitus **(Table 2)**.

*IIEF questionnaire*: In all cases of ED, this questionnaire is used to assess severity of erectile dysfunction **(Table 3)**.

**TABLE 1: Differential diagnosis for ED in DM.**

| Vascular | Neurological | Endocrine | Psychological | Local/Structural |
|---|---|---|---|---|
| Atherosclerosis | Diabetes | Hypogonadism | Depression | Peyronie disease |
| Hypertension | Multiple sclerosis | Hyperprolactinemia | Performance anxiety | Penile trauma |
| Peripheral vascular disease | Spinal cord injury | Hyper and hypothyroidism | | Phimosis<br>Paraphimosis |
| | Cerebrovascular accident | Obesity | | |

**TABLE 2: Drugs associated with erectile dysfunction in men with diabetes mellitus.**

| | |
|---|---|
| Diuretics | Spironolactone, thiazides |
| Antihypertensives | Methyldopa, clonidine, beta blockers, calcium channel blockers |
| Cardiac drugs | Digoxin |
| Antidepressants | SSRI, TCA, lithium |
| Cytotoxic agents | Methotrexate |
| Hormones | Estrogen, corticosteroids |
| H2 antagonists | Cimetidine, ranitidine |

**TABLE 3: IIEF questionnaire.**

| IIEF 5 score | Severity of ED |
|---|---|
| 22–25 | No ED |
| 17–21 | Mild ED |
| 12–16 | Mild-to-moderate |
| 8–11 | Moderate |
| 1–7 | Severe |

Investigations to diagnoses sexual dysfunction in diabetes

**Routine investigations:**
- Complete hemogram
- Liver and kidney function tests

**Biochemical investigations to assess endocrine function:**
- Serum testosterone
- FSH and LH levels

**Radiological investigations (in males):**
- Penile Doppler ultrasonography
- Combined intracavernosal injection and stimulation test
- Dynamic infusion cavernosometry, cavernosography
- Penile angiography
- Nocturnal penile tumescence and rigidity test

**Diabetes related investigations:**
- Fasting blood sugar/post prandial blood sugar
- HbA1c
- Fundoscopy
- Urine routine

**Investigations to assess cardiac and vascular function:**
- ECG, 2D ECHO
- Lipid profile
- Thyroid profile
- Vascular Doppler if indicated

**FIG. 1:** Clinical approach to SD in DM.

## CLINICAL EXAMINATION

The following parameters are to be specifically examined in cases of erectile dysfunction:

Built, behavior, BMI, secondary sexual characteristics, all peripheral pulses, fundoscopy and neuropathy assessment, genital examination (including bulbocavernosus reflex) and cardiovascular examination.

### Laboratory Examination (Fig. 1)

Lab investigations in case of erectile dysfunction in males in diabetes is represented in tabular form below **(Fig. 1)**:

- *ED and CV disease*: Cardiovascular disease constitute the main cause of mortality and morbidity in patients with DM. The main factor associated with CV disease, atherosclerosis is also associated with ED.Multiple studies in literature has confirmed correlation between ED and CV disease. ED can also present before onset of CAD, usually 2–5 years, providing opportunity for early diagnosis of silent CAD and stroke. Hence, cardiovascular examination and investigations to search silent CAD has to be included in work up for ED case especially in diabetes cases, to pick up the complications early in the natural disease progression.
- *ED and DKD*: The correlation between diabetic kidney disease and ED dysfunction has been established in a diabetic patient. The pathophysiology of vascular and endothelial damage affecting glomerular capillaries is similar to that of penile vessels in case of ED. Hence, it is also important to look for renal function in case of ED with diabetes.
- *ED and serum testosterone level*: The master hormone modulating erectile function is testosterone. Hypogonadism with low testosterone levels are associated with obesity, metabolic syndrome, insulin resistance forming a vicious cycle and resulting in erectile dysfunction in diabetes. Upto 40% cases of type 2 diabetes are associated with low testosterone and 90% experiencing ED. Measuring serum testosterone and gonadotropins is recommended in cases with clinical findings suggestive of hypogonadism.
- *Penile Doppler in ED*: Peak systolic velocity less than 30 cm/sec indicated arterial dysfunction. End diastolic velocity is indicator of venogenic impotence. Its value >5 cm/s indicates venous dysfunction. A good diastolic reversal virtually rules out venous insufficiency.

## PATHOPHYSIOLOGY

The understanding of pathophysiology of erectile dysfunction is crucial for appropriate treatment. ED in diabetes is caused by multiple factors: Vascular, neuropathic, endocrine and sociopsychological factors. Treatment of ED should address all these factors to have favorable response to treatment. The pathophysiological mechanism involved in ED in diabetic patient is represented in below **Flowchart 1**.

## TREATMENT AND PREVENTION

Most commonly used therapy for ED is oral therapy with phosphodiesterase inhibitors. Associated comorbidities and risk factors should be addressed to improve erectile dysfunction.

- *Oral phosphodiesterase inhibitors*: They act by increasing cGMP levels in penile tissues leading leading to relaxation of smooth muscles. These drugs are the first line option for treatment of erectile dysfunction. They are usually used as on demand before sexual activity. However, who do poorly with on demand PDE inhibitor, respond well to daily regimen.

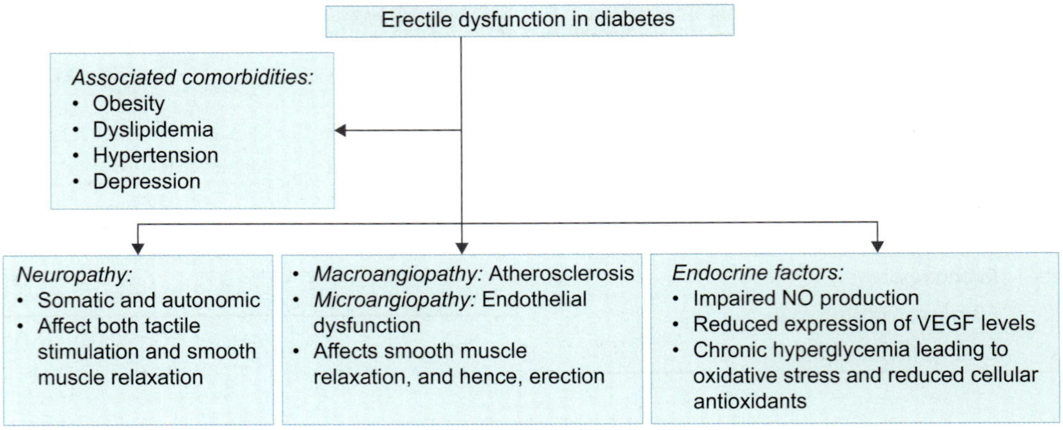


**FLOWCHART 1:** Erectile dysfunction in diabetes mellitus.

*Dosage of PDE5 inhibitors in ED*:

| | |
|---|---|
| Sildenafil | 50–100 mg empty stomach |
| Vardenafil | 10–20 mg empty stomach |
| Tadalafil | 10–20 mg 30 min before sexual activity |

## Contraindications

High or intermediate risk for CAD, nitrate use, retinitis pigmentosa, anterior ischemic optic neuropathy.

- *Injection therapies*:

| | |
|---|---|
| Intracavernous alprostadil | • PGE1 analogue<br>• Acts by increasing cAMP concentration and decreases intracellular calcium and hence promoting relaxation of smooth muscle |
| Intracavernous phentolamine + papaverine | • *Phentolamine*: Alpha 1 antagonist and papaverine—phosphodiesterase inhibitor<br>• This combination is indicated with treatment failure of alprostadil |
| Transurethral alprostadil | • Medicated urethral system for erection [MUSE]<br>• Drug delivered in suppository formulation |

Injection therapies are associated with small risk of priapism (1%), penile ache (5%), rarely penile fibrosis.

*Contraindications*: History priapism, sickle cell disease, multiple myeloma, thrombocytopenia.

*MUSE*: Urethritis, urethral stricture.

- *Testosterone therapy*: It is indicated in patients of erectile dysfunction with low levels of testosterone. In metanalysis of 16 studies, improvement in erectile dysfunction was more common in men with hypogonadism who were treated with testosterone than in those who received placebo (57% vs. 16.7%).

## Formulation

Testosterone levels should be reevaluated after 1–3 months and then annually.

*Adverse effects*: Gynecomastia, sleep apnea, development of LUTS due to BPH, erythrocytosis, elevation in liver enzyme levels, and reduced fertility.

- *Penile devices*: Vacuum erection devices can be used when other treatment fails or are contraindicated.
- *Penile prosthesis*: Surgically implanted is the last resort if less invasive measures fails to treat the condition.
- *Psychotherapy*: Sensate focus technique, sensory awareness exercises, therapy for interpersonal difficulties. These therapies, address the psychogenic and social factors associated with ED.

## Points to Ponder

- Erectile dysfunction is common in diabetics and contributes to morbidity of diabetic patients.
- Pathophysiology of ED in diabetes involves atherosclerosis, endothelial dysfunction, neuropathy, oxidative stress due to tissue hyperglycemia.
- ED in diabetes correlates with cardiovascular disease and can present 2–5 years before onset of CV disease. Hence, men presenting with ED should be evaluated for cardiovascular disease.
- ED is managed with lifestyle changes, PDE5 inhibitors, glycemic management.
- Injectable therapy is considered in cases of treatment failure with oral medication.
- A comprehensive multidisciplinary approach to treatment is need of the hour to manage ED and ensure sexual health of diabetic patients.

## MULTIPLE CHOICE QUESTIONS

1. **Which of the following is not pathophysiological mechanism involved in ED in diabetes mellitus?**
   A. Somatic neuropathy
   B. Increased NO and cGMP levels
   C. Increased oxidative stress
   D. Endothelial dysfunction
2. **Which of the following about MUSE therapy is false?**
   A. It involves intracavernous injection of alprostadil
   B. It is contraindicated in urethral stricture
   C. It is indicated when oral PDE5 inhibitors are contraindicated or there is treatment failure
   D. It is associated with risk of penile ache
3. **Tadalafil acts by:**
   A. Stimulating PDE 5
   B. Increasing cGMP levels
   C. Decreasing nitric oxide level
   D. Increasing cAMP levels
4. **PDE 5 inhibitors are contraindicated to use with:**
   A. Nitrates
   B. Calcium channel blockers
   C. Beta blockers
   D. Aspirin
5. **Which of the following statements is true?**
   A. S testosterone level is to be measured in all cases of erectile dysfunction
   B. Erectile dysfunction can be used to predict cardiovascular event in case of diabetes
   C. ED and diabetic kidney disease do not correlate with each other
   D. Severity of ED is not affected by glycemic control

### Answers

1. (B); 2. (A); 3. (B); 4. (A); 5. (B)

## SUGGESTED READINGS


1. Lewis RW, Fugl-Meyer KS, Corona G, et al. Definitions/epidemiology/risk factors for sexual dysfunction. J Sex Med. 2010;7(4 Pt 2):1598-607.
2. Corona G, Giorda CB, Cucinotta D, et al.; Gruppo di studio SUBITO-DE. Sexual dysfunction at the onset of type 2 diabetes: the interplay of depression, hormonal and cardiovascular factors. J Sex Med. 2014;11(8):2065-73.
3. Fedele D, Coscelli C, Santeusanio F, et al. Erectile dysfunction in diabetic subjects in Italy. Gruppo Italiano Studio Deficit Erettile nei Diabetici. Diabetes Care. 1998;21(11):1973-7.
4. Kouidrat Y, Pizzol D, Cosco T, et al. High prevalence of erectile dysfunction in diabetes: a systematic review and meta-analysis of 145 studies. Diabet Med. 2017;34(9):1185-92.
5. Francis ME, Kusek JW, Nyberg LM, et al. The contribution of common medical conditions and drug exposures to erectile dysfunction in adult males. J Urol. 2007;178(2):591-6.
6. Hatzimouratidis K, Hatzichristou D. How to treat erectile dysfunction in men with diabetes: from pathophysiology to treatment. Curr Diab Rep. 2014;14(11):545.
7. Roger VL, Go AS, Lloyd-Jones DM, et al. American Heart Association Statistics Committee and Stroke Statistics Subcommittee. Heart disease and stroke statistics—2012 update: a report from the American Heart Association. Circulation. 2012;125(1):e2-e220.
8. Gandaglia G, Briganti A, Jackson G, et al. A systematic review of the association between erectile dysfunction and cardiovascular disease. Eur Urol. 2014;65(5):968-78.
9. Montorsi P, Ravagnani PM, Galli S, et al. Association between erectile dysfunction and coronary artery disease. Role of coronary clinical presentation and extent of coronary vessels involvement: the COBRA trial. Eur Heart J. 2006;27(22):2632-39.
10. Vlachopoulos C, Jackson G, Stefanadis C, et al. Erectile dysfunction in the cardiovascular patient. Eur Heart J. 2013;34(27):2034-46.

# CHAPTER 21

# An Approach to a Case of Management of Common Endocrine Disorder in Pregnancy

*Rupak Chatterjee, Upoma Saha, Rajat Kanti Goswami*

**CASE VIGNETTE**

A 24-year-old primigravida in her third trimester is referred from the antenatal OPD with an isolated TSH report of 6.63 μU/mL and FBS report of 112 mg/dL. She is clinically asymptomatic. On examination, BP is 110/60 mm Hg, PR 70 beats/min, body weight is 65 kg. There is no clinically palpable goiter. There is no blood report prior to her pregnancy and there were no known comorbidities. How will you approach this case?

## PROVISIONAL DIAGNOSIS

Primary hypothyroidism in pregnancy with gestational diabetes mellitus.

## DIFFERENTIAL DIAGNOSIS

### Thyroid Dysfunction

- Hashimoto thyroiditis
- Iodine deficiency related hypothyroidism
- Thyroiditis in pregnancy

### Hyperglycemia

- Previously diagnosed diabetes mellitus (DM) (Pregestational)
- Medication induced hyperglycemia
- Other secondary hyperglycemia
- Thyroid disorders and DM constitute commonly encountered endocrine disorders in pregnancy.

## PATHOPHYSIOLOGY

### Thyroid Disorders

- Thyroid hormones play a crucial role in early embryogenesis for fetal brain development, embryo growth, and tissue differentiation.
- In pregnancy, physiological hormone alterations and increased metabolic demands lead to altered thyroid physiology. Thyroid gland increases by 10–40% in size during pregnancy.
- Raised estrogen levels result in increased hepatic production of serum thyroxine-binding globulin (TBG), which reach a plateau during the 20th week. This leads to gradual high total triiodothyronine (T3) and thyroxine (T4) serum concentrations up to the 20th week (1.5 of threshold). Also, hCG resembles thyroid-stimulating hormone (TSH) structurally, stimulating TSH receptors resulting in elevation of thyroid hormone production and reduced serum TSH concentrations via negative feedback. Therefore, TSH is completely suppressed in 20% of pregnant women, while another 2% may develop temporary hyperthyroxinemia. Furthermore, the development of the placenta, which results in the degradation of T3 and T4, the increase in plasma volume, and the increase in renal clearance, leads to elevated T4 production (50% approximately) and a similar increase in total daily iodine requirements.
- Thyroid hormones are converted into active forms (T4 to T3) via deiodinase, whose concentration and activity are upregulated by the placenta.

All together, the pathophysiological changes may lead to gestation-induced thyroid disorders or deregulation of pre-existing thyroid dysfunction **(Fig. 1)**.

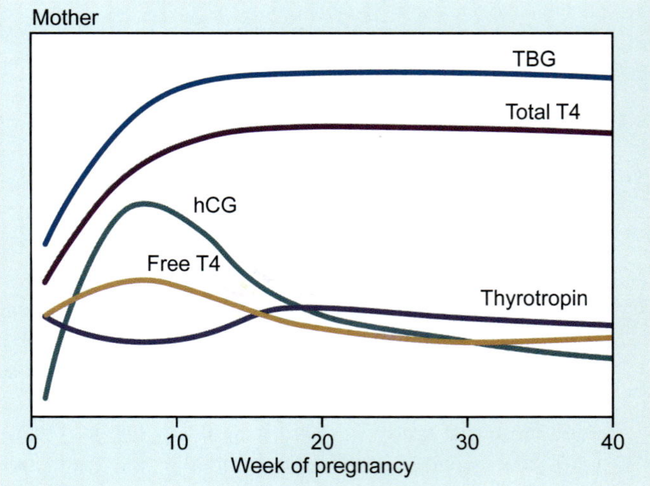


**FIG. 1:** Thyroid hormonal changes with pregnancy.
*Source*: Williams Textbook of Endocrinology, 14th Edition.

**TABLE 1: Physiological changes in pregnancy and effect on thyroid function**

| Physiologic change | Thyroid related consequence |
|---|---|
| Increased serum thyroxine-binding globulin | Increased total T4 and T3, increased T4 production |
| Increased plasma volume | Increased T4 and T3 pool size, increased T4 production, increased cardiac output |
| D3 expression in placenta and uterus | Increased T4 production |
| First trimester increase in hCG | Increased free T4, decreased basal thyrotropin, increased T4 production |
| Increased renal I-clearance | Increased iodine requirements |
| Increased T4 production, fetal T4 synthesis during second and third trimesters | |
| Increased oxygen consumption by fetoplacental unit, gravid uterus and mother | Increased basal metabolic rate, increased cardiac output |

Pregnancy affects the entire spectrum of thyroid hormone economy **(Table 1)**.

## HYPERTHYROIDISM IN PREGNANCY

Total serum T3, T4 rise to 1.5 times that of nonpregnant women, due to increase in thyroglobulin concentration in first trimester, followed by increase in T4 until new equilibrium is reached. hCG cross-reacts with TSH receptor alpha subunit, resulting in small and transient rise in T4 in first semester, with partial TSH suppression.

During pregnancy, autoimmunity is suppressed, affecting patients with Graves disease. TSH-R antibodies are increased in first trimester and decreased in second and third trimester.

Increase in BMR in second trimester, coupled with decreased peripheral vascular resistance and resting tachycardia, mimic thyrotoxicosis. It is pertinent to keep this in mind while treating hyperthyroid pregnant patient.

## PATHOPHYSIOLOGY OF DM IN PREGNANCY

- Hyperglycemia during pregnancy may be classified as overt or pregestational diabetes mellitus (PGDM) and gestational diabetes mellitus (GDM).
- GDM is defined as "onset or recognition of diabetes or impaired glucose tolerance occurred during pregnancy."
- Pregnancy is characterized by a high risk of developing glucose metabolism disorders, considering that insulin resistance increases from the 24th to 28th gestational week. GDM complicates 7–8% of pregnancies.
- Fetal glucose need is met through maternal glucose transport via the placenta due to the concentration gradient between them. As the pregnancy progresses, a rise in fetal glucose requirements results in increased maternal hepatic glucose production and transport. Simultaneously, the pancreatic β-cells are increased in mass to promote insulin production and prevent excessive glucose delivery to the fetus. Failure of this process leads to hyperglycemia, usually between the 24th and 28th gestational weeks.
- GDM has been implicated for adverse effects both for the mother as well as the fetus. Maternal or pregnancy related complications include: Preeclampsia, spontaneous miscarriage, preterm birth, dystocia, and increased cesarian section rates. Later, they are also prone to develop cardiovascular disease, type 2 diabetes mellitus (T2DM) and GDM in a subsequent pregnancy. Fetal complications include: Macrosomia, birth trauma, shoulder dystocia, hypoglycemia, hyperbilirubinemia, preterm birth, and stillbirth. Babies have a higher risk of obesity, metabolic syndrome and T2DM in later life.

## CLINICAL APPROACH AND INVESTIGATIONS

### Hypothyroidism

There is no consensus on whether universal screening and assessment of thyroid function should be performed during pregnancy. The gold standard test is TSH, accompanied by free T4 levels. Free thyroid hormones are preferred to total, since it is largely affected by thyroglobulin concentration. Primary hypothyroid in pregnancy is defined as the presence of elevated TSH with reduced serum free T4 levels in pregnancy. Subclinical hypothyroidism is defined by fT4 concentrations within normal range with elevated TSH. Untreated hypothyroidism may be associated with adverse pregnancy outcomes such as miscarriage, preeclampsia, gestational diabetes, placental abruption and preterm labor. The trimester-specific cut-offs for TSH levels are as mentioned in **Table 2**.

In euthyroid women, routine testing for thyroglobulin and anti-TPO antibodies is not recommended.

In absence of trimester-specific TSH reference range, an upper reference limit of 4.0 mU/L may be used. However, it is always recommended to use trimester specific reference intervals from local population data.

### Hyperthyroidism

Subclinical hyperthyroidism is defined by decreased TSH concentration with normal fT4 levels. Overt hyperthyroidism (decreased TSH, elevated fT4) is rare during pregnancy, of which Graves' disease is the most common cause. Untreated overt hyperthyroidism may lead to complications like preeclampsia, maternal heart failure and thyroid storm, foetal thyrotoxicosis, preterm birth, low birth weight, miscarriage and stillbirth.

It is worth noting that low serum TSH concentration during pregnancy could be the result of physiological gestational changes or indicate hyperthyroidism. Suggestive of hyperthyroidism is the clinical evidence of autoimmunity or thyroid receptor antibodies (TRAb or TSI) or a goiter. A high index of clinical suspicion is required for early detection in pregnancy due to limited means of investigation (Tc99 uptake scan being contraindicated). Then

**TABLE 2: Trimester-specific cut off for TSH levels.**

| | Endocrine Society American Thyroid Association | European Thyroid Association |
|---|---|---|
| Trimester | TSH (mU/L) | |
| First | 0.1–2.5 | 0.1–2.5 |
| Second | 0.2–3.0 | 0.2–3.0 |
| Third | 0.3–3.0 | 0.2–3.5 |

T3 thyrotoxicosis is suspected, total T3 concentration should be monitored as an index of thyroid function.

## CLINICAL APPROACH AND INVESTIGATIONS OF GDM

The main risk factors for developing GDM are advanced maternal age, obesity, abnormal weight gain in pregnancy, first-degree relative with T2DM, a history of GDM, macrocosmia (newborn > 4 kg), perinatal complications, and polycystic ovary syndrome.

One step approach of diagnosis is recommended by IADPSG (International Association of Diabetes and Pregnancy Study Groups) based on HAPO (Hyperglycemia and Adverse Pregnancy Outcome) study. Two step approach is based on Carpenter-Couston interpretation of O'Sullivan-Mahan criteria. **(Table 3)**

Diabetes in Pregnancy Study Group India (DIPSI) protocol: 75 g anhydrous glucose dissolved in 250–300 mL of water to be ingested by pregnant woman irrespective of last meal, followed by plasma glucose estimation after 2 hours. A 2 hours plasma glucose level ≥140 mg/dL is diagnostic of GDM. 2 hours value ≥200 mg/dL is considered as diabetes mellitus (overt) and ≥120 mg/dL as decreased glucose tolerance.

## TREATMENT AND PREVENTION (FLOWCHART 1)

### Hypothyroidism (Table 4)

- Replacement therapy with levothyroxine (LT4) should be provided to pregnant women with overt hypothyroidism to reduce the risk of fetomaternal complications.
- Full replacement therapy is achieved with LT4 at 1.6 µg/kg/day. If patient was previously hypothyroid before pregnancy, a dosage increase of 25–30% is required from 5th to 6th weeks' gestation.
- Levothyroxine replacement dosage should be adapted to reach and maintain serum trimester specific TSH concentrations.
- Thyroid function tests should be repeated every 4–6 weeks.
- After delivery, thyroid function returns to normal in 6–8 weeks postpartum. Some women decrease the T4 dosage to preconception level, while a majority of them may quit LT4.

### Hyperthyroidism

- Treatment of hyperthyroidism due to Graves' disease or toxic thyroid nodule involves antithyroid drugs and aims to maintain maternal fT4 concentration in the upper limit of normal.
- Propylthiouracil and methimazole/carbimazole are recommended during the first and second/third trimester respectively.
- Methimazole/carbimazole had potential teratogenic effects, such as aplasia cutis and other congenital malformations, since it crosses the placenta; and therefore, it is avoided in first trimester.

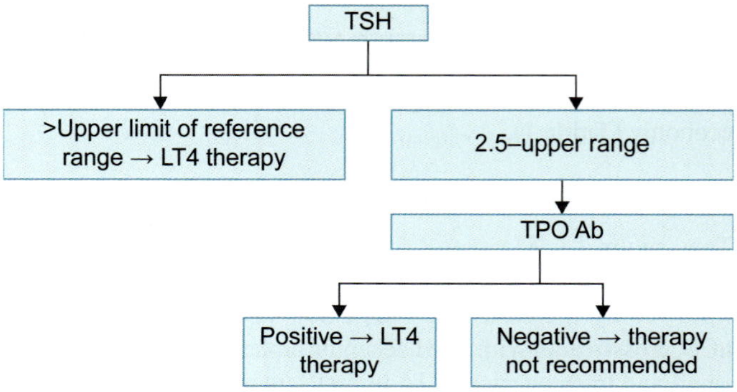


**FLOWCHART 1:** Treatment of subclinical hypothyroidism.

**TABLE 3: Diagnosis of gestational diabetes mellitus (GDM).**

| **Diagnosis of pre-existing diabetes** | | | | | | |
|---|---|---|---|---|---|---|
| **Glycemic index** | | | | **Threshold** | | |
| Fasting plasma glucose | | | | ≥126 mg/dL | | |
| Random plasma glucose | | | | ≥200 mg/dL | | |
| HbA1c | | | | ≥6.5% | | |
| **Diagnosis of GDM** | | | | | | |
| **2-step approach** | | | | **1-step approach** | | |
| **Glycemic index** | **Threshold (mg/dL)** | | | **Glycemic index** | **Threshold (mg/dL)** | |
| 50 g OGCT | 1 hour | ≥130–140 | | 75 g OGCT# | | |
| | | NDDG | Carpentar-Couostan | | | |
| 100 g OGTT* | Fasting | ≥105 | ≥95 | | Fasting | ≥92 |
| | 1 hour | ≥190 | ≥180 | | 1 h | ≥180 |
| | 2 hours | ≥165 | ≥155 | | 2 h | ≥153 |
| | 3 hours | ≥145 | ≥140 | | | |

*Two or more values for diagnosis.
#One value for diagnosis.

(OGCT: oral glucose challenge; OGTT: oral glucose tolerance test; NDDGL national diabetes data group)

*Source*: Paschou SA, Blesta E, Papazisi M et al. Screening and management of major endocrinopathies during pregnancy : an update. Endocrine. 2023;80(1):10-19.

**TABLE 4: Antithyroid drugs in pregnancy**

| Antithyroid drug | Initial dose | Typical dose in an average patient | Usual frequency |
|---|---|---|---|
| Methimazole | 5–30 mg/day | 10–20 mg/day | Once daily |
| Carbimazole | 10–40 mg/day | | Once daily |
| Propylthiouracil | 100–600 mg/day | 200–400 mg/day | Split into two or three daily doses |

- A woman, on ATD for Graves disease, if currently euthyroid, may attempt to suspend therapy temporarily with close monitoring of thyroid function tests during the first trimester; or may consider propylthiouracil as alternate drug.
- To avoid deleterious foetal complications, particularly foetal hypothyroidism, the aim is to maintain maternal fT4 concentration at or just above the pregnancy-specific upper normal limit, using the lowest effective dose of antithyroid drugs.
- Beta-blockers like propranolol may be used to control adrenergic symptoms for a short period of 2–4 weeks, however, the risk of fetal bradycardia, intrauterine growth retardation and neonatal hypoglycemia needs to be well considered and kept in mind.
- If thyroidectomy is needed, second trimester is the most suitable period for surgery.

## MANAGEMENT (TABLE 5)

According to American Diabetes Association (ADA) guidelines, therapeutic options for GDM are dietary changes, physical exercise, and insulin therapy. Notably, metformin is not recommended as a first-line agent by ADA. On the contrary, the National Institute for Health and Care Excellence (NICE) guidelines recommend using metformin as a first-line agent in women whose diabetes is not adequately controlled by diet, before the institution of insulin therapy.

- *Medical nutrition therapy and exercise*: The first therapeutic step is conservative, based on mild exercise, such as walking for at least 30 min/day if not contraindicated, together with a low-glycemic diet, consisting of three main meals and three snacks. The total caloric intake starts from 1,800 kcal/day, consisting of 35–45% carbohydrates, 20–25% proteins, and 30–40% fat.
- *Pharmacological therapies*:
  - *Insulin*:
    - Insulin initiation is recommended if 10–20% or more of glucose concentrations are abnormal after 2 weeks of appropriate diet and exercise.
    - In women with elevated fasting and postprandial glucose concentrations, the recommended starting total dosage is 0.7–1.0 U/kg/day, administered by multiple injections combining long- or intermediate-acting and short-acting insulin.
    - NPH, detemir, regular, lispro, aspart and insulin degludec (recently approved) are safe to use during pregnancy.
  - *Metformin*: Oral and noninsulin injectable antidiabetic agents are generally contradicted as they cross the placenta Metformin crosses the placenta to the fetus, and its concentrations are similar to or higher than those in the pregnant woman; as a result, some safety issues remain. It may also act as an endocrine disruptor, affecting the expression of gonad-related genes. Metformin may also inhibit mitochondrial activity and result in nutrient restriction, negatively affecting the function, growth, or differentiation of fetal or placental tissues. These issues need to keep in mind while prescribing metformin.

**TABLE 5: Glycemic targets.**

| Blood glucose parameters | Values (mg/dL) |
|---|---|
| Fasting | <95 |
| 1 hour postprandial | <140 |
| 2 hours postprandial | <120 |

General recommendations for women with PGDM are similar to those with GDM. However, glycemic targets are slightly different (≤100 in the fasting state, ≤130 at 60 minutes postprandially, and ≤140 mg/dL at 120 minutes). Contaminant medication, such as statins, should be interrupted during gestation, even if dyslipidemia is present, while only safe for pregnancy antihypertensive agents should be used to avoid adverse fetal outcomes.

### Points to Ponder

- ❑ Gestational diabetes mellitus (GDM) is the most prevalent endocrine disease during pregnancy, followed by thyroid disorders.
- ❑ Endocrine parameters that must be examined during pregnancy are glucose metabolism, thyroid function, and calcium and vitamin D.
- ❑ Endocrine disorders may be classified as pre-existing and gestation-induced.
- ❑ Endocrine disorders and their management during pregnancy pose therapeutic challenges for endocrinologists and obstetricians due to their potentially harmful maternal and fetal health effects.

## MULTIPLE CHOICE QUESTIONS

1. **What is the likely diagnosis in this patient based on her TSH report?**
   A. Hyperthyroidism
   B. Subclinical hypothyroidism
   C. Overt hypothyroidism
   D. Euthyroidism
2. **What is the most appropriate next step to confirm the diagnosis of subclinical hypothyroidism in this patient?**
   A. Repeat TSH after delivery
   B. Perform free T4 and anti-TPO antibody testing
   C. Start levothyroxine therapy immediately
   D. Perform thyroid ultrasound
3. **What is the main risk associated with untreated subclinical hypothyroidism in pregnancy?**
   A. Hypertension
   B. Maternal weight gain
   C. Adverse fetal outcomes such as developmental delay
   D. Polyhydramnios
4. **How should the patient's fasting blood sugar (FBS) of 112 mg/dL be interpreted?**
   A. Normal for pregnancy
   B. Diagnostic of gestational diabetes mellitus (GDM)
   C. Requires an oral glucose tolerance test (OGTT) for confirmation
   D. Requires dietary modifications without further testing
5. **What would be the treatment goal if subclinical hypothyroidism is confirmed in this patient?**
   A. Normalize TSH levels to <10 μU/mL
   B. Maintain TSH levels within the trimester-specific reference range
   C. Achieve complete suppression of TSH
   D. Focus solely on fetal outcomes without adjusting TSH

### Answers

1. (B); 2. (B); 3. (C); 4. (C); 5. (B)

## REFERENCE

1. Thyroid Disease in Pregnancy. ACOG Practice Bulletin Obstet Gynecol. 2020;135(6):e261-e4.

CHAPTER 22

# A Case-based Approach to Dehydration

*Bhagirath B Solanki*

**CASE VIGNETTE**

A 37-year-old male presented with diarrhea and low grade fever for last 10–12 hours. Diarrhea are 18–20 times since onset and are loose, watery, mixed with mucus-pus, occasional streaks of blood, tenesmus and abdominal discomfort. He had watery vomiting three times in last 2 hours which are nonbloody and nonprojectile but associated with nausea. His complaints increased thirst, leg cramps, fatigue, and dizziness. He passed scanty high colored urine three times in last 6 hours. He is not suffering from any medical diseases and no addictions as well no other member of family/community suffered similar complaints. On examination temperature—99.8°F, pulse—118 beats/min, RR—17 breaths/min, BP—104/78 mm Hg with orthostatic drop. $SpO_2$—97% on room air. He is conscious, restless and moderately dehydrated. Per abdomen had vague lower abdominal tenderness, CVS—tachycardia and RS—normal. ECG—sinus tachycardia and RBS—105 mg%.

## PROVISIONAL DIAGNOSIS

Acute infectious gastroenteritis with moderate dehydration.

## DIFFERENTIAL DIAGNOSIS

This patient is suffering from acute gastroenteritis (AGE) with moderate dehydration resulting in hypotension and may be impending hypovolemic shock/AKI. In > 90% cases these are GI infections of acute onset with duration of hours to days and caused by infectious agents like bacteria, viruses, parasites and fungi (immunocompromised host). Clinical picture of watery diarrhea and vomiting is toxin mediated etiology while presence of blood-mucus in stool and associated with high fever, abdominal pain, bloating indicates inflammatory etiology. This clinical distinction usually becomes the basis for empiric antibiotics therapy. Remaining 10% cases are due to medications (magnesium containing antacids, laxatives, NSAIDs, antibiotics, antidepressants, colchicines, ferrous sulphate, alpha glucosidase inhibitor, chemo therapeutic agents) algid malaria, toxic ingestion (capsaicin, mushrooms, sea food), food allergy/anaphylaxis, herbal medicines, partial bowel obstruction, colonic ischemia, intestinal diverticulitis and GVHD. These are evident in the appropriate clinical settings. Tuberculosis, HIV-AIDS, IBD and GI malignancies causes insidious onset diarrhea of days to weeks duration with relevant clinical presentation pertaining to the disease concerned, but many a time their initial presentation mimics the acute watery diarrhea. Diarrhea is caused by feco-oral route of transmission via contaminated food or water and incubation period is from 1–3 hours to 3–5 days. Acute infection occurs when the ingested pathogen overcomes the host's defenses like gastric acidity, digestive enzymes, peristalsis, mucus secretions, suppressive gut flora and mucosal local immunity.

## PATHOPHYSIOLOGY

The pathophysiology in this case likely involves *bacterial invasion of the intestinal mucosa*, leading to an *inflammatory response* characterized by the release of cytokines and chemokines. This results in:

- *Mucosal damage*: Disruption of the epithelial barrier allows leakage of blood, mucus, and immune cells into the stool.
- *Increased fluid secretion*: Inflammation triggers excessive fluid and electrolyte loss, causing diarrhea and dehydration.
- *Systemic effects*: The body's response to dehydration and infection includes tachycardia, orthostatic hypotension, and fatigue.

These combined processes explain the patient's symptoms and clinical findings.

## CLINICAL APPROACH

Look for the signs of dehydration and it's severity to estimate the extent of fluid loss in a patient **(Table 1)**.

## INVESTIGATIONS

- *ECG*: Normal or sinus tachycardia or sometimes Changes related to $K^+$ CBC—hemoconcentration, raised WBC count as a SIRS/sepsis
- *RFT*: Normal or will shows features of AKI
- *Urine*: High specific gravity and low FENa
- *Stool*: Pus cells, blood, ova, cysts, motile organisms, lactoferrin, bacteriological studies, immunoassay for bacteria/viruses
- *USG abdominal*: Normal or signs of colitis

TABLE 1: Assessment of dehydration severity.

| Examination | Mild hypovolemia | Moderate hypovolemia | Severe hypovolemia |
|---|---|---|---|
| Mental status | Alert | Restless, irritable | Lethargic or unconscious |
| Tears | Moist, slightly dry | Dry | Very dry |
| Eyes | Normal | Sunken | Very sunken and dry |
| Mouth and tounge | Moist, slightly dry | Dry | Very dry |
| Thirst | Increased thirst | Thirsty, drinks eagerly | Drinks poorly or not able to drink |
| Skin pinch | Goes back rapidly | Goes back slowly | Goes back very slowly |
| Pulse | Normal | Rapid, weak | Very fast, weak or nonpalpable |
| Systolic blood pressure | Normal | Normal to orthostatic, >10 mm Hg change | Hypotension |
| Urine output | Decreased | Moderately decreased | Markedly decrease, anuria |
| *Extent of volume loss* | | | |
| | <5% of body weight | From 5 to 10% of body weight | >10% of body weight |
| *Estimated fluid deficit* | | | |
| | <50 mL/kg | 50–100 mL/kg | >100 mL/kg |

Sigmoidoscopy with biopsy, flexible endoscopy with duodenal aspirates and CT abdomen may be reserved for persistent diarrhea.

## TREATMENT AND PREVENTION

Check the signs of dehydration **(Table 1)** and decide about volume loss. If the patient is able to take orally, ORS and plenty of oral fluids are advised. IV fluids are administered as per the volume status of the patient.

### Oral Rehydration Solution

Principle of oral rehydration solution (ORS) contains a precise mix of sodium and glucose in 1:1 molar ratio. Absorption of glucose and sodium occurs through SGLT-1 receptor. The presence of glucose in ORS facilitates the absorption of sodium and water in the intestines, promoting rapid rehydration. Excess amount of either of the two can lead to osmotic diarrhea and further worsen the condition. Older (Standard) formula with more amount of glucose also caused hypernatremia.

### Intravenous Fluids

IV fluids are started with a large bore needle via a peripheral venous access preferably at two different sites. In presence of severe dehydration and shock when peripheral IV access is difficult, a central line can be considered. Type of IV fluid—Ringer's lactate (preferred) or normal saline (acceptable). Rate of IV fluid—30 mL/kg in first 30 minutes then slow down. Goal of IV fluid—200 mL/kg over 24 hours with 100 mL/kg in the first 4 hours. Reassure the patient regularly in first 6 hours and monitor for rehydration. Look for resolution of dehydration (urine output of at least 0.5 mL/kg/h) to decide about the escalation/continuation/de-escalation of IV fluids. One should keep in mind about the signs of fluid overload in patients with cardiac, renal and other medical conditions.

### Antibiotics

Appropriate antimicrobials are started according to the organism isolated in stool sample. Broad way to empiric treatment is according to geography, outbreak pattern and resistance development information. Accordingly, many physician uses a quinolone–ciprofloxacin 500 mg BID for 3–5 days, if febrile diarrhea and in suspected giardiasis an imidazole derivative—metronidazole, tinidazole is considered. Antibiotic coverage is indicated for immune compromised, have mechanical heart valves, vascular grafts and elderly even if causative organisms are discovered or not.

### Points to Ponder

- Diarrhea is passage of unusually loose or watery stools at least three times in 24 hours. It poses the threat of electrolyte disturbances, hypovolemia, shock, AKI and thrombo-occlusive episodes which increases in the morbidity and mortality.
- Clinical signs of dehydration, pulse, BP and thirst and urine output helps in assessment of volume status of the patients. ORS/ORT is sufficient for mild dehydration while moderate-to-severe dehydration requires IV fluids.
- Ringer's lactate is the choice of solution and normal saline is acceptable.
- Antibiotics are administered as per the evidence of organism in the stool examination and empiric treatment is based on clinical judgment.
- Strict public health measures about safe drinking water, sewerages, sanitation, food safety, health education and individual practice of hand wash is having the central role in prevention of feco-orally transmissible diseases.

## MULTIPLE CHOICE QUESTIONS

1. **What is the most likely etiology of this patient's condition?**
   A. Viral gastroenteritis
   B. Bacterial dysentery
   C. Amobic dysentery
   D. Food intolerance
2. **What is the most appropriate initial step in management for this patient?**
   A. Immediate administration of antibiotics
   B. Oral rehydration therapy (ORT) and electrolyte replacement
   C. Antidiarrheal medication
   D. IV proton-pump inhibitors
3. **Which investigation would be most helpful in confirming the diagnosis?**
   A. Complete blood count (CBC)
   B. Stool microscopy, culture, and sensitivity
   C. Abdominal ultrasound
   D. Serum electrolyte levels
4. **What finding on stool microscopy would support bacterial dysentery?**
   A. Presence of trophozoites
   B. Presence of leukocytes and erythrocytes
   C. Absence of leukocytes and erythrocytes
   D. Fat globules
5. **What is the primary goal of treatment in this patient?**
   A. Eradicate the infectious agent
   B. Prevent dehydration and electrolyte imbalance
   C. Reduce abdominal tenderness
   D. Control fever and vomiting

### Answers

1. (B); 2. (B); 3. (B); 4. (B); 5. (B)

## SUGGESTED READINGS


1. Camilleri M, Murray J. Diarrhea and constipation. Harrison's Principles of internal medicine. 21st edition. McGraw Hill. 2022. pp. 297-302.
2. Charles R, LaRocque R. Acute infectious diarrheal diseases and bacterial food poisoning. Harrison's Principles of internal medicine. 21st edition. McGraw Hill. 2022. pp. 1061-6.
3. World Health Organization. Updated guideline: paediatric emergency triage, assessment and treatment: care of critically-ill children. World Health Organization. Geneva. 2016. https://iris.who.int/handle/10665/204463 (Accessed on 28 July 2024).
4. Stefano G. Probiotics for Prevention and Treatment of Diarrhea. J Clin Gastroenterol. 2011:45 Suppl:S149-53.
5. Siri Ancha, Christine A, Devin C, et al. Diarrhea. The Washington Manual of Medical Therapeutics. 37th edition. Lippincott Williams & Wikins; 2022. pp. 631-3.

CHAPTER 23

# An Approach to a Case of Hypomagnesemia

*Sanjay Tandon, Arjun Tandon*

**CASE VIGNETTE**

A 55-year-old male presents to the clinic with complaints of persistent fatigue, generalized muscle cramps, and occasional palpitations over the past few weeks. He reports a history of chronic alcohol use and recent episodes of gastrointestinal disturbances, including diarrhea. He also mentions tingling in his hands and feet and occasional muscle twitching. Physical examination reveals slight tremors and hyperreflexia. Laboratory investigations reveal abnormalities in electrolyte levels.

## DIFFERENTIAL DIAGNOSIS

The patient's presenting symptoms and history necessitate consideration of several differential diagnoses, including:

- *Electrolyte imbalances*: Hypomagnesemia, hypokalemia, hypocalcemia.
- *Endocrine disorders*: Hyperparathyroidism, hypothyroidism.
- *Gastrointestinal disorders*: Chronic diarrhea, malabsorption syndromes (e.g., Crohn's disease, celiac disease).
- *Renal disorders*: Chronic kidney disease, tubular dysfunction.
- *Neurological disorders*: Seizure disorders, neuromuscular disorders.
- *Cardiovascular conditions*: Arrhythmias secondary to electrolyte imbalances.

## CLINICAL APPROACH

### Signs and Symptoms

The clinical manifestations of hypomagnesemia vary widely, depending on the severity and chronicity of the deficiency.

- *Mild hypomagnesemia*: Often asymptomatic or presents with nonspecific symptoms such as fatigue, weakness, and anorexia. Patients may not recognize these symptoms as related to an electrolyte disturbance, leading to delayed diagnosis.
- *Neuromuscular symptoms*: Include muscle cramps, tremors, carpopedal spasm, tetany, and in severe cases, seizures. Chvostek's and Trousseau's signs may be positive. Neuromuscular symptoms are often the most prominent and distressing for patients. Seizures and tetany occur due to increased neuronal excitability resulting from reduced magnesium levels.
- *Cardiovascular symptoms*: Palpitations, arrhythmias (e.g., atrial fibrillation, ventricular arrhythmias), and hypertension. Hypomagnesemia can precipitate life-threatening arrhythmias, particularly in patients with underlying heart disease. Torsades de pointes, a form of polymorphic ventricular tachycardia, is a particularly dangerous arrhythmia associated with severe hypomagnesemia.
- *CNS symptoms*: Include irritability, depression, confusion, and in severe cases, delirium or coma. The CNS manifestations are due to the role of magnesium in neurotransmitter release and neuronal stability. Severe deficiency can lead to profound neurological disturbances, including altered mental status and coma.
- *Other symptoms*: Hypokalemia and hypocalcemia are commonly associated with hypomagnesemia due to its effect on renal potassium and parathyroid hormone secretion. Hypomagnesemia-induced hypokalemia occurs because magnesium is a cofactor for the renal outer medullary potassium channel (ROMK), which is involved in potassium retention in the kidneys.

### Classification of Hypomagnesemia

#### *Mild Hypomagnesemia (1.2–1.7 mg/dL)*

- *Symptoms*:
  - Fatigue
  - Muscle cramps
  - Nausea
  - Anorexia
- *Signs*:
  - Slightly increased deep tendon reflexes (DTRs)
  - Mild tremors or fasciculations

#### *Moderate Hypomagnesemia (0.6–1.2 mg/dL)*

- *Symptoms*:
  - More pronounced muscle weakness
  - Paresthesia (tingling or numbness)
  - Mood changes (anxiety, depression)
  - Sleep disturbances

- *Signs*:
  - Increased DTRs
  - Positive Chvostek's sign (facial twitching upon tapping)
  - Positive Trousseau's sign (carpal spasm upon occlusion of the brachial artery)

### Severe Hypomagnesemia (< 0.6 mg/dL)

- *Symptoms*:
  - Severe muscle weakness
  - Arrhythmias (e.g., torsades de pointes)
  - Seizures
  - Altered mental status (confusion, lethargy)
- *Signs*:
  - Significant DTRs
  - Ataxia
  - Respiratory depression
  - Hypocalcemia or hypokalemia (often accompanying electrolyte imbalances)

## DIAGNOSIS

Diagnosis involves a comprehensive clinical evaluation, including a detailed history and physical examination, and laboratory tests.

### Clinical Evaluation

A thorough clinical assessment is the first step in diagnosing magnesium disorders:

- *History taking*:
  - Symptom review: Fatigue, muscle weakness, cramps, arrhythmias, and neurological symptoms.
  - Medical history: Assess for gastrointestinal disorders, renal diseases, or chronic medication use (e.g., diuretics, proton pump inhibitors).
- *Physical examination*:
  - Check for signs of magnesium deficiency such as:
    - Muscle twitching or spasms.
    - Neurological deficits (e.g., seizures).
    - Cardiac arrhythmias (detected via ECG).

### Laboratory Tests

- *Serum magnesium levels*:
  - Normal range: 1.7–2.3 mg/dL (0.85–1.15 mmol/L).
  - Sensitivity and specificity:
    - Sensitivity: Approximately 75% for detecting hypomagnesemia.
    - Specificity: Around 85%, but may be falsely normal in patients with low intracellular magnesium despite normal serum levels.
- *24-hour urinary magnesium excretion*:
  - Useful for determining renal handling of magnesium.
  - Normal range: 100–400 mg/day.
  - Sensitivity and specificity:
    - Sensitivity: 70% for identifying magnesium deficiency.
    - Specificity: 80% for distinguishing between renal and gastrointestinal causes of magnesium loss.
- *Ionized magnesium*:
  - Measures the biologically active form of magnesium.
  - Sensitivity and specificity:
    - More accurate for assessing true magnesium status than serum levels alone.
    - Higher sensitivity in cases of critical illness.
- *Additional electrolyte tests*:
  - Calcium and potassium levels: Often measured alongside magnesium due to interdependencies.
  - Parathyroid hormone (PTH): Evaluates for secondary causes of magnesium disorders.

### Advanced Diagnostic Tools

#### Magnesium Load Test

The magnesium load test is a diagnostic procedure used to assess the body's ability to absorb and retain magnesium. It is particularly useful in diagnosing magnesium deficiency, especially when serum magnesium levels may not reflect total body magnesium status.

#### Indications

- Suspected magnesium deficiency despite normal serum magnesium levels.
- Patients with conditions that predispose them to magnesium loss (e.g., chronic diarrhea, malabsorption syndromes, renal issues).
- Monitoring response to magnesium supplementation.

#### Procedure

- *Preparation*: Ensure the patient has not taken magnesium supplements or medications that may affect magnesium levels for at least one week prior to the test.
- *Baseline assessment*: Obtain baseline serum magnesium and urinary magnesium levels to evaluate pre-test status.
- *Administration of magnesium*:
  - Administer a magnesium supplement, typically in the form of magnesium sulfate or magnesium oxide, either orally or intravenously.
  - The dose may vary but is often around 1 g (or equivalent) for oral administration.
- *Urinary collection*: Collect urine over a 24-hour period following magnesium administration to measure urinary magnesium excretion.
- *Follow-up testing*: Repeat serum magnesium levels may also be obtained after the test period to assess the immediate impact of the magnesium load.

#### Interpretation of Results

- *Increased urinary excretion*: A high percentage of the administered magnesium excreted in urine (usually >70%) suggests adequate renal function and a positive response to the magnesium load, indicating that magnesium stores were low prior to the test.
- *Low urinary excretion*: If less than 50–70% of the administered magnesium is excreted, it may indicate:
  - Renal retention: Suggesting magnesium deficiency or an adaptive response to low magnesium status.
  - Renal failure: In cases of renal impairment, the kidneys may be unable to excrete magnesium efficiently.

### Sensitivity and Specificity

The magnesium load test is generally considered a useful tool for detecting chronic magnesium deficiency. However, sensitivity and specificity can vary based on the population studied and underlying conditions.

### Limitations

- The test may not be practical in all clinical settings due to the need for careful monitoring and patient compliance.
- Factors such as acute illness, hydration status, and dietary intake can influence results.

## Bone Biopsy (Rarely Used)

- Direct measurement of magnesium in bone, typically reserved for research or extreme cases.
- Limited clinical utility due to invasiveness.

## PATHOPHYSIOLOGY (FIGS. 1 AND 2)

The pathophysiology of hypomagnesemia is complex and involves multiple organ systems, primarily due to magnesium's role as a crucial intracellular ion involved in various biochemical processes, including enzyme activation, bone health, DNA synthesis, cardiovascular stability and maintaining electrical potentials across cell membranes.

The deficiency leads to a cascade of disturbances in neuromuscular, cardiovascular, and central nervous system functions, often exacerbated by concurrent electrolyte imbalances. The underlying causes are diverse, ranging from gastrointestinal and renal losses to chronic alcoholism, chronic diarrhea, malabsorption syndromes and endocrine disorders.

Hypomagnesemia frequently coexists with other electrolyte imbalances, such as hypokalemia and hypocalcemia, due to its role in renal potassium handling and PTH secretion. These associated electrolyte disorders further complicate the clinical picture and require concurrent management.

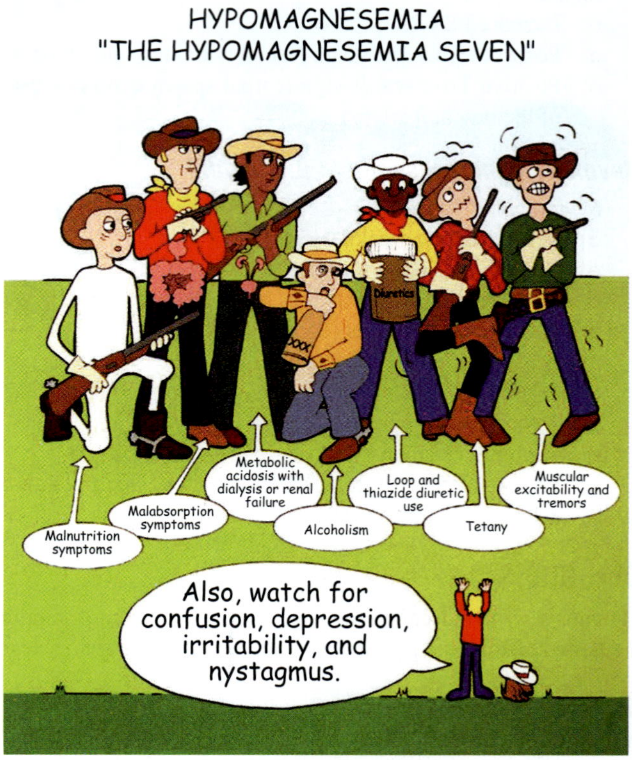


**FIG. 1:** Seven key symptoms of hypomagnesemia.

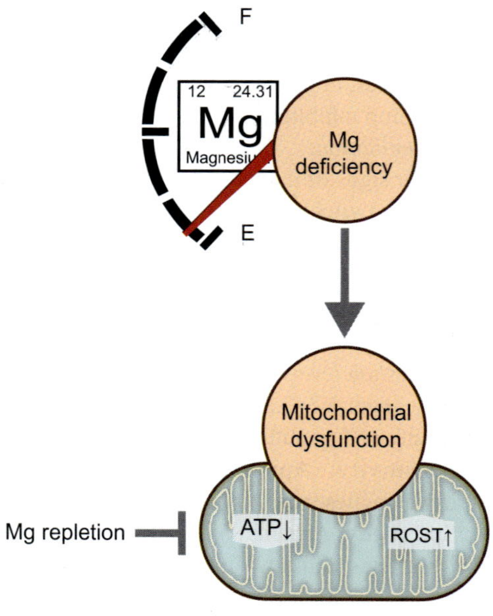


**FIG. 2:** Hypomagnesemia pathophysiology.

*Source*: With permission from Liu M, Liu H, Feng F, et al. Magnesium deficiency causes a reversible, metabolic, diastolic cardiomyopathy. J Am Heart Assoc. 2021;10(12).

## TREATMENT

The treatment of hypomagnesemia involves correcting the underlying cause and replenishing magnesium stores.

- *Mild-to-moderate hypomagnesemia*: Oral magnesium supplements, such as magnesium oxide or magnesium chloride, are often sufficient. Dietary sources rich in magnesium, including green leafy vegetables, nuts, seeds, and whole grains, should be encouraged. Oral supplementation is preferred for stable patients as it is safe, convenient, and effective.
- The recommended dietary allowance (RDA) for magnesium varies by age and gender:
    - Adult men: 400–420 mg/day
    - Adult women: 310–320 mg/day
    - Pregnant women: 350–360 mg/day
    - Older adults: Needs may increase due to absorption changes.
    - Typical supplement doses:
        - Magnesium oxide: 250–500 mg (elemental magnesium) daily.
        - Magnesium citrate: 200–400 mg daily.
        - Magnesium glycinate: 100–400 mg daily.
        - Magnesium chloride: 200–400 mg daily.
        - Magnesium malate: 300–600 mg daily.
- *Severe or symptomatic hypomagnesemia*: Intravenous magnesium sulfate is indicated. The initial dose is typically 1–2 g (8–16 mEq) administered over 5–60 minutes, followed by a continuous infusion if necessary. Continuous cardiac monitoring is recommended during IV magnesium administration due to the risk of arrhythmias. Intravenous therapy is reserved for patients with severe deficiency, symptomatic patients, or those unable to tolerate oral supplements.

- *Monitoring and follow-up*:
    - During IV magnesium administration
    - Serum magnesium levels:
        - Check every 6–12 hours based on clinical status and dosage.
        - Target levels typically range from 1.7 to 2.5 mg/dL during treatment.
    - Vital signs monitoring:
        - Monitor heart rate, blood pressure, and respiratory rate continuously.
        - Assess for hypotension and bradycardia.
    - Neuromuscular function:
        - Evaluate for signs of muscle weakness or respiratory distress.
        - Monitor deep tendon reflexes (DTRs).

*Signs of magnesium toxicity*:
- *Clinical signs*:
    - CNS effects: Drowsiness, confusion, decreased reflexes.
    - Neuromuscular effects: Muscle weakness, respiratory depression.
    - Cardiovascular effects: Bradycardia, hypotension, and potentially cardiac arrest.
    - Gastrointestinal effects: Nausea and vomiting.

*Post-administration monitoring*:
- *Continued monitoring*: Continue to monitor serum magnesium levels for 24 hours postinfusion to detect any rebound effects or delayed toxicity.
- *Renal function*: Assess renal function daily to adjust future magnesium doses appropriately.

## Points to Ponder

- *Interdependence of electrolytes*: Hypomagnesemia often coexists with hypokalemia and hypocalcemia, necessitating a comprehensive approach to electrolyte management.
- *Chronic alcoholism*: A significant risk factor for hypomagnesemia due to poor dietary intake and gastrointestinal losses.
- *Medication-induced hypomagnesemia*: Awareness of common medications that can induce hypomagnesemia, such as diuretics and proton pump inhibitors, is crucial.
- *Special populations*: Elderly patients and those with multiple comorbidities are at higher risk and require vigilant monitoring.
- *Prevention and education*: Educating patients on the importance of dietary magnesium and regular follow-up can help prevent recurrent hypomagnesemia.

## MULTIPLE CHOICE QUESTIONS

**1. Which of the following is a common symptom of hypomagnesemia?**
A. Hyperkalemia
B. Hypotension
C. Muscle cramps
D. Hypercalcemia

**2. What is the typical range for normal serum magnesium levels?**
A. 0.5–1.0 mg/dL
B. 1.7–2.3 mg/dL
C. 2.5–3.0 mg/dL
D. 3.0–3.5 mg/dL

**3. Which sign is associated with hypomagnesemia and neuromuscular irritability?**
A. Positive Babinski's sign
B. Positive Chvostek's sign
C. Negative Tinel's sign
D. Positive Romberg's sign

**4. Which of the following laboratory findings would most likely be seen in a patient with severe hypomagnesemia?**
A. Elevated serum calcium
B. Hypokalemia
C. Hyperphosphatemia
D. Elevated parathyroid hormone (PTH)

**5. A life-threatening arrhythmia associated with severe hypomagnesemia is:**
A. Atrial fibrillation
B. Torsades de pointes
C. Bradycardia
D. Sinus tachycardia

### Answers

1. (C); 2. (B); 3. (B) 4. (B); 5. (B)

## SUGGESTED READINGS


1. Rude RK, Shils ME. Magnesium deficiency: Clinical manifestations and management. The New England Journal of Medicine. 2012.
2. Jameson JL, Fauci AS, Kasper DL. Electrolyte and acid-base disorders (20th ed.). In Harrison's Principles of Internal Medicine. 2018.
3. Shechter M, Shalmon G. Magnesium and cardiovascular disease: Pathophysiological and clinical implications. Journal of the American College of Cardiology. 2016.
4. Schenker S, Halsted CH. Chronic alcoholism and electrolyte imbalances: A focus on magnesium. Alcohol Research: Current Reviews. 2015.
5. Grober U, Schmidt J. Drug-induced magnesium deficiency: Mechanisms and implications. The Lancet. 2014.
6. Elin RJ, Hosking DJ. The magnesium load test: Diagnostic utility in clinical practice. Clinical Chemistry. 2013.
7. Polderman KH, Girbes AR. Magnesium treatment in critical illness: Overview and recommendations. Critical Care Medicine. 2017.
8. Barbagallo M, Dominguez LJ. Neuromuscular effects of magnesium deficiency in clinical practice. Journal of Neurology, Neurosurgery & Psychiatry. 2014.
9. Quamme GA. Renal regulation of magnesium homeostasis. Kidney International. 2015.
10. Rosanoff A, Weaver CM, Rude RK. Dietary magnesium: Health benefits and recommendations. The American Journal of Clinical Nutrition. 2016.
11. Reddy KS, Naik N. The role of magnesium deficiency in cardiovascular diseases: An Indian perspective. Indian Heart Journal. 2018.

CHAPTER

24

# An Approach to a Case of Recurrent Hyponatremia

*Anupama YJ, Sangram S Biradar*

## CASE VIGNETTE

Mrs P, a 75-year-old lady was brought to the psychiatrist with complaints of aggressive behavior, irritability and forgetfulness. She had nausea and vomiting for a few days prior to this. She was a patient with diabetes for the past 12 years and hypertension for the past 6 years. Her medications included glibenclamide, metformin, telmisartan and hydrochlorothiazide.

Clinical examination showed that she had BP of 130/70 mm Hg, no pedal edema and systemic examination was unremarkable. She had recent memory deficits and incoherent speech. No obvious neurological deficits noted. Computerized tomography of the brain did not show any abnormality. Her laboratory parameters revealed random blood sugar of 145 mg/dL, serum creatinine of 1.5 mg/dL, serum sodium of 122 mmol/L, potassium ($K^+$) of 3.6 mmol/L. She was treated in the hospital with hypertonic saline. She was discharged with a prescription of haloperidol 5 mg/day and anticholinergics to control her restlessness. She remained well for a few days, after which her symptoms recurred. She became stuporous and she was taken back to the same doctor. Serum creatinine was 2.2 mg% and serum $Na^+$ was 115 mmol/L at this time. 3% saline was started again and the patient had a transient increase in serum $Na^+$ the next day to 120 mmol/L. But over the next few days, serum $Na^+$ dropped to 112 mmol/L. She was referred to the nephrologist for renal evaluation. On examination, the patient had dry oral mucosa, BP was 110/80 mm Hg, and pulse was 110 beats/min, regular. She was noted to have rigidity of all limbs. Urine $Na^+$ was 8 mmol/L. She was evaluated to be volume depleted and intravenous hydration was started. She was hydrated with intravenous normal saline at 100 mL/h for the next 12 hours. Haloperidol, telmisartan and hydrochlorothiazide were withdrawn. Repeat serum $Na^+$ was 120 mmol/L, hydration was continued for next 24 hours at 75 m/h. At the end of day 3, serum creatinine was 1.1 mg%, $Na^+$ was 130 mmol/L, and $K^+$ was 4.5 mmol/L. Blood pressure was 160/100 mm Hg and she was put on calcium channel blockers. Her sensorium improved and the memory improved. She started recognizing relatives and speaking relevantly. Rigidity reduced and the hydration was adequate. She was discharged in a stable state.

## PROVISIONAL DIAGNOSIS

Hypovolemic hyponatremia secondary to diuretic use (hydrochlorothiazide) and inadequate sodium intake.

## DIFFERENTIAL DIAGNOSIS

- Syndrome of inappropriate antidiuretic hormone secretion (SIADH).
- Drug-induced hyponatremia (haloperidol, hydrochlorothiazide, telmisartan).
- Adrenal insufficiency.
- Acute kidney injury with volume depletion.
- Hyponatremia due to poor oral intake and overhydration.

## CLINICAL APPROACH

Hyponatremia can be due to a variety of causes. Renal and extrarenal loss of salt and water stimulate secretion of antidiuretic hormone (ADH) which is an appropriate response by the body and may lead to hyponatremia. Syndrome of inappropriate secretion of ADH also may occur due to a variety of causes and may result in hyponatremia. Chronic heart failure, cirrhosis and nephrotic syndrome may result in a low circulating blood volume and hyponatremia is seen in these conditions too.

Generally, acute hyponatremia often presents with devastating symptoms whereas chronic hyponatremia (hyponatremia > 48 hours) may be asymptomatic. Mild-to-moderate hyponatremia (serum sodium >125–134 mmol/L) may not need treatment.

Diagnosis of the cause of hyponatremia depends on assessment of serum osmolality. True hyponatremia is almost always hypo osmolar. Thereafter, determining the volume status of the patient will lead to ascertaining the probable cause for hyponatremia **(Flowchart 1)**.

Patients could be hypovolemic, euvolemic or hypervolemic. In hypovolemic hyponatremia, low urine sodium is indicative of hypovolemia due to extrarenal loss of salt and water as in vomiting and diarrhea. Urine sodium > 20 mmol/L in the presence of hypovolemia indicates a renal loss of sodium and water. Similarly hypervolemic hyponatremia may be due to extrarenal causes or renal causes. Hypervolemia can be due to cardiac failure, renal failure or cirrhosis. In patients who appear to be euvolemic, hyponatremia is more often due to conditions

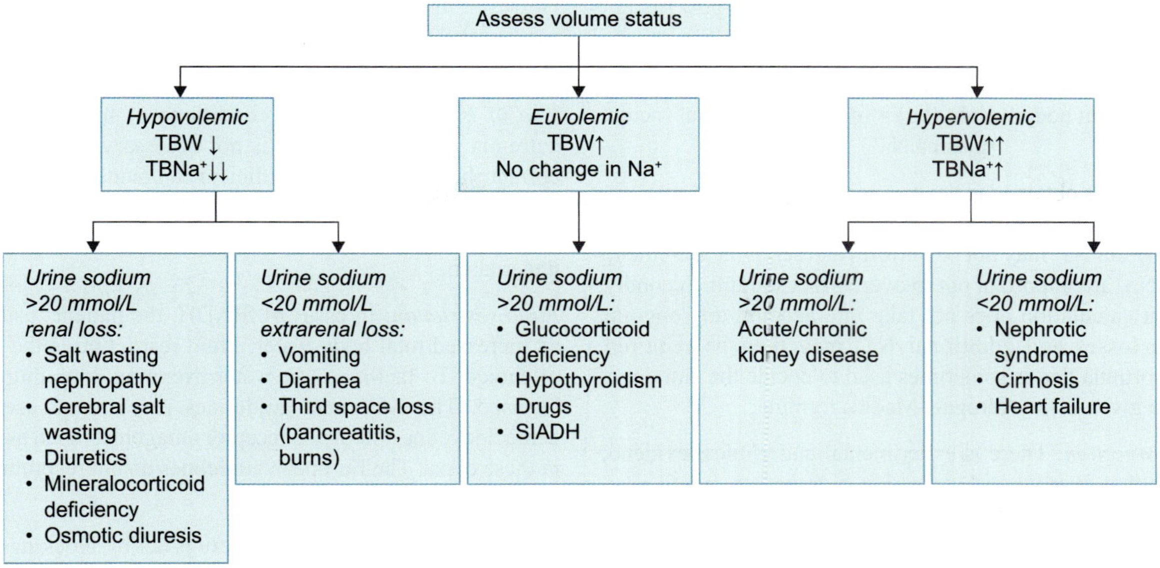


**FLOWCHART 1:** Approach to the diagnosis of hyponatremia.

like syndrome of inappropriate secretion of antidiuretic hormone (SIADH). SIADH can be due to a variety of causes like drugs, malignancies, neurologic causes, pulmonary diseases, etc. Other causes for euvolemic hyponatremia include cortisol deficiency, hypothyroidism or diuretics.

Many commonly used drugs may cause hyponatremia by various mechanisms. Drugs causing hyponatremia are enumerated in **Box 1**. Diuretics can cause hyponatremia, and among them, thiazide groups of drugs are the most common culprits. They impair sodium absorption in the distal tubule and impair the diluting capacity of the tubule. Other diuretics such amiloride, spironolactone, furosemide, torsemide may also rarely cause hyponatremia. Angiotensin-converting enzyme inhibitors, angiotensin receptor blockers, proton pump inhibitors, antidiabetic drugs such as gliclazide, glimeperide, and levodopa may all rarely cause hyponatremia. It is prudent to review all the medications that the patient is taking currently, when confronted with hyponatremia.

**BOX 1: Drugs causing hyponatremia.**

- *Drugs affecting sodium and water homeostasis*:
  - *Diuretics*: Thiazides, indapamide, amiloride, spironolactone, loop diuretics
- *Drugs affecting water homeostasis*:
  - Increased hypothalamic production of antidiuretic hormone (ADH) or potentiate the effect of ADH:
    - Antidepressants: Tricyclic antidepressants (amitriptyline, protriptyline, desipramine)
    - Selective serotonin reuptake inhibitors
    - Monoamine oxidase inhibitors
    - Antipsychotic drugs: Phenothiazines (thioridazine, trifluoperazine), haloperidol
    - Antiepileptic drugs: Carbamazepine, sodium valproate
    - Anticancer agents: Vinca alkaloids, cisplatin, carboplatin, intravenous cyclophosphamide, melphalan, ifosfamide
    - Nonsteroidal anti-inflammatory drugs
  - Reset osmostat:
    - Antidepressants: Venlafaxine, quetiapine
    - Antiepileptic drugs: Carbamazepine
  - Exogenous ADH (desmopressin) and oxytocin
- *Rare and miscellaneous causes*:
  - Antihypertensive agents: Angiotensin-converting enzyme inhibitors, angiotensin receptor blockers, amlodipine
  - Antibiotics: Trimethoprim-sulfamethoxazole, ciprofloxacin, cefoperazone/sulbactam
  - Antiarrhythmic drugs: Amiodarone
  - Theophylline
  - Proton pump inhibitors

*Source*: Adapted from Liamis G, et al. (2008).

## PATHOPHYSIOLOGY

Recurrent hyponatremia arises from repeated triggers like diuretic use, excessive water intake, or chronic conditions such as SIADH. Hydrochlorothiazide inhibits sodium reabsorption in the distal tubule, causing sodium and water loss, leading to volume depletion and increased ADH secretion. Inadequate sodium intake worsens the deficit, and water retention further dilutes serum sodium, perpetuating hyponatremia.

## TREATMENT AND PREVENTION

It must be remembered that hyponatremia is due to a disorder of water balance in the body. There is primarily an excess of total body water and deficit of total body $Na^+$. The removal of the excess water and addition of $Na^+$ is the cornerstone of therapy. Hypertonic saline, isotonic saline, fluid restriction, intravenous furosemide are all used in varying combinations in the treatment and the success of treatment depends on the appropriateness of the treatment chosen. The presence or absence of symptoms and acuteness of hyponatremia are important guides to the rate of correction of $Na^+$ deficit.

*Hypertonic saline*: Use of hypertonic saline must be governed by the calculation of sodium deficit in the body.

$$Na^+ \text{ deficit} = \text{volume of distribution of plasma} \times Na^+ \text{ deficit per liter} = 0.5 \times \text{lean body weight (kg)} \times (\text{desired serum } Na^+ - \text{actual plasma } Na^+)$$

The value that is obtained is the $Na^+$ required to raise the plasma $Na^+$ concentration to a safe level of 120 mEq/L. However, the rate of rise in serum $Na^+$ may not be uniform and serial measurements of serum $Na^+$ are important not to overcorrect sodium. Secondly, this deficit calculation does not take into account any ongoing isosmotic losses and additional $Na^+$ may then be required. Another formula that is sometimes used to decide the amount of fluid to be given is the Adrogue–Madias formula.

*Rate of correction*: There is experimental and clinical evidence to suggest that overly rapid correction of hyponatremia to near-normal sodium levels can be harmful and may lead to osmotic demyelination syndrome. This is a neurologic condition and is said to occur because the astrocytes in the brain have an impaired ability to respond to a sudden increase in tonicity of extracellular fluid that occurs after the sodium is rapidly corrected. The patient may have altered sensorium, delirium, impaired memory. Sometimes, the patient may develop quadriparesis and pseudobulbar palsy, and be in a "locked-in" state. Hence, generally one is advised to correct sodium by not > 10–12 mEq/L over the first 24 hours and < 18 mEq/L over the first 2 days. However in acute, severe hyponatremia, there is evidence to suggest that rapid correction may be done for the first 6 hours and then slowed down.

*Use of isotonic saline*: In conditions of hypovolemic hyponatremia, hypertonic saline is not necessary. Isotonic saline to correct the fluid deficit is sufficient to counter the hypovolemic stimulus to ADH secretion and hyponatremia may be corrected. Correction of the underlying cause for hypovolemia must also be undertaken.

*Fluid restriction*: In cases of SIADH, the patients usually have an increased total body water. Fluid restriction is the treatment of choice. To facilitate free water excretion, loop diuretics may be used. The American guidelines recommend use of urea, demeclocycline and/or V2-receptor antagonists such as tolvaptan in these cases. The European guidelines do not recommend these alternative agents.

*V2 receptor antagonists*: These drugs act by blocking the ADH action on the cells of collecting tubules. This results in reduced urinary concentration and excretion of dilute urine. Tolvaptan is readily and easily available and can be used in SIADH, and hypervolemic hyponatremia as in cardiac failure and cirrhosis. However, the rate of rise of serum $Na^+$ is unpredictable.

In cases of glucocorticoid deficiency, mineralocorticoid deficiency and hypothyroidism, specific therapy to correct the endocrine disturbance should be instituted.

## Points to Ponder

- Hyponatremia is a common disorder of water balance. Patients may be asymptomatic or may have severe symptoms affecting the nervous system.
- Approach to diagnosis depends on assessment of volume status and urinary $Na^+$ and osmolality. Treatment should be tailored according to the presentation of the patient and includes treating the underlying cause as well as correction of sodium deficit.
- Many commonly used drugs may cause hyponatremia. When a patient presents with recurrent hyponatremia, review of all the drugs that the patient is currently taking, may help to unravel the cause.

## MULTIPLE CHOICE QUESTIONS

**1. What is the most likely cause of recurrent hyponatremia in this patient?**
A. Overhydration
B. Excessive sodium intake
C. Diuretic use and volume depletion
D. Hyperglycemia

**2. Which drug was most likely contributing to the patient's hyponatremia?**
A. Metformin
B. Telmisartan
C. Hydrochlorothiazide
D. Haloperidol

**3. What was the primary intervention that led to the patient's improvement?**
A. Administration of hypertonic saline
B. Withdrawal of hydrochlorothiazide and telmisartan
C. Use of haloperidol
D. Starting calcium channel blockers

**4. What was the key clinical finding that indicated volume depletion?**
A. BP of 160/100 mm Hg
B. Urine sodium of 8 mmol/L
C. Random blood sugar of 145 mg/dL
D. Serum creatinine of 1.5 mg%

**5. What was the most appropriate long-term management strategy for this patient?**
A. Re-initiation of diuretics at a lower dose
B. Periodic hydration monitoring and withdrawal of offending drugs
C. Long-term haloperidol therapy
D. Increasing sodium intake with supplements

### Answers

1. (A); 2. (A); 3. (C); 4. (B); 5. (B)

## SUGGESTED READINGS


1. Rose BD, Post TW. Hypoosmolal states-Hyponatremia. In: Rose BD, Post TW (Eds). Clinical Physiology of Acid-Base and Electrolyte Disorders, 5th edition. McGraw Hill; 2001.
2. Hoorn EJ, Zietse R. Diagnosis and Treatment of Hyponatremia: Compilation of the Guidelines. J Am Soc Nephrol. 2017;28(5):1340-9.
3. Kashkouli A, Berl T, Sands JM. Disorders of water metabolism. In: Editors. Johnson RJ, Floege J, Tonelli M (Eds). Comprehensive Clinical Nephrology, 7th edition. Elseviers Publications; 2023.
4. Liamis G, Milionis H, Elisaf M. A review of drug-induced hyponatremia. Am J Kidney Dis. 2008;52(1):144-53.
5. Sahay M, Sahay R. Hyponatremia: A practical approach. Indian J Endocrinol Metab. 2014;18(6):760-71.
6. Verbalis JG, Goldsmith SR, Greenberg A, et al. Diagnosis, evaluation, and treatment of hyponatremia: Expert panel recommendations. Am J Med. 2013;126(Suppl 1):S1-S42.
7. Spasovski G, Vanholder R, Allolio B, et al. Hyponatraemia Guideline Development Group: Clinical practice guideline on diagnosis and treatment of hyponatraemia. Nephrol Dial Transplant. 2014;29(Suppl2): i1–i39.

CHAPTER 25

# An Approach to a Case of Refractory Ascites

*Atul Mehrotra, S Anita Nambiar*

**CASE VIGNETTE**

Mr X, a 60-year-old male patient, is hepatitis B positive, with alcohol use > 60 g for more than the last 30 years. He has a history of ascites for the last 2 years. The ascites was initially responding well to diuretic usage on two tablets of Lasilactone and sodium restriction. In the last 6 months, he has been admitted twice with the complication of hepatic encephalopathy. On evaluation, the potential cause was found to be hypokalemia that was diuretic induced. On lowering the dose of diuretic, he recovered but on the lower dose the ascites could not be controlled. Each time the diuretic dose was increased, he landed up in hepatic encephalopathy. He has now come for evaluation of his ascites and further management.

He had no history of hematemesis or melena. His current presentation was with abdominal distension and shortness of breath.

On physical examination, he had a blood pressure of 110/70 mm Hg, a heart rate of 104 beats/min, respiratory rate of 26 breaths/min, normal body temperature, and $SpO_2$ of 96% in room air. There was mild pallor. On abdominal examination, he had tense ascites (grade 3) and abdominal distension with pitting edema in the lower extremities. The rest of the examination was within normal range.

Laboratory values on admission were as follows: WBC 4,090 cells/cc; hemoglobin 7.8 g/dL; MCV 74 fL; MCH 22 pg; PLT 136,000; albumin 2.6 g/dL; SGOT 13 U/L; SGPT 12 U/L; BUN 50 mg/dL; serum creatinine 0.78 mg/dL; Na 130 mmol/L; K 2.9 mmol/L; and Cl 90 mmol/L. No abnormalities were found on chest X-ray.

## PROVISIONAL DIAGNOSIS

The provisional diagnosis for this case appears to be decompensated cirrhosis with refractory ascites (RA) and hepatic encephalopathy due to a combination of chronic hepatitis B and alcoholic liver disease.

## DIFFERENTIAL DIAGNOSIS

In a patient of ascites, the first priority is to determine the etiology of ascites. This further determines the management. A routine ultrasound of the abdomen to confirm the presence of ascites in a patient with abdominal distension is the primary test. This should be accompanied with a Doppler study of the hepatic venous system to rule out hepatic venous obstruction–a cause of ascites that is often overlooked. Doppler also helps in assessing the hepatic venous gradient which is important and a decisive test to determine the source of ascites, whether sinusoidal or not. Diagnostic paracentesis is the first test that needs to be done. Serum-ascites albumin gradient (SAAG) (a measure of sinusoidal pressure) and ascites total protein are two tests that taken together are very useful and inexpensive **(Table 1)**. Three main causes of ascites—cirrhosis, peritoneal pathology such as tuberculosis or malignancy, and heart failure—can be easily diagnosed by combining these two.

When the considered source is likely to be peritoneal (such as carcinomatosis or tuberculosis), laparoscopy with peritoneal biopsy, culture, and histological examination is needed.

## CLINICAL APPROACH

### Definition

Refractory ascites is ascites that cannot be mobilized or early recurrence of which (after therapeutic paracentesis) cannot be satisfactorily prevented by medical therapy. It can be divided into:

- *Diuretic-resistant ascites*: Lack of response to dietary sodium restriction and intensive diuretic treatment. It is pertinent to add that failure to respond to the dosage of diuretics

**TABLE 1: Serum-ascites albumin gradient (SAAG): A measure of sinusoidal pressure in assessing portal hypertension.**

| | | |
|---|---|---|
| Cirrhosis | High SAAG > 1.1 g/dL | Low ascites protein < 2.5 g/dL |
| Peritoneal disease | Low SAAG < 1.1 g/dL | High ascites protein > 2.5 g/dL |
| Heart failure | High SAAG > 1.1 g/dL | High ascites protein > 2.5 g/dL |

considered to be intensive (being 160 mg/day of furosemide or 40 mg/day of torsemide and 400 mg/day of spironolactone or 30 mg/day of amiloride along with low sodium diet for a period of ≥7 days) is important to label a patient to have refractory ascites
- *Diuretic-intractable ascites*: Development of a diuretic-induced complication that precludes the use of an effective diuretic dosage

## Causes

About 75% of the patients presenting as ascites have cirrhosis as its underlying cause. It is a major complication of cirrhosis seen in 50% of the patients over a 10-year follow-up period and is associated with a 50% mortality over a 2-year period. Other major causes of ascites are malignancy 10%, heart failure 3%, tuberculosis 2%, and pancreatitis among others.

Among the various liver disorders causing ascites, cirrhosis is the foremost and may be due to chronic hepatitis C, chronic hepatitis B, nonalcoholic fatty liver disease (NAFLD renamed as MASLD), history of high alcohol intake, chronic heart failure with liver congestion, long-term usage of drugs like anabolic steroids and methotrexate, autoimmune hepatitis, genetic disorders like hemochromatosis and Wilson's disease, primary biliary cholangitis, and diseases leading to blockage of bile ducts.

A detailed history to evaluate and rule out the above causes forms an essential part of the approach to the patient. Main symptoms of refractory ascites are:
- Progressive painless non-reducing abdominal swelling
- Weight gain
- Abdominal tenderness
- Dyspnea

Refractory ascites may be associated with complications such as:
- Hepatorenal syndrome (HRS)
- Bacterial infections
- Hepatic encephalopathy
- Hernias
- Pleural effusion

Major signs to look for which are red flags:
- Thorough general physical examination to evaluate for hypovolemia, presence of jaundice, pedal edema
- Tense abdominal distension—grade 3 ascites
- May lead to umbilical hernia
- Abdominal tenderness
- Neurological examination to evaluate for confusional state which may suggest the development of hepatic encephalopathy, flaps, and tremors
- Detailed examination of the chest to look for pleural effusion
- Cardiovascular evaluation to rule out chronic heart failure as cause of ascites
- Muscle wasting

*Diagnostic evaluation*: Routine blood tests CBC, liver function test, kidney function test, serum amylase, serum lipase, serum electrolytes, gamma GT, and coagulation profile form the basic blood evaluation for ascites. Apart from this, viral markers such as hepatitis B and hepatitis C need to be evaluated.

Routine ultrasound of the whole abdomen including Doppler study, CT scan, upper GI endoscopy is recommended **(Figs. 1A and B)**. Detailed testing of the ascitic fluid which includes cell count, albumin culture, lactose dehydrogenase, glucose, ADA, amylase, cytology and tuberculosis smear and culture is also done.

The SAAG value is to be calculated as per the following formula:

$$\text{SAAG} = (\text{Albumin serum}) - (\text{Albumin ascites})$$

## PATHOPHYSIOLOGY

Ascites is mainly because of portal hypertension and renal sodium retention.

Increased resistance to portal flow at sinusoidal level leads to the development of sinusoidal portal hypertension and backward transmission of this increased pressure in splanchnic capillaries and excess localization of fluid in peritoneal cavity, further associated with the development of peripheral mainly splanchnic arterial vasodilation and increase in the blood flowing in the splanchnic area as well as a further increase in portal pressure and reduction of central or essential volemia. Another suggestive mechanism is renal sodium retention related to portal hypertension and subtle hypovolemia. Minimal activation of the renin–angiotensin–aldosterone system (RAAS) and continued renal sodium retention is a prerequisite to ascites formation, and increased hydrostatic pressure without sodium retention will not result in ascites. These lead to a continuous escape of fluid from hepatic sinusoids and splanchnic capillaries to the interstitial space, initially compensated by an increased return of fluids to the systemic circulation mediated through the lymphatic system and thoracic duct as cirrhosis progresses escape becomes greater

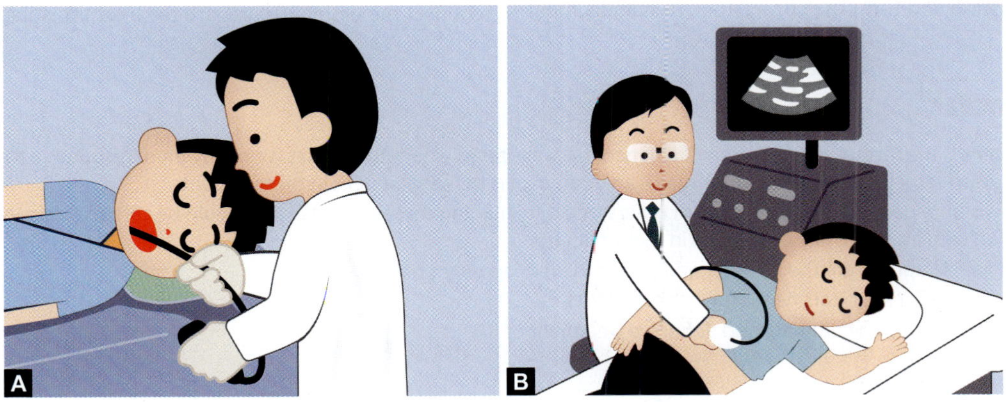


**FIGS. 1A AND B:** Upper GI endoscopy and routine ultrasound of the whole abdomen for refractory ascites.

than return leading to progressively increasing ascites and further activation of renal mechanisms of sodium and water reabsorption.

## TREATMENT AND PREVENTION

Management strategies for RA include a step-wise approach of dietary sodium restriction, medical management using non-selective beta-blockers, use of diuretics—both loop and mineralocorticoid, large-volume paracentesis (LVP), insertion of transjugular intrahepatic portosystemic shunt in suitable patients, Alfapump, peritoneovenous shunt (PVS), and permanent indwelling peritoneal catheter. Liver transplant remains the only long-term curative treatment.

### Dietary Sodium Restriction

Dietary sodium should be restricted to 2 g/day and increasing the urinary sodium excretion using diuretic therapy inducing a negative sodium balance. Patient education regarding dietary sodium restriction is the cornerstone in managing sodium restrictive therapy. To pursue dietary sodium restriction, it is important to calculate the sodium balance. For this, weight chart and 24-hour sodium excretion measurement are required. A patient on 2 g/day sodium intake and not excreting any sodium will be in a net positive balance of 88 mmol/day. This would lead to net weekly ascites accumulation of approximately 4.5 L. If the patient is excreting 88 mol/day of sodium, then his ascites volume should not change and if he is excreting > 88 mol/day, it should lead to weight loss. Severe sodium restriction or loss can cause malnutrition, which in turn leads to sarcopenia, hyponatremia, and renal dysfunction.

### Large-volume Paracentesis

It is largely a safe and effective outpatient procedure in managing large-volume ascites in comparison to diuretic therapy. It has a lower incidence of renal dysfunction, electrolyte disturbances, and much less disturbances of systemic and hemodynamic state. However, there is no difference in the survival rate. It is usual to remove 4–6 L of ascitic fluid by paracentesis in a single session. LVP has minimal complication risks even in the presence of coagulopathy. Since there is significant loss of proteins with LVP, intravenous human albumin supplementation (HAS) by infusion is usually recommended to prevent paracentesis-induced circulatory dysfunction (PICD) from developing.

### Medical Management

Nonselective beta-blockers (NSBB) are used in the management of portal hypertension and form the cornerstone in management. They work by reducing the heart rate and consequently the cardiac output. The beta-2 action causes splanchnic vasoconstriction, thereby reducing the portal flow and also by reducing the flow in collateral vessels. Labetalol and carvedilol, two NSBBs, have additional alpha-blocker effects and thereby cause hepatic vasodilation and a further reduction in portal pressure. In patients with compensated cirrhosis and significant portal hypertension, use of NSBB has been significantly able to reduce decompensation. However, due to significant vasodilation, they may impair cardiac systolic function and reduce renal perfusion pressure, leading to the kidneys not being able to autoregulate renal perfusion in response to its fall. Therefore, use in RA may lead to development of hepatorenal syndrome and hence should not be used in RA. There are conflicting reports on the use of midodrine because although it is beneficial in preventing PICD, it may have a higher mortality rate. Most patients with RA undergoing hyponatremia trials have suggested using Vaptans with diuretics to reduce the frequency of LVP. A couple of case studies have suggested using sodium-glucose cotransporter-2 (SGLT-2) inhibitors on account of their diuretic property in diabetics with cirrhosis, but further trials are needed.

Transjugular intrahepatic portosystemic shunt (TIPS) effectively lowers intrahepatic portal pressure while functioning as a side-to-side portocaval shunt and is effective in managing RA by lowering portal pressure and helping in the return of splanchnic volume to central circulation. This helps in gradual suppression of activated renin–angiotensin–aldosterone and sympathetic nervous systems, thereby reducing the renal sodium retention. This takes about 3–6 months to significantly clear ascites. It is usually recommended in the lower age group where it gives the best results and is contraindicated above the age of 70 years.

The automated low flow ascites pump (alfapump), a rechargeable and programmable device, is implanted subcutaneously and slowly pumps the ascites from peritoneal cavity via a catheter to the bladder and into the urine. It still needs further study and evaluation.

The ultimate and definitive treatment for RA is liver transplantation. However, ascites may persist for some time as it takes time to restore the hemodynamics.

In the current patient based on the above-mentioned management strategies, we would consider, apart from blood transfusion, correction of sodium and potassium by infusion and large-volume paracentesis with albumin infusion first. Subsequently, we may consider TIPS as a management modality for the long-term benefit of the patient. Also, we may consider to counsel the patient to prepare for liver transplant.

#### Points to Ponder

- Refractory ascites is the further deterioration of a patient with ascites in whom the ascites is not any more responsive to diuretic therapy. However, restriction of sodium still remains an integral part of management in these patients.
- Though large-volume paracentesis remains the cornerstone of managing these patients, one should be careful not to induce PICD. Regular infusion with albumin may be needed in these patients.
- TIPS insertion and Alfapump are the newer modalities in the management of RA.
- The recent use of SGLT-2 inhibitors needs further evaluation.
- Liver transplant remains to be ultimate and definitive treatment of RA.

## MULTIPLE CHOICE QUESTIONS

1. **What is the primary cause of refractory ascites in patients with chronic liver disease?**
   A. Hepatorenal syndrome
   B. Portal hypertension
   C. Spontaneous bacterial peritonitis
   D. Hepatic encephalopathy
2. **Which of the following criteria is most commonly used to define refractory ascites?**
   A. Ascites that resolves with low-dose diuretics
   B. Ascites that recurs within 6 months of treatment
   C. Ascites that is unresponsive to sodium restriction and maximal diuretic therapy
   D. Ascites associated with spontaneous bacterial peritonitis
3. **What is the first-line intervention for managing refractory ascites when diuretic therapy fails?**
   A. Liver transplantation
   B. Low-sodium diet
   C. Paracentesis
   D. Transjugular intrahepatic portosystemic shunt (TIPS)
4. **Which medication is commonly recommended for refractory ascites to help reduce portal pressure?**
   A. Furosemide
   B. Spironolactone
   C. Nonselective beta-blockers (e.g., Propranolol)
   D. Albumin infusion
5. **In patients with refractory ascites, which of the following complications is most concerning after repeated large-volume paracentesis?**
   A. Electrolyte imbalance
   B. Bowel obstruction
   C. Renal dysfunction
   D. Variceal bleeding

### Answers

1. (B); 2. (C); 3. (C); 4. (C): 5; (C)

## SUGGESTED READINGS


1 Salerno F, Guevara M, Bernardi M, et al. Refractory ascites: pathogenesis, definition and therapy of a severe complication in patients with cirrhosis: Liver Int. 2010;30:937-47.

2 Wong F. Management of refractory ascites. Clin Mol Hepatol. 2023;29:16-32.

3 Adebayo D, Shuet Fong SF, Wong F, et al. Refractory Ascites in Liver Cirrhosis. Am J Gastroenterol. 2019;114(1):40-7.

CHAPTER 26

# A Case-based Approach to Acute Abdomen for Physicians

*Sudeshna Guha Thakurta Ghosh*

**CASE VIGNETTE**

A 62-year-old female nondiabetic, nonhypertensive presented with acute abdominal pain in right upper abdomen and central part for 2–3 days increased for 1 day. Pain is associated with nausea, no fever. From history differential diagnosis (d/d);

- Acute cholecystitis
- Acute hepatitis
- Cholangitis
- Duodenal ulcer
- Pancreatitis
- Liver abscess
- Right lower lobe pneumonia

## PROVISIONAL DIAGNOSIS

*Acute cholecystitis*: Likely due to the right upper abdominal pain, associated nausea, and lack of fever, suggesting gallbladder inflammation.

## DIFFERENTIAL DIAGNOSIS

- *Acute hepatitis*: Possible due to right upper quadrant pain and nausea, though typically with fever and jaundice.
- *Cholangitis*: Should be considered due to pain and nausea, especially if fever develops later.
- *Duodenal ulcer*: Can present with upper abdominal pain and nausea, but typically associated with a history of peptic ulcers.
- *Pancreatitis*: Needs consideration due to abdominal pain, nausea, and potential vomiting, with amylase/lipase elevation.
- *Liver abscess*: Consider if pain is associated with fever, nausea, and tenderness over the liver.
- *Right lower lobe pneumonia*: Referred pain from the diaphragm, though unlikely without respiratory symptoms.

## CLINICAL APPROACH

The cornerstone of accurate diagnosis is a detailed history that includes full description of patient's pain and associated symptoms. For this we have to know the anatomy which is depicted in **Figure 1**.

After history taking, we get an idea about the disease process, now we should proceed for examination. The objective of abdominal examination includes assessment of patients' general condition and localization. The patients' general appearance and vital signs will guide to the d/d. Patients with peritonitis tend to lie still, whilst renal colic seem unable to stay still.

All vitals are stable, icterus present, patient looks toxic tenderness over right hypochondrium and epigastric region. It is essential to evaluate abdominal pain with a focus on six key features:

1. *Onset*: Abdominal pain can have an acute, rapid, or gradual onset, which aids in diagnosis.
2. *Localization*: Knowledge of anatomy helps in distinguishing potential causes (refer to **Fig. 2**).
3. *Character*: Understanding the type of pain—such as hunger pain, colicky pain, shooting, or burning pain—is crucial.
4. *Intensity*: Pain intensity varies between individuals. Pain from conditions like a distended gallbladder or abscess typically presents as constant, dull aching. Intense pain can indicate conditions like acute pancreatitis, renal colic, myocardial infarction, or visceral perforation.
5. *Progression*: Tracking the progression of pain from onset is key to making a correct diagnosis.
6. *Radiation and referral*: Abdominal pain can radiate through splanchnic, cerebrospinal, phrenic, obturator, and genito-femoral nerves.

| Right upper quadrant (RUQ) | |
|---|---|
| Pulmonary | Lower lobe pneumonia, emboli |
| Biliary | Colic, cholecystitis, cholangitis |
| Hepatic | Hepatitis, abscess |
| Renal | Colic, pyelonephritis, nephrolithiasis |
| GI | • Duodenitis, duodenal ulcer<br>• Retrocecal appendicitis |
| Pancreas | Pancreatitis |

| Epigastric | |
|---|---|
| Cardiac | ACS, MI |
| Biliary | Colic, cholecystitis, cholangitis |
| Pancreas | Pancreatitis |
| Vascular | AAA, dissection |
| GI | • Gastritis, early appendictis<br>• Epigastric hernia |

| Right upper quadrant (RUQ) | |
|---|---|
| Cardiac | ACS, MI, myocarditis, pericarditis |
| Pulmonary | Lower lobe pneumonia, emboli |
| Pancreas | Pancreatitis |
| Splenic | Splenic infarction, rupture |
| GI | Gastritis |
| Renal | Colic, pyelonephritis, nephrolithiasis |

| Right lumbar (RL) | |
|---|---|
| Vascular | • AAA, dissection<br>• Mesenteric ischemia |
| Renal | Colic, pyelonephritis |
| Others | Psoas abscess |

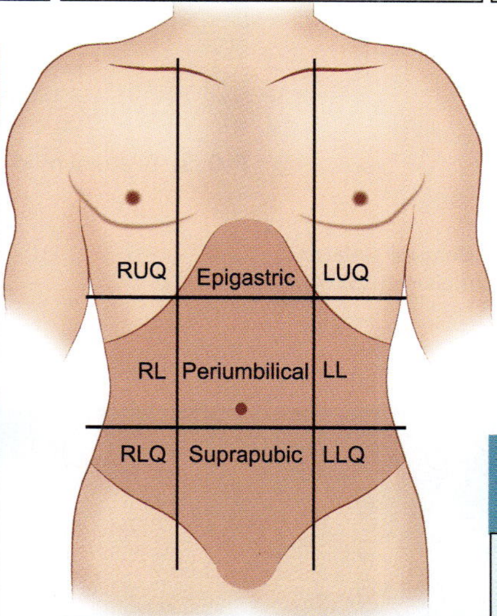


| Left lumbar (LL) | |
|---|---|
| Vascular | • AAA, dissection<br>• Mesenteric ischemia |
| Renal | Colic, pyelonephritis, nephrolithiasis |
| Others | Psoas abscess |

| Periumbilical | |
|---|---|
| Vascular | AAA, dissection |
| GI | • Early appendicitis<br>• Intestinal obstruction<br>• Gastroenteritis |

| Left lower quadrant (LLQ) | |
|---|---|
| GI | • Cecal obstruction, left diverticulitis constipation<br>• Ulcerative colitis, Crohn's disease |
| GU | Epididymo-orchitis, testicular torsion ureteric colic, nephrolithiasis, UTI ectopic pregnancy, PID |
| GYN | Tubo-ovarian pathology, endometriosis |
| Others | • Hernia, psoas abscess<br>• Mesenteric lymphadenitis |

| Suprapubic | |
|---|---|
| GI | Appendicitis, diverticulitis, constipation ulcerative colitis, Crohn's disease |
| GI | Urinary retention, UTI, cystitis |
| GYN | Ectopic pregnancy, PID Tubo-ovarian pathology, endometriosis |
| Others | Hernia |

| Right lower quadrant (RLQ) | |
|---|---|
| GI | • Appendicitis, cecal obstruction<br>• Ileitis, right diverticulitis, constipation, ulcerative colitis, nephrolithiasis, UTI |
| GYN | • Ectopic pregnancy, PID<br>• Tubo-ovarian pathology, endometriosis |
| Others | • Hernia, psoas absecess<br>• Mesenteric lymphadenitis |

**FIG. 1:** Anatomical localization of pain.

(AAA: abdominal aortic aneurysm; ACS: acute coronary syndrome; GI: gastrointestinal; GU: gastric ulcer; GYN: gynecology; LUQ: left upper quadrant; MI: myocardial infarction; PID: pelvic inflammatory disease; UTI: urinary tract infection)

*Source*: Karrar S. Abdominal pain – International emergency medicine education project [Internet]. International Emergency Medicine Education Project [cited Jan 25 2021]. Available from: https://iem-student.org/abdominal-pain/

## INVESTIGATION

Imaging and laboratory studies play a crucial role in evaluating abdominal pain. The selection of investigations depends on the clinical scenario and may include CBC, CRP, ESR, LFT, serum amylase, lipase, glucose, RFT, and urine analysis. A plain X-ray is useful for detecting perforation or foreign bodies. Ultrasound is commonly used due to its non-invasive nature and lack of radiation, but if the results are inconclusive, a CT scan of the abdomen is recommended. The patient, with an Hb of 13.2 g%, TLC of 15,100, and elevated ESR (48) and CRP (82.2), presents with acute cholecystitis, jaundice, and elevated lipase (210 IU) and amylase (480 IU). She has hepatomegaly with fatty changes on ultrasound. Additional lab findings include a random blood sugar of 218, HbA1c of 6.9, serum bilirubin of 4.9, SGPT of 346, SGOT of 230, and albumin of 3.8. Her blood urea is 24, and serum creatinine is 0.8 mg/dL. The working diagnosis is acute cholecystitis with jaundice, and a contrast-enhanced CT abdomen is planned for further evaluation **(Figs. 3 to 5)**.

## PATHOPHYSIOLOGY

Acute cholecystitis is inflammation of the gallbladder, often caused by obstruction of the cystic duct, typically due to gallstones. This obstruction leads to bile stasis, increased pressure within the gallbladder, and bacterial overgrowth. The

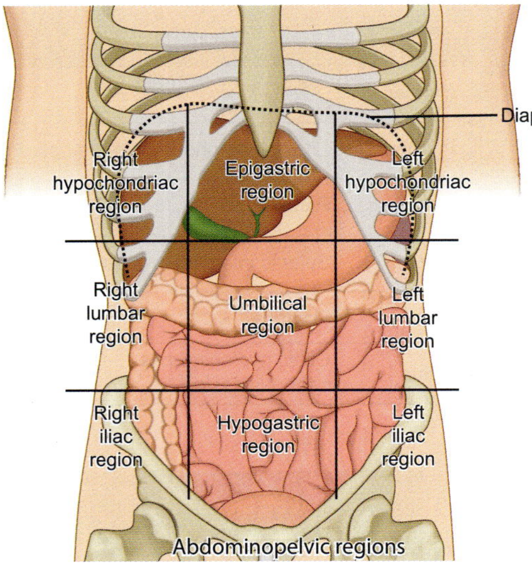


**FIG. 2:** Nine regions of abdomen.

*Source*: Wijayagoonawardana P, Sheikh Y, Jones J, et al. Abdominal surfaceanatomy. Radiopaedia.org [Accessed on 10 Dec 2024]. https://doi.org/10.53347/rID-6234

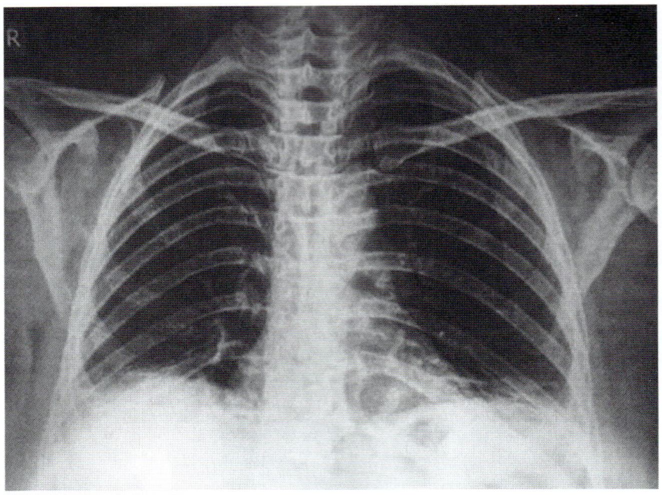


**FIG. 3:** Bilateral mild pleural effusion.

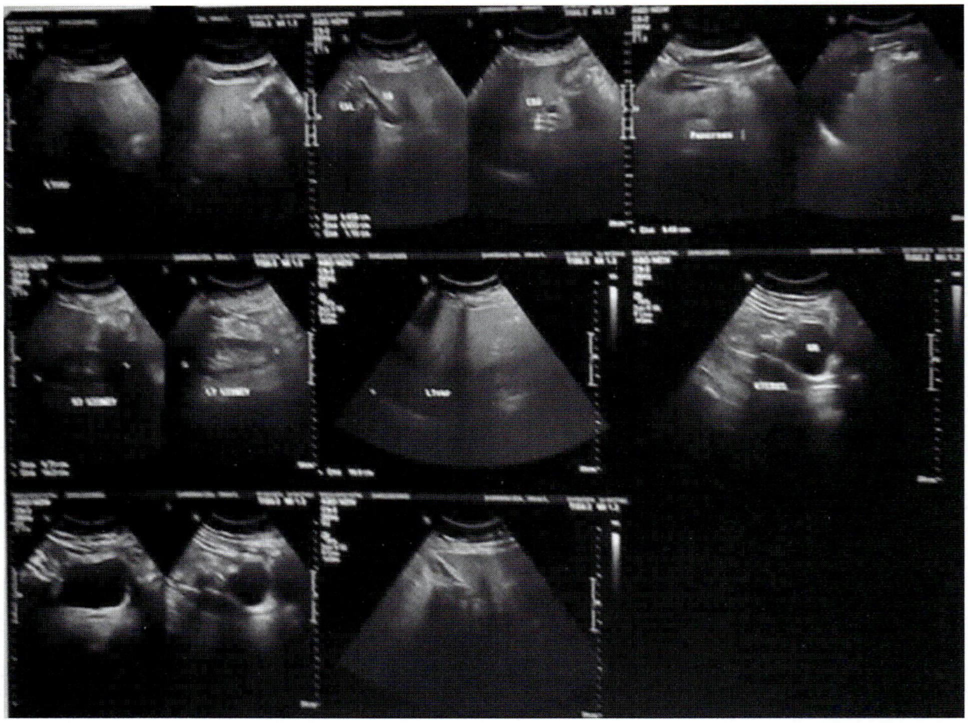

**FIG. 4:** Sludge in GB, mild ascites.

resulting inflammation triggers an immune response, causing pain, fever, and leukocytosis. If untreated, the condition may progress to gallbladder necrosis, perforation, or sepsis. The primary pathophysiological mechanisms involve mechanical obstruction, ischemia, and infection.

## TREATMENT AND PREVENTION

The management of abdominal pain begins with immediate assessment and investigation. Key interventions include analgesics, fluid resuscitation, antiemetics, nasogastric suction, and antibiotics, tailored based on the patient's history, examination, and lab findings. Early analgesia alleviates suffering, while rapid diagnosis and treatment are essential for life-threatening conditions such as airway compromise due to recurrent vomiting, oxygen requirement, or signs of circulatory failure. In our case, conservative management was effective, and the patient recovered and was discharged with advice to consult a surgeon for further evaluation.

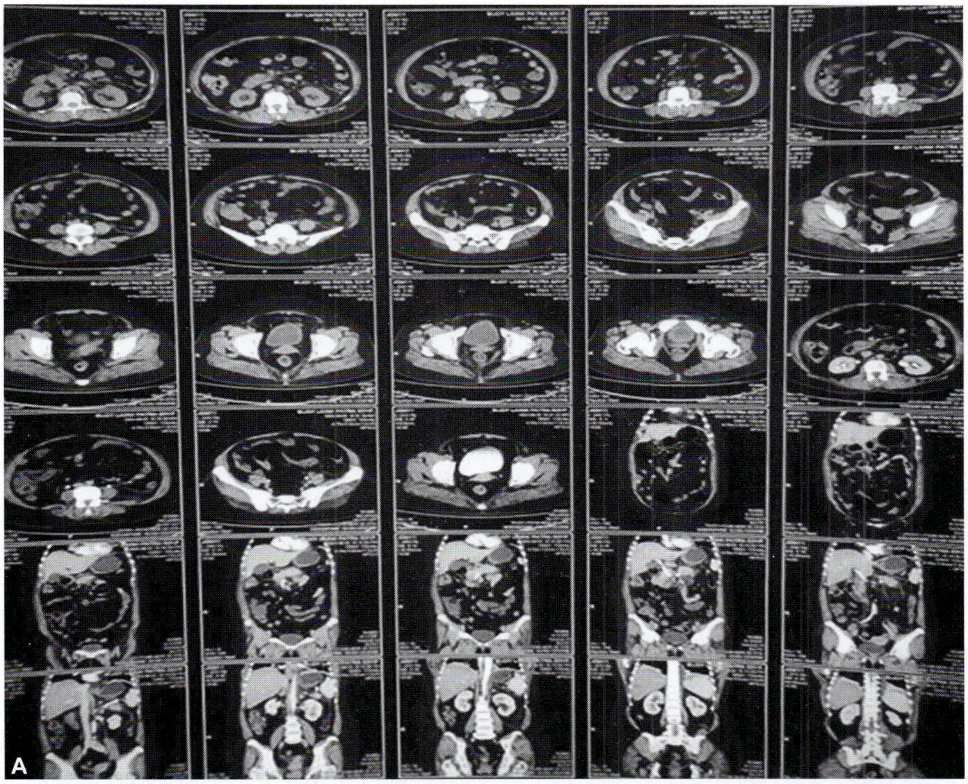

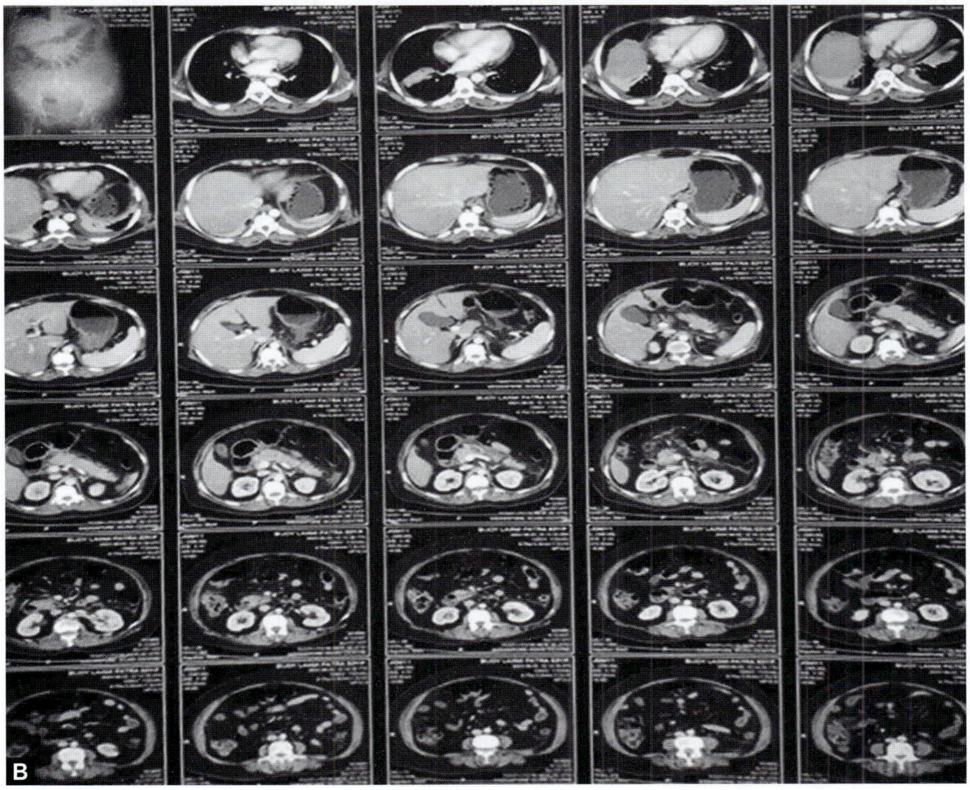

**FIGS. 5A AND B:** Diffuse hepatomegaly with fatty change, moderate acute pancreatitis.

## Points to Ponder

- Proper history taking.
- Detail clinical examination
- Related investigations.

Above 3 lines of evaluation can lead to correct diagnosis in 80–90% cases.

## MULTIPLE CHOICE QUESTIONS

1. **Which of the following is most likely given the patient's right upper abdominal pain and nausea without fever?**
   A. Acute hepatitis
   B. Acute cholecystitis
   C. Pancreatitis
   D. Right lower lobe pneumonia
2. **Which condition is characterized by right upper quadrant pain, nausea, and is most often associated with gallstones?**
   A. Acute hepatitis
   B. Cholangitis
   C. Acute cholecystitis
   D. Liver abscess
3. **In this patient with acute abdominal pain and nausea, which of the following would be the most likely initial diagnostic tool?**
   A. CT abdomen
   B. Ultrasound abdomen
   C. MRI abdomen
   D. Endoscopic retrograde cholangiopancreatography (ERCP)
4. **Which of the following symptoms does not typically align with acute cholecystitis?**
   A. Fever
   B. Right upper quadrant pain
   C. Nausea
   D. Diarrhea
5. **What is a common cause of acute cholecystitis in patients with gallstones?**
   A. Bile duct obstruction
   B. Hepatitis infection
   C. Duodenal ulcer
   D. Pneumonia

### Answers

1. (B); 2. (C); 3. (B); 4. (D); 5. (A)

## SUGGESTED READINGS

1. Natesan S, Lee J, Volkamer H, et al. Evidence-based medicine approach to abdominal pain. Emerg Med Clin N Am. 2016;34(2):165-90.
2. Kendal JL, Moreira ME. Evaluation of the adult with abdominal pain in the emergency department (homepage on the Internet]. UpToDate; 2020 [cited 2021 Jan 25]. Available from: https://www.uptodate.com/contents/evaluation-of-the-adult-with abdominal-pain-in-the-emergency-department.
3. McNamara R, Dean AJ. Approach to acute abdominal pain. Emerg Med Clin N Am. 2011;29(2):159-73.
4. Penner RM, Fishman MB. Evaluation of the adult with abdominal. Massachusetts: UpToDate; 2020.
5. Shian B, Larson ST. Abdominal wall pain: Clinical evaluation, differential diagnosis, and treatment. Am Fam Physician. 2018;98(7):429-36.
6. Koop H, Koprdova S, Schürmann C. Chronic abdominal wall pain. Dtsch Arztebl Int. 2016;113(4):51-7.
7. Fatovich D. Acute medical emergencies. 2nd ed. London: BMJ Books; 2004.
8. Karrar S. Abdominal pain - International emergency medicine education project homepage on the Internet]. International Emergency Medicine Education Project [cited 2021 Jan 25]. Available from: https://iem-student.org/abdominal-pain/
9. Cartwright SL, Knudson MP. Evaluation of acute abdominal pain in adults. Am Fam Physician. 2008;77(7):971-8.
10. Suleiman S, Johnston DE. The abdominal wall: An overlooked source of pain. Am Fam Physician. 2001;64(3):431.

CHAPTER

27

# A Case-based Approach to Hepatitis B Virus Management

*Shrikant Mukewar*

**CASE VIGNETTE**

A 35-year-old male, incidentally, detected as HBsAg positive, shows no clinical signs of chronic liver disease. He is HBeAg positive, anti-HBe negative, with an HBV DNA level of 11,410,980 IU/mL. Laboratory tests and imaging are normal, and there is no significant medical or family history of HBV, HCC, or other risk factors.

A study by Keeffe EB et al. found that in HBeAg-positive patients, the prevalence of significant histologic disease increases with ALT levels: 26.9% for ALT 1–1.5× ULN, 52.6% for ALT 1.5–2× ULN, and 76.5% for ALT >2× ULN ($p < 0.001$). Similarly, in HBeAg-negative patients, the prevalence increases with ALT levels: 20.0% for ALT 1–1.5× ULN, 44.4% for ALT 1.5–2× ULN, and 58.1% for ALT >2× ULN ($p = 0.04$).

## PROVISIONAL DIAGNOSIS

Chronic hepatitis B infection in the immune-tolerant phase (HBeAg-positive, normal ALT, high-HBV DNA levels).

## DIFFERENTIAL DIAGNOSIS

- Acute hepatitis B infection (unlikely due to normal liver function and absence of acute symptoms).
- Hepatitis C (not supported by test results).
- Alcoholic liver disease (no history or clinical evidence).
- Nonalcoholic fatty liver disease (no clinical signs or imaging findings).
- Autoimmune hepatitis (normal liver function tests and absence of specific markers).

## CLINICAL APPROACH

The EASL 2017 guideline recommends antiviral therapy for HBeAg-positive chronic HBV patients over 30, even with normal ALT levels and no significant liver damage. The AASLD 2018 guideline sets ALT ULN at 35 U/L for males and 25 U/L for females. For adults over 40 with normal ALT, high HBV DNA (1,000,000 IU/mL), and significant liver biopsy findings, treatment is recommended. The immune-tolerant phase, with high viral load and normal ALT, may require treatment for elderly patients or those with significant liver disease, as 1.9% may develop HCC over 10 years. Tenofovir plus emtricitabine offers greater viral suppression than tenofovir alone, though with no significant benefits in HBeAg loss, seroconversion, or HBsAg clearance. Treatment may involve a liver biopsy to diagnose necroinflammation tenofovir disoproxil fumarate (TDF) or entecavir (ETV), due to their efficacy and safety profiles.

## PATHOPHYSIOLOGY

Hepatitis B virus (HBV) infection leads to chronic liver inflammation and potential liver damage. In the immune-tolerant phase, high HBV DNA levels and positive HBeAg indicate active viral replication without significant liver inflammation, reflected by normal ALT levels. Over time, chronic infection may progress to cirrhosis and hepatocellular carcinoma (HCC), especially with persistent high viral loads. The immune response is usually insufficient to clear the virus, maintaining a high level of viral replication.

## TREATMENT AND PREVENTION

### Comparison of Oral versus Pegylated Interferon Treatment

Oral NUCs require indefinite use, show potent antiviral activity, and are safe in decompensated cirrhosis and pregnancy (class B). Pegylated interferon (PEG-IFN) is used for about 12 months with no antiviral resistance and modest HBeAg loss. Interferon therapy significantly reduces hepatic events, cirrhotic complications, HCC, and liver-related mortality. Combination therapy with PEG-IFN and TDF achieves superior HBsAg loss (9.1% at 72 weeks) compared to TDF alone (0%) or PEG alone (2.8%).

### Treatment Duration and Stopping Rules

The duration of treatment varies, with stopping rules for PEG-IFN at 48 weeks and NUCs depending on HBsAg loss, HBeAg status, and viral suppression. The REVEAL study demonstrates that high HBV viral load is associated with increased incidence of cirrhosis over a 13-year follow-up period. Wan YM et al. showed that for HBeAg-negative CHB patients without cirrhosis, stopping NUCs treatment after at least 4 years leads to 100% HBV DNA relapse within 96 weeks, necessitating close monitoring, with outcomes of 0% HBsAg loss if continued, 10% HBsAg loss if stopped, 41% sustained remission, and 14% requiring retreatment without hepatic decompensation.

## Prevention of Cirrhotic Complications

Antiviral therapy with entecavir significantly lowers the risk of spontaneous bacterial peritonitis (SBP) in cirrhotic patients ($p < 0.001$) but shows no significant difference in hepatic encephalopathy ($p = 0.393$). It also significantly reduces esophageal variceal bleeding incidence (29.1% vs. 65.8%, $p < 0.001$) and is an independent factor in reducing bleeding risk (HR 11.3, $p < 0.001$). The mean annual increase in variceal grade is lower in the antiviral group ($1.0 \pm 1.3$ vs. $1.7 \pm 1.2$, $p = 0.003$), with prolonged nonbleeding duration noted. Entecavir and adefovir reduce bleeding rates more effectively than lamivudine. HBV treatment reduces liver transplant risk, with treated responders showing the highest transplant-free survival rates ($p < 0.0003$). Over 5 years, antiviral therapy with lamivudine or entecavir significantly improves transplant-free survival ($p = 0.0098$).

NUCs treatment significantly lowers the 5-year cumulative incidence of HCC in CHB patients in Hong Kong (aHR 0.55), Taiwan (aHR 0.31), and Japan, indicating effective cancer prevention across populations.

## HBV Drug Resistance

Lamivudine (LAM) shows the highest resistance rates (70% at 2 years, 67% at 5 years), followed by adefovir (ADV) with 29% at 5 years, and telbivudine (TBV) with 11% at 3 years. Entecavir has very low resistance (1.2% at 5 years), while tenofovir (TDF) and tenofovir alafenamide (TAF) exhibit no resistance even after 5 years. Choosing antivirals with lower resistance profiles is crucial for long-term management of chronic hepatitis B (CHB).

## Efficacy of Antiviral Treatment

Tenofovir and TAF are the most effective treatments for CHB, achieving undetectable HBV DNA at week 48 or 52 in up to 76% of HBeAg-positive and 93% of HBeAg-negative patients. Entecavir is also highly effective, especially in HBeAg-negative patients (90% undetectable HBV DNA), while PEG-IFN shows the lowest efficacy for long-term undetectable HBV DNA levels.

## Head-to-head Antiviral Studies in Decompensated Cirrhosis

Four studies involving 607 patients with decompensated cirrhosis showed that entecavir significantly reduced the risk of HCC compared to adefovir (RR 0.4; 95% CI 0.2–0.8) and reduced all-cause mortality compared to lamivudine (RR 0.4; 95% CI 0.3–0.7). Other comparisons included adefovir versus lamivudine and telbivudine versus lamivudine.

### Points to Ponder

- Immune-tolerant phase in chronic hepatitis B is characterized by high viral load but normal liver function tests (e.g., ALT levels).
- The risk of developing significant liver damage and HCC increases with prolonged viral replication and high HBV DNA.
- The EASL and AASLD guidelines suggest antiviral therapy even for patients with normal ALT levels if there are signs of significant liver damage or high viral load.
- Monitoring ALT levels and HBV DNA is crucial in assessing the progression of liver disease and the need for antiviral therapy.
- Antiviral medications such as tenofovir and entecavir are commonly used due to their potent viral suppression and low risk of resistance.

## MULTIPLE CHOICE QUESTIONS

**1. What is the most likely phase of chronic hepatitis B in a patient with HBeAg positive, normal ALT levels, and high HBV DNA?**

A. Acute phase
B. Immune-tolerant phase
C. Immune-active phase
D. Cirrhosis phase

**2. Which of the following is recommended for antiviral therapy in HBeAg-positive chronic hepatitis B patients over 30 years of age?**

A. Only if ALT levels are elevated
B. Only if HBV DNA is above 100,000 IU/mL
C. Even with normal ALT levels and no significant liver damage
D. Only if the patient is symptomatic

**3. What is the risk of developing hepatocellular carcinoma (HCC) in patients with chronic hepatitis B over a 10-year period in the immune-tolerant phase?**

A. 1.9%
B. 5%
C. 10%
D. 20%

**4. Which of the following antiviral treatments is commonly used for chronic hepatitis B due to its efficacy and safety profile?**

A. Interferon alpha
B. Tenofovir and emtricitabine
C. Ribavirin
D. Acyclovir

**5. What is the recommended liver biopsy approach in the management of chronic hepatitis B infection?**

A. Only in symptomatic patients
B. To diagnose necroinflammation in high viral load cases
C. Routine biopsy for all patients
D. Not required for immune-tolerant phase

### Answers

1. (B); 2. (C); 3. (A); 4. (B); 5. (B)

## SUGGESTED READINGS


1. Datta S. An overview of molecular epidemiology of hepatitis B virus (HBV) in India. Virology Journal. 2008;5:1-2.
2. Batham A, Narula D, Toteja T, et al. Systematic review and meta-analysis of prevalence of hepatitis B in India. Indian pediatrics. 2007;44(9):663.
3. Schweitzer A, Horn J, Mikolajczyk RT, et al. Estimations of worldwide prevalence of chronic hepatitis B virus infection: a systematic review of data published between 1965 and 2013. The Lancet. 2015;386(10003):1546-55.
4. Jeng WJ, Papatheodoridis GV, Lok ASF. Hepatitis B. Lancet. 2023;401(10381).
5. Lampertico P, Agarwal K, Berg T, et al. EASL 2017 Clinical Practice Guidelines on the management of hepatitis B virus infection. Journal of hepatology. 2017;67(2):370-98.
6. Peng CY, Chien RN, Liaw YF. Hepatitis B virus-related decompensated liver cirrhosis: benefits of antiviral therapy. Journal of hepatology. 2012;57(2):442-50.
7. Keeffe EB, Dieterich DT, Han SH, et al. A treatment algorithm for the management of chronic hepatitis B virus infection in the United States: 2008 update. Clinical gastroenterology and hepatology. 2008;6(12):1315-41.
8. Terrault NA, Lok AS, McMahon BJ, et al. Update on prevention, diagnosis, and treatment of chronic hepatitis B: AASLD 2018 hepatitis B guidance. Hepatology. 2018;67(4):1560-99.
9. Konerman MA, Lok AS. Interferon treatment for hepatitis B. Clinics in Liver Disease. 2016;20(4):645-65.
10. Marcellin P, Ahn SH, Ma X, et al. Combination of tenofovir disoproxil fumarate and peginterferon α-2a increases loss of hepatitis B surface antigen in patients with chronic hepatitis B. Gastroenterology. 2016;150(1):134-44.
11. Iloeje UH, Yang HI, Su J, et al. Predicting cirrhosis risk based on the level of circulating hepatitis B viral load. Gastroenterology. 2006;130(3):678-86.
12. Marcellin P, Gane E, Buti M, et al. Regression of cirrhosis during treatment with tenofovir disoproxil fumarate for chronic hepatitis B: a 5-year open-label follow-up study. The Lancet. 2013;381(9865):468-75.
13. Li CZ, Cheng LF, Li QS, et al. Antiviral therapy delays esophageal variceal bleeding in hepatitis B virus-related cirrhosis. World Journal of Gastroenterology: WJG. 2013;19(40):6849.
14. Jonas MM, Lok AS, McMahon BJ, et al. Antiviral therapy in management of chronic hepatitis B viral infection in children: A systematic review and meta-analysis. Hepatology. 2016;63(1):307-18.

CHAPTER

# 28

# An Approach to a Case of Chronic Abdominal Pain

*Vijay Karthik Bhogaraju, Kutty Sharada Vinod*

## CASE VIGNETTE

A 65-year-old woman presented with crampy upper abdominal pain that developed shortly after eating, especially after lunch, over the past 8 months. This discomfort would persist for up to 2 hours before gradually subsiding. She reported an unintended weight loss of 15 kg in the last 6 months, going from 68 to 53 kg. She reported that she developed food aversion in the past 2 months due to the significant post-prandial pain. While the reduced food intake reduced her pain frequency, it also left her feeling perpetually fatigued. She was concerned that she had cancer, and hence presented to her physician for a consult. She denied any symptoms of dysphagia, changes in bowel habits, jaundice, back pain, or urinary complaints. Her medical history included 5 years of chronic stable angina managed with antiplatelet therapy and beta-blockers, 7 years of diabetes controlled on oral medications, as well as a history of systemic hypertension and dyslipidemia for which she is on an angiotensin receptor blockers and statins. On examination, there was tenderness in the epigastric area, with a noticeable bruit heard upon auscultation in this region. An abdominal ultrasound and upper GI endoscopy appeared normal. A contrast-enhanced MRI abdominal angiography and aortography revealed significant atherosclerotic stenosis in the celiac artery and superior mesenteric artery branches, with evidence of collateral branch formation from the inferior mesenteric artery **(Fig. 1)**. A diagnosis was considered by the treating physician and an abdominal scan was performed.

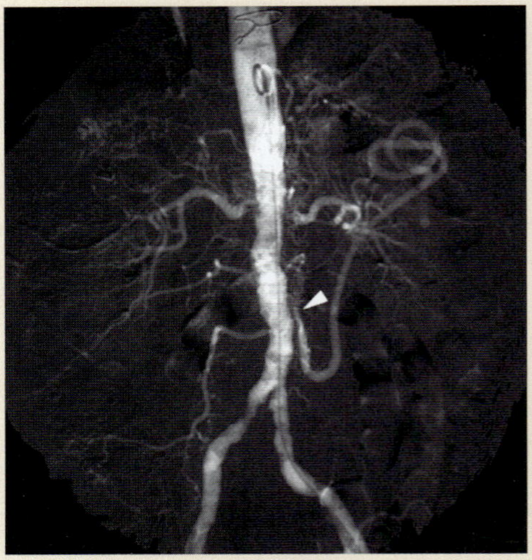

**FIG. 1:** Contrast-enhanced MRI showed significant atherosclerotic stenosis in the celiac and superior mesenteric arteries, with collateral formation from the inferior mesenteric artery (arrowhead).

## PROVISIONAL DIAGNOSIS

Chronic mesenteric ischemia.

## DIFFERENTIAL DIAGNOSIS

- Gastrointestinal malignancy
- Chronic cholecystitis
- Chronic pancreatitis
- Inflammatory bowel disease
- Peptic ulcer disease
- Abdominal tuberculosis

### Gastrointestinal Malignancy

- *Clinical*: Commonly presents with progressive abdominal pain, significant weight loss, and may cause GI bleeding.
- *Imaging*: CT scan reveals mass lesions, often with lymphadenopathy and metastasis in advanced cases.

### Chronic Cholecystitis

- *Clinical*: Causes dull right upper quadrant pain, exacerbated by meals, with a positive Murphy's sign on exam.
- *Imaging*: Ultrasound shows gallbladder wall thickening and gallstones.

### Chronic Pancreatitis

- *Clinical*: Persistent epigastric pain radiating to the back, often worsens after eating.
- *Imaging*: CT reveals pancreatic calcifications and ductal dilation.

### Inflammatory Bowel Disease (IBD)

- *Clinical*: Recurrent abdominal pain, diarrhea, and systemic symptoms like fever and weight loss.

- *Imaging*: CT/MRI shows bowel wall thickening and skip lesions in Crohn's disease and continuous bowel involvement with ulcerative colitis; confirmed with colonoscopy and biopsy.

### Peptic Ulcer Disease (PUD)

- *Clinical*: Burning pain in the epigastric area, often meal-related, with possible GI bleeding.
- *Imaging*: Upper GI endoscopy shows mucosal ulcers.

### Abdominal Tuberculosis

- *Clinical*: Chronic abdominal pain, fever, weight loss, and ascites.
- *Imaging*: CT shows mesenteric lymphadenopathy, bowel thickening, and ascites; biopsy confirms granulomas. Ascitic fluid examination would reveal a low SAAG ascites with raised ADA.

## CLINICAL APPROACH

Chronic abdominal pain is defined as continuous or intermittent abdominal pain persisting for at least 3 months, with a significant impact on daily activities and quality of life. The complexity of diagnosis and management is particularly challenging in the Indian healthcare system due to diverse disease patterns, variable healthcare accessibility, cultural and socioeconomic factors and traditional medicine practices.

The prevalence is 8–10% in 18–30 years, 15–18% in 31–45 years, 12–15% in 46–60 years and 10–12% in >60 years of age. Almost 60–65% of patients are found to be female and there is a marked female predominance noted in functional disorders. The Indian diet with excessive spices, higher carbohydrates and reduced fiber intake along added with a sedentary lifestyle, elevated stressors predisposes our population to various causes of chronic abdominal pain. In the coming years, climate change and increasing pollution will bring renewed challenges to the diagnosis and management of chronic abdominal pain.

### Etiology includes Functional and Organic Causes

- *Functional gastrointestinal disorders (40–50%)*:
  - Irritable bowel syndrome
  - Functional dyspepsia
  - Functional abdominal pain syndrome
- *Organic causes (30–40%)*:
  - Infectious causes:
    - Abdominal tuberculosis:
      - Peritoneal
      - Intestinal
      - Mesenteric lymphadenitis
    - Parasitic infections:
      - Amebiasis
      - Giardiasis
      - Helminthic infections
  - Inflammatory conditions:
    - Inflammatory bowel disease:
      - Crohn's disease
      - Ulcerative colitis
    - Chronic pancreatitis:
      - Tropical pancreatitis
      - Alcohol-induced
  - Structural disorders:
    - Adhesions
    - Partially obstructed hernias
    - Gallbladder disease
    - Chronic appendicitis
- *Others (10–20%)*:
  - Endometriosis
  - Chronic pelvic inflammatory disease
  - Adenomyosis
  - Diabetic gastropathy

## HISTORY AND EXAMINATION

### History

#### *Pain Characteristics (SOCRATES Approach)*

- *S*ite
- *O*nset
- *C*haracter
- *R*adiation
- *A*ssociated symptoms
- *T*iming
- *E*xacerbating/Relieving factors
- *S*everity

#### *Dietary History*

- Meal patterns
- Food triggers
- Cultural dietary practices
- Fasting habits
- Spice consumption

#### *Psychosocial Assessment*

- Stress factors
- Family dynamics
- Work environment
- Social support
- Economic factors

### Physical Examination

#### *General Examination*

- Nutritional status
- Pallor
- Lymphadenopathy
- Vital signs
- BMI

### Abdomen

- *Inspection*:
  - Scars
  - Sinuses
  - Distension
  - Visible peristalsis
  - Surface abnormalities (dilated veins/pulsatile masses/obvious lumps)
- *Palpation*:
  - Superficial tenderness
  - Deep tenderness
  - Masses
  - Organomegaly
  - Palpable bruits/hums

- *Percussion*:
  - Dullness (shifting)
  - Organomegaly
  - Fluid thrill
- *Auscultation*:
  - Bowel sounds
  - Bruits
  - Hums
  - Friction rubs

## Investigations

### First Line Investigations

- *Blood investigations*:
  - Complete blood count with differential counts
  - ESR/CRP
  - Liver function tests
  - Renal function tests
  - Blood sugar levels
  - Serum electrolytes
  - Thyroid function tests
- *Stool examination*:
  - Routine microscopy (Ova/cyst/blood)
  - Culture and sensitivity
- *Imaging*:
  - Chest X-ray
  - Ultrasonography of abdomen and pelvis
  - X-ray abdomen (if indicated)

### Second Line Investigations

- *Endoscopic procedures*:
  - Upper GI endoscopy
  - Colonoscopy
  - Capsule endoscopy
  - ERCP (when indicated)
- *Advanced imaging*:
  - CT abdomen with contrast
  - MRI abdomen
  - MR enterography
  - MRCP
- *Specialized tests (case-to-case basis)*:
  - TB-specific tests
  - Inflammatory markers
  - Autoimmune markers
  - Tumor markers

### Third Line Investigations

- Diagnostic laparoscopy
- Specialized motility studies
- Nuclear medicine studies
- Biochemical markers

## General Principles: Management

- Pain control and symptomatic management
- Dietary modifications
- Lifestyle changes
- Regular follow-up
- Quality of life assessment

## Specific Management Strategies

### Functional Disorders

- *Lifestyle modifications*:
  - Regular exercise
  - Stress management
  - Sleep hygiene
  - Dietary modifications
- *Pharmacological treatment*:
  - Antispasmodics
  - Prokinetics
  - Low-dose antidepressants
- *Psychological interventions*:
  - Cognitive behavioral therapy
  - Mindfulness training
  - Biofeedback measures

## Organic Causes

- *Infectious conditions*:
  - Appropriate antimicrobial therapy and appropriate duration
  - Monitoring of treatment response
  - Prevention of complications
- *Inflammatory conditions*:
  - Disease modifying anti-inflammatory drugs
  - Biological agents
  - Surgical intervention when indicated
- *Structural disorders*:
  - Surgical correction when indicated
  - Prevention of complications

# PATHOPHYSIOLOGY

Functional and organic causes of chronic abdominal pain differ significantly in their pathophysiological mechanisms. Functional gastrointestinal disorders (FGIDs), lacks identifiable structural or biochemical abnormalities and is associated with dysfunctions in the gut-brain axis. In contrast organic conditions have identifiable physical causes for pain.

## Functional Abdominal Pain Mechanisms

- *Gut-brain axis dysfunction*: Disturbances in the gut-brain interaction (psychological, genetic, and environmental factors) leads to altered visceral sensation and motility, contributing to pain perception.
- *Central and peripheral sensitization*: Functional abdominal pain involves central and peripheral sensitization, where neuroplasticity increase the perception of pain. Due to central sensitization, few patients also experience heightened sensitivity to pain stimuli known as visceral hyperalgesia.
- *Psychosocial factors*: Psychological stressors, anxiety, and depression are frequently associated with functional abdominal pain.

## Organic Abdominal Pain Mechanisms

- *Inflammation and structural abnormalities*: Organic abdominal pain is often caused by identifiable physical conditions such as inflammation, infections, or structural abnormalities in the gastrointestinal tract. These conditions stimulate nociceptors, leading to pain.

- *Peripheral sensitization and neuroimmune interactions*: Peripheral sensitization occurs by the direct activation of nociceptors by inflammatory mediators or mechanical factors. These cytokines and chemokines may modulate pain pathways via neuroimmune mechanisms and lead to persistence of pain.

## TREATMENT AND PREVENTION

### Pharmacological Approaches

- *Stepwise pharmacotherapy*: Begin with nonopioid analgesics, progressing to weak and strong opioids.
- *Targeted therapies*: Emerging and experimental treatments focus on specific receptors and pathways, such as serotonin, α-2 adrenergic, transient receptor potential vanilloid-1 channels and cannabinoid receptor agonists.

### Nonpharmacological Interventions

- *Cognitive-behavioral therapy (CBT)*: CBT helps in cognitive restructuring and behavioral modification, which can alter pain perception and improve psychological well-being
- *Traditional therapy*: Therapies like acupuncture have shown promise in reducing symptoms and improving quality of life in patients with chronic abdominal pain, particularly those with IBS.

### Multidisciplinary and Integrative Approaches

- *Biopsychosocial model*: This model emphasizes a holistic approach, integrating pharmacotherapy, psychotherapy, and other interventions to address the multifaceted nature of chronic pain
- *Patient-centered care*: Tailoring treatment to individual patient needs and experiences.

### Integrated Multimodal Approaches

- *Pre-emptive analgesia*: Initiating pain management before surgical procedures
- *Digital monitoring*: Allows for early identification of risk factors and personalized interventions
- *Psychoeducational support*: Addressing psychological through education and coping strategies

### Risk Factor Identification

- *Preoperative assessment*: Identifying patients at high risk for chronic pain through comprehensive evaluations.
- *Surgical technique modifications*: Adjusting surgical methods to minimize tissue damage.

### Points to Ponder

- ❑ Majority of patients with chronic abdominal pain, suffer from functional disorders.
- ❑ A detailed history and physical examination identifies sinister causes for chronic abdominal pain.
- ❑ *Constitutional symptoms* [unintentional weight loss (>10% in 6 months), fever, night sweats, fatigue], *gastrointestinal signs* (hematochezia, melena, progressive dysphagia, persistent vomiting, changes in bowel habits), *other signs* (family history of GI malignancy, age >50 years with new-onset symptoms, unexplained iron deficiency anemia, palpable mass, lymphadenopathy) should provoke further evaluation.
- ❑ Functional and organic abdominal pain can coexist, and needs individualized treatment strategies.
- ❑ Role of intestinal microbiota in modulating pain perception is an emerging area of interest, in both functional and organic conditions.

## MULTIPLE CHOICE QUESTIONS

**1. A 68-year-old female smoker presents with postprandial abdominal pain and 20-kg weight loss. Which vessel is most commonly involved in chronic mesenteric ischemia?**

A. Celiac artery
B. Superior mesenteric artery
C. Inferior mesenteric artery
D. Splenic artery

**2. Which best describes the pathophysiology of chronic mesenteric ischemia?**

A. Acute thrombosis
B. Progressive atherosclerosis
C. Vasculitis
D. Embolic occlusion

**3. A patient with suspected chronic mesenteric ischemia needs imaging. Which is the gold standard?**

A. CT angiography
B. MR angiography
C. Duplex ultrasound
D. Digital subtraction angiography

**4. Which finding is least consistent with chronic mesenteric ischemia?**

A. Food fear
B. Weight loss
C. Bloody diarrhea
D. Postprandial pain

**5. Best initial management for chronic mesenteric ischemia?**

A. Conservative management
B. Endovascular revascularization
C. Anticoagulation only
D. Antiplatelet therapy only

### Answers

1. (B)
*Explanation*: SMA is most commonly affected. Classic triad: postprandial pain, weight loss, and abdominal bruit.

2. (B)
*Explanation*: CMI typically results from progressive atherosclerotic narrowing of mesenteric vessels.

3. (A)
*Explanation*: CTA offers detailed vascular anatomy and degree of stenosis while being less invasive than conventional angiography.
4. (C)
*Explanation*: Bloody diarrhea suggests acute ischemia or other conditions. CMI typically presents with postprandial pain and food fear.
5. (B)
*Explanation*: Endovascular intervention is preferred first-line treatment due to lower morbidity compared to open surgery.

## SUGGESTED READINGS


1. Thomson AB, Barkun AN, Armstrong D, et al. The prevalence of clinically significant endoscopic findings in primary care patients with uninvestigated dyspepsia: the Canadian Adult Dyspepsia Empiric Treatment - Prompt Endoscopy (CADET-PE) study Aliment Pharmacol Ther. 2003;17(12):1481-91.
2. Shih MP, Hagspiel KD. CTA and MRA in Mesenteric Ischemia: Part 1, Role in Diagnosis and Differential Diagnosis. AJR Am J Roentgenol. 2007;188(2):452-61.
3. Lukic S, Mijac D, Filipovic B, et al. Chronic Abdominal Pain: Gastroenterologist Approach. Dig Dis. 2022;40(2):181-6.
4. Jha DK, Pathiyil MM, Sharma V. Evidence-based approach to diagnosis and management of abdominal tuberculosis. Indian J Gastroenterol. 2023;42(1):17-31.
5. Häuser W, Morlion B, Vowles KE, et.al. European* clinical practice recommendations on opioids for chronic noncancer pain. Eur J Pain. 2021;25(5):949-68.
6. Patel R, Waheed A, Costanza M. Chronic Mesenteric Ischemia. In: StatPearls. Treasure Island (FL): StatPearls Publishing; 2023.
7. Xhepa G, Vanzulli A, Sciacqua LV, et al. Advancements in Treatment Strategies for Chronic Mesenteric Ischemia: A Comprehensive Review. J Clin Med. 2023;12(22):7112.
8. Mealie CA, Ali R, Manthey DE. Abdominal Examination. In: StatPearls. Treasure Island (FL): StatPearls; 2024.

CHAPTER 29

# An Approach to a Case of Intractable Hiccups

*Srikant Behera*

**CASE VIGNETTE**

A 45-year-old, male patient presented to your OPD with history of hiccups for 6 months. He is on treatment for chest discomfort, dyspepsia, nausea, and gastroesophageal reflux for 1 year. Except for the hiccups, the patient had no significant prior medical history and no abnormality findings, including a blood test, electrocardiography, and chest X-ray. He has visited multiple physicians his hiccups and received multiple medications. But he did not get relieved from his hiccups.

## PROVISIONAL DIAGNOSIS

Intractable hiccups.

## DIFFERENTIAL DIAGNOSIS

Though the diagnosis of hiccups is relatively easy, but it may get confused with coughing or gagging. Intractable hiccups are usually manifestation of other diseases. There is a long list of differentials, and these include but are not limited to ear, nose and throat, CNS, cardiovascular, gastrointestinal, infectious, intrathoracic, metabolic and psychogenic disorders. Also, many medications can lead to hiccups. Hiccups may occur during anesthesia, sedation, endoscopy, and postsurgical procedures.

## CLINICAL APPROACH (FLOWCHART 1)

A hiccup is an abrupt contraction of the inspiratory muscles that happens repeated for several times per minute. This results in sudden rush of air in to the lungs causing the glottis to close and creates a distinctive sound. Hiccups occur due to powerful involuntarily spasm of the diaphragm and its being followed by sudden inspiration with a closed glottis. Hiccups can be *acute*—lasting for less than 48 hours, *persistent*—lasting over 2 days, or *intractable*—lasting >1 month. Intractable hiccups can lead to malnutrition, weight loss, dehydration, fatigue, depression, insomnia, and reduced quality of life. Intractable hiccups are rare, affecting males and females equally, though males are affected by hiccups more commonly.

*Hiccup reflex arc* ***(Fig. 1)***: Hiccups reflex arc is formed by (a) afferents from pharyngeal plexus and thoracic sympathetic chain via phrenic, vagus, and sympathetic nerves (T6–T12) to hiccups centre; (b) the hiccup centre lies in the midbrain involving the periaqueductal gray and subthalamic nuclei, (c) efferents—the motor fibres run from the brain stem hiccup centre via the phrenic nerve, vagus nerve, and accessory nerve to the intercostal muscles, anterior scalene muscle, the hemidiaphragms, and the laryngeal musculature. Efferent motor fibres in the recurrent laryngeal branch of the vagus nerve cause glottal closure. The phrenic nerve and vagus nerve give supply to both afferent and efferent pathways: to and from the hemidiaphragms and the laryngeal musculature. The central processing area is in the medulla oblongata, the periaqueductal gray, subthalamic nuclei, phrenic nerve nuclei, reticular formation, and hypothalamus. This hiccups arc is different from pathways for rhythmic breathing. Multiple neurotransmitters including GABA, dopamine, serotonin, glutamate, glycine, histamine, epinephrine, acetylcholine, etc., are involved in hiccups reflex.

## PATHOPHYSIOLOGY (FIG. 2)

Hiccups occur due to powerful involuntarily spasm of the diaphragm and its being followed by sudden inspiration with a closed glottis. There is spontaneous, myoclonic contraction of the diaphragm and in many cases the intercostal musculature contractions. Pathophysiologically hiccups occur due to irritation of its reflex arc. The activation of the reflex arc leads to release and stimulation of various neurotransmitters and neuroreceptors like dopamine, serotonin, opioid, calcium channel, and GABA pathways in the brain hiccup centre. Hiccups usually involve unilateral diaphragmatic contraction, mostly involving left side. The afferent impulses are carried by the vagus nerve, phrenic nerves, or sympathetic nerve fibres (thoracic outflow T6–T12). The efferent response of the reflex is being carried by the phrenic nerve to the diaphragm to contract unilaterally or sometimes bilaterally. The activation of accessory nerves leads to contraction of intercostal muscles.

## ETIOLOGY

Due to the far-reaching reflex arc and myriads of neurotransmitters involved in its pathophysiology, there are many causes of intractable hiccups. Anything, either a lesion along its pathway or drugs or systemic conditions that irritates the afferent, efferent, or

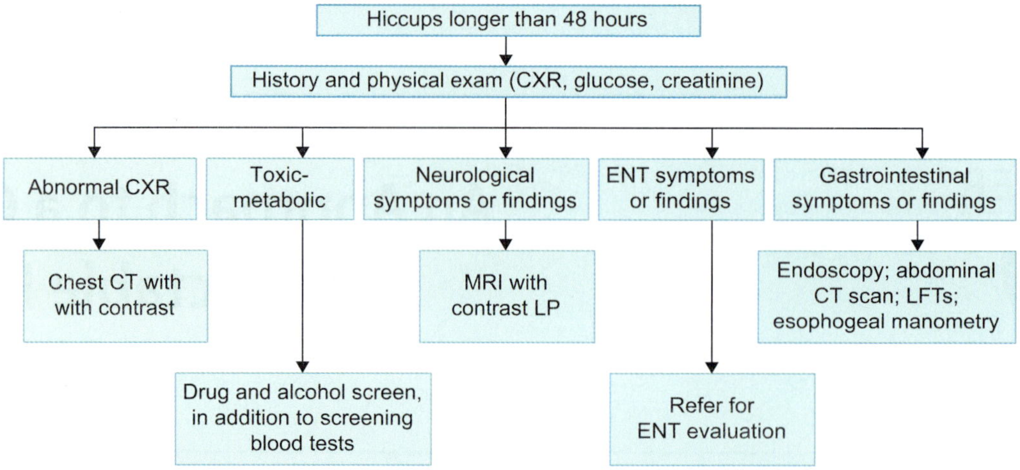


**FLOWCHART 1:** Approach to intractable hiccups.

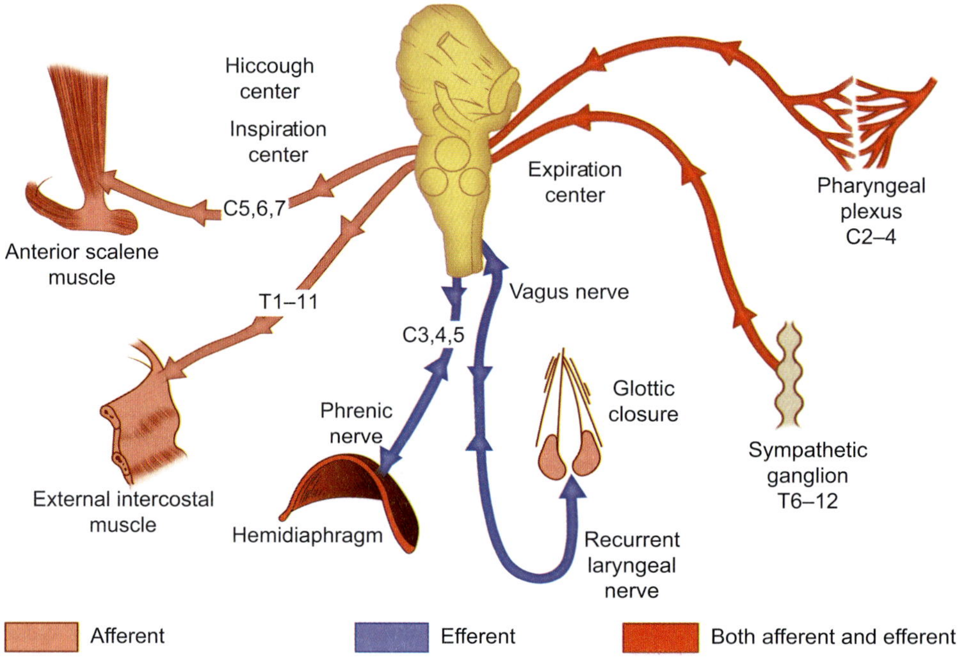


**FIG. 1:** Schematic diagram showing neural pathways of hiccup. Afferent pathways from pharyngeal plexus and thoracic sympathetic chain. Efferent pathways from brainstem hiccup centre to external intercostal muscles, anterior scalene muscle, hemidiaphragm, and laryngeal musculature via phrenic nerve, vagus nerve, and accessory nerve. The phrenic nerve and vagus nerve give supply to both afferent and efferent pathways: to and from the hemidiaphragms and the laryngeal musculature.

central processing area can trigger hiccups. They can result from a variety of causes. Hiccups are more common in diseases affecting the gastrointestinal or central nervous systems. In particular, hiccups are often caused by gastrointestinal disorders such as gastroesophageal reflux. Up to 20% cases with Parkinson's diseases, and about 10% patients with GERD suffer from hiccups. Other causes include medication side-effects, cardiovascular disorders, central nervous system disorders, ear, nose, and throat disorders, psychogenic disorders, or metabolic disorders.

- *Abdominal cause*: Gastric stasis and distension (the far more common cause), gastroesophageal reflux disorder (GERD), intra-abdominal inflammation, intra-abdominal hemorrhage, tumor, subdiaphragmatic abscess/collection, pancreatis disorders, hepatobiliary diseases, abdominal aortic aneurysm, etc.
- *CNS causes:* Trauma, infection, tumor, stroke, seizures, uremia, chemicals, thrombosis, vascular insufficiency, etc., by disrupting the normal control over hiccup reflex.
- *Pulmonary and cardiothoracic diseases:* Mass lesion, pneumonia, pulmonary embolism, diaphragmatic tumor, compression of phrenic nerve, irritation of diaphragm, irritation of phrenic nerves, esophageal dysfunction, coronary disease, pericarditis
- *Ear, nose, and throat diseases:* Goiter, neck cyst, pharyngitis, laryngitis, etc.
- *Metabolic:* Electrolyte imbalance (hyponatremia, hypomagnesemia, hypercalcemia, etc.), uremia, hyperglycemia, adrenal insufficiency.
- Toxin/recreational drugs: alcohol

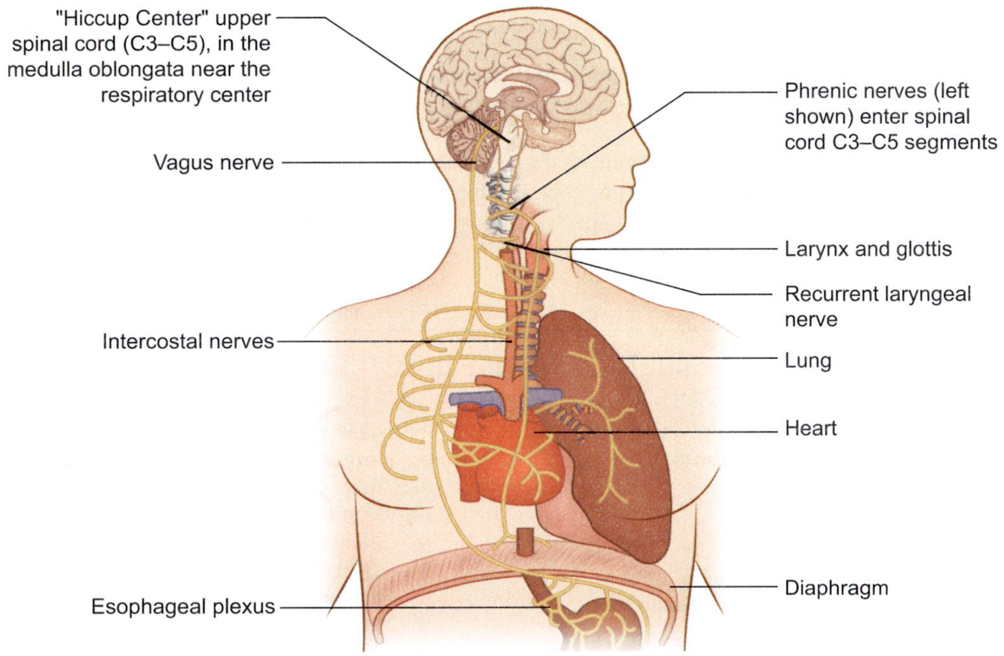


**FIG. 2:** Schematic representation of pathophysiology of intractable hiccups.

- *Drugs:* Corticosteroids, antibiotics, benzodiazepines, opioids, chemotherapeutics, anti-Parkinson medications, anti-psychotics, etc.
- *Postsurgery/postprocedures:* Anesthesia, postoperative or postprocedures (endoscopy, epidural injections, etc.)
- Patients with cancer or chemotherapy
- *Psychogenic*: Anorexia nervosa, stress, schizophrenia, conversion reaction, etc.

## EVALUATION

Though acute hiccups are typically benign and usually do not require a workup, intractable hiccups should be evaluated thoroughly to find the underlying etiology to identify a treatable cause. A thorough review of cardiovascular, pulmonary, gastrointestinal, and neurologic symptoms, including recent medications, toxins, procedures, or injuries, will guide the next step in work up and what anatomic area should be focused on. Investigations: routine investigations (CBC, LFT, RFT, serum electrolytes), other specific investigations as indicated. It is reasonable to obtain lab work for evaluation of electrolyte abnormalities or to rule out infectious and neoplastic processes not identified on history and physical exam. Laboratory studies such as electrolytes, calcium, blood urea nitrogen (BUN), creatinine, lipase, and liver tests can be useful. Imaging: Chest X-ray, ultrasound of abdomen, CT scan/MRI of brain; toxicology screening, endoscopy, gastroscopy, ENT evaluation, etc. A chest radiograph may identify intrathoracic sources of hiccups such as pneumonia, empyema, diaphragmatic hernia, adenopathy or aortic disease.

## TREATMENT AND PREVENTION

Many often hiccups remit spontaneously over a short time period, but in some cases, they may persist for a prolonged period without remission. The etiology of hiccups should be evaluated, and the underlying cause to be treated if identified. At present, there is no recommended specific treatment for hiccups as per the available evidences. Multiple pharmacological as well as nonpharmacological interventions have been tried to manage persistent and intractable hiccups. Various drugs, e.g., metoclopramide, phenytoin, diazepam, quinine, droperidol, chlorpromazine, methylamphetamine, baclofen, haloperidol, etc., have been tried for the management of intractable hiccups. Other drugs used for the treatment of intractable hiccups are amitriptyline, baclofen, carbamazepine, gabapentin, pregabalin, nifedipine, and valproic acid. The nonpharmacological interventions used for the management of intractable hiccups are swallowing dry granulated sugar, swallowing boiled rice, hypnosis, acupuncture, breath holding, drinking ice cold water, drinking from the wrong side of the cup, attention diversion, etc. Vinegar as intranasal spray also has been used as for resolution of hiccups (0.1 mL intranasal vinegar). Digital rectal massage has also been reported to abort in a case of intractable hiccups. There are various proposed surgical treatment options for intractable hiccups: (a) continuous cervical epidural block with use of local anesthetic agent (ropivacaine) continuously through a catheter at the level of C3–C5; (b) phrenic nerve block with bupivacaine and epinephrine.

The pathophysiology of intractable hiccups is complex. Multiple pharmacological, surgical intervention as well as nonpharmacological modalities have been tried to address this issue. A detailed investigations into the etiological diagnosis and to target the therapy accordingly would-be better choice to treat intractable hiccups. Literature shows intractable hiccups as part of or a presenting sign of lesions somewhere affecting the reflex arc of the hiccup neural pathways. The commonly used drugs for the management of intractable hiccups are baclofen or gabapentin, metoclopramide, chlorpromazine, and haloperidol. The evolving surgical interventions involving blocks within or near to the phrenic nerve are also used in some cases. A variety of nonpharmacological and nonmedical approaches have been reported to be effective in managing intractable hiccups.

## Points to Ponder

- Hiccups persisting for more than a month is termed as intractable hiccups.
- GERD is a common cause of intractable hiccups, and antacids, antihistamines or proton pump inhibitors are used as first-line therapy especially when no other cause is identifiable.
- Hiccups are often terminated by maneuvers which stimulate the vagus nerve or increase the partial pressure of $CO_2$.
- GABA agonists and dopamine antagonists are usually prescribed for intractable hiccups.
- Intractable hiccups unrelieved by medications may require invasive surgical procedures such as vagal nerve stimulator or stellate or phrenic nerve block.

## MULTIPLE CHOICE QUESTIONS

**1. What is the primary symptom that the 45-year-old patient has been experiencing for 6 months?**

A. Chest discomfort
B. Dyspepsia
C. Hiccups
D. Nausea

**2. What tests did not reveal any abnormalities in this patient?**

A. Abdominal ultrasound
B. Blood test
C. Colonoscopy
D. MRI

**3. Despite visiting multiple physicians, what was the outcome regarding the patient's primary complaint?**

A. Significant improvement
B. Complete resolution
C. No relief from hiccups
D. Development of new symptoms

**4. A 50-year-old male presented to ER with hiccups, i.e., on going for last 3 months. He is on chemotherapy for urothelial cancer. Which of the drug combinations is significantly associated with hiccups?**

A. Promethazine + Methotrexate
B. Cisplatin + Dexamethasone
C. Ondansetron + Vincristine
D. Pembrolizumab + Methylprednisolone

**5. In a healthy 30 years individual developed intractable seizure after an ENT procedure. Which of the following medications is most effective in treating the condition?**

A. Lidocaine
B. Ketamine
C. Chlorpromazine
D. Dexamethasone

### Answers

1. (C); 2. (B); 3. (C); 4. (B); 5. (C)

## SUGGESTED READINGS

1. Moretto EN, Wee B, Wiffen PJ, et al. Interventions for treating persistent and intractable hiccups in adults. Cochrane Database Syst Rev. 2013;2013(1):CD008768.
2. Bhatti MA, Sheikh AS, Fatima M, et al. Treatment Approaches for Persistent and Intractable Hiccups: A Systematic Review and Recommendations. Journal of Population Therapeutics and Clinical Pharmacology. 2024;31(3):1757-67.
3. Rouse S, Wodziak M. Intractable Hiccups. Curr Neurol Neurosci Rep. 2018;18(8):51.
4. Rajagopalan V, Sengupta D, Goyal K, et al. Hiccups in neurocritical care. J Neurocritical Care. 2021;14(1):18-28.

CHAPTER 30

# An Approach to a Case of Diabetic Patient Who Presents with Epigastric Pain

*Rohit Raina, Preeti Singh Dhoat, Amandeep Kaur, Niket Verma*

**CASE VIGNETTE**

A 50-year-old female with, known case of type 2 diabetes mellitus on irregular medications and uncontrolled blood glucose levels presents to you with symptoms of epigastric pain, bloating, early satiety and occasional episodes of emesis. What will you suspect?

## PROVISIONAL DIAGNOSIS

- Dyspepsia
- *Helicobacter pylori* infection
- Diabetic gastroparesis

### Dyspepsia in Diabetic Patients

Dyspeptic symptoms are a frequent finding in patients with diabetes and they are part of the so-called diabetic enteropathy (DE), which includes the GI manifestations of DM, presenting as dyspepsia, nausea, vomiting, constipation and fecal incontinence. When organic dyspepsia, medication side effects and DG are excluded, the clinical management is analog to that of nondiabetic patients, except for a more important therapeutic role of prokinetics in patients with DM.

### *H. pylori* Infection in Patients with Diabetes

Hyperglycemia has been suggested as a predisposing factor for *H. pylori* colonization. A recent case–control serological study demonstrated a significantly higher prevalence of *H. pylori* infection in patients with DM, who had positive antibody titers in 50.7% of cases, compared to 38.2% of controls. Among patients with DM, *H. pylori* infection has been shown to be higher in patients with gastroparesis, and bacterial eradication reduced symptoms such as upper abdominal pain and distention, early satiety and anorexia, thus suggesting a pathogenetic role of *H. pylori* in DG and reaffirming the therapeutic role of its eradication.

### Diabetic Gastroparesis

Diabetic gastroparesis was first coined as 'Gastroparesis diabeticorum' by Kssender to describe asymptomatic gastric retention in diabetic patients. Diabetic gastroparesis affects 20–50% of the diabetic population, especially type 1 diabetes and long-standing type 2 diabetes mellitus. It is a relatively common complication associated with diabetes, however, goes unrecognized many a times. About one-third of the patients with gastroparesis have diabetes. The mean age of onset is 34 years and prevalence increases with increasing age. Most studies have shown a higher prevalence of gastroparesis in women than in men. It refers to a syndrome of objectively delayed gastric emptying of solids in the absence of a mechanical obstruction. Management requires a holistic, all round approach.

## DIFFERENTIAL DIAGNOSIS

Refer to **Table 1**.

## CLINICAL APPROACH

### Clinical Presentation

Patients usually present with nausea, vomiting, abdominal pain, postprandial fullness, bloating, alternating constipation and diarrhea. Weight loss can be seen in severe cases. Some patients present with wide glycemic fluctuations.

Gastroparesis can be clinically differentiated based on severity with a gastroparesis cardinal symptom index (GCSI) **(Table 2)** score ranging from 0 to 5.

**TABLE 1: Summarizing differential diagnosis with their relevant evaluations.**

| Differential diagnosis | Evaluation |
|---|---|
| Functional dyspepsia | Milder symptoms. Delayed gastric emptying may be present. Diagnosis of exclusion |
| Rumination syndrome | History of passive regurgitation of unpleasant tasting substances without preceding nausea |
| Cyclical vomiting syndrome | Episodic bouts of emesis with intervening asymptomatic periods |
| Gastric outlet obstruction | Has to be ruled out using UGIE or barium studies |
| Drugs | To be ruled out through proper history |
| Hypothyroidism | Thyroid profile. Other clinical signs of hypothyroidism |

TABLE 2: Gastroparesis cardinal symptom index (GCSI).

| Symptom subscale | Symptom | None | Very mild | Mild | Moderate | Severe | Very severe |
|---|---|---|---|---|---|---|---|
| Nausea/Vomiting | Nausea | 0 | 1 | 2 | 3 | 4 | 5 |
| | Retching | 0 | 1 | 2 | 3 | 4 | 5 |
| | Vomiting | 0 | 1 | 2 | 3 | 4 | 5 |
| Fullness/Early satiety | Stomach fullness | 0 | 1 | 2 | 3 | 4 | 5 |
| | Not able to finish meal | 0 | 1 | 2 | 3 | 4 | 5 |
| | Fullness after eating | 0 | 1 | 2 | 3 | 4 | 5 |
| | Loss of appetite | 0 | 1 | 2 | 3 | 4 | 5 |
| Bloating/Distention | Bloating | 0 | 1 | 2 | 3 | 4 | 5 |
| | Belly visibly larger | 0 | 1 | 2 | 3 | 4 | 5 |

## Gastroparesis Severity Based on Severity of Illness

- *Grade 1*: Mild intermittent symptoms that are controlled with diet modification and avoidance of exacerbating agents
- *Grade 2*: Moderately severe symptoms but no weight loss, require prokinetic agents plus antiemetics for control
- *Grade 3*: Refractory to medications, unable to maintain oral nutrition and frequent emergency room visits. Require IV fluids, enteral/parenteral nutrition, and surgery.

## Physical Examination

Physical examination is nonspecific for gastroparesis. Abdominal distension, succussion splash, orthostatic hypotension, and postprandial hypotension may be seen in a few cases.

## Establishing the Diagnosis

Upper GI endoscopy excludes strictures, mass or ulcer. Drugs causing delayed gastric emptying have to be ruled out. Exclude infectious, metabolic and immunological causes by CBC, LFT, KFT, urinalysis, ESR, thyroid function test, rheumatoid factor and ANA.

## Radiological Tests

Gastric scintigraphy, stable isotope gastric emptying breath testing, wireless motility capsule, single photon emission computed tomography and electrogastrography are few radiological tests used to diagnose gastroparesis.

## Gastric Scintigraphy (Fig. 1)

Gastric scintigraphy is the gold standard for diagnosis of gastroparesis. Incorporation of radioisotope tracer into a standard meal (99-m technetium sulfur colloid labeled low fat egg white meal) and tracing its passage into stomach using gamma camera is done. Drugs causing delayed gastric emptying (opiates, anticholinergics, prokinetics, GLP-1 agonists) is to be stopped 2–3 days prior. Patients must refrain from smoking and alcohol consumption. Blood glucose levels should be < 275 mg/dL on the day of testing. Patient should be overnight fasting. Most commonly used meal: 255 kcal low fat test meal consisting of egg beaters labeled with Tc-99, two slices of bread, strawberry jam (30 g) and water (120 mL).

- *Interpretation*: Considered positive if >10% gastric retention after 4 hours of food ingestion

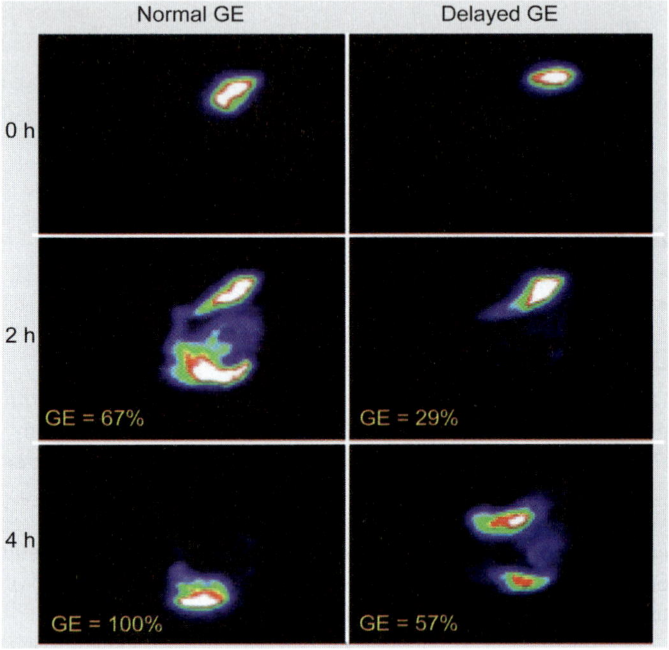


**FIG. 1:** Represents severely delayed gastric emptying with 57% retention of radionuclide labeled meal after 4 hours of ingestion.

- *Mild*: 10–15% retention after 4 hours
- *Moderate*: 16–35% retention after 4 hours
- *Severe*: >35% retention after 4 hours

## Stable Isotope Gastric Emptying Breath Testing

Stable isotopes, i.e., 13C octanoic acid or 13C spirulina platensis are used and breath excretion of $13CO_2$ measured. There must be no radiation exposure. These are safe in pregnancy, lactating mothers and children.

## Wireless Motility Capsule

Wireless motility capsule (2 cm long wireless transmitting capsule) is used that has ability to record and transmit data on pH, pressure and temperature. Gastric emptying is reflected by an abrupt change in pH as the capsule moves from stomach to duodenum. It can be continuously monitored upto 5 days. Normal gastric emptying is interpreted by rise in pH by 4 units.

### Nondelayed Gastric Emptying

It occurs with type 2 diabetes mellitus, early in the course of the disease. There is impairment of nitric oxide mediated gastric accommodation which leads to higher gastric pressure and thereby rapid gastric emptying of liquids. These symptoms are quite similar to those with delayed gastric emptying (diabetic gastroparesis). Management includes avoiding liquids with meals and for 30 minutes post meals, addition of dietary fiber and GLP-1 analogs.

## PATHOPHYSIOLOGY (TABLES 3 AND 4)

- Etiology of gastroparesis **(Table 3)**.
- Pathogenesis of diabetic gastroparesis **(Table 4)**.

**TABLE 3: Etiology of gastroparesis.**

| Category | Major causes |
|---|---|
| Idiopathic | |
| Metabolic | • Diabetes mellitus<br>• Hypothyroidism |
| Infectious | • EBV<br>• Parvovirus<br>• Varicella |
| Rheumatological | • Systemic sclerosis<br>• SLE<br>• Dermatomyositis/Polymyositis |
| Neuropsychiatric | • Rumination syndrome<br>• Anorexia nervosa/bulimia |
| Surgical | • Vagotomy<br>• Fundoplication |
| CNS disorders | CVA |

**TABLE 4: Pathogenesis of diabetic gastroparesis.**

| Etiology | Mechanism |
|---|---|
| Extrinsic denervation of stomach | Delayed gastric emptying |
| Loss of nitric oxide synthetase in enteric nerves | • Impaired inhibitory input which includes:<br>○ Decreased gastric accommodation, and possible accelerated gastric emptying of liquids<br>○ Uncoordinated antral contractility resulting in delay in gastric emptying of solids<br>○ Pylorospasm, which in the presence of antral hypomotility, may impair gastric emptying |
| Altered function of immune cells such as type 2 macrophages | Loss of cytoprotective factors resulting in damage to interstitial cells of Cajal (also termed as Cajalopathy) |
| Loss of interstitial cells of Cajal (also termed as Cajalopathy) | Decreased smooth muscle contractility and arrhythmias |
| Smooth muscle atrophy | Decreased IGF-1 levels with resultant loss of ICC |

## TREATMENT AND PREVENTION (TABLE 5)

### Nutritional Management

Daily calorie requirement should be calculated. Fats and fibers should be minimized as they impair emptying. Multiple small low fat meals 4–5 times per day are recommended. Carbonated drinks to be avoided. Patients should not lie down after meals, should walk for 1–2 hours after meals.

### Glycemic Management

Glucose levels are to be maintained below 180 mg/dL. Oral agents are not recommended for patients with significant diabetic gastroparesis. Hyperglycemia delays gastric emptying even in the absence of neuropathy or myopathy. Basal insulin is initiated at a dose of 0.2–0.3 U/kg/day for patients with T2DM and 0.15 U/kg/day for patients with type 1 diabetes mellitus. Prandial insulin may be administered after meals to prevent postprandial hyperglycemia (full meal couldn't be taken/postprandial emesis).

### Pharmacological Treatment

It includes prokinetics **(Table 6)**, antiemetics, and analgesics (rarely).

### Antiemetics

Phenothiazines are both dopamine and cholinergic receptor antagonists. They act on area prostrema. 5HT3 receptor antagonists like ondansetron, granisetron, dolasetron act on chemoreceptor trigger zone and peripheral afferent nerve fibers within vagus nerve. Antihistaminics and tricyclic antidepressants (TCA) can also used as a adjuvant therapy.

### Other Therapies

- *Intrapyloric botulinum injection*: It affects pylorospasm.
- *Pyloroplasty*: Surgically or endoscopically (G-POEM)
- *Gastric electrical stimulation*: It improves nausea, vomiting, nutritional status and quality of life in patients with refractory diabetic gastroparesis.

**TABLE 5: Lifestyle and behavioral modification.**

| | |
|---|---|
| Hydration | • Maintain adequate hydration<br>• Liquid diets if unable to take solid diets |
| Meal volume/portion | Small frequent meals divided throughout the day instead of 1–2 heavy meals |
| Fat intake | Maintain 20–30% from fats |
| Dietary fiber | Avoid high-fiber diets which limit gastric motility |
| Address micronutrient deficiency | Balance your micronutrient intake before feeding on empty calories |
| Miscellaneous | • *Avoid foods that lower LES pressure*: Caffeine, peppermint, chocolate<br>• Avoid smoking, alcohol<br>• Chew and eat slowly over 20–30 minutes<br>• Do not lie down immediately after food |

TABLE 6: Prokinetics.

| Prokinetics | Metoclopramide | Domperidone | Levosulpiride | Erythromycin |
|---|---|---|---|---|
| Dose | 10 mg 4 times a day (maximum 40 mg/day) | 10 mg TDS (maximum 30 mg/day) | 25 mg TDS | • *IV*: 3 mg/kg TDS<br>• *Oral*: 200–250 mg TDS before meals |
| Side effects | Anxiety, depression, hyperprolactinemia, QT prolongation, dystonia, tardive dyskinesia | Increased risk of arrhythmia | GI dosage: 75 mg/day | Diarrhea, QT prolongation, ototoxicity |

## Surgical Interventions

It include venting gastrostomy or jejunostomy and gastrectomy.

## Novel Drugs for Diabetic Gastroparesis

- *Ghrelin agonists*: Relamorelin (currently in phase 3 trials)
- *Motilin agonists*: Erythromycin, clarithomycin, azithromycin are used in treatment of gastroparesis, on an off-label basis.
- *Newer 5HT4 agonists*: Prucalopride, velusetrag, ATI-7505, naronapride, felcisetrag and renzapride.
- *Pistacia lentiscus (mastic gum)*: A novel patented drug formulation in pure vegan capsule formulation was compared with levosulpiride in patients with diabetic gastroparesis and its long-term safety and effectiveness was also studied in a 24-week interim analysis post intervention. Mastic gum in dose of 500 mg per oral twice daily was found to have significantly improve gastric emptying time and GCSI score in patients with DG.

## Points to Ponder

- ❑ Diabetic gastroparesis should be suspected in patients with diabetes with symptoms of early satiety, nausea, vomiting, and abdominal pain.
- ❑ GCSI score is an important clinical bedside tool for diagnosis of the severity of gastroparesis.
- ❑ Gastric scintigraphy is the gold standard for diagnosis of gastroparesis.
- ❑ Management involves a holistic approach with nutritional, behavioral and pharmacological interventions.
- ❑ *Pistacia lentiscus* (mastic gum)—a novel patented drug formulation in a pure vegan capsule is currently under research.

## MULTIPLE CHOICE QUESTIONS

1. **GCSI score stands for:**
   A. Gastroparesis symptom clinical index
   B. Gastroparesis symptom cardinal index
   C. Gastroparesis severity cardinal index
   D. Gastroparesis severity clinical index
2. **Identify the test?**

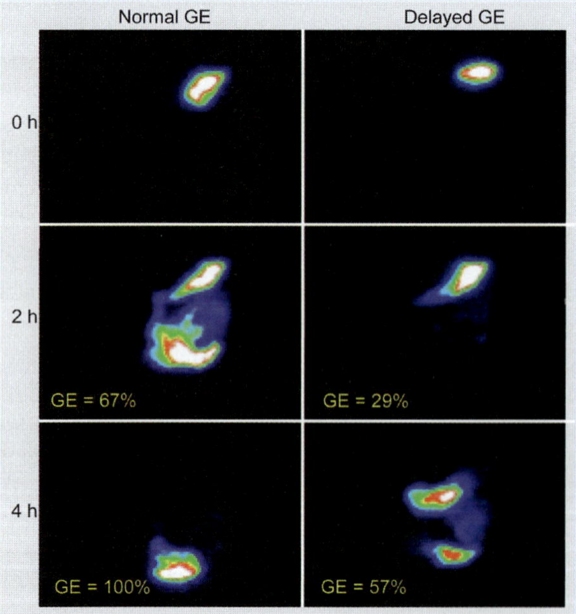


   A. Electrogastrography
   B. Wireless motility capsule
   C. Gastric scintigraphy
   D. Stable isotope gastric emptying breath analysis
3. **Gold standard investigation for diagnosis of gastroparesis is:**
   A. Electrogastrography
   B. Wireless motility capsule
   C. Gastric scintigraphy
   D. Stable isotope gastric emptying breath analysis
4. **Which of the following is true regarding nutritional management in diabetic gastroparesis?**
   A. Prolonged fasting recommended to avoid distressing symptoms
   B. Patients should lie down after food, and avoid walking postmeals
   C. Multiple small low fat meals 4–5 times a day recommended
   D. Caffeine recommended to alleviate the symptoms
5. **Which of the following class of drugs is not used in treatment of diabetic gastroparesis?**
   A. Prokinetics
   B. Antiemetics
   C. TCAs
   D. Beta blockers

## Answers

1. (B); 2. (C); 3. (C); 4. (C); 5. (D)

## SUGGESTED READINGS


1. Gotfried J, Priest S, Schey R. Diabetes and the Small Intestine. Curr Treat Options Gastroenterol. 2017;15:490-507.
2. Devrajani BR, Shah SZ, Soomro AA, et al. Type 2 diabetes mellitus: A risk factor for *Helicobacter pylori* infection: A hospital based case-control study. Int J Diabetes Dev Ctries. 2010;30:22-6.
3. Bener A, Ağan AF, Al-Hamaq AO, et al. Prevalence of *Helicobacter pylori* infection among Type 2 Diabetes Mellitus. Adv Biomed Res. 2020;9:27.
4. Huang J. Analysis of the Relationship between *Helicobacter pylori* infection and diabetic gastroparesis. Chin Med J. 2017;130:2680-5.
5. Bharucha AE, Batey-Schaefer B, Cleary PA, et al. Delayed gastric emptying is associated with early and long-term hyperglycemia in Type 1 diabetes mellitus. Gastroenterology. 2015;149:330-9.
6. Koch KL. Diabetic gastropathy: gastric neuromuscular dysfunction in diabetes mellitus: a review of symptoms, pathophysiology, and treatment. Dig Dis Sci. 1999;44:1061-75
7. Stanghellini V, Tosetti C, Paternico A, et al. Risk indicators of delayed gastric emptying of solids in patients with functional dyspepsia. Gastroenterology. 1996;110:1036-42.
8. Revicki DA, Rentz AM, Dubois D, et al. Gastroparesis Cardinal Symptom Index (GCSI): Development and Validation of a Patient Reported Assessment of Severity of Gastroparesis Symptoms. Quality of Life Research. 2004;13(4):833-44.
9. Singh A, Kant R, Raina R, et al. Efficacy of *Pistacia lentiscus* Plant (Rumi Mastagi) in Comparison to Levosulpiride in Patients with Diabetic Gastroparesis: A Double-Blind Non-Inferior Randomised Control Trial Study. Indian J Endocrinol Metab. 2024;28(1):35-42.
10. Kant R, Singh A, Raina R, et al. Real-world safety and effectiveness of *Pistacia lentiscus* (mastic gum) in patients with diabetic gastroparesis: 24-week interim analysis postintervention. Indian J Pharmacol. 2024; 56(1):4-9.

CHAPTER

31

# An Approach to a Case of Bloody Diarrhea

*Sushil Kumar, Manuj Kumar Sarkar*

**CASE VIGNETTE**

A 25-year-old male presented to the emergency department with complaints of 8–10 episodes blood-streaked stools per day associated with cramps and lower abdominal pain and tenesmus from the past 5 days. It was not associated with fever, vomiting, or weight loss. Patient had a history of consuming undercooked chicken at a local restaurant seven days ago. There was no significant travel history, and he had not taken any antibiotics or any other medications recently. His past medical and surgical history was unremarkable, with no known gastrointestinal or systemic illnesses. Physical examination revealed mild dehydration, with dry mucous membranes and general examination revealed a heart rate of 102 beats/min, regular rhythm; temperature 37.5°C, a blood pressure of 110/72 mm Hg, and a respiratory rate of 16 breaths/min. Abdominal examination revealed a soft abdomen on palpation with mild tenderness in the left lower quadrant, with no rebound tenderness or guarding; no organomegaly; and bowel sounds were normal on auscultation.

## PROVISIONAL DIAGNOSIS

Based on the acute onset of symptoms, dietary history of consuming undercooked poultry, and the presence of bloody diarrhea, the provisional diagnosis of acute infectious colitis, likely due to a bacterial pathogen, was made. The most likely causative organisms include *Escherichia coli O157:H7, Shigella, Salmonella,* or *Campylobacter*. The absence of systemic symptoms such as fever does not rule out a bacterial etiology, as *Campylobacter* infections may present without fever.

## DIFFERENTIAL DIAGNOSIS

Bloody diarrhea can result from a variety of infectious and noninfectious causes. The differential diagnoses include:

- *Infectious causes*:
  - *Bacterial*:
    - *Escherichia coli O157: H7* (Shiga toxin-producing *E. coli* or STEC): Often linked to undercooked meat and presents with bloody diarrhea, abdominal cramps, and occasionally hemolytic uremic syndrome (HUS).
    - *Shigella:* A highly infectious organism causing dysentery characterized by fever, abdominal pain, and bloody diarrhea.
    - *Salmonella:* Can cause gastroenteritis with diarrhea that may be bloody, particularly in severe cases.
    - *Campylobacter jejuni:* Often from contaminated poultry, presenting with fever, crampy abdominal pain, and diarrhea which can be bloody.
  - *Parasitic*:
    - *Entamoeba histolytica:* Causes amebic dysentery with bloody diarrhea, often seen in areas with poor sanitation.
  - *Viral*:
    - Although viral causes like cytomegalovirus (in immunocompromised hosts) may cause bloody diarrhea, they are less common in immunocompetent individuals.
- *Inflammatory bowel disease (IBD)*:
  - *Ulcerative colitis (UC)*: Typically presents with chronic diarrhea, bloody stools, and abdominal pain, with exacerbations and remissions.
  - *Crohn's disease*: Can present similarly to UC but with more systemic involvement, perianal disease, and segmental bowel involvement.
- *Ischemic colitis:* More common in older adults or those with cardiovascular risk factors. Presents with sudden-onset lower abdominal pain and bloody diarrhea.
- *Malignancy:* Colorectal cancer or bleeding polyps, though less likely in younger individuals without a significant family history, must be considered.

## CLINICAL APPROACH

Diarrhea is defined as stool weight > *200 g/day*, but this definition has limited value in clinical practice. A more useful definition, which is employed by the World Health Organization, is *three or more loose or watery stools per day or more frequently than an individual's baseline*. Diarrhea may be further defined as *acute* if <2 weeks, *persistent* if 2–4 weeks, and *chronic* if >4 weeks in duration.

Initially there was no blood in stool but presence of blood in stool within 5 days signifies bacterial infection and if blood presents in stool after 1 week it is least likely to be due to a bacterial infection. However, most of patients do not know the exact timing of the appearance of the blood in the stools. Painless bloody diarrhea is unlikely to be infectious in origin and is mostly due to inflammatory bowel disease. Bloody diarrhea generally signifies one of four bacterial infections namely *Shigella, Campylobacter*, *Salmonella*, and Enterohemorrhagic *Escherichia coli* (EHEC) O157:H7.

*Campylobacter* is generally contracted from undercooked poultry while *Salmonella* is associated with the ingestion of poultry, eggs, and milk products; these are associated with fever, pain abdomen and sometimes bloody diarrhea The route of transmission of EHEC is usually undercooked ground beef and infection may be complicated by the development of *thrombotic thrombocytopenic purpura (TTP)* and *hemolytic uremic syndrome (HUS)*. While the primary risk factors for *C. difficile* remain antibiotic usage and hospitalization, the incidence of community-associated *C. difficile* infection is also rising, and it is also important to note that *C. difficile* is a common cause of flares in patients with IBD.

*Entamoeba histolytica* common in developing country causes intestinal amebiasis symptoms range from mild diarrhea to severe bloody dysentery with abdominal pain and in developed countries it is mainly seen among immigrants from and travelers to endemic countries. Sexually active homosexuals are also at an increased risk of this infection.

Patients with *IBD* present with bloody diarrhea as the most common symptom—*ulcerative colitis (UC)* is confined to the colon and involves the mucosa and sub mucosa. Mild UC may present with up to four episodes of diarrhea with or without blood and severe cases have more frequent episodes of bloody diarrhea (>6–8); and is often associated with severe weakness, pain abdomen, fever and weight loss.

*Crohn's disease* is characterized by transmural inflammation that can involve any site along that gastrointestinal tract while sparing the rectum. Both these diseases can include extra intestinal manifestations involving the joints (seronegative spondyloarthropathies, ankylosing spondylitis, sacroiliitis); skin (pyoderma gangrenosum, erythema nodosum); and eyes (episcleritis, uveitis), amongst others diarrhea in ulcerative colitis is typically bloody and can occur with or in the absence of abdominal pain. Patients with rectal involvement may relate a sensation of incomplete stool voiding known as tenesmus. Gastrointestinal symptoms are variable in Crohn's disease and largely depend on the area affected.

*Ischemic colitis* often present with bloody diarrhea within 24 hours of onset of abdominal pain three clinical stages have been described:

1. *Hyperactive phase*: Occurs immediately after occlusion or hypoperfusion characterized by severe abdominal pain with bloody diarrhea. Blood loss is usually mild and does not require transfusion and symptoms resolve with conservative measures.
2. *Paralytic phase*: Pain diminishes but it becomes more diffuse and continuous all over the abdomen with tenderness and distension.
3. *Shock phase*: Characterized by massive fluid, electrolyte, and protein loss which occurs through a gangrenous mucosa. Severe dehydration with shock may be present which requires rapid surgical intervention.

### Laboratory Testing

Laboratory evaluations should only be used to obtain data that will help manage patients in the short term, make rapid and correct diagnoses, and optimize management. Laboratory testing includes fecal leukocytes or fecal lactoferrin latex agglutination assay with high sensitivity or specificity and stool culture in for bacterial infections.

## PATHOPHYSIOLOGY

The mechanisms behind bloody diarrhea are diverse and they are primarily linked to the insult caused to intestinal mucosa by the causative organisms. Bacterial toxins are one of the most commonly seen causes of the same and they function by causing mucosal damage and toxin release which leads to inflammation and capillary damage in the intestinal tract causing ulceration and bleeding. In cases of protozoal invasion, the primary mechanism is invasive tissue destruction that initiates ulceration and inflammation which clinically manifests as bloody diarrhea. Inflammatory bowel disease as the name suggests is characterized by chronic inflammation that damages the colonic mucosa which leads to bleeding. Lastly, ischemic colitis which stems from injury due to hypoperfusion causes sloughing of the intestinal mucosa leading to bleed. This highlights the multitude of ways that an insult to the intestinal mucosa can result in bloody diarrhea. The same has been summarized in the **Table 1**.

## TREATMENT AND PREVENTION

### Treatment (Flowchart 1)

The mainstay of treatment for acute diarrhea is hydration. Most deaths from diarrhea occur because of dehydration, therefore, the most important part of the clinical assessment of such patients are their fluid status followed by treatment of hypovolemia and electrolyte disturbances. Severely dehydrated patients require intravenous fluid while those who are alert and only mildly dehydrated loperamide is not given to patients with high fevers or blood in stool antiemetics are safe and make symptoms more tolerable. Empirical antibiotics may be considered for patients with severe symptoms, immunocompromised status, or specific bacterial infections confirmed by testing.

TABLE 1: Causes and mechanisms of intestinal ulceration and bleeding.

| Cause | Mechanism | Intestinal response | Outcome |
|---|---|---|---|
| Bacterial toxins | Mucosal invasion and toxin release | Inflammation and capillary damage | Ulceration and bleeding |
| Protozoal invasion | Invasive tissue destruction | Ulceration and inflammation | Bloody diarrhea |
| IBD | Chronic inflammation | Ulceration on colonic mucosa | Bleeding |
| Ischemic colitis | Hypoperfusion injury | Mucosal sloughing | Ulceration and bleeding |

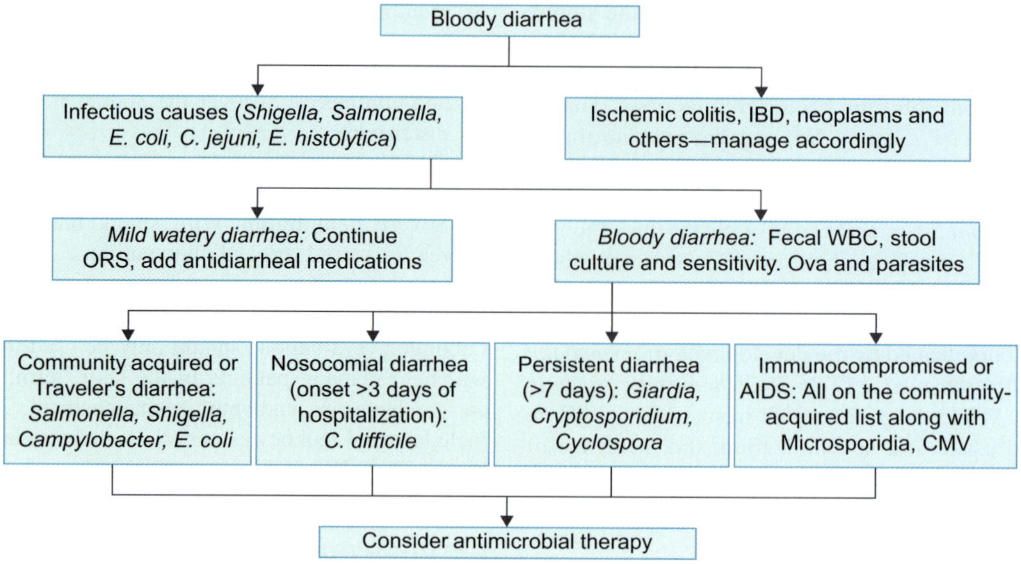


**FLOWCHART 1:** Bloody diarrhea management pathway: Differentiation of infectious versus noninfectious causes, diagnostics, and therapy-based on severity and patient profile.

## Prevention

Improvements in hygiene of water and food to limit feco-oral spread of enteric pathogens would be necessary for reduction of diarrheal diseases significantly in developing countries. Travelers can limit their risk of diarrhea by eating fresh, hygienic, only hot and cooked food and should avoid vegetables, salads, unpeeled fruits and drinking only boiled or treated water.

A new typhoid conjugate vaccine was recently prequalified and recommended by WHO. At present there are no effective commercially available vaccines against *E. coli, Shigella, Campylobacter, Norovirus* or intestinal parasites.

### Points to Ponder

- Bloody diarrhea presenting within 5 days is most likely to be of infectious origin; most commonly due to *Salmonella, Shigella, Campylobacter,* and *E. coli.*
- If blood is present in stools after 1 week of onset of diarrhea, then an infectious cause is least likely.
- Painless bloody diarrhea is unlikely to be infectious in origin and is mostly caused due to inflammatory bowel disease.
- Antimotility agents (e.g., loperamide) should be avoided in infectious causes of diarrhea.

## MULTIPLE CHOICE QUESTIONS

1. **Which of the following scenarios are least likely to indicate a bacterial infection?**
   A. Fever and abdominal cramps associated with diarrhea
   B. Bloody diarrhea appearing within 5 days of symptom onset
   C. Blood appearing in stools after 1 week of onset of symptoms
   D. Diarrhea following intake of poorly cooked meat
2. **A 37-year-old woman presents with complaints of chronic bloody diarrhea, abdominal pain, and weight loss over the past few months. She experiences frequent episodes, with blood visible in her stools. General examination, and systemic examination was otherwise normal. The patient only complained of multiple joint pains over the last few months. She denied any complaints of fever over the last few months. What is the most likely diagnosis?**
   A. Ischemic colitis
   B. Ulcerative colitis
   C. Amebic dysentery
   D. *Clostridioides difficile* infection
3. **A 27-year-old male returns from a trip where he consumed various street foods. He now presents with abdominal pain, bloody diarrhea, and tenesmus. He has mild dehydration and fever. Which of the following medications should be avoided in this case?**
   A. Oral rehydration solution
   B. Antimicrobial therapy
   C. IV fluids
   D. Loperamide
4. **A 65-year-old man with a history of atherosclerosis presents with sudden onset of severe lower abdominal pain followed by bloody diarrhea. Physical examination shows diffuse abdominal tenderness and mild distension. His blood pressure is low, and he appears dehydrated. What is the best next step in managing this patient?**
   A. Immediate surgical consultation
   B. Conservative management with hydration
   C. Empirical antibiotic therapy
   D. Stool culture for bacterial pathogens

**5. A 27-year-old female presents with 5–6 episodes of watery diarrhea from 2 days. On examination she is conscious, pulse rate is 102 beats/min, regular; blood pressure is 98/70 mm Hg; temperature is 37.5°C; respiratory rate is 16 breaths/min. Which of the following treatment options is least likely to be considered?**

A. Oral rehydration solution
B. IV antibiotics
C. IV fluids
D. Loperamide

## Answers

1. (C); 2. (B); 3. (D); 4. (A); 5. (B)

## SUGGESTED READINGS

1. Podolsky DK, Camilleri M, Fitz JG, et al., (Eds.). Yamada's Textbook of Gastroenterology, 2 Volume Set. 6th ed. Hoboken, NJ: Wiley-Blackwell; 2015.
2. Shane AL, Mody RK, Crump JA, et al. IDSA 2017 clinical practice guidelines for the diagnosis and management of infectious diarrhea. Clinical Infectious Diseases. 2017;65:e45-e80.
3. Loscalzo IE. Harrison's principles of internal medicine, twenty-first edition vol 1 & 2 (SET). 21st ed. Columbus, OH: McGraw-Hill Education; 2022.
4. Holtz LR, Neill MA, Tarr PI. Acute bloody diarrhea: a medical emergency for patients of all ages. Gastroenterology. 2009;136(6):1887-98.
5. Riddle MS, DuPont HL, Connor BA. ACG Clinical Guideline: Diagnosis, treatment, and prevention of acute diarrheal infections in adults. Am J Gastroenterol. 2016;111(5):602-22.

# CHAPTER 32

# A Case-based Discussion on Febrile Neutropenia

*Rajesh Bhawani*

## CASE VIGNETTE

A 22-year-old male with a history of epilepsy controlled on carbamazepine for 9 months, presented to the emergency department with fever (38.8°C), chills, and malaise for the past 2 days. He reported no recent travel, sick contacts, or other systemic symptoms. On examination, the patient appears unwell with a temperature of 38.8°C. There are no localizing signs of infection on initial assessment. Complete blood counts revealed severe neutropenia with an absolute neutrophil count (ANC) of 146 cells/mm$^3$. Two sets of blood cultures were sent prior to starting antibiotics along with other routine workup. Based on the clinical presentation and laboratory findings, the patient was diagnosed with carbamazepine-induced febrile neutropenia. Patient was managed with guideline based empirical antibiotics and supportive management, clinically improved and discharged in hemodynamically stable condition.

Guidelines continue to evolve based on emerging resistance patterns and clinical trial data, emphasizing the importance of staying updated with recommendations from organizations such as the Infectious Diseases Society of America (IDSA), the European Society for Medical Oncology (ESMO), and the American Society of Clinical Oncology (ASCO).

Carbamazepine is an antiepileptic and mood stabilizing drug known to occasionally induce hematologic adverse effects, including neutropenia and febrile neutropenia. Neutropenia is defined as an ANC < 1,500 cells/mm$^3$, while febrile neutropenia occurs when there is fever (often defined as a single oral temperature of ≥38.3°C or a sustained temperature of ≥38.0°C for >1 hour) in the setting of neutropenia, which is a serious complication requiring prompt evaluation and management **(Fig. 1)**.

Carbamazepine-induced neutropenia and febrile neutropenia are believed to be immune-mediated, although the exact mechanism remains unclear.

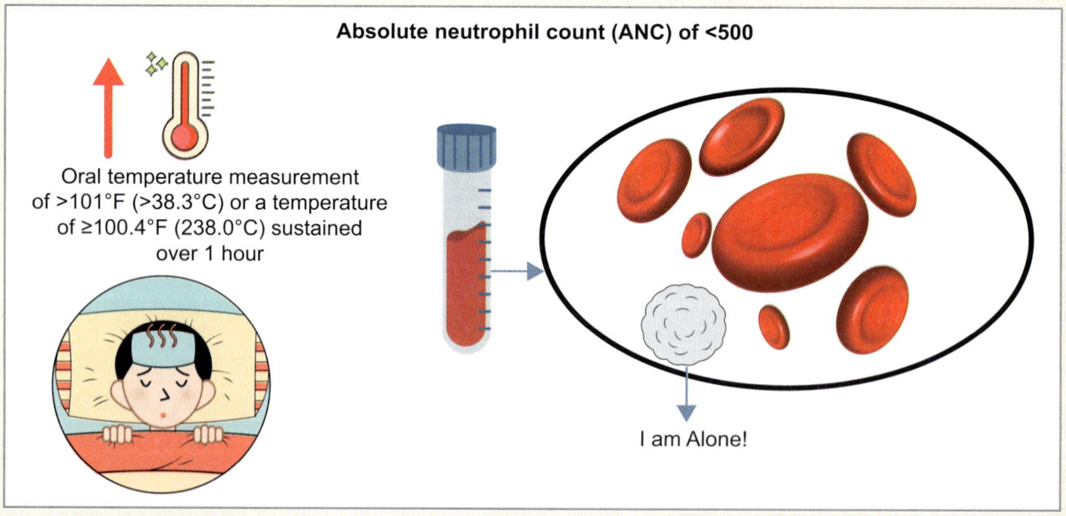


**FIG. 1:** Febrile neutropenia.

## PROVISIONAL DIAGNOSIS

Carbamazepine-induced febrile neutropenia in a 22-year-old male with a history of epilepsy, presenting with fever, chills, and severe neutropenia (ANC of 146 cells/mm$^3$) after 9 months of carbamazepine therapy.

## DIFFERENTIAL DIAGNOSIS

- *Infections*:
  - Bacterial infections: Commonly gram-positive (e.g., *Staphylococcus aureus*, *Streptococcus*) and gram-negative bacteria (e.g., *Escherichia coli*, *Pseudomonas aeruginosa*).
  - Fungal infections: *Candida* species, *Aspergillus*, and other fungi.
  - Viral infections: Herpes simplex virus, cytomegalovirus (CMV), and other viruses.
  - Parasitic infections: Less common, but possible in immunocompromised patients.
- *Noninfectious causes*:
  - Drug reactions: For example, antibiotics, other anticonvulsants.
  - Autoimmune diseases: Conditions like systemic lupus erythematosus (SLE) or vasculitis.
  - Oncologic causes: Tumor lysis syndrome, leukemia, or other malignancies affecting bone marrow function.
  - Metabolic causes: Severe metabolic disturbances or endocrine disorders (e.g., adrenal insufficiency).
  - Inflammatory conditions: Rheumatoid arthritis or inflammatory bowel disease.
- *Other considerations*:
  - Sepsis syndrome
  - Bone marrow disorders: Primary bone marrow pathology (e.g., aplastic anemia, myelodysplastic syndromes).
  - Central line infections: Infections related to indwelling catheters or ports used for chemotherapy.

Diagnostic steps often include a thorough clinical assessment, blood cultures, imaging studies, and possibly other laboratory tests. Identifying the underlying cause is crucial for effective management and treatment.

## CLINICAL APPROACH

Patients typically present with fever (defined as a single oral temperature ≥ 38.3°C or a sustained temperature ≥ 38.0°C for > 1 hour), often accompanied by chills, malaise, and signs of infection such as hypotension or localized symptoms (e.g., respiratory symptoms).

### Diagnostic Workup

- *Blood culture*: Obtain at least two sets of blood cultures from separate sites before starting antibiotics.
- *Imaging*: Consider imaging studies (e.g., chest X-ray or CT scan) based on clinical findings to identify the source of infection.
- *Other cultures*: Obtain cultures from other suspected sites of infection (e.g., urine, sputum).

### Risk Stratification

#### MASCC Score

The Multinational Association for Supportive Care in Cancer (MASCC) score helps stratify patients into low-risk and high-risk categories based on clinical parameters:

- *Low risk (MASCC score ≥ 21)*: Consider outpatient management with oral antibiotics.
- *High risk (MASCC score < 21)*: Hospitalization for intravenous antibiotics and supportive care.

## PATHOPHYSIOLOGY

Neutropenia, defined as an absolute neutrophil count (ANC) < 500 cells/mm$^3$ or < 1,000 cells/mm$^3$ with a predicted decline to < 500 cells/mm$^3$, increases the risk of infections due to impaired neutrophil function **(Fig. 2)**. Chemotherapy-induced neutropenia disrupts mucosal barriers, allowing opportunistic pathogens to enter the bloodstream, leading to FN. It is hypothesized that carbamazepine or its metabolites may cause direct toxic effects on bone marrow progenitor cells or induce an immune response that leads to neutropenia.

Risk stratification is crucial in managing FN to guide appropriate management decisions. High-risk factors typically include:

- Profound neutropenia (ANC < 100 cells/mm$^3$)
- Prolonged neutropenia (expected to last > 7 days)
- Age ≥ 65 years
- Presence of significant comorbidities (e.g., diabetes, renal impairment)
- Clinical instability (e.g., hypotension, altered mental status)
- Recent stem cell transplantation or receipt of allogeneic hematopoietic cell transplant.

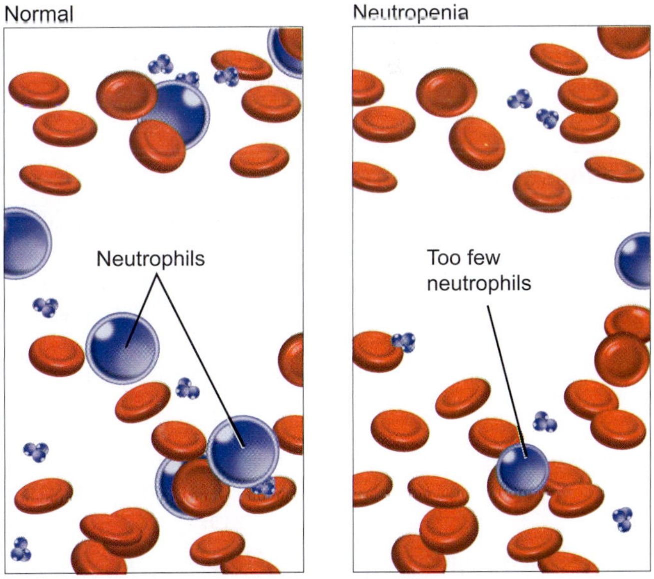


**FIG. 2:** Difference between normal neutrophil count versus neutropenia.

## TREATMENT AND PREVENTION

Effective management of febrile neutropenia relies on timely risk stratification, empirical antibiotic therapy tailored to local resistance patterns, close monitoring for clinical response, and consideration of outpatient management for selected low-risk patients.

### Empirical Antibiotic Therapy

Prompt initiation of empirical antibiotic therapy is recommended upon suspicion of FN to cover both gram-positive and gram-negative bacteria. Common regimens include:

- *Antipseudomonal beta-lactams*: Such as piperacillin-tazobactam or cefepime
- *Combination therapy*: With an aminoglycoside (e.g., gentamicin, amikacin) or a fluoroquinolone (e.g., ciprofloxacin) for additional gram-negative coverage

  In patients with penicillin allergy, alternatives like aztreonam or a fluoroquinolone can be considered.
- *De-escalation*: Adjustment of antibiotics based on culture results and clinical response within 48–72 hours to minimize antimicrobial resistance.

### Monitoring

- *ANC monitoring*: Daily monitoring of ANC until recovery (ANC ≥ 500 cells/mm³) to guide management decisions.
- *Clinical response*: Assess clinical improvement (e.g., resolution of fever and other signs of infection) to guide duration of antibiotic therapy.

### Outpatient Management

Selected low-risk FN patients, who are clinically stable and have adequate support at home, may be candidates for outpatient management with oral antibiotics. Fluoroquinolones (e.g., ciprofloxacin) or other oral agents with antipseudomonal activity are commonly used for this purpose.

### Duration of Therapy

The duration of antibiotic therapy is generally based on clinical response, with a minimum of 7–10 days recommended for most patients. Discontinuation of antibiotics should be considered when the patient is clinically stable, afebrile for at least 48–72 hours, and has evidence of neutrophil recovery.

### Supportive Care

- *Growth factor support*: Consider granulocyte colony-stimulating factor (G-CSF) for patients at high risk of prolonged neutropenia (e.g., ANC < 100 cells/mm³).
- *Fluids and nutritional support*: Ensure adequate hydration and nutritional support to maintain patient comfort and immune function.

### Antifungal Prophylaxis

*High-risk patients*: Consider antifungal prophylaxis (e.g., fluconazole, micafungin) for prolonged neutropenia (> 7 days) or in settings with high rates of fungal infections.

### Discharge Planning and Outpatient Management

- *Transition to oral antibiotics*: Consider outpatient oral antibiotics (e.g., fluoroquinolones with or without amoxicillin-clavulanate) for low-risk patients meeting discharge criteria (e.g., stable clinical condition, tolerating oral intake).
- *Follow-up*: Schedule close follow-up to monitor for signs of treatment failure or complications postdischarge.

## GUIDELINES AND RECOMMENDATIONS

- *Infectious Diseases Society of America (IDSA)*: The IDSA guidelines provide comprehensive recommendations for the management of FN, emphasizing the importance of timely empirical antibiotic therapy and risk stratification based on MASCC score.
- *European Society for Medical Oncology (ESMO)*: The ESMO guidelines also endorse similar principles for the management of FN, focusing on individualized patient assessment and treatment strategies.

### Points to Ponder

- ❑ *Drug monitoring*: Regular blood count monitoring is crucial for patients on carbamazepine due to the risk of neutropenia.
- ❑ *Early recognition*: Prompt identification of febrile neutropenia is essential to initiate timely empirical antibiotic therapy.
- ❑ *Supportive care*: Supportive management plays a critical role in stabilizing patients with drug-induced febrile neutropenia.
- ❑ *Patient history*: A thorough medication history is vital in cases of unexplained febrile neutropenia to identify potential drug-related causes.
- ❑ *Follow-up*: Regular follow-up is necessary after discharge to monitor recovery of neutrophil counts and prevent recurrence.

## MULTIPLE CHOICE QUESTIONS

**1. What is the most likely cause of febrile neutropenia in this 22-year-old male?**

A. Viral infection
B. Carbamazepine-induced neutropenia
C. Bacterial pneumonia
D. Fungal infection

**2. What was the patient's absolute neutrophil count (ANC) at the time of presentation?**

A. 500 cells/mm³
B. 250 cells/mm³
C. 146 cells/mm³
D. 900 cells/mm³

**3. Which of the following is a common first step in the management of febrile neutropenia?**
- A. Immediate antiviral therapy
- B. Empirical antibiotic treatment
- C. Blood transfusion
- D. Steroid therapy

**4. How long had the patient been on carbamazepine therapy before presenting with febrile neutropenia?**
- A. 3 months
- B. 6 months
- C. 9 months
- D. 12 months

**5. What was the patient's condition upon discharge?**
- A. He was in critical condition and required intensive care.
- B. He remained febrile but was discharged with oral antibiotics.
- C. He was hemodynamically stable with clinical improvement.
- D. He had persistent severe neutropenia without clinical improvement.

## Answers

1. (B); 2. (C); 3. (B); 4. (C); 5. (C)

## SUGGESTED READINGS

1. Pirmohamed M, James S, Meakin S, et al. Adverse drug reactions as cause of admission to hospital: prospective analysis of 18 820 patients. BMJ. 2004;329(7456):15-9.
2. Aronson JK. Meyler's Side Effects of Drugs: The International Encyclopedia of Adverse Drug Reactions and Interactions. 16th ed. Amsterdam: Elsevier; 2016.
3. Freifeld AG, Bow EJ, Sepkowitz KA, et al. Clinical practice guideline for the use of antimicrobial agents in neutropenic patients with cancer: 2010 update by the Infectious Diseases Society of America. Clin Infect Dis. 2011;52(4):e56-93.
4. Klastersky J, Paesmans M, Rubenstein EB, et al. The Multinational Association for Supportive Care in Cancer risk index: A multinational scoring system for identifying low-risk febrile neutropenic cancer patients. J Clin Oncol. 2000;18(16):3038-51.
5. Klastersky J, de Naurois J, Rolston K, et al. Management of febrile neutropaenia: ESMO Clinical Practice Guidelines. Ann Oncol. 2016;27(suppl 5):v111-8.
6. Talcott JA, Siegel RD, Finberg R, et al. Risk assessment in cancer patients with fever and neutropenia: A prospective, two-center validation of a prediction rule. J Clin Oncol. 1992;10(8):316-22.
7. Taplitz RA, Kennedy EB, Bow EJ, et al. Antimicrobial prophylaxis for adult patients with cancer-related immunosuppression: ASCO and IDSA Clinical Practice Guideline Update. J Clin Oncol. 2018;36(17):3043-54.
8. Cornely OA, Bohme A, Buchheidt D, et al. Primary prophylaxis of invasive fungal infections in patients with hematologic malignancies. Recommendations of the Infectious Diseases Working Party of the German Society for Haematology and Oncology. Haematologica. 2009;94(1):113-22.
9. Kern WV, Cometta A, De Bock R, et al. Oral versus intravenous empirical antimicrobial therapy for fever in patients with neutropenia who are receiving cancer chemotherapy. N Engl J Med. 1999;340(5):382-9.

CHAPTER 33

# An Approach to a Case of Bleeding Patient

*Abha Gupta, Priyank Rastogi*

## CASE VIGNETTE

A 19-year-old college going male patient presented with large hematoma over left arm. One day back he had represented his college team in a cricket match and was hit by cricket ball on his left arm while fielding. Detailed history revealed that he had developed a similar hematoma seven years back over his forehead after sustaining an injury while playing in his school. There was no history of easy bruisability, epistaxis or intake of aspirin or nonsteroidal anti-inflammatory drugs (NSAIDs). He had no history of prior surgeries or use of any medications. His maternal uncle had passed away 20 years back from decompensated chronic liver disease due to transfusion related hepatitis B infection. On further enquiring, it was revealed that that his maternal uncle also used to experience similar bleeding episodes.

The patient was subjected to laboratory investigations and given initial treatment with paracetamol and ice packs. Clues from the clinical assessment and results of lab investigations helped in identification of the bleeding disorder.

## PROVISIONAL DIAGNOSIS

- *Hemophilia A or B* (X-linked recessive bleeding disorder)
- Likely *factor VIII deficiency (hemophilia A)* or *factor IX deficiency (hemophilia B)*, considering the family history, recurrent hematomas, and the absence of other bleeding symptoms like easy bruising or epistaxis.

## DIFFERENTIAL DIAGNOSIS

The differentials in such a case are summarized in **Box 1**. These consist of defects in any of the three mechanisms involved in process of hemostasis as described below:

1. *Constriction of blood vessels*: When endothelial injury occurs, a brief intense vasoconstriction occurs in the vessel which is a reflexive contraction that causes a decrease in blood flow to the area.
2. *Platelet aggregation and plugging*: In the second step, platelets encounter the area of vessel injury and begin to clump together and bind to the exposed collagen and endothelial lining. The process is assisted by von Willebrand factor (VWF), a glycoprotein in the blood plasma.
3. *Activation of coagulation cascade*: This is mediated by clotting factors (or coagulation factors) which prompt reactions that activate still more coagulation factors. The process is complex and is initiated along two basic pathways. The extrinsic pathway is triggered by trauma. This is mediated via coagulation factor VII. The intrinsic pathway begins in the bloodstream and is triggered by internal damage to vessel wall. This is mediated by coagulation factors VIII, IX, XI, XII, prekallikrein (PK) and high-molecular-weight kininogen (HMWK). Both of these merge into a third pathway, referred

**BOX 1: Differential diagnosis of bleeding disorders.**

*Disorders of vessel wall*:
- Hereditary hemorrhagic telangiectasia, scurvy, Ehlers–Danlos syndromes

*Platelet disorders*:
- *Quantitative (thrombocytopenia)*:
  - *Congenital thrombocytopenia*: Wiskott–Aldrich syndrome
  - *Impaired bone marrow production*: Infections and hematological malignancies
  - *Increased platelet destruction*: ITP (antibodies against platelet membrane glycoproteins IIb and IIIa cause removal of platelets by monocyte macrophage system), systemic lupus erythematosis (antibody to platelet glycoprotein Ib), drugs and nonimmune conditions such as infections, hypersplenism, DIC, TTP (widespread hyaline micro thrombi formed due to deficiency of ADAMTS13 in arterioles and capillaries)
- *Qualitative (decreased platelet function)*:
  - *Inherited*: Glanzmanns thrombasthenia, Bernard–Soulier syndrome and von Willebrand disease
  - *Acquired*: Drugs like antiplatelet therapy, uremia and in myeloproliferative disorders

*Coagulation disorders*:
- *Inherited*: Hemophilia A (factor VIII deficiency), hemophilia B (factor IX deficiency), hemophilia C, von Willebrand disease (due to increased factor VIII destruction) and congenital fibrinogen deficiency
- *Acquired*: Liver disease (liver failure leads to decreased levels of coagulation factors V, VII, IX, X, XI and prothrombin and vitamin K deficiency), vitamin K deficiency (leading to defective function of vitamin k dependent coagulation factors II, VII, IX, X), DIC and anticoagulant therapy

to as the common pathway. This is mediated by coagulation factors I, II, V and X.

In all, there are a total of 12 known clotting factors secreted primarily by the liver and the platelets. The liver requires the fat-soluble vitamin K to produce some of them (factor II, VII, IX and X). All these factors combine to form fibrin clot thereby achieving hemostasis. In human body, this process is balanced by the counterregulatory pathway consisting of platelet activation inhibitors, coagulation cascade inhibitors and fibrinolytic pathway. Disorder of any of these mechanisms can result in bleeding disorders in this case and a diligent clinical approach can help in arriving at the cause of bleeding in this case.

## CLINICAL APPROACH

### Detailed History

A careful and meticulous history as summarized in **Box 2** should be elicited with respect to the following points:

- *Site of bleeding*: It gives an important clue as to the cause of bleeding like bleeding into muscles or joints is usually seen in coagulation disorders while bleeding from nose or under skin and menorrhagia may be suggestive of platelet disorders.
- *Duration and frequency*: Recurrent Bleeding episodes since childhood may suggest congenital bleeding disorders
- *Severity of bleeding*: Small pin point bruises/purpura occur in thrombocytopenia while large deep hematomas form in coagulopathies.
- *Past history*: Previous history of uncontrollable bleeding during previous surgical procedures or dental extraction may lead to suspicion of an antecedent cause. Recent viral infections hint at immune thrombocytopenic purpura.
- *Drug history*: One should enquire about the intake of antiplatelet drugs like aspirin and clopidogrel or anticoagulants like warfarin or novel oral anticoagulants (NOACS) like apixaban, rivaroxaban, and dabigatran. Frequently one encounters cases where patients are on long term anticoagulants start experiencing bleeding episodes. In such cases, the history of concomitant intake of other drugs interacting with metabolism of oral anticoagulants becomes very important and critical step in management of such patients.
- *Family history*: Some inherited bleeding disorders have a specific mode of inheritance and doing pedigree analysis of such patients may help in identification of such disorders. For example, hemophilia A and B are transmitted in an X-linked recessive fashion are thus males are usually affected by the disease while females act as carriers.
- History of other comorbid conditions affecting liver and kidney help in arriving at the cause of bleeding.

**BOX 2: Important points in history.**

- *Personal history of bleeding episodes*:
  - Frequency
  - Severity (including need for any medical or surgical treatments)
  - Anatomic location
  - Spontaneous or provoked
- *Drug history*:
  - Aspirin or NSAIDs
  - Oral anticoagulants
- *Past history*:
  - History of excessive bleeding after trauma or surgical and dental procedures
  - History of menorrhagia or excessive postpartum bleeding in women
  - History of blood transfusion
  - History of thrombotic events
- *Family history*:
  - Similar bleeding events
  - Known heritable bleeding disorder
  - History of consanguinity (especially important in autosomal recessive disorders)
- *Personal history*:
  - Symptoms of any conditions associated with coagulopathy (e.g., liver disease, malignancy or autoimmune disease)
  - History of recurrent miscarriage in women

## PHYSICAL EXAMINATION

During physical examination, the skin and mucous membranes should be inspected for presence of bruising and petechiae. Bleeding in such superficial mucosal surfaces is commonly seen with platelet disorders. Bleeding in deeper sites like joints and muscles is usually seen in coagulation disorders. Hence, joints should be examined for presence of swelling and tenderness as in cases of hemarthrosis in hemophilia. Other findings suggestive of potential underlying causes of bleeding should also be explored (e.g., jaundice and telangiectasia in liver disease). Abdominal examination may reveal splenomegaly which is usually present in cases of thrombocytopenia due to hypersplenism.

## INVESTIGATIONS

These consist of initial screening tests and some specialized ones depending on the possible cause of bleeding suspected from history and examination.

The screening tests include:

- *Complete blood count/peripheral blood film*: This may reveal thrombocytopenia. Peripheral smear may show associated hematological malignancies. Giant platelets may be seen in Bernard–Soulier syndrome. If there is thrombocytopenia with normal smear, patient may be tested for HIV and hepatitis C infection. Thrombocytopenia with fragmented red blood cells on smear raises the suspicion of thrombotic thrombocytopenic purpura or hemolytic uremic syndrome.
- *Bleeding time (BT)*: It (normal value 3–9 minutes) detects a platelet function abnormality and can be prolonged in cases with thrombocytopenia and defective platelet function. The test is getting obsolete now due to concerns regarding variable results and many centers instead prefer standardized platelet function assays like PFA-100.
- *Prothrombin time (PT)*: Its normal value is 10–14 seconds and assesses the extrinsic coagulation pathway. Thus, it is usually prolonged in cases of factor VII deficiency
- *Activated partial thromboplastin time (APTT)*: The intrinsic pathway of coagulation is assessed by APTT (normal value 25–38 seconds). Thus, it is usually prolonged in cases

of deficiency of coagulation factors VIII, IX, XI, XII, prekallikrein (PK) and HMWK.

- *Thrombin time (TT)*: The generation of fibrin is detected by the thrombin time (normal value 15–19 seconds) as it assesses fibrinogen function and polymerization and is prolonged by low or dysfunctional fibrinogen, fibrin degradation products, direct thrombin inhibitors and valproic acid therapy.

### Specialized Investigations

These include mixing studies in the case of abnormal PT or aPTT for further information on the nature of the defect (coagulation factor deficiency or coagulation factor inhibitor or lupus anticoagulant); coagulation factor assays to confirm and assess the severity of the coagulation factor deficiency such as in hemophilia A or B; and platelet aggregation studies to confirm platelet qualitative defects and investigations for von Willebrand disease (VWD).

The laboratory diagnosis of VWD is based on VWF antigen concentration (VWFAg) and VWF function tests, combined with FVIII coagulant activity. Ristocetin cofactor activity which measures platelet agglutination in the presence of VWF induced by ristocetin is an indirect test for VWF function and can be helpful in diagnosis of VWD. Investigations for factor XIII deficiency and alpha 2-antiplasmin deficiency are warranted in cases where no other cause can be found. Factor XIII deficiency may be diagnosed by a clot solubility test. Some cases of bleeding disorder have normal baseline screening test results. Repeated testing may be required in such cases to diagnose mild cases of VWD because of the fluctuating levels of VWF in the plasma. If all investigations are still found normal, the patient should be investigated for blood vessel wall abnormalities. Diagnosis of such disorders needs a high level of suspicion and other presenting features of these disorders need to be screened. Blood vessel disorders can be hereditary like hereditary hemorrhagic telangiectasia and Ehlers–Danlos syndromes (EDS), or acquired like scurvy.

In this case, the boy had bleeding episodes in deep tissues like muscles which indicates defect in coagulation pathway and a previous history of similar episodes as well in childhood implying an inheritable disorder. His maternal uncle had a history of blood transfusions and hepatitis B could well have been transmitted during one such transfusion. The fact that maternal uncle had a possibility of bleeding disorder while mother was unaffected implies that the disorder could have an X-linked inheritance pattern. On laboratory testing the tests for platelet function were found to be normal but the coagulation tests were abnormal. The PT was normal while aPTT was prolonged. All these findings indicate that this case was of inherited coagulation disorder (X-linked inheritance) most likely hemophilia A or B. Further assays for factor VIII and factor IX established the diagnosis.

Thus, with careful history, examination and use of appropriate investigations, a correct diagnosis can be established. A simplified diagnostic algorithm for diagnosis of such cases is presented in **Flowchart 1**.

## PATHOPHYSIOLOGY

*Hemophilia A* is a genetic disorder caused by a deficiency in *factor VIII* in the blood coagulation pathway. This leads to improper clot formation after injury, resulting in uncontrolled bleeding and formation of large hematomas, particularly after trauma. It is inherited in an X-linked recessive manner, making it more common in males. *Hemophilia B* (caused by a deficiency in factor IX) shares similar symptoms. Both types of hemophilia have a history of easy bruising, spontaneous bleeding, and excessive bleeding from injuries. Hemophilia can also be diagnosed by measuring the levels of factor VIII or IX in the blood.

## TREATMENT AND PREVENTION

### General and Supportive Management

All patients with history of bleeding episodes should be advised to avoid medications like aspirin and NSAIDs which can impair hemostatic mechanisms. Comorbid conditions like severe hypertension which may pose a problem during bleeding episode should be actively managed. Dental care and hygiene also needs to be stressed upon in such patients.

### Management of Vessel Wall Disorders

In vessel wall disorders, tests for hemostasis are usually normal. In case of hereditary disorders like EDS and Marfan syndrome with defective collagen, assessment tools for hypermobility are available. Genetic testing is required only in rare types of EDS. Management of bleeding is supportive in such cases.

Hereditary hemorrhagic telangiectasia (Osler–Weber–Rendu disease) is a hereditary disorder of vascular malformation where arteriovenous malformations (AVMs) are found in nose, lungs, brain, gastrointestinal tract and liver. It caused by pathogenic DNA variants in genes involved in the TGF-β/BMP signaling cascade. These patients commonly present with epistaxis, GI bleeding and small reddish violet lesions on face and mucosal surfaces. In such cases, estrogen containing medications can be helpful. Bevacizumab has been found to block vessel growth and appears to be a promising treatment.

Bleeding due to defect in vessel wall can also occur in scurvy where lack of vitamin C is the cause of defective collagen (due to lack of vitamin C dependent synthesis of hydroxyproline, an essential constituent of collagen). Treatment involves vitamin C supplementation which can cure the disease.

### Management of Platelet Disorders

Quantitative platelet disorders can be easily suspected based on decreased platelet counts. They include acquired disorders like infections (dengue fever), drugs like antibiotics (penicillin group), heparin, phenytoin, furosemide and others. Treatment of causative infection is usually required apart from supportive treatment in such cases. Immune thrombocytopenic purpura (ITP) is an acquired disorder in which there is immune-mediated destruction of platelets. It presents as a chronic disease with history of mucocutaneous bleeding and a low platelet count. Spontaneous remission is seen in some patients. The mainstay of treatment includes steroids while in severe cases mycophenolate mofetil, intravenous immunoglobulin (IVIG) therapy, Rho(D) immune globulin may be used. Rituximab, anti-CD20 (B-cell) antibody and TPO receptor agonists (romiplostim and eltrombopag) are effective in the treatment of refractory ITP. Splenectomy remains a treatment option in refractory cases. Therapeutic plasma exchange (TPE) remains the mainstay of

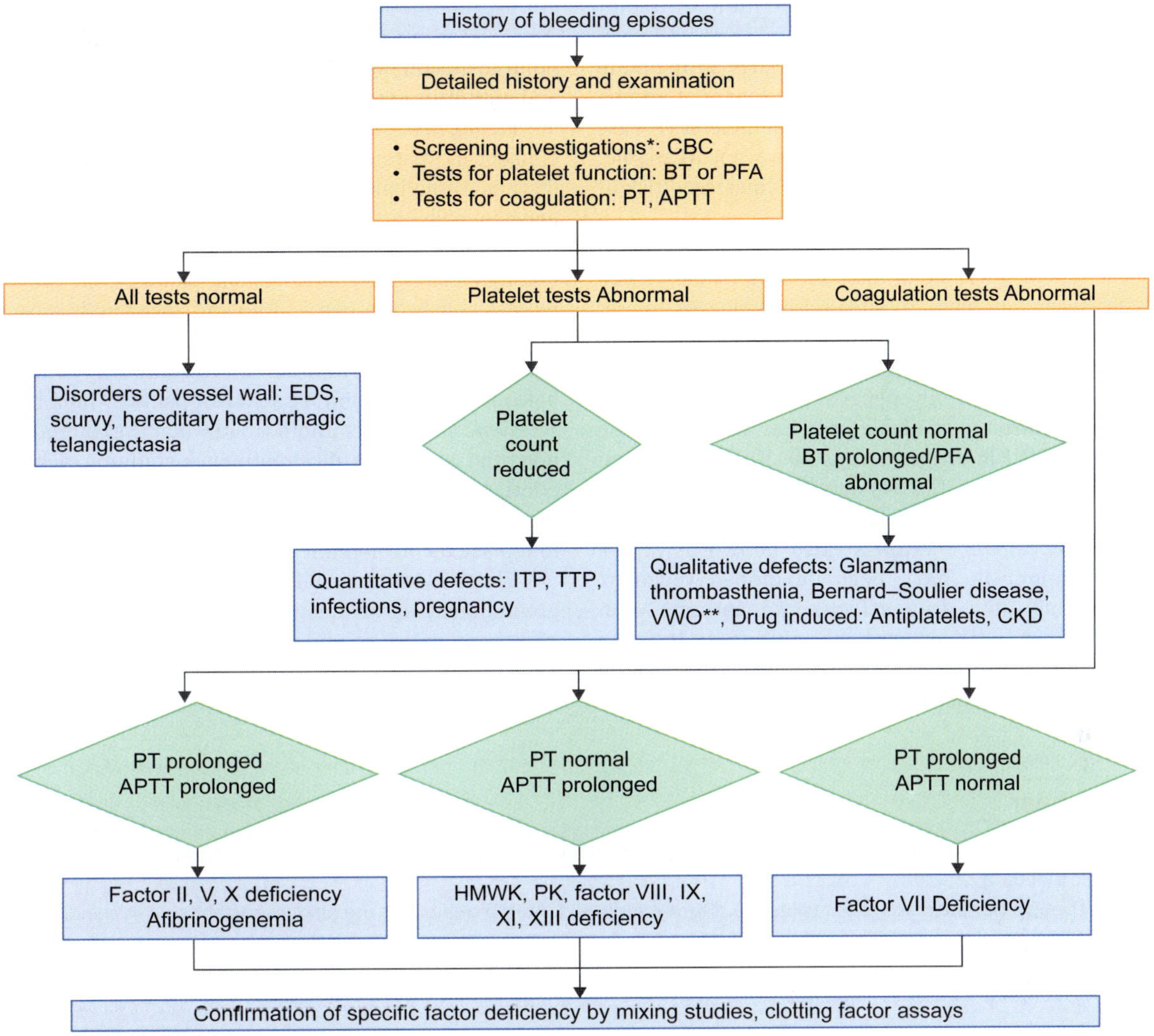


*All screening tests may be abnormal in DIC.

**In VWD, APTT may also be prolonged due to factor VIII derangement.

**FLOWCHART 1:** Simplified approach to bleeding disorders.

treatment of thrombotic thrombocytopenic purpura (TTP) while other treatment alternatives include glucocorticoids, rituximab, caplacizumab (anti-VWF nanobody).

Qualitative platelet disorders include the common acquired and rare inherited disorders. Common acquired causes like uremia and medications like antiplatelets are to be managed accordingly. Inherited disorders include Glanzmann's thrombasthenia (absence of the platelet GPIIb/IIIa receptor) and Bernard–Soulier syndrome (absence of the platelet GPIb-IX-V receptor). Both are inherited in an autosomal recessive fashion and common presentation is that of bleeding symptoms since childhood. Another class of platelet dysfunction includes secretion defects where platelets are unable to secrete their granule content. Treatment of bleeding episodes in such conditions includes use of antifibrinolytic agents like tranexamic acid. This may be given in conjunction with desmopressin (DDAVP) which increases plasma VWF and factor VIII levels. Platelet transfusion (preferably single donor platelets to avoid the risk of alloimmunization) is required in severe bleeding.

## von Willebrand Disease

It is the most common inherited bleeding disorder worldwide. VWF serves a dual role in hemostasis. It acts as the major adhesion molecule which attaches the platelet to the exposed subendothelium; and also as the binding protein for factor VIII (FVIII) thereby increasing its half-life in circulation. Thus although most of the symptoms of VWD due to VWF deficiency are "platelet-like" (mucocutaneous bleeds) but in more severe VWD, symptoms are similar to those found in FVIII deficiency (hemophilia A). DDAVP results in release of VWF and FVIII from endothelium and is the mainstay of treatment.

## Management of Coagulation Disorders

Common coagulation disorders encountered in clinical practice consist of hemophilia A and B as in the case history discussed above. Hemophilia is an X-linked recessive hemorrhagic disease due to mutations in the *F8* gene (hemophilia A or classic hemophilia) or *F9* gene (hemophilia B). Male subjects are clinically affected while women are usually carriers. Treatment of hemophilia bleeds requires prompt initiation of factor replacement and avoidance of antiplatelet drugs. The FVIII half-life of 8–12 hours requires injections twice a day to maintain therapeutic levels, whereas the FIX half-life is longer at around 24 hours and hence, once-a-day injection is sufficient. In case of emergencies where factor concentrates are not available, cryoprecipitate can be used. However, it carries increased risk of blood borne infections.

Engineered clotting factors where clotting factors are fused to polyethylene glycol, IgG1-Fc or albumin have recently been developed. These agents have an added advantage of longer half-life thus requiring fewer weekly injections to maintain circulation levels >1% and are also called as *extended half-life clotting factors*. For example, glycopegylated extended half-life FVIII and FIX are currently available in India. The usual dose of glycopegylated FVIII in active bleed is 40–50 IU/kg with an additional dose administered after 24 hours if required and a dose of 50 IU/kg every 4 days for prophylaxis in adult patients.

*Nonfactor replacement therapies* (also known as *factor mimetics*) for hemophilia have been developed recently. Emicizumab is one such drug effective in patients with severe hemophilia A with or without inhibitors. It is an antibody which binds to both FIXa and FX bringing them in close contact resulting in activation of FX by FIXa thereby eliminating the need of factor VIII in treatment of hemophilia A. It is administered subcutaneously once weekly. Other nontransfusion therapies in hemophilia consist of desmopressin and antifibrinolytics like tranexamic acid.

*Hemostasis rebalancing therapy* is another interesting concept in treatment of hemophilia. Generally, in human body there is a fine balance between procoagulant and anticoagulant agents which gets tilted toward anticoagulants in hemophilia as there is a deficiency in procoagulant pathway. It is postulated that by blocking the anticoagulant pathway, the fine balance can be reestablished in hemophilia and adequate hemostasis can be achieved. The drugs currently under development in this category include fitusiran (inhibits antithrombin), concizumab and befovacizumab (inhibit tissue factor pathway inhibitor).

*Gene therapy* is another area being explored and has the potential to change the treatment paradigm of hemophilia. It consists of transfer of functional gene responsible for clotting factor production using the adeno-associated viral vector (AAV) to replace the hemophilic patients own defective gene.

Thus in summary, with the availability of existing and newer ground breaking treatment modalities, bleeding disorders can be effectively managed and treated provided the initial assessment using appropriate tests is diligently performed to diagnose the disorder.

### Points to Ponder

- In cases presenting with bleeding symptoms, a thorough history and physical examination are essential prerequisites for identification of pathologic bleeding.
- Performing the appropriate diagnostic evaluation after excluding identifiable causes is the next important step in evaluation of such patients.
- A comprehensive knowledge of the pathophysiologic processes contributing to impaired hemostasis in any given bleeding disorder paves the way for proper treatment and avoids investigations and therapies that are irrelevant.

## MULTIPLE CHOICE QUESTIONS

**1. What is the most likely cause of recurrent hematomas in this patient with a family history of similar bleeding episodes?**

A. Vitamin K deficiency
B. Hemophilia A or B
C. Liver cirrhosis
D. Platelet dysfunction

**2. Which of the following is the primary defect in hemophilia A?**

A. Factor IX deficiency
B. Factor VIII deficiency
C. Factor VII deficiency
D. Factor XIII deficiency

**3. What is the inheritance pattern of hemophilia A?**

A. Autosomal dominant
B. X-linked recessive
C. Autosomal recessive
D. Mitochondrial inheritance

**4. Which of the following would be the most appropriate initial test to confirm the diagnosis of hemophilia?**

A. Complete blood count (CBC)
B. Prothrombin time (PT)
C. Activated partial thromboplastin time (aPTT)
D. Liver function tests (LFTs)

**5. In a patient with hemophilia A, what treatment would be used to manage a bleeding episode?**

A. Antiplatelet agents
B. Fresh frozen plasma (FFP)
C. Factor VIII replacement therapy
D. Vitamin K supplements

### Answers

1. (B); 2. (B); 3. (B); 4. (C); 5. (C)

## SUGGESTED READINGS


1. Loscalzo J, Fauci A, Kasper D, et al. Harrison's Principles of Internal Medicine. 21e. McGraw-Hill Education. https://accessmedicine.mhmedical.com/content.aspx?bookid=3095&sectionid=259856983
2. Srivastava A, Santagostino E, Dougall A, et al. WFH Guidelines for the Management of Hemophilia. 3rd edition. Haemophilia. 2020;26(Suppl 6):1-158.
3. Ellsworth P, Ma A. Factor mimetic and rebalancing therapies in Hemophilia A and B: The end of factor concentrates? Hematology Am Soc Hematol Educ Program. 2021;(1):219-25.
4. Bashawri LA, Ahmed MA. The approach to a patient with a bleeding disorder: for the primary care physician. J Family Community Med. 2007;14(2):53-8.
5. Kruse-Jarres R, Singleton TC, Leissinger CA. Identification and basic management of bleeding disorders in adults. J Am Board Fam Med. 2014;27(4):549-64.
6. Gopinath R, Sreekanth Y, Yadav M. Approach to bleeding patient. Indian J Anaesth. 2014;58(5):596-602.

CHAPTER

34

# An Approach to a Case of Leukemoid Reaction

*Smita Gupta, Neeraj Kapoor, Piyush Kumar Gupta*

**CASE VIGNETTE**

A 23-year-old woman with no previous medical condition presented with chief complaints of fever for a 5-day duration. Fever was continuously high associated with chills, rigors, and myalgia. She had no significant previous history, occupational or personal history. She denied any contact with pets and working in paddy fields. Her systemic clinical examination revealed no abnormality with provisional investigations: Total leukocyte count: 2,100 cells/$mm^3$ (normal range: 4,000–11,000/$mm^3$), platelet count: 100,000 cells/$mm^3$ (normal range: 150,000–450,000 cells/$mm^3$), serum lactate dehydrogenase (LDH) enzyme: 1,000 international units/liter (IU/L) (normal range: 140–290 IU/L), serum creatinine: 0.8, serum urea: 32, total serum bilirubin: 0.7 (direct: 0.5, indirect: 0.2), SGOT: 28, SGPT: 26. Ultrasound of abdomen showed mild hepatosplenomegaly. She was admitted to the hospital and was managed symptomatically with antipyretics and fluid therapy.

In her diagnostic workup, nonstructural antigen-1 (NS-1) by enzyme-linked immunosorbent assay (ELISA) and dengue real-time reverse transcriptase-polymerase chain reaction (RT-PCR) were positive confirming diagnosis as a case of dengue infection. Following confirmation of the diagnosis of dengue fever, we continued to manage her symptomatically. She was afebrile following 48 hours of admission; however, she developed an-icteric hepatitis, features of the capillary leak in the form of ascites, and pleural effusion. There were no bleeding manifestation except mild pruritis. Platelets were not transfused, only IV fluids given.

On day 6 of her illness, she had an elevated leukocyte count of 23,000 cells/$mm^3$, platelet count of 120,000 cells/$mm^3$ and liver transaminases of >1,500 IU/L (both alanine and aspartate aminotransferases). Her leukocyte counts further increased to 58,000 cells/$mm^3$ within 2 days, and peripheral blood smear (PBS) revealed the predominance of neutrophils with both mature and immature cells. Leukemoid reaction (LR) was suspected, and as it is a diagnosis of exclusion testing for CML (BCR-ABL), was performed, which came out to be negative. LR diagnosis was confirmed after ruling out all other differentials in the presence of a high LAP score of 300 IU/L (normal: <130 IU/L). She was managed symptomatically with adequate fluid and nutrition support. On her day 12 of illness, the leukocyte count and liver transaminases returned to normal limits, and she was subsequently discharged after complete clinical recovery.

## PROVISIONAL DIAGNOSIS

Dengue fever with leukemoid reaction (LR).

## DIFFERENTIAL DIAGNOSIS

- *Severe infection*:
  - Bacterial sepsis
  - Severe pneumonia
  - Abscess formation (e.g., hepatic and lung)
  - Tuberculosis
- *Inflammatory conditions*:
  - Severe rheumatoid arthritis flare
  - Systemic lupus erythematous
  - Inflammatory bowel disease (e.g., severe ulcerative colitis or Crohn's disease)
- *Tissue damage*:
  - Major trauma or burns
  - Extensive surgical procedures
  - Acute pancreatitis
- *Malignancies*:
  - Solid tumors (e.g., metastatic cancer)
  - Hematologic malignancies (e.g., chronic myeloid leukemia, chronic neutrophilic leukemia, myeloproliferative disorders)
- *Other conditions*:
  - Severe hemolysis (e.g., sickle cell crisis, autoimmune hemolytic anemia)
  - Medications or toxins (e.g., corticosteroids, lithium)
  - Stress leukocytosis (e.g., in response to major physiological stress like myocardial infarction)
  - Myeloproliferative disorders

It is important to differentiate leukemoid reaction from hematological malignancies (like CML, CNL). The following points must be noted to differentiate leukemoid reaction from leukemias **(Table 1)**.

Döhle *bodies* are round, oval, elongated, or triangular, blue, gray-blue, or gray-green cytoplasmic inclusions (shown by arrow in **Fig. 1**). These are RNA containing structures derived from rough ER.

**TABLE 1: Differences between leukemoid reaction and leukemias.**

| Clinical parameters | Leukemoid reaction | Leukemia |
|---|---|---|
| Basis | Physiological process | Pathological process |
| Causes | Stressor like infection or any inflammatory process | Carcinogens |
| Pathogenesis | Activation of normal hematopoiesis and exit of increased number of white blood cells in peripheral blood | Transformation of normal hematopoietic cells into highly dividing tumor cells |
| Hemoglobin level | Usually normal | Usually low |
| Duration | Acute, temporary and reversible | Chronic |
| Genetic defect | No defect | Defect |
| Splenomegaly | Absent | Present |
| Peripheral blood | Mature and immature granulocyte with left shift | Immature cells, pancytopenia |
| Bone marrow | Myeloid hyperplasia and normal morphology | Increase in blast and immature cells |
| LAP score | High (>100) | Low (<10) |
| Toxic granules and Döhle bodies | Present | Absent |

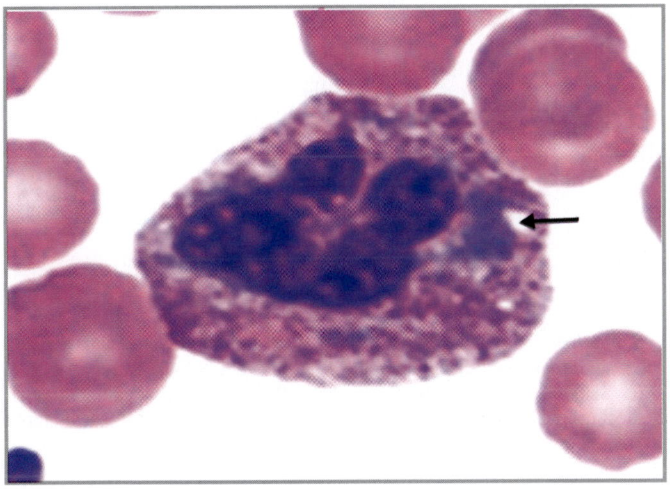

**FIG. 1:** Döhle bodies

*Toxic granulation*: Purple to dark-blue granules, resembling primary granules in segmented neutrophils, bands, and metamyelocytes.

## CLINICAL APPROACH

- *History and physical examination*:
  - Detailed history focusing on the onset, duration, and progression of symptoms, any recent infections, trauma, or surgery, and a review of medications.
  - Thorough physical examination to identify signs of infection, inflammation, or trauma.
- *Laboratory tests*:
  - *Complete blood count (CBC) with differential*: To assess WBC count and identify the presence of immature cells.
  - *Blood cultures*: To identify potential infectious organisms.
  - *Inflammatory markers*: Such as C-reactive protein (CRP) and erythrocyte sedimentation rate (ESR).
  - *Other tests*: Based on clinical suspicion, such as liver function tests, renal function tests, coagulation profile, and lactate dehydrogenase (LDH).
- *Imaging*:
  - *Chest X-ray or CT scan*: To identify infections, tumors, or other causes of the leukemoid reaction.
  - *Ultrasound or CT of the abdomen*: If abdominal pathology is suspected.
- *Further diagnostic procedures*:
  - *Peripheral blood smear*: To differentiate between leukemoid reaction and leukemia by examining the morphology of white blood cells.
  - *Bone marrow biopsy*: If malignancy is strongly suspected or the diagnosis remains unclear after initial tests.

## PATHOPHYSIOLOGY

Dengue virus infection can cause systemic manifestations including fever, hepatosplenomegaly, and myalgia. It induces a capillary leak syndrome resulting in ascites and pleural effusion. In some cases, an immune response leads to leukemoid reaction (marked increase in leukocytes) with predominance of neutrophils. This reaction is an extreme response to infection or stress and can mimic leukemia but is not associated with the *BCR-ABL* fusion gene. The elevated liver transaminases and other laboratory abnormalities are consistent with hepatic involvement during the acute phase of dengue fever.

## TREATMENT AND PREVENTION

- *Address the underlying cause*: Treatment of leukemoid reaction depends on the underlying cause.
  - *Infections*: Empirical broad-spectrum antibiotics tailored to the likely pathogens, adjusted based on culture results.
  - *Inflammatory conditions*: Anti-inflammatory medications, such as corticosteroids or disease-specific treatments (e.g., immunosuppressants for autoimmune diseases).
  - *Tissue damage*: Surgical intervention if required, along with supportive care and management of complications.
- Supportive care
- *Regular monitoring* of WBC count, vital signs, and other relevant parameters.
- *Measures to reduce white blood cells include:*
  - Leukapheresis
  - Hydration
  - Urine alkalinization

## Points to Ponder

- *Differentiating from leukemia*: Careful evaluation to rule out hematologic malignancies, as the management differs significantly.
- *Polypharmacy and toxins*: Consider the role of medications and toxins in causing leukemoid reactions.
- *Monitoring for complications*: Be vigilant for potential complications of the underlying condition or the leukemoid reaction itself, such as disseminated intravascular coagulation (DIC).

## MULTIPLE CHOICE QUESTIONS

**1. What is the most likely cause of leukemoid reaction (LR) in this patient?**

A. Chronic myelogenous leukemia (CML)
B. Dengue fever
C. Acute myeloid leukemia (AML)
D. Tuberculosis

**2. Which of the following lab findings is most consistent with dengue fever?**

A. High total leukocyte count
B. Severe thrombocytosis
C. Positive NS1 antigen and RT-PCR for dengue
D. Elevated blood urea nitrogen (BUN)

**3. In a patient with dengue fever, what is a common complication associated with capillary leak syndrome?**

A. Hyperkalemia
B. Ascites and pleural effusion
C. Hypotension and shock
D. Hyperglycemia

**4. A leukemoid reaction is characterized by an elevated leukocyte count with predominance of which type of cells?**

A. Lymphocytes
B. Eosinophil's
C. Neutrophils
D. Basophils

**5. Which of the following is the most important test for diagnosing dengue infection?**

A. Peripheral blood smear
B. Dengue NS1 antigen and RT-PCR
C. Liver function tests
D. Complete blood count (CBC) with differential

### Answers

1. (B); 2. (C); 3. (B); 4. (C); 5. (B)

## SUGGESTED READINGS

1. Krumbhaar EB. Leukemoid blood pictures in various clinical conditions. AMJ Med J. 1926;172:519-33.
2. Leukemoid reaction response to chemotherapy and radiotherapy in a patient with cervical carcinoma. Ann Hematol. 2003;82:316-7.
3. Au WY, Ma SK, Kwong YL. Disseminated hepatosplenic mycobacterial infection masking myeloproliferative diseases as leukemoid reaction: a diagnostic pitfall. Leuk Lymphoma. 2001;805-8.
4. Ganti AK, Potti A, Mehdi S. Uncommon syndromes and treatment manifestations of malignancy: case 2. Metastatic non-small-cell lung cancer presenting with leukocytosis. J Clin Oncol. 2003;168-70.
5. McKee Jr. LC. Excess leukocytosis (leukemoid reactions) associated with malignant diseases. South Med J. 1985;78:1475-82.
6. Sakka V, Tsiodras S, Giamarellos-Bourboulis EJ, Giamarellou H. An update on the etiology and diagnostic evaluation of a leukemoid reaction. Eur J Intern Med. 2006;17(6):394-8.
7. Alfraij A, Al-Enazi N. A case report of leukemoid reaction in a child with severe diabetic ketoacidosis (DKA) and cerebral edema: When rarity and complexity meet. Clin Case Rep. 2024;12(6):e9017.
8. Reddy S, Agrawal S, Kumar S, et al. The Leukemoid Reaction in Severe Alcoholic Hepatitis: A Case Report. Cureus. 2024;16(2):e54039.

CHAPTER 35

# An Approach to a Case of Multiple Granuloma in Spleen

*Santosh Kumar Swain, Khemeswar Agasti*

## CASE VIGNETTE

A 44-year-old male from rural Odisha was recently diagnosed with diabetes, presenting with fever and altered sensorium for 7 days. He was diagnosed with diabetes 20 days before presentation, though he had not yet commenced any antidiabetic treatment.

On examination, the patient appeared disoriented, pale, icteric and displayed splenomegaly on abdominal palpation. His vitals were unstable with a fever of 101.4°F and blood pressure was low owing to septic shock. On this background, a provisional diagnosis of sepsis was made and the patient was put on vasopressor support, injection insulin, metronidazole, and ceftriaxone.

On day 2, his routine investigations revealed anemia with hemoglobin of 9.8 g/dL, a TLC of 14.6 × 103/μL (neutrophil 88%, lymphocyte 10%, monocyte 1.8%, basophil 0.2%, eosinophil 0%), thrombocytopenia (TPC = 1.03 × 103/μL), and deranged liver function tests (total bilirubin—3.1 mg/dL, direct bilirubin—1.7 mg/dL, AST—242 IU/L, ALT—124 IU/L), normal renal function (urea 32 mg/dL, creatinine 0.8 mg/dL). His HbA1c was 8.4%. On day 6, an ultrasound of his abdomen suggested splenomegaly with multiple small punctate hypoechoic focal lesions (granulomatous lesions, micro abscess), and CECT of abdomen on day 8, showed tiny nodules and some showing honeycombing of abscess, some showing calcification in the splenic lesion **(Fig. 1)**. By day 8, the patient was afebrile. Moreover, there was no improvement in his liver function tests, hence the antibiotics were switched to meropenem and teicoplanin. Additionally, the blood culture sent on day 3 returned negative by day 6.

Due to the patient's deteriorating condition, a subsequent blood culture was performed on day 7, which tested positive for *Burkholderia pseudomallei* by day 10 and was sensitive to ceftazidime, imipenem, and co-trimoxazole.

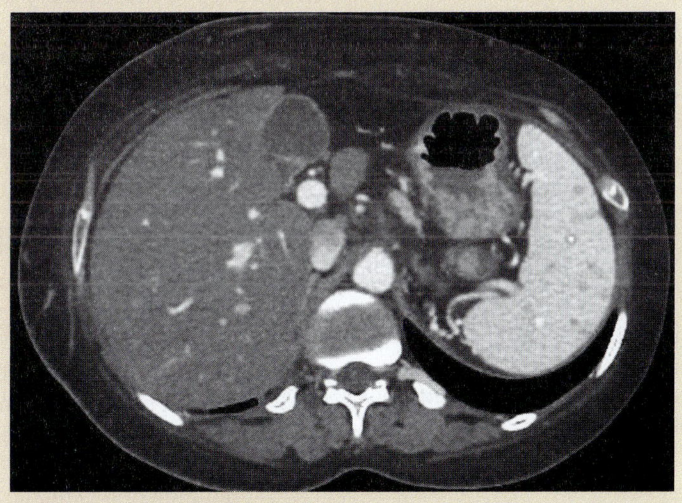

**FIG. 1:** Spleen studded with many tiny hypodense nodules, some of which have a punctate hyperdense center that perhaps signifying central calcification.

## PROVISIONAL DIAGNOSIS

The diagnosis of *melioidosis* was confirmed on day 10, and appropriate antibiotics were initiated based on the culture sensitivity, the patient was shifted to the ICU and gradually patient improved and was discharged.

## DIFFERENTIAL DIAGNOSIS

The presence of multiple granulomas in the spleen may indicate a range of infectious, inflammatory, or neoplastic conditions. The primary differential diagnoses include:

- *Infective causes*:
  - *Tuberculosis*: Granulomas are commonly seen in splenic involvement of miliary tuberculosis, hematogenous spread of disease to the spleen and *Mycobacterium avium* complex (MAC).
  - *Fungal infections: Histoplasmosis* and other fungal infections like *Pneumocystis carinii pneumonia* can cause granulomatous inflammation in the spleen.
  - *Melioidosis: Burkholderia pseudomallei* also causes granulomatous lesion in spleen.
  - *Brucellosis*: A zoonotic infection commonly associated with granulomatous inflammation in the spleen.
  - *Q fever*: *Coxiella burnetii* can lead to chronic infections with granuloma formation.
- *Noninfectious/Inflammatory causes*:
  - *Sarcoidosis*: A multisystem inflammatory disease that often manifests with noncaseating granulomas in the spleen and other organs.
  - *Autoimmune diseases*: Conditions like systemic lupus erythematosus (SLE) and rheumatoid arthritis can lead to secondary granulomatous involvement.
- *Neoplastic and miscellaneous causes*:
  - *Lymphoma*: Certain lymphomas can cause granulomatous reactions within the spleen.
- *Granulomatous disease of unknown origin/idiopathic granulomatous splenitis*: Inspite of extensive diagnostic efforts, in some cases no underlying cause can be identified, thus leading to a diagnosis of idiopathic granulomatous splenitis.
- *Primary masses*:
  - Hemangioma
  - Hemangiosarcoma
  - Lymphangioma
  - Splenic infarction
- *Secondary metastasis*: Most commonly from melanoma, lymphoma, breast or lung cancer.
- *Langerhans cell histiocytosis*: This condition can be a differential diagnosis for splenic granulomas.

## CLINICAL APPROACH

A structured clinical approach is essential for accurate diagnosis and management of multiple granulomas in the spleen:

- *Detailed history*:
  - Assess the patient's travel history for visits to regions endemic for tuberculosis or fungal infections.
  - Inquire about occupational exposure to animals (for brucellosis) or recent tick bites (for Q fever).
  - Review of systems for symptoms of autoimmune or systemic inflammatory diseases (fever, joint pain, skin lesions).
- *Physical examination*:
  - Assess for splenomegaly, hepatomegaly, or lymphadenopathy.
  - Search for signs of systemic involvement, such as skin nodules or respiratory symptoms.
- *Laboratory investigations*:
  - *Complete blood count (CBC)*: Evaluation for anemia, leukopenia, or thrombocytopenia, which may indicate underlying systemic involvement.
  - *Erythrocyte sedimentation rate (ESR) or C-reactive protein (CRP)*: To assess the inflammatory state.
  - *Serologic tests*: For infections like tuberculosis, brucellosis, or fungal pathogens.
  - *Autoimmune markers*: ANA, rheumatoid factor, ACE levels (for sarcoidosis).
- *Radioimaging*:
  - *Ultrasound*: Initial investigation to assess splenic size and detect granulomas.
  - *CT scan or MRI*: Provides better visualization of the splenic lesions and evaluates other organ involvement.
- *Biopsy*:
  - *Fine-needle aspiration (FNA)* or *core biopsy* of the spleen is essential for histopathological diagnosis. Special stains (acid-fast for TB, fungal stains) and cultures may be necessary to identify causative agents.

## PATHOPHYSIOLOGY

The patient presents with sepsis due to *melioidosis*, caused by *Burkholderia pseudomallei*. The pathogen commonly affects individuals in rural areas and can lead to *acute systemic infection* with *fever, septic shock, liver dysfunction, and splenomegaly*. The presence of *granulomatous lesions*, microabscesses, and *honeycombing in splenic lesions* suggests disseminated infection. In untreated or inadequately treated cases, it can result in organ dysfunction, septic shock, and death. The *hyperglycemia* observed in the patient could exacerbate infection due to impaired immune function in diabetic individuals. *Burkholderia pseudomallei* can also cause *abscess formation*, particularly in the liver and spleen, with characteristic calcification and nodular lesions seen on imaging.

## TREATMENT AND PREVENTION

Management of multiple granulomas in the spleen is determined by the underlying cause:

- *Infectious etiologies*:
  - *Tuberculosis*: For infectious causes such as tuberculosis, prolonged antitubercular therapy as per guidelines is recommended, typically involving a combination of rifampin, isoniazid, pyrazinamide, and ethambutol for a duration of 6–9 months.
  - *Fungal infections*: Treatment with antifungal agents like amphotericin B or itraconazole based on the specific pathogen.
  - *Brucellosis*: Doxycycline combined with rifampin for 6 weeks is the standard therapy.
  - *Melioidosis*: Ceftrazidime or meropenem
- *Sarcoidosis*: For splenic sarcoidosis, corticosteroids are the first-line treatment for symptomatic patients, with immunosuppressive agents like methotrexate or azathioprine reserved for refractory cases.

- *Autoimmune diseases*: Immunosuppressive agents, including corticosteroids, are used to manage granulomas secondary to systemic autoimmune diseases.
- *Surgical management*: Splenectomy is rarely required but may be considered for diagnostic purposes or in cases of severe splenomegaly with hypersplenism, or refractory disease.

## Points to Ponder

- *Thorough diagnostic evaluation*: Identifying the cause of granulomas is critical, as treatment varies significantly based on the underlying condition (e.g., infectious vs. autoimmune).
- *Biopsy is crucial*: While imaging can suggest granulomas, definitive diagnosis requires histological confirmation via biopsy.
- *Infectious causes predominate*: Tuberculosis remains a leading cause of splenic granulomas, particularly in endemic regions. Re-emerging infections like melioidosis are also increasingly recognized as important contributors.
- *Long-term follow-up*: Patients with granulomatous diseases often require long-term follow-up to monitor treatment response and recurrence, especially in chronic infectious or inflammatory conditions.
- The unique environmental and demographic conditions of some regions of India, including heavy rainfall, cyclonic activity, extensive paddy cultivation, and high prevalence of diabetes, may position it as a potential hotspot for melioidosis. Thus, there's a dire necessity for the creation of awareness among clinicians and capacity building of existing laboratories for early diagnosis and management of this neglected tropical disease.
- This chapter provides an overview of how to assess, diagnose, and manage patients presenting with multiple granulomas in the spleen. The key to successful management lies in identifying the underlying etiology and tailoring treatment accordingly.

## MULTIPLE CHOICE QUESTIONS

1. **Which of the following is the most likely diagnosis in this patient?**
   A. Malaria
   B. Typhoid fever
   C. Melioidosis
   D. Leptospirosis
2. **What is the most characteristic feature of *Burkholderia pseudomallei* infection seen on ultrasound?**
   A. Hepatic abscesses
   B. Splenic granulomas
   C. Renal enlargement
   D. Gallbladder thickening
3. **What is the most common complication associated with diabetes in the context of sepsis?**
   A. Diabetic ketoacidosis
   B. Impaired immune function
   C. Hyperosmolar hyperglycemic state
   D. Hypoglycemic coma
4. **Which antibiotic is most effective for treating *Burkholderia pseudomallei* infection?**
   A. Amoxicillin
   B. Ceftazidime
   C. Ciprofloxacin
   D. Doxycycline
5. **What is the most likely cause of the patient's elevated liver enzymes (AST, ALT)?**
   A. Hepatitis B
   B. Liver metastasis
   C. Septicemia with liver involvement
   D. Alcoholic liver disease

### Answers

1. (C); 2. (B); 3. (B); 4. (B); 5. (C)

## SUGGESTED READINGS


1. Williams O, Fatima S. Granuloma. In: StatPearls. StatPearls Publishing; 2024. Accessed September 12, 2024. http://www.ncbi.nlm.nih.gov/books/NBK554586/
2. Weerakkody Y. Splenic granulomatous disease | Radiology Reference Article | Radiopaedia.org. Radiopaedia. doi:10.53347/rID-41220.
3. Dash P, Prusty SK, Pattnaik SS, et al. Solid Organ Abscess by Melioidosis: An Emerging Infection Among Diabetics in Odisha, India. Cureus. 2022;14(12):e32975.
4. Kobayashi K, Einama T, Fujinuma I, et al. A rare case of isolated splenic sarcoidosis: A case report and literature review. Molecular and Clinical Oncology. 2021;14(2):1-1.
5. Elzein FE, Elzein S, Albalawi R. Splenic calcification in systemic lupus erythematosus. BMJ Case Rep. 2017;2017:bcr2017222206.
6. Kim N, Auerbach A, Manning MA. Algorithmic Approach to the Splenic Lesion Based on Radiologic-Pathologic Correlation. RadioGraphics. 2022;42(3):683-701.

CHAPTER 36

# An Approach to a Case of Delirium in the ICU

*Naresh Kumar Midha, Deepak Kumar, Ashutosh Chaturvedi*

**CASE VIGNETTE**

Mrs S is a 72-year-old female with hypertension, type 2 diabetes mellitus, and chronic kidney disease (stage 3). She is admitted to ICU for septic shock with underlying urosepsis.

## PRESENTATION

Mrs S was admitted to the ICU with altered mental status, fever, and hypotension. Upon admission, she was diagnosed with septic shock due to a urinary tract infection and was started on broad-spectrum antibiotics, intravenous fluids, and vasopressors. Initially, she was alert but disoriented to time and place.

### Clinical Course

On the third day of ICU admission, Mrs S's condition began to deteriorate despite the stabilization of her vital signs. She became agitated, attempting to remove her IV lines and Foley catheter, and was disoriented to person, place, and time. Her speech was not comprehensive, and she exhibited fluctuating levels of consciousness, alternating between lethargy and hyperactivity.

### Provisional Diagnosis

Delirium secondary to septic encephalopathy in the context of urosepsis, complicated by underlying hypertension, type 2 diabetes mellitus, and chronic kidney disease.

### Differential Diagnoses

*Delirium*: Delirium is common in elderly ICU patients, particularly those with underlying chronic conditions such as hypertension, diabetes, and chronic kidney disease. The acute onset of fluctuating mental status, disorientation, and agitation with underlying infection and critical illness strongly suggest delirium. Delirium is usually precipitated by septic shock, medication effects, and metabolic imbalances.

*Septic encephalopathy*: Sepsis can lead to encephalopathy, characterized by altered mental status due to the systemic inflammatory response.

*Uremic encephalopathy*: In CKD patients, Uremic encephalopathy may present with confusion, agitation, and altered consciousness, especially if renal function worsens during critical illness.

*Cerebrovascular event (stroke or transient ischemic attack)*: A cerebrovascular event could present with acute changes in mental status, especially in an elderly patient with cardiovascular risk factors like hypertension and diabetes. A stroke or TIA should be considered if focal neurological deficits are identified.

*Hypoxia-related encephalopathy*: Despite stabilization of vital signs, periods of hypoxia can occur in critically ill patients, leading to brain dysfunction. Hypoxia leads to delirium is not uncommon.

*Central nervous system (CNS) infection*: Although Mrs S's altered mental status is likely due to sepsis, the possibility of a CNS infection, such as meningitis or encephalitis, should be considered, particularly if fever and neurological symptoms persist despite treatment for urosepsis.

### Pathophysiology

The pathophysiology of delirium remains incompletely understood. However, it is widely accepted that delirium is a multifactorial condition, with various contributing factors that can lead to its development in critically ill patients.

#### *Neuroinflammation*

Neuroinflammation plays a key role in delirium, often triggered by systemic inflammation during critical illness. Underlying sepsis or cerebrovascular events can lead to microglial activation, proinflammatory cytokine release (e.g., IL-1$\beta$, IL-6, TNF-$\alpha$), blood-brain barrier disruption, and altered neurotransmission, resulting in cognitive disturbances.

#### *Neurotransmitter Imbalance*

Delirium is linked to disruptions in key neurotransmitter systems. Acetylcholine, essential for attention and cognition, is often depleted, especially in cases involving anticholinergic drugs or dementia. Elevated dopamine levels contribute to hyperactive delirium, while serotonin, GABA, and glutamate pathway disturbances further play a role in its development.

### *Oxidative Stress*

Critically ill patients often experience oxidative stress due to ischemia-reperfusion injury, sepsis, or metabolic derangements. Oxidative stress leads to neuronal damage and apoptosis, which can exacerbate delirium.

### *Neuroendocrine Dysregulation*

Critical illness triggers neuroendocrine changes, especially in the HPA axis, leading to excessive release of cortisol, which impairs hippocampal function and contributes to delirium. Melatonin dysregulation further disrupts consciousness and circadian rhythms.

### *Risk Factors*

Several risk factors predispose critically ill patients to delirium. These can be broadly categorized into predisposing (baseline) and precipitating (acute) factors.

## Clinical Approach

A detailed history, including baseline cognitive function, medication use, recent surgeries, and any acute changes in mental status, is crucial in diagnosing delirium. A comprehensive neurological examination should be performed to assess the level of consciousness, attention, orientation, and cognitive function.

## Screening Tools

*Confusion assessment method for the ICU (CAM-ICU)*: The CAM-ICU is a widely used and validated tool for diagnosing delirium in critically ill patients. It assesses four key features: sudden onset and fluctuating course, inattention, disorganized thinking, and altered consciousness.

*Richmond agitation-sedation scale (RASS)*: The RASS is used to assess the level of sedation and agitation in ICU patients, aiding in the detection of delirium, particularly the hyperactive subtype.

*Intensive care delirium screening checklist (ICDSC)*: The ICDSC is another validated tool that scores patients on eight delirium-related criteria, including altered level of consciousness, inattention, disorientation, hallucinations, and psychomotor agitation.

## Utility of MRI Brain and EEG

Magnetic resonance imaging (MRI) brain scans can diagnose structural problems like strokes or abscesses, aiding treatment decisions and providing information about long-term cognitive outcomes. While not typically part of standard delirium care, an MRI is valuable for excluding other significant differential diagnoses.

Electroencephalogram (EEG) can be a valuable tool in assessing delirium. Generalized theta or delta slowing on EEG in a delirium patient is associated with longer hospital stays, poor functional outcomes, and high mortality. EEG also helps exclude non-convulsive seizures related to delirium **(Flowchart 1)**.

## Treatment and Prevention

Delirium cannot be treated with a single medication. Clinicians should prioritize addressing underlying predisposing factors and emphasize non-pharmacologic approaches. In some instances, medications may be required to manage hyperactive behavior in

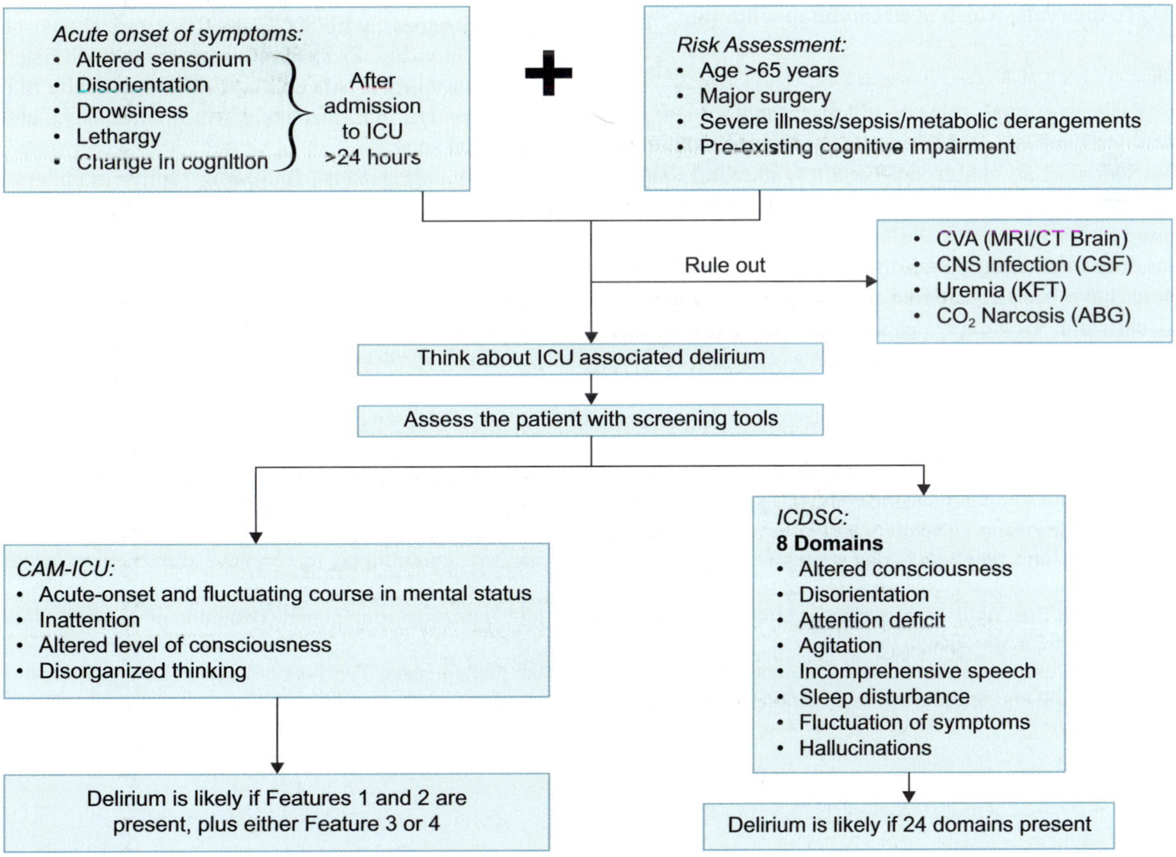


**FLOWCHART 1:** Clinical approach to delirium in the ICU

delirious patients, but it is essential to understand that it does not cure delirium itself.

Treatment of symptomatic delirium in ICU can be divided into pharmacological and non-pharmacological strategies.

## Pharmacological Treatment

Before considering pharmacological treatment for ICU-associated delirium, it is crucial to address and correct the precipitating risk factors. The initial and most important step is to identify and alleviate these factors. The use of benzodiazepines (particularly lorazepam and midazolam), opioids, and anticholinergic drugs is independently linked to a higher risk of delirium.

## Dexmedetomidine

Dexmedetomidine, a selective α-2 adrenoreceptor agonist, aids in sleep-wake cycle regulation with sedation. In two double-blind, randomized trials, it reduced delirium risk by 23% in mechanically ventilated patients compared to midazolam. A recent Cochrane analysis suggests dexmedetomidine may also shorten delirium duration, mechanical ventilation time, and ICU stay.

## Antipsychotics

Antipsychotic drugs like quetiapine and haloperidol have been widely used and studied for managing delirium in critically ill patients. Various studies showed a positive outcome with quetiapine. Although it shortened delirium duration and reduced agitation, no large RCTs have confirmed significant treatment benefits. Key side effects of antipsychotic drugs include metabolic dysfunction, extrapyramidal symptoms, hyperglycemia, and prolonged QTc intervals, which need careful monitoring.

## Thiamine

Thiamine plays a crucial role in glucose metabolism and neurotransmitter synthesis. A 2021 systematic review and meta-analysis by Sedhai et al. analyzed 18 studies, showing that IV thiamine supplementation reduced ICU delirium odds by 42% and decreased mortality in critical illness.

Various drugs, including statins, melatonin, rivastigmine, and valproic acid, have been considered in various RCTs for ICU-associated delirium. However, despite rigorous methodology and outcome assessments, none of these medications showed significant improvements over placebo.

## Nonpharmacological Interventions

The key elements of this non-pharmacological approach are outlined in the ABCDEF bundle, as detailed below:

- *Assess, prevent, and manage pain*: Critically ill patients often experience pain both at rest and during routine procedures. If pain is not effectively managed, it can lead to delirium. Therefore, it is important to assess pain in all adult ICU patients regularly.
- *Both spontaneous awakening trials (SATs) and spontaneous breathing trials (SBTs)*: Spontaneous awakening trials (SATs) involve pausing intravenous narcotics and sedatives, resuming at half the previous dose if necessary. Spontaneous breathing trials (SBTs) provide minimal ventilator support, significantly reducing ventilator time compared to standard care.
- *Choice of appropriate sedative*: Effective management of pain, anxiety, and delirium is crucial in the ICU, requiring patient-centered goals and standardized assessments. Several validated scales, like the Richmond Agitation–Sedation Scale (RASS) and Riker Sedation–Agitation Scale, guide sedation assessment. The MENDS trial found dexmedetomidine led to more delirium- and coma-free days than lorazepam in mechanically ventilated patients.
- *Delirium—early identification and prevention*: Early detection and risk factor modification is essential in managing delirium. The Confusion Assessment Method for the ICU (CAM-ICU) is the most extensively used assessment tool for delirium. It evaluates four features: acute mental status change, inattention, disorganized thinking, and altered consciousness, with 80% sensitivity and 95.9% specificity.
- *Early mobility*: From passive exercises to assisted walking, early mobility is safe and feasible for critically ill patients. It reduces delirium, mechanical ventilation days, and ICU and hospital stays.
- *Family engagement*: Involving family members in patient care enhances ICU team performance and communication, offers valuable insights into the patient's condition, and ensures care remains focused on the patient's goals. This approach may also reduce family stress by encouraging clear, simplified, and deliberate communication.

## Points to Ponder

*Delirium prevalence and impact*: Delirium affects over 50% of ICU patients, significantly increasing the risk of death, prolonged hospital stays, and post-ICU cognitive impairment, including ICU-acquired dementia.

1. *Complex pathophysiology*: Delirium arises from multifactorial causes, including neuroinflammation, neurotransmitter imbalances, oxidative stress, and neuroendocrine dysregulation, with these mechanisms contributing to cognitive disturbances in critically ill patients.
2. *Diagnostic Tools*: The Confusion Assessment Method for the ICU (CAM-ICU) is a crucial tool for early detection of delirium, offering 80% sensitivity and 95.9% specificity.
3. *Pharmacological and non-pharmacological management*: Effective delirium management involves both pharmacological treatments, like dexmedetomidine and antipsychotics, and non-pharmacological interventions, such as early mobility, pain management, and family engagement.

## SUGGESTED READINGS


1. Ali M, Cascella M. ICU Delirium. 2024 Mar 13. In: Stat Pearls [Internet]. Treasure Island (FL): Stat Pearls Publishing; Jan 2024. PMID: 32644706.
2. Gotur DB. Delirium in the Critically Ill. J Med Sci Health. 2018;4(1): 5-14.
3. Wilson JE, Mart MF, Cunningham C, et al. Delirium. Nat Rev Dis Primers. 2020;6(1):90.
4. Mart MF, Roberson SW, Salas B, et al. Prevention and Management of Delirium in the Intensive Care Unit. Semin Respir Crit Care Med. 2021;42(1):112-26.
5. Stollings JL, Kotfis K, Chanques G, et al. Delirium in critical illness: clinical manifestations, outcomes, and management. Intensive Care Med. 2021;47(10):1089-103.
6. Ankravs MJ, McKenzie CA, Kenes MT, et al. Precision-based approaches to delirium in critical illness: A narrative review. Pharmacotherapy. 2023;43(11):1139-53.

CHAPTER 37

# A Case-based Approach to Toxidrome in Emergency Care

*Shambo Samrat Samajdar*

**CASE VIGNETTE**

A 66-year-old female was brought to the emergency department (ED) with altered mental status, confusion, and agitation, which developed over the past 3 days. Her past medical history included hypertension, major depression, and chronic alcohol use. Her current medication list consisted of venlafaxine 150 mg daily and losartan 50 mg twice daily. Recently, she had been taking terbinafine for a skin infection. The patient's husband reported that she had been using an over-the-counter antihistamine, promethazine, at a higher-than-recommended dose for several days.

On examination, she presented with tachycardia (heart rate 120 beats/min), hypertension (blood pressure 180/102 mm Hg), dilated pupils, dry skin, and a low-grade fever of 36.7°C. Neurological examination revealed a Glasgow Coma Scale (GCS) score of E4M6V3, indicating moderate impairment. A toxidrome approach was utilized to guide the diagnosis, which revealed features consistent with an anticholinergic toxidrome.

## PROVISIONAL DIAGNOSIS

Anticholinergic toxicity secondary to promethazine overdose in the context of polypharmacy and chronic alcohol use.

## DIFFERENTIAL DIAGNOSIS

When encountering a patient with altered mental status and other signs of potential toxidrome, consider the following differential diagnoses:

- *Central nervous system disorders*: Stroke, intracranial hemorrhage, seizure, encephalitis.
- *Metabolic disorders*: Hypoglycemia, hyponatremia, hypercalcemia, hepatic or renal failure.
- *Infections*: Sepsis, meningitis, or other systemic infections.
- *Medication or substance-induced conditions*: Poisoning, withdrawal syndromes, or drug interactions.
- *Cardiac disorders*: Hypertensive encephalopathy, arrhythmias, or acute coronary syndrome.

## CLINICAL APPROACH

### Signs and Symptoms

The clinical manifestations of various toxidromes can differ significantly depending on the substance involved. Common toxidromes encountered in emergency care include:

- *Anticholinergic toxidrome*: Characterized by altered mental status (agitation, hallucinations, or delirium), dry skin, hyperthermia, tachycardia, mydriasis, urinary retention, and decreased bowel sounds.
- *Cholinergic toxidrome*: Presents with excessive salivation, lacrimation, urination, diarrhea, gastrointestinal cramps, emesis (SLUDGE syndrome), miosis, bradycardia, and muscle fasciculations.
- *Opioid toxidrome*: Typically includes pinpoint pupils, respiratory depression, bradycardia, and altered consciousness.
- *Sympathomimetic toxidrome*: Features include tachycardia, hypertension, hyperthermia, mydriasis, and diaphoresis.
- *Sedative-hypnotic toxidrome*: Involves central nervous system depression, respiratory depression, bradycardia, and hypotension.

**Table 1** is summarizing common toxidromes.

## DIAGNOSTIC APPROACH

A systematic approach to evaluating a suspected toxidrome involves:

### History Taking

- *Medication and substance use history*: Obtain a thorough history of prescribed and over-the-counter medications, supplements, recreational drugs, and recent changes in dosing.
- *Timeline of symptom onset*: Rapid onset may suggest acute intoxication, while a gradual onset may indicate chronic exposure.
- *Possible access to toxins*: Consider occupational or environmental exposures.

### Physical Examination

- *Vital signs monitoring*: Identify abnormalities in heart rate, blood pressure, respiratory rate, temperature, and oxygen saturation.
- *Neurological examination*: Assess level of consciousness, pupillary responses, and presence of neuromuscular abnormalities.

**TABLE 1: Characteristics of common toxidromes in emergency care.**

| Toxidrome | Examples | Mental status | HR | BP | RR | T | Pupil size | Bowel sounds | Diaphoresis | Other |
|---|---|---|---|---|---|---|---|---|---|---|
| Sympathomimetic | Cocaine, amphetamine | Agitation | ↑ | ↑ | ↑ | ↑ | ↑ | ↑ | ↑ | Tremor, seizures |
| Anticholinergic | Diphenhydramine, atropine | Delirium | ↑ | ↑ | ± | ↑ | ↑ | ↓ | ↓ | Flushing, urinary retention, dry mucus membranes |
| Cholinergic | Organophosphates | Somnolence | ± | ± | ± | nc | ↓ | ↑ | ↑ | DUMBBELLS (Diarrhea, Urination, Miosis, Bradycardia, Bronchospasm, Emesis, Lacrimation, Lethargy, Salivation) |
| Opioid | Heroin, oxycodone | Somnolence | ↓ | ↓ | ↓ | ↓ | ↓ | ↓ | nc | |
| Sedative-hypnotic | Benzodiazepines, barbiturates | Somnolence | ↓ | ↓ | ↓ | ↓ | ± | ↓ | nc | Ataxia, hyporeflexia |
| Serotonin toxicity | Sertraline, citalopram | Normal or agitation | ↑ | ↑ | ↑ | ↑ | ↑ | ↑ | ↑ | Clonus, hyperreflexia, tremor, seizures |
| Sympatholytic | Clonidine | Somnolence | ↓ | ↓ | ↓ | ↓ | ↓ | ↓ | ↓ | |

(HR: heart rate; BP: blood pressure; RR: respiratory rate; T: temperature; nc: no change; ↑: increased; ↓: decreased; ±: variable)

- *Skin examination*: Evaluate for diaphoresis, dry skin, or flushed appearance.

## Laboratory Investigations

- *Electrolyte and glucose levels*: To rule out metabolic causes of altered mental status.
- *Arterial blood gas (ABG)*: Evaluate for acid-base disturbances.
- *Toxicology screen*: Perform a urine drug screen and serum toxicology tests as indicated.
- *ECG and imaging*: Assess for cardiac rhythm disturbances or structural abnormalities (e.g., brain CT).

**Table 2** is summarizing the drugs commonly associated with electrocardiogram (ECG) changes in cases of poisoning.

## Role of ECG in Diagnosing Toxidromes

The electrocardiogram (ECG) is a vital tool in the assessment of suspected toxidromes, as it can reveal characteristic cardiac effects of various toxins. For example, QRS interval prolongation is often associated with sodium channel blockade, commonly seen in tricyclic antidepressant overdoses. QTc interval prolongation, on the other hand, may indicate an increased risk of torsades de pointes and is seen with drugs such as antipsychotics and certain antidepressants. Bradycardia or heart block can result from toxicity involving cholinergic agents, beta-blockers, or calcium channel blockers. By providing rapid and noninvasive evaluation, the ECG helps to identify life-threatening arrhythmias, guides antidotal therapy, and supports the diagnosis of specific toxidromes, allowing for timely and appropriate management in emergency settings.

**TABLE 2: Drugs commonly associated with ECG changes.**

| Bradycardia/Heart block | QRS interval prolongation | QTc interval prolongation |
|---|---|---|
| *Cholinergic agents*:<br>• Physostigmine<br>• Neostigmine<br>• Organophosphates, carbamates<br>*Sympatholytic agents*:<br>• β Receptor antagonists<br>• Clonidine<br>• Opioids<br>*Other*:<br>• Digoxin<br>• $Ca^{2+}$ channel blockers<br>• Lithium | • Antiarrhythmics (Class 1)<br>• Bupropion<br>• Chloroquine/hydroxychloroquine<br>• Cocaine<br>• Diphenhydramine<br>• Lamotrigine<br>• Propranolol<br>• Tricyclic antidepressants | • Antiarrhythmics (Class 1a, 1c, III)<br>• Atypical antipsychotics (ziprasidone, quetiapine)<br>• Fluoroquinolones<br>• Loperamide<br>• Macrolides<br>• Ondansetron<br>• Phenothiazines<br>• SNRIs (venlafaxine, desvenlafaxine)<br>• SSRIs (citalopram, escitalopram)<br>• Tricyclic antidepressants<br>• Typical antipsychotics (haloperidol, droperidol) |

# MANAGEMENT

## General Management Principles

- *Stabilization*: Follow the "ABCDE" approach in emergency care (Airway, Breathing, Circulation, Disability, Exposure).

- *Airway and breathing*: Ensure airway patency and adequate ventilation. Administer supplemental oxygen if needed.
- *Circulation*: Treat hypotension with fluid resuscitation and vasopressors as indicated.
- *Disability (neurological assessment)*: Monitor for seizures or coma and treat accordingly.
- *Exposure*: Remove contaminated clothing and decontaminate skin if necessary.

- *Decontamination*:
  - *Activated charcoal*: May be used within 1–2 hours of ingestion if the substance is known to bind to charcoal.
  - *Gastric lavage or whole-bowel irrigation*: Consider for life-threatening ingestions if within an appropriate time frame.
- *Antidotal therapy*: **Table 3** is summarizing antidotal therapies and their poisoning indications.
  - *Anticholinergic toxidrome*: Use of physostigmine, an acetylcholinesterase inhibitor, may be indicated.
  - *Cholinergic toxidrome*: Administer atropine and pralidoxime.
  - *Opioid toxidrome*: Naloxone is the antidote of choice.
  - *Sympathomimetic toxidrome*: Use benzodiazepines for sedation and seizure control.

**Table 4** outlines the essential phases in the management of a poisoned patient, emphasizing the need for simultaneous stabilization, evaluation, and treatment interventions.

## CASE-SPECIFIC MANAGEMENT (ANTICHOLINERGIC TOXIDROME)

- *Identify and discontinue offending agents*: In this case, promethazine was identified as the culprit and discontinued.
- *Symptomatic treatment*:
  - *Cooling measures*: For hyperthermia, initiate external cooling with ice packs and cold saline.
  - *Benzodiazepines*: For agitation and seizures, administer benzodiazepines such as lorazepam.
  - *Bladder catheterization*: May be needed for urinary retention.

**TABLE 3: Antidotal therapies and poisoning indications.**

| Antidote | Poisoning indication(s) |
|---|---|
| N-acetylcysteine | Acetaminophen |
| Atropine sulfate | Pesticide poisoning (carbamate and organophosphate) |
| Calcium | Calcium channel blockers, fluoride |
| Calcium disodium EDTA | Chronic lead poisoning |
| Cyproheptadine | Serotonin toxicity |
| Dantrolene | Anesthetic-induced malignant hyperthermia |
| Deferoxamine | Iron overload (acute and chronic) |
| Digoxin immune Fab | Cardiac glycoside toxicity |
| Dimercaprol (BAL) | Lead, mercury, arsenic poisoning |
| Fomepizole | Ethylene glycol, methanol poisoning |
| Flumazenil | Benzodiazepine overdose |
| Glucagon hydrochloride | Beta-blocker and calcium channel blocker toxicity |

Continued

Continued

| Antidote | Poisoning indication(s) |
|---|---|
| Glucarpidase | Methotrexate toxicity |
| Hydroxocobalamin | Cyanide poisoning |
| Idarucizumab | Dabigatran toxicity |
| Leucovorin | Methotrexate toxicity |
| L-Carnitine | Valproic acid toxicity (off-label use) |
| Lipid emulsion | Local anesthetic toxicity |
| Methylene blue | Methemoglobinemia |
| Naloxone | Opioid overdose |
| Octreotide | Sulfonylurea-induced hypoglycemia |
| Physostigmine | Anticholinergic delirium |
| Pralidoxime (2-PAM) | Organophosphate pesticide poisoning |
| Protamine | Heparin toxicity |
| Prothrombin complex concentrate | Vitamin K antagonist toxicity |
| Prussian blue | Thallium, cesium toxicity |
| Pyridoxine | Hydrazine, isoniazid poisoning |
| Sodium bicarbonate | Salicylate, tricyclic antidepressant toxicity |
| Succimer (DMSA) | Lead poisoning (on label); mercury and arsenic (off-label) |
| Vitamin K1 (phytonadione) | Vitamin K antagonist toxicity (warfarin, coumarin, etc.) |

**TABLE 4: Management steps for a poisoned patient.**

| Phase | Components | Description |
|---|---|---|
| Stabilization | Airway | Ensure airway is clear and open to maintain adequate oxygenation |
| | Breathing | Assess and support respiratory function; administer supplemental oxygen if needed |
| | Circulation | Monitor blood pressure and heart rate; manage hypotension or shock with fluids/vasopressors |
| Clinical evaluation | Toxidrome recognition | Identify characteristic signs and symptoms that suggest a specific class of toxin (e.g., anticholinergic, opioid) |
| | Laboratory tests | Obtain laboratory tests such as toxicology screens, blood gases, electrolytes, and ECG |
| Treatment | Supportive care | Provide general medical care, including hydration, oxygen, and symptom management |
| | Decontamination | Administer activated charcoal, perform gastric lavage, or skin decontamination, as appropriate |
| | Enhanced elimination | Consider methods like urinary alkalinization, hemodialysis, or multiple-dose activated charcoal |
| | Antidote administration | Use specific antidotes to neutralize toxins (e.g., naloxone for opioids, atropine for organophosphates) |

- *Monitoring and follow-up*:
  - *Frequent reassessment of vital signs*: Monitor for changes in blood pressure, heart rate, and temperature.
  - *Neurological monitoring*: Regularly assess consciousness and neurological status.
  - *Toxidrome resolution*: Symptoms should gradually resolve over hours to days as the offending agent is metabolized and eliminated.

## PATHOPHYSIOLOGY

The pathophysiology of toxidromes involves interactions between toxins and various physiological systems, including the nervous, cardiovascular, and respiratory systems. For example, anticholinergic toxidrome arises from competitive inhibition of acetylcholine at muscarinic receptors, leading to:

- *Central nervous system effects*: Agitation, hallucinations, and delirium result from impaired cholinergic neurotransmission in the brain.
- *Cardiovascular effects*: Tachycardia and hypertension develop due to decreased parasympathetic tone.
- *Gastrointestinal and urinary symptoms*: Reduced smooth muscle tone leads to decreased bowel sounds and urinary retention.

Other toxidromes similarly affect specific receptor sites or ion channels, leading to characteristic clinical presentations.

## ANTICHOLINERGIC TOXIDROME AND THE ROLE OF ANTICHOLINERGIC BURDEN

In this case, the patient presented with classic signs of anticholinergic toxidrome, including confusion, agitation, dilated pupils, dry skin, and urinary retention. Anticholinergic toxidrome occurs due to the competitive antagonism of acetylcholine at muscarinic receptors in the central and peripheral nervous systems. The effects manifest as a constellation of symptoms that may range from mild delirium to life-threatening conditions involving seizures or cardiovascular complications.

### Understanding Anticholinergic Burden

The concept of anticholinergic burden is crucial in evaluating the cumulative effects of medications with anticholinergic properties, especially in older adults who may be more susceptible to these adverse effects. The Anticholinergic Risk Scale (ACB) quantifies the anticholinergic activity of individual medications by assigning scores ranging from 1 to 3 based on the drug's known anticholinergic effects. A total ACB score of 3 or more is considered clinically significant, increasing the risk of adverse effects such as cognitive impairment, falls, and delirium.

In this patient's case, the use of promethazine (ACB score of 3) contributed significantly to the overall anticholinergic burden. The coadministration of terbinafine and venlafaxine could have potentiated the anticholinergic effects of promethazine, leading to the presentation of anticholinergic toxidrome. The patient's polypharmacy situation exemplifies the need for careful evaluation of anticholinergic load in clinical settings to prevent drug-induced disorders.

## ROLE OF CLINICAL PHARMACOLOGY REVIEW AND RECONCILIATION FEEDBACK

Clinical Pharmacology Review and Reconciliation Feedback (CPRRF) is a systematic approach that aids in the identification and prevention of drug-induced disorders. It involves:

- *Thorough medication history review*: Identifying medications that contribute to the anticholinergic burden.
- *Reconciliation of medication lists*: Ensuring all medications are reviewed for their necessity, potential interactions, and cumulative effects.
- *Feedback and recommendations*: Providing referring clinicians with guidance on optimizing the medication regimen, including deprescribing anticholinergic drugs when possible and considering safer alternatives. In this case, early application of CPRRF could have facilitated timely identification of the high anticholinergic burden, thereby preventing the development of anticholinergic toxidrome.

## HOW TO CALCULATE THE ANTICHOLINERGIC BURDEN?

To calculate the anticholinergic burden for a patient, identify each medication the patient is currently taking and assign the corresponding ACB score based on the **Table 5** above. Sum the scores to determine the total ACB score for the patient. A higher total score indicates a greater risk of anticholinergic-related adverse effects, warranting consideration of medication adjustments or deprescribing strategies.

**TABLE 5: Anticholinergic risk scale (ACB) and scoring.**

| Score: 3 points | Score: 2 points | Score: 1 point |
|---|---|---|
| • Amitriptyline | • Amantadine | • Carbidopa-levodopa |
| • Atropine products | • Baclofen | • Entacapone |
| • Benztropine | • Cetirizine | • Haloperidol |
| • Chlorpheniramine | • Cimetidine | • Methocarbamol |
| • Cyproheptadine | • Clozapine | • Mirtazapine |
| • Dicyclomine | • Cyclobenzaprine | • Paroxetine |
| • Diphenhydramine | • Desipramine | • Pramipexole |
| • Fluphenazine | • Loperamide | • Quetiapine fumarate |
| • Hydroxyzine hydrochloride and pamoate | • Loratadine | • Ranitidine |
| • Hyoscyamine products | • Nortriptyline | • Risperidone |
| • Imipramine | • Olanzapine | • Selegiline |
| • Meclizine | • Prochlorperazine | • Trazodone |
| • Oxybutynin | • Pseudoephedrine and triprolidine | • Ziprasidone |
| • Perphenazine | • Tolterodine tartrate | |
| • Promethazine | | |
| • Thioridazine | | |
| • Tizanidine | | |
| • Trihexyphenidyl | | |

For instance, if a patient is taking promethazine (3 points), cetirizine (2 points), and paroxetine (1 point), the total ACB score would be 6 points.

A total score of 6 indicates a significant anticholinergic burden, which could predispose the patient to adverse effects such as delirium, cognitive decline, and falls. This situation would require clinical evaluation to consider alternative therapies with lower anticholinergic activity.

## Points to Ponder

- *Early recognition of toxidromes is critical*: Timely identification improves patient outcomes and guides appropriate interventions.
- *Assess anticholinergic burden (ACB)*: High ACB scores increase the risk of cognitive impairment and adverse effects.
- *Use clinical pharmacology review and reconciliation feedback (CPRRF)*: Systematic medication reviews can prevent drug-induced toxicities.
- *Thorough medication history is essential*: Accurate history aids in identifying causative agents and informing treatment.
- *Deprescribing reduces anticholinergic burden*: Especially important in older adults to minimize adverse drug effects.

## MULTIPLE CHOICE QUESTIONS

**1. What is the most likely cause of this patient's altered mental status and associated symptoms?**

A. Serotonin syndrome
B. Anticholinergic toxicity
C. Neuroleptic malignant syndrome
D. Delirium tremens

**2. Which of the following medications is most likely contributing to this patient's condition?**

A. Venlafaxine
B. Terbinafine
C. Promethazine
D. Losartan

**3. Which of the following is a hallmark feature of anticholinergic toxicity?**

A. Hypothermia
B. Pupil constriction
C. Hyperreflexia
D. Tachycardia and dry skin

**4. Which of the following is the most appropriate management for this patient's condition?**

A. Administration of activated charcoal
B. Intravenous fluids and benzodiazepines
C. Administration of physostigmine
D. Immediate intubation and mechanical ventilation

**5. What is the most likely underlying mechanism of this patient's altered mental status and confusion?**

A. Inhibition of serotonin reuptake
B. Blockade of muscarinic acetylcholine receptors
C. Increased dopamine release
D. Excessive catecholamine release

### Answers

1. (B); 2. (C); 3. (D); 4. (C); 5. (B)

## SUGGESTED READINGS


1. Johnson AR, Brown KM. Principles of Clinical Toxicology. In: Brunton LL, Knollmann BC. eds. Goodman & Gilman's: The Pharmacological Basis of Therapeutics, 14th Edition. McGraw-Hill Education; 2023. Accessed October 27, 2024. https://accessmedicine.mhmedical.com/content.aspx?bookid=3191&sectionid=268044850.
2. Samajdar SS, Sharma J, Mukherjee S, et al. Clinical Pharmacological Principles in Emergency Geriatric Care: Toxidrome Approach. J Indian Acad Geriatr. 2023;19(4):282-4.
3. Samajdar SS, Das S, Sarkar S, et al. Association between Polypharmacy and Cardiovascular Autonomic Function among Elderly Patients in an Urban Municipality Area of Kolkata, India: A Record-Based Cross-Sectional Study. Geriatrics (Basel). 2022;7(6):136.
4. Samajdar SS, Tripathi SK. Clinical Pharmacological Reconciliation, Review, and Feedback in Ensuring Patient Safety: A Commentary. J Clin Pharmacol. 2023;63(9):1074-1075.

# CHAPTER 38

# An Approach to a Case of Acute Flaccid Paralysis in ICU

*Kiran Vadapalli*

**CASE VIGNETTE**

A 30-year-old male athlete was admitted in the intensive care unit (ICU) with a history of rapidly progressive weakness initially of both lower limbs followed by upper limbs over the past 1 week. He also complained of difficulty in breathing over the past 2 days. He had an episode of acute gastroenteritis 2 weeks prior. On examination, he has flaccid weakness of all four limbs, with power 1/5 in both lower limbs and 2/5 in both upper limbs, and all deep tendon reflexes are absent. He has shallow breathing and paradoxical abdominal movement on inspiration.

## PROVISIONAL DIAGNOSIS

The clinical diagnosis of the above presentation is Guillain–Barré syndrome (GBS). Other possible conditions that can present as acute flaccid paralysis include botulinum toxicity, tick paralysis, myasthenia gravis, hypokalemic paralysis, high cervical transverse myelitis.

## DIFFERENTIAL DIAGNOSIS

Other possible conditions that can present as acute flaccid paralysis include Botulinum toxicity, tick paralysis, myasthenia gravis, hypokalemic paralysis, high cervical transverse myelitis.

## CLINICAL APPROACH

Acute inflammatory demyelinating polyneuropathy aka GBS, is an autoimmune disease in which an infection or vaccination triggers autoantibody production. These autoantibodies by molecular mimicry cause demyelination of peripheral nerves. Key features include ascending paresis/paralysis, sensory disturbances, bulbar and diaphragmatic weakness. Cranial nerve involvement and autonomic dysfunction are common. Acute motor axonal neuropathy (AMAN), acute, motor and sensory, axonal neuropathy (AMSAN) and Miller Fisher syndrome are other common variants of GBS. Tick paralysis (neurotoxin secreted by some ticks during blood meal) presents as subacute ascending symmetrical flaccid paralysis with no sensory involvement following a tick bite. In tick paralysis, cranial nerve involvement and autonomic symptoms are rare. Botulism is characterized by descending paralysis, early cranial nerve involvement and is associated with ingestion of contaminated food or wound infection. Paralytic poliomyelitis albeit rare in vaccinated individuals can present as fever followed by asymmetric flaccid muscle weakness and occasional respiratory paralysis with preserved sensorium and cognition. Nerve conduction studies (NCS) can be normal in early illness hence clinical diagnosis may be essential in the management. NCS in acute inflammatory demyelinating polyneuropathy (AIDP) reveals prolonged distal latencies, conduction blocks, reduced conduction velocities and prolonged or absent F waves. Cerebrospinal fluid (CSF) analysis reveals albumin-cytological dissociation (raised protein with normal cell counts) usually after 1st week of illness. Antibody testing can be used to identify specific types of GBS. Reduced vital capacity and negative inspiratory force indicate respiratory muscle weakness necessitating intubation and mechanical ventilation. Features of respiratory distress like tachypnoea, hypoxemia, hypercarbia, use of accessory muscles and respiratory acidosis on arterial blood gas (ABG) point toward impending respiratory failure. These features are indicative of diaphragmatic weakness are observed in neurological conditions presenting with acute flaccid paralysis.

## TREATMENT AND PREVENTION

Management includes ICU admission for monitoring respiratory function clinically or with validated scores along with serial ABG's. Cardiovascular monitoring is with continuous ECG and BP monitoring. Treatment includes intravenous immunoglobulin (IVIg) is first line therapy typically 2 g/kg total dose, administered over 5 days (e.g., 0.4 g/kg/day for 5 days). Plasmapheresis or plasma exchange stands as an alternative to IVIG. Usually involves 4–6 exchanges over 7–14 days. Typically, IVIG and plasmapheresis are not used together as there is no additional benefit compared to using one alone in Guillain–Barré syndrome. Physical therapy, speech, swallowing and occupational therapy should accompany definitive therapy for good outcomes.

GBS variants occur due to antibodies against gangliosides (nodal proteins like GM1, GD1A, GQ1b, etc.). But a subset of patients with AIDP presentation with atypical features (aggressive severe onset, rapid progression, sensory ataxia and tremor, severe neuropathic pain, autonomic dysfunction etc.) were found to have antibodies against paranodal proteins (NF155, CNTN1, CASPR1 etc.,). Identification of these patients is essential because they are usually refractory to IVIg and may have partial response to PLEX or steroids, with a very good response to early rituximab therapy.

## Points to Ponder

- Diagnostic lucidity is essential as many overlapping conditions may present as acute flaccid muscle weakness.
- Broad differentials need to be considered and evaluated to confirm the diagnosis. Respiratory assessment should be performed periodically, and any respiratory distress may necessitate early intubation and mechanical ventilation.
- Regular periodic neurological assessment should be done to recognize rapidity of progression of the disease.
- Apart from definitive therapy, infection control practices, early enteral nutrition, stress ulcer prophylaxis, thromboprophylaxis, physical therapy and rehabilitation and multidisciplinary care are essential in caring for such patients.

## MULTIPLE CHOICE QUESTIONS

**1. What is the most likely diagnosis for this patient?**
A. Myasthenia gravis
B. Guillain–Barré syndrome (GBS)
C. Multiple sclerosis
D. Acute poliomyelitis

**2. Which of the following is a common precipitating factor for the suspected diagnosis?**
A. Recent viral or bacterial infection
B. Excessive physical activity
C. Long-term steroid use
D. Head trauma

**3. What is the most critical initial management for this patient in the ICU?**
A. Intravenous immunoglobulin (IVIg) or plasmapheresis
B. High-dose corticosteroids
C. Aggressive physiotherapy
D. Airway support and monitoring for respiratory failure

**4. Which diagnostic test is most specific to confirm the suspected diagnosis?**
A. Serum creatinine kinase levels
B. Nerve conduction studies and electromyography
C. MRI of the spine
D. Blood culture

**5. What is the most likely cause of shallow breathing and paradoxical abdominal movements in this patient?**
A. Upper airway obstruction
B. Weakness of respiratory muscles
C. Pulmonary embolism
D. Diaphragmatic paralysis due to spinal cord injury

### Answers

1. (B); 2. (A); 3. (D); 4. (B); 5. (B)

## SUGGESTED READINGS

1. Bellanti R, Rinaldi S. Guillain–Barré syndrome: a comprehensive review. Eur J Neurol. 2024;31(8):e16365.
2. Tisavipat N, Flanagan EP. Current perspectives on the diagnosis and management of acute transverse myelitis. Expert Rev Neurother. 2023;23(4):389-411.
3. Vanhorebeek I, Latronico N, Van den Berghe G. ICU-acquired weakness. Intensive Care Med. 2020;46(4):637-53.
4. Claytor B, Cho SM, Li Y. Myasthenic crisis. Muscle Nerve. 2023;68(1):8-19.

CHAPTER 39

# An Approach to a Case of SARI in the Elderly

*Nandini Chatterjee*

**CASE VIGNETTE**

A 70-year-old man presented with history of fever for the last 5 days with cough and expectoration. He came to the emergency with breathing difficulty since this morning on examination temperature 101.7°F, pulse 120 beats/min, respiratory rate 34 breaths/min, BP 100/65 mm Hg.

Chest scattered rhonchi bilaterally along with coarse crepitations at the lower right infra scapular area.

Other systemic examinations were noncontributory.

## PROVISIONAL DIAGNOSIS

The patient is experiencing influenza-like illness (ILI), defined by the World Health Organization as an acute respiratory infection with a fever of 38°C or higher and a cough, starting within the past 10 days. If hospitalization becomes necessary, the illness is reclassified as a severe acute respiratory infection (SARI).

**When do the patients require hospitalization?**

The red flag signs are to be promptly recognized **(Fig. 1)**, e.g.:
- Difficulty in breathing or shortness of breath
- Persistent pain or pressure in the chest or abdomen
- Persistent dizziness, confusion, inability to arouse
- Seizures

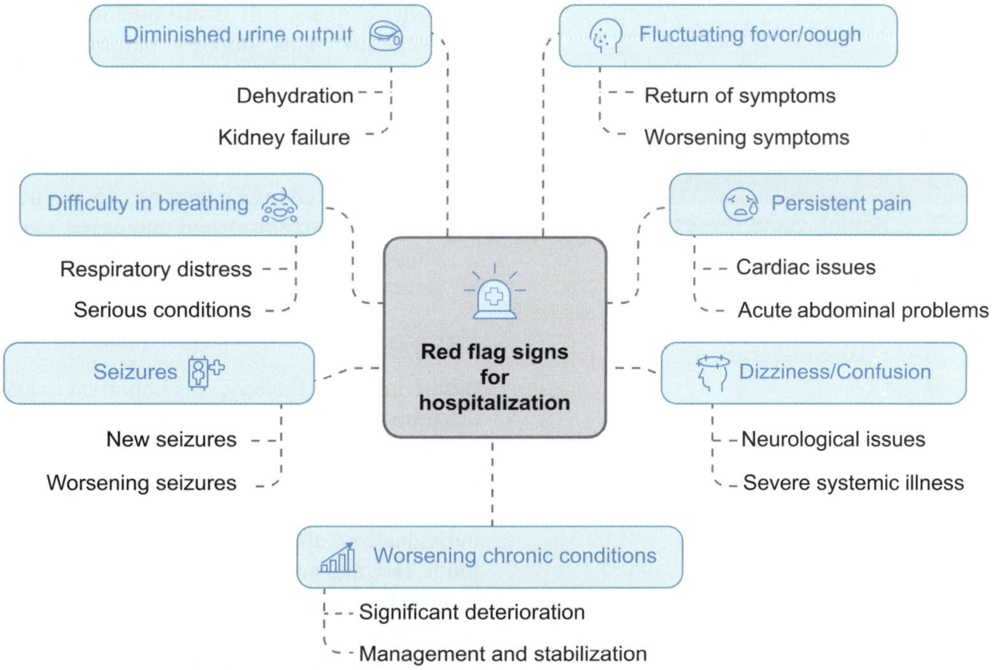


**FIG. 1:** Red flag signs for hospitalization in patients with severe acute respiratory infection (SARI).

- Diminished urine output
- Fever or cough that improve but then return or worsen
- Worsening of chronic medical conditions

CURB-65 is a score for assessment of pneumonia patients and ascertain whether they require admission:

- Confusion (based upon a specific mental test or new disorientation to person, place, or time)
- Urea (blood urea nitrogen in the United States) >7 mmol/L (20 mg/dL)
- Respiratory rate ≥30 breaths/min
- Blood pressure (systolic <90 mm Hg or diastolic <60 mm Hg)
- Age ≥65 years

A score of 1 is assigned for each criterion. If the patient scores 2 or more, hospitalization is required, while scores of 3–5 typically indicate the need for intensive care unit admission.

The physicians' discretion is important here. The patients aged greater than 65 years are especially vulnerable.

## DIFFERENTIAL DIAGNOSIS

Differential diagnosis for ILI is as follows in **(Table 1)**.

Noninfectious causes are essential mimickers that must be ruled out. Additionally, besides typical respiratory pathogens, diseases such as malaria, dengue, scrub typhus, leptospirosis, and even hepatitis viruses can sometimes present similarly to an acute respiratory infection.

## CLINICAL APPROACH

- Clinical evaluation
- History is suggestive of the diagnosis.
- One has to look for red flag signs to ascertain prognosis and take decision regarding need for hospitalization:
    - Higher function
    - Respiratory rate
    - Pulse
    - BP
    - Cyanosis
    - Oxygen saturation
    - Systemic examination

Typically, ILI is mild and self-limiting, so investigations are often unnecessary. However, if the patient fails to improve or develops red flag signs, the following tests should be conducted:

- CBC with PBS
- MPDA
- NS1 antigen
- RT-PCR for COVID-19
- Sputum for stain and culture
- Urine RE/ME
- Chest X-ray PA view
- Blood/Urine culture
- LFT/RFT/Electrolytes/ABG
- Typhidot IgM, scrub typhus IgM/*Leptospira* IgM
- Test for influenza (PCR from nasopharyngeal, oropharyngeal swab) is done if results will change clinical management or for surveillance

**TABLE 1: Influenza-like illness (ILI): Infectious versus noninfectious causes.**

| Infections | Noninfectious causes |
|---|---|
| • Influenza virus A/B<br>• Rhinovirus<br>• Respiratory syncytial virus<br>• Adenovirus<br>• Parainfluenza<br>• COVID-19<br>• HSV<br>• Streptococcus pneumoniae<br>• Mycoplasma<br>• Legionella<br>• Malaria<br>• Dengue<br>• Scrub typhus<br>• Leptospirosis<br>• Hepatitis | • Acute hypersensitivity pneumonitis<br>• SLE pneumonitis<br>• Lung malignancy |

## PATHOPHYSIOLOGY

- *Pathogen entry and initial infection*: Pathogens usually enter the respiratory tract through inhaled droplets, direct contact, or fomites, and then attach to and invade the epithelial cells lining the tract using specific host cell receptors.
- *Immune response and inflammation:* The initial immune response activates innate immune cells (like macrophages and neutrophils) and releases proinflammatory cytokines (e.g., IL-1, IL-6, TNF-α). This causes inflammation, increasing vascular permeability, leading to edema and immune cell infiltration in the lungs, along with the release of reactive oxygen species (ROS) and proteases that further damage tissues.
- *Damage to respiratory epithelium*: The pathogen and inflammatory response damage the respiratory epithelial cells, causing cell death and disrupting the mucociliary escalator. This impairs pathogen clearance, increases susceptibility to secondary infections, and allows fluids and proteins to leak into the alveolar space.
- *Altered gas exchange*: Fluid accumulation in the alveoli and interstitial spaces impairs oxygen and carbon dioxide exchange, leading to reduced blood oxygen levels (hypoxemia) and increased carbon dioxide levels (hypercapnia). This can result in respiratory distress and potentially lead to organ failure **(Fig. 2)**.

## TREATMENT

Before initiating therapy, it is important to assess the duration of the illness to determine the therapeutic window. Additionally, the disease severity—whether mild or severe, progressive, or complicated—must be evaluated. Treatment should be tailored based on the specific etiology of SARI, requiring an individualized approach. Mild ILI should be managed with oral fluids, rest, and home isolation. Acetaminophen or ibuprofen may be used for symptom relief, but salicylates, including aspirin, are contraindicated.

*Patients at higher risk of complications are*:

- *Age*: <2 years, >65 years
- *Comorbidity*: Hypertension, diabetes mellitus, COPD/asthma, chronic kidney disease, chronic liver disease, malignancy or connective tissue disorders

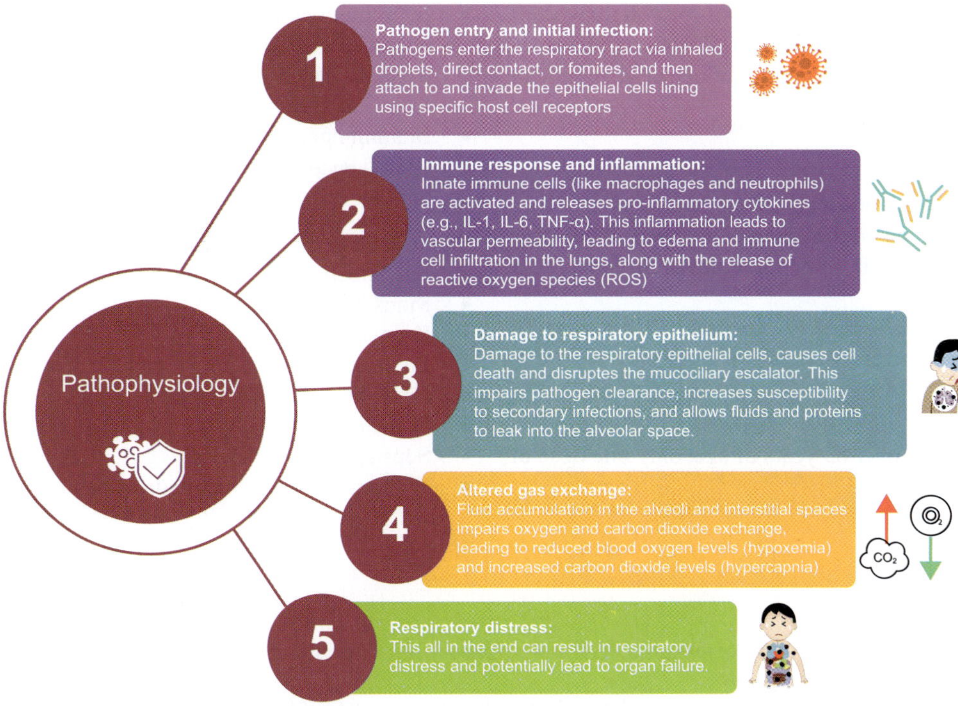


**FIG. 2:** Pathophysiology of severe acute respiratory infection (SARI).

- *Addiction*: Smoking, alcoholism
- Pregnancy

*For SARI patients*:
- Admission in ITU
- IV fluids are to be started.
- Oxygen therapy is given if $SO_2$ <90%, and mechanical ventilation if not corrected by $O_2$, drowsiness, or respiratory failure
- Ibuprofen/paracetamol/nutrition/electrolyte balance/circulation are to be maintained.
- For hospitalized patients with suspected or confirmed influenza, initiation of antiviral treatment with oral or enterically administered oseltamivir is recommended as soon as possible. Dosage 75 mg BD for 5 days.
- If the clinical course remains severe or progressive, the duration of the antiviral treatment is recommended to be extended longer.
- All patients at higher risk for influenza complications or worsening of comorbidities also to be given oseltamivir.

Combination antiviral therapy is generally not recommended for severe influenza. However, for patients with severe influenza complicated by pneumonia, otitis media, or sinusitis, a treatment regimen including both an antibiotic and an antiviral agent is advised. *However, the specific treatment is to be given if etiology is ascertained with investigations.*

If a bacterial infection is detected, antibiotics such as ampicillin/sulbactam, amoxicillin/clavulanate, third-generation cephalosporins, and respiratory quinolones, which are effective against *Staphylococcus aureus, Streptococcus pneumoniae, Streptococcus pyogenes, Moraxella catarrhalis*, and *Haemophilus influenzae*, should be used. Systemic corticosteroids are not recommended for treating severe influenza, except in cases where their therapeutic benefit is well-established, such as in asthma, COPD, and adrenal insufficiency.

## PREVENTION

- Regular hand washing with proper drying of the hands
- Good respiratory hygiene—covering mouth and nose when coughing or sneezing, using tissues and disposing of them correctly
- Early self-isolation of those feeling unwell, feverish and having other symptoms of influenza
- Avoiding close contact with sick people
- Avoid touching one's eyes, nose or mouth.

### Immunization

The national guidelines for adult immunization recommend influenza and pneumonia vaccinations for individuals over 65 years of age.

### For Influenza

There are two types of vaccines:
1. *Inactivated vaccine*: Trivalent and quadrivalent (preferred), available in split virion and subunit types. Administered via IM injection in the deltoid, 0.5 mL once a year.
2. *Live attenuated vaccine*: Intranasal spray (LAIV4).

### Timing

For adults, only one annual dose of the influenza vaccine is recommended. In India, the peak influenza season occurs during the monsoon, so the vaccine should be administered before the monsoon, ideally in April–May. For adults aged ≥65 years, the recommended vaccines include the quadrivalent high-dose inactivated influenza vaccine (HD-IIV4), quadrivalent recombinant influenza vaccine (RIV4), or quadrivalent adjuvanted inactivated influenza vaccine (aIIV4). If these are not available, any other age-appropriate influenza vaccine can be used.

## Pneumococcal Vaccine

There are two types of pneumococcal vaccines:

1. *PPSV23 (pneumococcal polysaccharide vaccine):* It contains capsular polysaccharides from 23 serotypes of *Streptococcus pneumoniae*.
2. *PCV13 (pneumococcal conjugate vaccine)*: It contains 13 serotypes of *Streptococcus pneumoniae*.

## Dosing

- In healthy individuals over 65 years of age, only one dose of PPSV23 is recommended.
- In immunocompetent individuals with comorbidities, one dose of PPSV23 should be given, followed by PCV13 after 5 years, based on shared clinical decision-making, only if there is a high risk of pneumococcal infection.
- In immunocompromised patients with comorbidities, PCV13 should be given first, followed by PPSV23 after 8 weeks, and another dose of PPSV23 after 5 years.

### What are the Complications of SARI?

- Ear infections
- Sinus infections
- Bronchitis
- Pneumonia
- Encephalopathy/Encephalitis
- Myocarditis
- Sepsis, MOF, shock
- Worsening of chronic medical conditions

## Points to Ponder

- *Pathogens:* SARIs are caused by viruses like influenza, RSV, and coronaviruses. Understanding the specific pathogen is crucial for targeted treatment and control measures.
- *Global burden*: High morbidity and mortality, particularly affecting healthcare systems during peak seasons especially in low-resource settings.
- *Preparedness:* Requires stockpiling, healthcare training, and community awareness for outbreaks.
- *Surveillance*: Timely diagnosis is vital for managing SARIs. Systems like WHO's SARI surveillance enable early detection and response.
- *At-risk populations*: Especially impacts children, elderly, and immunocompromised individuals. Prevention strategies often focus on these high-risk populations to reduce severe outcomes.
- *Vaccination*: Influenza vaccines are crucial for prevention. Expanding vaccination coverage, especially in vulnerable groups, is a priority for reducing the incidence and severity of SARIs.
- *Treatment challenges*: Limited effective antivirals; supportive care remains primary. Managing SARIs involves supportive care, oxygen therapy, and sometimes antiviral medications, depending on the pathogen.
- *Antimicrobial stewardship*: Essential to manage bacterial superinfections and reduce resistance. Implementing antimicrobial stewardship programs is essential to prevent antibiotic resistance, growing global health concern.
- *COVID-19 impact*: Boosted research on SARIs and highlighted preparedness gaps.

## MULTIPLE CHOICE QUESTIONS

**1. What is a common clinical sign of severe acute respiratory infection?**
A. Bradycardia
B. Hyperthermia
C. Hypertension
D. Hypoglycemia

**2. Which symptom is typically associated with severe acute respiratory infections?**
A. Persistent headache
B. Severe dyspnea
C. Abdominal pain
D. Joint pain

**3. Which of the following is a recommended preventive measure for severe acute respiratory infections?**
A. Frequent hand washing and respiratory hygiene
B. Increased dietary intake of carbohydrates
C. Regular use of antihypertensive medications
D. Avoidance of high-fat foods

**4. Which diagnostic test is most useful for identifying bacterial pathogens in severe acute respiratory infections?**
A. Sputum culture
B. Complete blood count (CBC)
C. Liver function test
D. Serum electrolytes

**5. What is the role of corticosteroids in treating severe acute respiratory infections?**
A. To treat bacterial infections
B. To reduce inflammation and immune response
C. To manage electrolyte imbalances
D. To enhance fluid balance

## Answers

1. (B); 2. (B); 3. (A); 4. (A); 5. (B)

## SUGGESTED READINGS

1. Janssens JP, Krause KH. Pneumonia in the very old. Lancet Infect Dis. 2004;4:112-24.
2. Stupka JE, Mortensen EM, Anzueto A, et al. Community-acquired pneumonia in elderly patients. Aging Health. 2009;5:763-74.
3. Shi T, Denouel A, Tietjen AK, et al. Global and Regional Burden of Hospital Admissions for Pneumonia in Older Adults: A Systematic Review and Meta-Analysis. J Infect Dis. 2020;222:S570-6.
4. Quan TP, Fawcett NJ, Wrightson JM, et al. Increasing burden of community-acquired pneumonia leading to hospitalisation, 1998–2014. Thorax. 2016;71:535-42.
5. Jain SK, Jain S, Trikha S. Study of Clinical, Radiological, and Bacteriological Profile of Community-Acquired Pneumonia in Hospitalized Patients of Gajra Raja Medical College, Gwalior, Central India. Int J Sci Stud. 2014;2:96-100.

CHAPTER 40

# An Approach to a Case of Extrapulmonary TB

*AR Balamurugan*

**CASE VIGNETTE**

A 28-year-old female was brought to the ER with a 15-day history of fever, abdominal pain, and vomiting. The fever was high-grade, with evening spikes and associated chills, relieved by antipyretics. The abdominal pain, which had worsened over the last 15 days, was dull and nonprogressive, located in the upper abdomen without radiation. She also reported loss of appetite, weight loss, and night sweats during fever episodes. There was no history of gastrointestinal, respiratory, neurological, or joint symptoms. She had no significant past medical history and no family history of similar illness. On examination, she was conscious, oriented, and afebrile with pallor but no jaundice or edema. Vital signs included a BP of 110/70 mm Hg, HR 120 beats/min, and normal oxygen saturation. Abdominal examination revealed tenderness in the right and left hypochondriac and epigastric regions. Investigations included normal chest X-ray, an ultrasound showing gallbladder wall edema and multiple hypoechoic splenic nodules, and CT showing hepatosplenomegaly, splenic lesions, and bilateral pyelonephritis. Cervical and inguinal lymphadenopathy was noted. The patient was treated with IV fluids, antibiotics (ceftriaxone and doxycycline), pantoprazole, ondansetron, and paracetamol.

## PROVISIONAL DIAGNOSIS

Extrapulmonary tuberculosis (TB) with possible involvement of the spleen, liver, and lymph nodes.

## DIFFERENTIAL DIAGNOSIS

- Extrapulmonary tuberculosis
- Infective endocarditis with systemic embolization
- Brucellosis
- Lymphoma
- Infectious mononucleosis
- Hepatosplenic schistosomiasis

## CLINICAL APPROACH

The clinical approach to a patient presenting with fever, abdominal pain, and weight loss includes a thorough history and physical examination to assess the onset, duration, and progression of symptoms.

A detailed history should focus on recent infections, travel history, contact with sick individuals, and any past medical history or risk factors for tuberculosis or other infections. On examination, assess for signs of systemic infection, lymphadenopathy, hepatosplenomegaly, and abdominal tenderness.

Laboratory tests should include complete blood count, liver function tests, renal function tests, and inflammatory markers (ESR, CRP). Imaging studies, including ultrasound and CT scans, are crucial for identifying hepatosplenomegaly, splenic lesions, and lymphadenopathy. A chest X-ray should be done to rule out pulmonary tuberculosis, and further investigations like tuberculosis PCR, acid-fast bacilli smear, or biopsy may be required for definitive diagnosis.

Extrapulmonary TB should be considered in patients with unexplained systemic symptoms and organ involvement, especially when there is evidence of granulomatous inflammation.

## PATHOPHYSIOLOGY

Extrapulmonary tuberculosis **(Fig. 1)** occurs when *Mycobacterium tuberculosis* spreads to sites outside the lungs, such as the spleen, liver, and lymph nodes. The infection causes granulomatous inflammation, leading to tissue damage and the formation of hypoechoic lesions in the spleen, hepatosplenomegaly, and lymphadenopathy. The associated fever, night sweats, and weight loss are systemic inflammatory responses due to the body's attempt to control the infection.

## TREATMENT AND PREVENTION

### Treatment

The treatment for extrapulmonary tuberculosis involves a combination of antitubercular drugs, typically including rifampin, isoniazid, pyrazinamide, and ethambutol for an initial intensive phase (usually for 2 months), followed by rifampin and isoniazid for a continuation phase (usually for 4–7 months). Supportive care, such as pain management, hydration, and nutritional support, may also be necessary. For coinfections, such as bacterial or viral infections, appropriate antibiotics or antivirals should be administered.

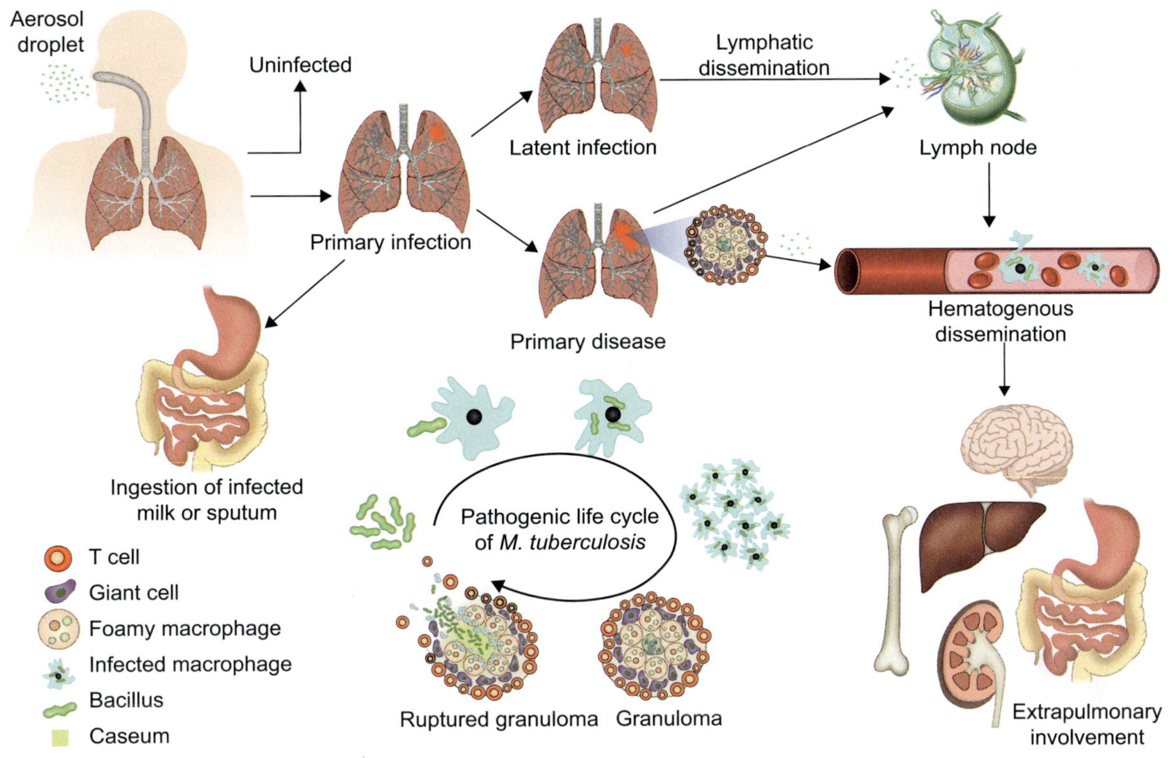


**FIG. 1:** Pathogenic life cycle and extrapulmonary dissemination of *M. tuberculosis*.

*Source*: Baykan AH, Sayiner HS, Aydin E, Koc M, Inan I, Erturk SM. Extrapulmonary tuberculosis: an old but resurgent problem. Insights Imaging. 2022;13(1).

## Prevention

Prevention of extrapulmonary TB focuses on early detection and treatment of pulmonary TB to reduce transmission. Vaccination with the BCG (Bacillus Calmette–Guérin) vaccine is recommended in high-risk populations to provide some protection against severe forms of TB. Preventive measures also include proper hand hygiene, wearing masks in high-risk environments, and screening at-risk individuals, such as those with close contact to TB patients or immunocompromised conditions. Regular follow-up for patients on TB treatment is crucial to ensure adherence and prevent complications.

### Points to Ponder

- *Clinical symptoms:* Extrapulmonary TB can present with nonrespiratory symptoms such as fever, weight loss, abdominal pain, and night sweats, often without the typical lung involvement.
- *Imaging findings*: Hepatosplenomegaly and splenic lesions on ultrasound or CT are significant findings suggesting extrapulmonary TB, especially in the absence of pulmonary symptoms.
- *Risk factors:* Extrapulmonary TB is more common in immunocompromised patients, but it can also affect otherwise healthy individuals, often after an initial primary infection.
- *Diagnosis:* The diagnosis of extrapulmonary TB relies on clinical suspicion, imaging, and laboratory tests (e.g., tuberculin skin test, biopsy, or PCR for *Mycobacterium tuberculosis*).
- *Treatment adherence:* As with pulmonary TB, adherence to a multidrug regimen for an adequate duration is crucial to ensure successful treatment and prevent relapse or drug resistance in cases of extrapulmonary TB.

## MULTIPLE CHOICE QUESTIONS

1. **What is the most likely diagnosis for a patient with fever, abdominal pain, weight loss, hepatosplenomegaly, and lymphadenopathy in the absence of respiratory symptoms?**
   A. Extrapulmonary tuberculosis
   B. Hepatocellular carcinoma
   C. Systemic lupus erythematosus
   D. Acute pancreatitis

2. **Which imaging finding is most consistent with extra-pulmonary tuberculosis in this case?**
   A. Bilateral lung infiltrates
   B. Hepatosplenomegaly with multiple hypoechoic splenic nodules
   C. Pericardial effusion
   D. Renal cysts

**3. Which laboratory finding is a strong indicator for extra-pulmonary tuberculosis?**

A. Negative sputum culture
B. Positive tuberculin skin test
C. Elevated liver enzymes
D. HLA-B27 positivity

**4. What is the first-line treatment for extrapulmonary tuberculosis?**

A. Intravenous antibiotics (ceftriaxone and doxycycline)
B. Rifampin, isoniazid, pyrazinamide, and ethambutol
C. Steroids
D. Antimalarial drugs

**5. Which of the following is not a common manifestation of extrapulmonary tuberculosis?**

A. Lymphadenopathy
B. Hepatosplenomegaly
C. Abdominal pain
D. Productive cough

## Answers

1. (A); 2. (B); 3. (B); 4. (B); 5. (D)

## SUGGESTED READINGS


1. Alavi SM, Sharifi M, Salami S. Epidemiology of extrapulmonary tuberculosis in Iran: A systematic review. Indian J Tuberc. 2019;66(4):515-24.
2. Sharma SK, Mohan A, Kadhiravan T. HIV-TB co-infection: epidemiology, diagnosis & management. Indian J Med Res. 2005;121(4):550-67.
3. Global Tuberculosis Report 2020 [Internet]. Who. int. [cited 2023 Nov 1]. Available from: https://www.who.int/publications-detailredirect/9789240013131. [Last Accessed December 2024]
4. Rieder HL. Epidemiologic basis of tuberculosis control. International Union Against Tuberculosis and Lung Disease; 1999. 5. Peto HM, Pratt RH, Harrington TA, LoBue PA, Armstrong LR. Epidemiology of extrapulmonary tuberculosis in the United States, 1993–2006. Clin Infect Dis. 2009;49(9):1350-7.
5. Treatment of tuberculosis: guidelines for national programmes [Internet]. Who. int. [cited 2023 Nov 1]. Available from: https://www.who.int/news/item/07-05-2010- treatment-of-tuberculosis-guidelines-for-national-programme [Last Accessed December 2024].

CHAPTER

41

# A Case-based Approach to Persistent Pyrexia in an Immunocompromised Individual

*Arup Kumar Kundu, Parthajit Das*

## CASE VIGNETTE

We report an interesting clinical presentation of a 55-year-old gentleman from Bhopal, Madhya Pradesh, India, who presented with intermittent high-grade fever with chills, cough with scanty expectorations, occasional chest discomfort and significant weight loss in the past 2 months. He denied any history of headache, shivering, skin rash, myalgia, burning micturition, hemoptysis, tachypnea, abdominal/chest pain or external bleeding. He is a known diabetic as well as hypertensive, which were well controlled with medications. There was no history of recent travel or contact with any sick individual or pet. Clinical examination revealed pallor, mild icterus, proptosis of left eye, hepatosplenomegaly and basal crackles in the lower chest in auscultation. He was also diagnosed with a demyelinating disease of the dorsal spine 8 months ago, for which prednisolone and mycophenolate mofetil were prescribed. However, mycophenolate was discontinued at a later date because of the development of pancytopenia. He was prescribed empirical antituberculous therapy elsewhere without any significant symptomatic relief. He needed hospital admission and was commenced on broad-spectrum intravenous antibiotics. Routine laboratory investigations revealed pancytopenia and features of chronic liver disease. Blood and urine culture were sterile. Tuberculosis, retroviral, Covid-19 screen were negative. Pulmonary function tests demonstrated restrictive pattern. Chest X-ray and HRCT thorax showed miliary reticulonodular opacities in the lungs bilaterally **(Fig. 1)**.

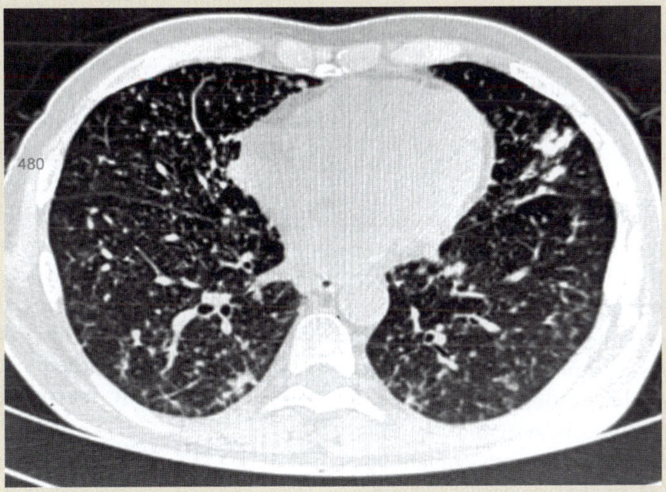


**FIG. 1:** HRCT thorax showing miliary shadows with multiple lung nodules.

The autoimmune screen was essentially within normal limits, apart from elevated serum ACE (angiotensin-converting enzyme) levels. Bronchoscopic alveolar lavage (BAL) fluid culture did not grow any significant bacteria or fungus, and the *GeneXpert* test for tuberculosis was negative. Bronchoscopy revealed granulomatous involvement of major bronchi **(Fig. 2)** and transbronchial lung biopsy showed epithelioid granulomas suggesting a granulomatous disease.

He remained pyrexial despite being on intravenous antibiotics for more than a week. PET-CT was performed, showing metabolically active mesenteric lymphadenopathy and splenomegaly, and gave an impression of chronic granulomatous disease (CGD). A corticosteroid trial was initiated after discussing the risks with other specialist doctors. He had a good initial clinical response to corticosteroid therapy, but the fever relapsed on corticosteroid withdrawal. Considering the clinical scenario, it was planned to revisit the history and clinical examination once again, which is a must in patients dealing with pyrexia of unknown origin (PUO). At this juncture, serum beta-D-glucan level was done, and it came elevated, and

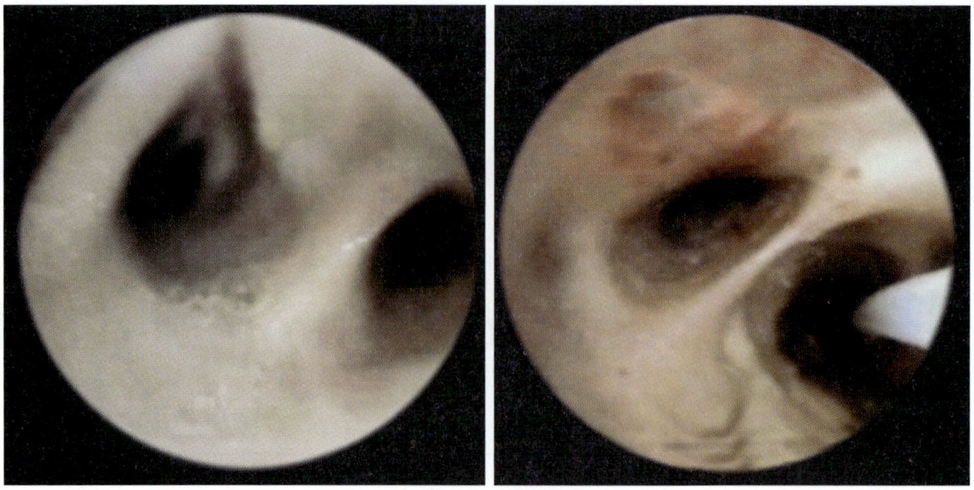

**FIG. 2:** Bronchoscopy showing granulomatous involvement of major bronchi.

subsequent urine tests confirmed elevated Histoplasma antigen. As the cause of pyrexia still remained unresolved, a bone marrow biopsy was done, and it showed normocellular marrow with granulomas and presence of fungal elements within. A multidisciplinary team input was sought involving an internist, infectious disease specialist, pulmonologist and rheumatologist, and empirical IV liposomal amphotericin B along with low-dose prednisolone was considered because of persistent and nagging pyrexia. Now, he responded well and was discharged in a stable condition after intravenous course of amphotericin B for 14 days. He also received oral isavuconazole for next 6 months with a remarkable clinical improvement.

## PROVISIONAL DIAGNOSIS

Disseminated infection with a possible fungal etiology (e.g., invasive aspergillosis or histoplasmosis).

## DIFFERENTIAL DIAGNOSIS

The major diagnostic dilemma in this case was establishing the etiology of persistent fever in a middle-aged, immunocompromised patient (suffering from diabetes mellitus, and was on corticosteroid and mycophenolate for a long duration) with significant weight loss, unilateral proptosis, hepatosplenomegaly, pancytopenia and miliary shadows. Various differential diagnoses were considered at different stages such as miliary tuberculosis, disseminated histoplasmosis, retroviral disease, sarcoidosis, systemic vasculitis, hypersensitivity pneumonitis, granulomatosis with polyangiitis (Wegener's granulomatosis), IgG4-related diseases, systemic lupus erythematosus (SLE) and lymphoproliferative diseases. Multidisciplinary team input and a thorough multilayered investigative algorithm were followed, and close differentials were excluded one by one in a stepwise manner.

He was finally diagnosed with 'Histoplasmosis' when blood culture grew *Histoplasma capsulatum*, bone marrow examination showed granulomas with a presence of fungal elements and urine examination confirmed Histoplasma antigen.

## CLINICAL APPROACH

In this type of puzzling scenario, a thorough history taking, appropriate clinical examination and a structured diagnostic approach are essential for prompt recognition of the underlying pathology or any infectious etiology, and an early institution of a comprehensive management plan with utmost priority concurrently. A detailed inquiry should include a past medical or surgical history, drug history including alternative medicines, over-the-counter (OTC) medicines, recreational drugs and vaccinations. A detailed travel history should review environmental, animal and sexual exposures. A relevant contact history with an infectious focus should be looked at. A focused clinical examination should be performed with a special attention towards the respiratory, cardiovascular and alimentary systems to identify the important sources of fever. The first round of diagnostic evaluations should be guided by the clues received from history and clinical examination, and subsequent investigations including infection screening, immunological assays, histopathology, and specialized radiological tests such as CT, MRI or FDG-PET should be customized as per the individual needs. A stepwise methodical therapeutic algorithm should be adopted to minimize costs and optimize treatment outcomes. However, when a diagnosis remains elusive, a specialist opinion from another medical discipline, such as infectious disease, rheumatology, hematology, pulmonology, gastroenterology etc. may be helpful.

## PATHOPHYSIOLOGY

Histoplasmosis is caused by *Histoplasma capsulatum*, a dimorphic fungus. Inhalation of microconidia from contaminated soil leads to fungal growth in alveolar macrophages. The fungus survives intracellularly by inhibiting phagolysosome acidification. It spreads via the lymphatic and hematogenous routes, forming granulomas in the lungs and other organs. In immunocompetent individuals, granulomas may calcify, whereas in immunocompromised hosts, uncontrolled fungal proliferation leads to disseminated disease.

## TREATMENT AND PREVENTION

Granulomatous diseases comprise a wide spectrum of heterogeneous disorders including infections such as tuberculosis, fungal infections and non-infectious diseases such as sarcoidosis, granulomatosis with polyangiitis, and eosinophilic granulomatosis with polyangiitis (Churg-Strauss syndrome), etc. Diseases such as sarcoidosis, IgG4-related diseases, systemic lupus erythematosus (SLE), lymphoproliferative diseases, tuberculosis, and histoplasmosis have significant similarities in terms of clinical presentations, laboratory investigations and radiological manifestations. The tuberculosis screening was repeatedly negative in this patient and hence was excluded. IgG4-related disease, systemic vasculitides, connective tissue diseases and lymphoproliferative diseases were also excluded following relevant investigations. This clinical case posed a significant diagnostic challenge to differentiate between sarcoidosis and histoplasmosis. Unilateral proptosis is more commonly found in sarcoidosis when compared with histoplasmosis. However, there are rare case reports of unilateral proptosis in patients with disseminated histoplasmosis. Wheat et al. reported 11 patients with suspected sarcoidosis who demonstrated laboratory evidence of histoplasmosis, confirmed by urine antigen, serologic tests, and/or immunodiffusion. All of these patients received corticosteroid therapy prior to the diagnosis of histoplasmosis. Reimann et al. also described a case of histoplasmosis which was mistakenly diagnosed as sarcoidosis. Bronchoscopic cultures could be negative for fungal infections because of significant rate of false negatives. Interestingly, Sharma reported cases of diffuse histoplasmosis in a sarcoidosis patient. Our patient had a good response with oral prednisolone and his symptoms relapsed upon steroid withdrawal. He was therefore kept on low dose of oral prednisolone. Although he had received multiple courses of antibiotics at other centers, he had a remarkable response with IV liposomal amphotericin B as per regional guidelines. He was also prescribed oral isavuconazole for the next six months with a complete clinical recovery. Corticosteroid therapy was withdrawn at a later stage.

It remains a matter of debate whether histoplasmosis in this patient was the primary infection or a secondary infection following strong immunosuppressive therapy, which he received for demyelinating spinal disease. Because of the identical disease manifestations, misdiagnosis can occur, and an inappropriate management plan can lead to significant morbidity. Multidisciplinary specialist input and a thorough, multilayered investigative strategy helped us to institute an appropriate plan, leading to affirmative clinical outcome for this patient.

### Points to Ponder

- Treating physicians should develop a focused diagnostic and therapeutic approach for the management of immunocompromised patients with persistent fever.
- A cautious investigative algorithm should be applied to investigate close mimickers such as miliary tuberculosis, disseminated histoplasmosis, retroviral disease, sarcoidosis, systemic vasculitis, IgG4-related diseases, systemic lupus erythematosus (SLE), and lymphoproliferative diseases etc. to avoid misdiagnosis and inappropriate treatment in immunocompromised host.
- The judicious use of modern diagnostic modalities, appropriate use of emerging antimicrobial agents, as well as immunosuppressive agents are the essential steps towards improved survival in this group of patients.
- The use of regional guideline-directed antimicrobial agents is strongly recommended to avoid drug resistance.

## MULTIPLE CHOICE QUESTIONS

1. **What was the initial imaging finding in this patient suggestive of a disseminated disease?**
   A Pleural effusion
   B. Miliary reticulonodular opacities on HRCT thorax
   C. Consolidation in the right lung
   D. Pulmonary embolism
2. **Which diagnostic test confirmed the diagnosis of histoplasmosis in this patient?**
   A. Serum beta-D-glucan level and urine Histoplasma antigen
   B. Blood culture
   C. Tuberculosis PCR
   D. Bone marrow biopsy alone
3. **What is the most likely cause of persistent pyrexia in this immunocompromised patient?**
   A. Viral infection
   B. Fungal infection (Histoplasmosis)
   C. Bacterial sepsis
   D. Tuberculosis
4. **What was the primary treatment for this patient's histoplasmosis?**
   A. Empirical antibiotics
   B. Liposomal amphotericin B followed by oral isavuconazole
   C. High-dose corticosteroids
   D. Empirical antituberculous therapy
5. **What key clinical feature led to suspicion of fungal infection in this patient?**
   A. Persistent pyrexia despite broad-spectrum antibiotics
   B. Positive blood culture
   C. Rapid resolution of symptoms with corticosteroids
   D. Presence of hepatosplenomegaly and pancytopenia

### Answers

1. (B); 2. (A); 3. (B); 4. (B); 5. (A)

## SUGGESTED READINGS

1. Klotz SA, Penn CC, Negvesky GJ, et al. Fungal and parasitic infections of the eye. Clin Microbiol Rev. 2000;13(4):662-85.
2. Wheat LJ, French MLV, Wall JL. Sarcoidlike manifestations of histoplasmosis. Arch Intern Med. 1989;149(11):2421-6.
3. Reimann HA, Price AH. Histoplasmosis in Pennsylvania; confusion with sarcoidosis. Pa Med J. 1949;52(4):367-71.
4. Sharma OP. Histoplasmosis: a masquerader of sarcoidosis. Sarcoidosis. 1991;8(1):10-3.

CHAPTER

42

# An Approach to a Case of Pregnant Lady with Hepatitis B

*Uppara Kadiyala Rakesh, Mohd Asif, Manuj Kumar Sarkar*

**CASE VIGNETTE**

A 30-year-old primigravida with 28 weeks' gestation presents with new-onset jaundice accompanied by fatigue, nausea, and yellowish discoloration of urine. She was under regular antenatal check-ups. Prenatal screening at 8 weeks confirmed chronic HBV (HBsAg positive), and the liver function test (LFT) was normal. Other past medical history, medications, or typical risk factors for liver disease (like blood transfusions or IV drug use), but she gave a history of tattooing done 3 years prior. At present (28 weeks' gestation), LFT: Total bilirubin—4 mg/dL, indirect 3 mg/dL and liver enzymes are normal, HBV DNA level is 250,000 IU/mL, HBeAg is positive, indicating high infectivity. There are no complications during the current pregnancy.

*Current concerns*: The patient is concerned about the risk of transmitting hepatitis B to her baby and the need for antiviral therapy during pregnancy.

## PROVISIONAL DIAGNOSIS

This 30-year-old primigravida with chronic hepatitis B virus (HBV) infection is presenting with new-onset jaundice, which could be indicative of acute exacerbation of chronic hepatitis B during pregnancy.

- The elevated bilirubin levels, positive HBeAg, and high HBV DNA suggest active viral replication and significant liver involvement.
- Given the absence of complications and normal liver enzymes, this presentation may reflect a subclinical hepatic flare associated with pregnancy, though further monitoring and assessment are necessary to rule out other potential causes, such as obstetric cholestasis or acute fatty liver of pregnancy.

## DIFFERENTIAL DIAGNOSIS

While hepatitis B is the most likely diagnosis, given the patient's history and test results, other conditions should be considered:

- *Chronic hepatitis B in pregnancy*:
  - The patient is positive for HBsAg and has high levels of HBV DNA and HBeAg positivity, which suggests active replication of the virus and a higher risk of vertical transmission to the newborn.
- *Hepatitis C and hepatitis E*:
  - Distinguishing feature: The presence of positive HBsAg and negative anti-HCV and anti-hepatitis E (if tested) would confirm chronic hepatitis B as the diagnosis.
- *Autoimmune hepatitis*:
  - Distinguishing feature: Autoimmune hepatitis typically presents with elevated ALT/AST, positive autoantibodies (e.g., antinuclear antibodies, antismooth muscle antibodies), and elevated immunoglobulin G (IgG). The patient's HBsAg positivity and negative autoimmune markers make this less likely.
- *Nonalcoholic fatty liver disease (NAFLD)*:
  - Distinguishing feature: NAFLD is often associated with obesity, diabetes, and metabolic syndrome. The absence of these risk factors makes it less likely in this case.
- *Hepatic complications of pregnancy*:
  - Distinguishing feature: Conditions like intrahepatic cholestasis of pregnancy (ICP) andacute fatty liver of pregnancy (AFLP) would present with symptoms such as pruritus and jaundice. This patient has no such symptoms.
- *HELLP (hemolysis, elevated liver enzymes, low platelet) syndrome*:
  - In HELLP syndrome, high blood pressure, anemia, and schistocytes on blood smear are present. It is also associated with elevated liver enzymes (AST/ALP), a low platelet count, and an elevated LDH level.

## CLINICAL APPROACH

- *Confirming the diagnosis*:
  - HBV testing: Confirm chronic hepatitis B with tests for HBsAg, HBV DNA, HBeAg, and liver function tests (ALT/AST).

- Liver ultrasound: If cirrhosis is suspected, assess liver architecture and the presence of any focal lesions that could indicate hepatocellular carcinoma (HCC).
- HBV DNA level: Confirm viral load (>200,000 IU/mL in the third-trimester indicates a higher risk of vertical transmission).
- Liver function tests (LFTs): Assess for liver injury (elevated ALT/AST, bilirubin).
- Assessment for co-infection: Test for HCV, HIV, or HDV co-infection, if clinically indicated.

- *Assessing risk of vertical transmission*:
  - HBeAg positivity: Positive HBeAg suggests a higher risk of vertical transmission.
  - HBV DNA levels: High HBV DNA levels (>200,000 IU/mL) further increase the risk of neonatal infection.
- *Obstetric considerations*:
  - Fetal monitoring: Ultrasound to monitor fetal growth and well-being, particularly if the patient has underlying liver disease that could affect placental function.
  - Monitor for signs of hepatic decompensation: Although the patient is asymptomatic, watch for signs of cirrhosis or preeclampsia.
  - Mode of delivery: Vaginal delivery is recommended unless there are obstetric complications or concerns regarding maternal liver function.

## PATHOPHYSIOLOGY OF HEPATITIS B IN PREGNANCY

In acute HBV infection, early markers like HBeAg, HBsAg, and HBV DNA appear, with IgM anti-HBc indicating diagnosis; recovery includes ALT normalization and seroconversion to anti-HBe and anti-HBs, signifying past infection. Chronic HBV is marked by prolonged HBsAg, HBeAg, and HBV DNA without anti-HBs, with HBsAg persistence beyond 6 months indicating chronicity **(Fig 1)**.

- *HBV infection mechanism*:
  - HBV transmission: The virus primarily infects hepatocytes through the hepatitis B surface antigen (HBsAg). It can be transmitted from mother to baby during childbirth, especially in women with high viral loads and positive HBeAg.
  - Immunologic factors: Pregnant women have a slightly suppressed immune system, which can allow for increased viral replication in HBV. Despite this, vertical transmission rates can be minimized with appropriate interventions.
- *Maternal impact **(Fig. 2)***:
  - Liver inflammation: Chronic HBV may cause liver inflammation, fibrosis, or cirrhosis over time. Pregnancy can exacerbate liver dysfunction, though pregnancy itself generally does not worsen HBV.
  - Flare of hepatitis: Pregnancy may trigger a flare of hepatitis in some women, especially in those with active HBV. Close monitoring is essential.
  - Increased risk of preeclampsia: Women with liver disease, including HBV, are at higher risk for pre-eclampsia or gestational hypertension.
- *Fetal impact*:
  - Risk of vertical transmission: The risk of mother-to-child transmission is highest when the mother is HBeAg positive and has high HBV DNA levels. This risk is approximately 20–30% without antiviral treatment.
  - Increased risk of preterm birth: Women with chronic hepatitis B may have a higher risk of preterm labor, though the exact relationship is not well-established.

## TREATMENT AND PREVENTION

### Antiviral Treatment during Pregnancy (Flowchart 1)

- *Indications*:
  - High HBV DNA levels (>200,000 IU/mL) antivirals initiated at 28 weeks' gestation.
  - Chronic hepatitis B with evidence of active liver disease (elevated ALT), HBeAg positivity, or co-existing liver conditions (e.g., cirrhosis).
- *Preferred treatment*:
  - Tenofovir disoproxil fumarate (TDF) (Category B in pregnancy) is the first-line therapy during pregnancy as it is safe, effective, and has a low risk of resistance. TDF has been shown to reduce maternal HBV DNA levels, lowering the risk of vertical transmission. An RCT by Pan CQ et al. shows that starting tenofovir earlier in pregnancy (at 16 weeks) prevents mother-to-child transmission of hepatitis B, even without using HBIG. This is particularly important in areas where HBIG may not be readily available. More robust studies are needed.

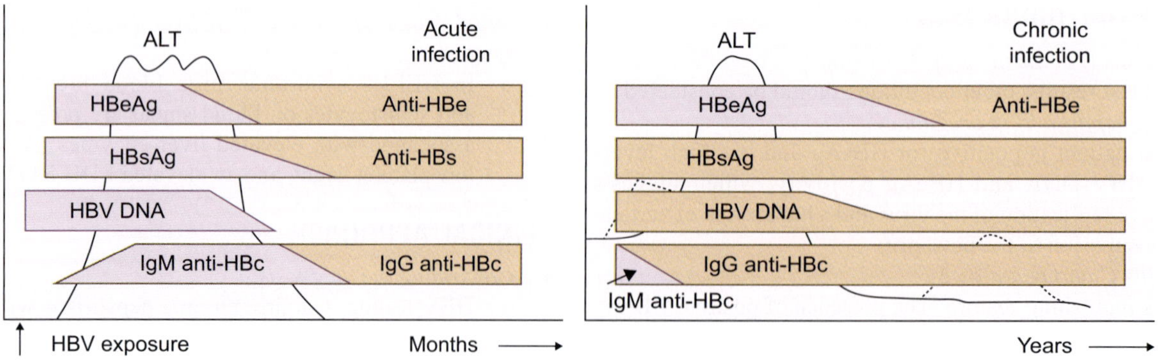


**FIG. 1**: Serologic responses to hepatitis B virus infection.
*Source*: 2024 UpToDate

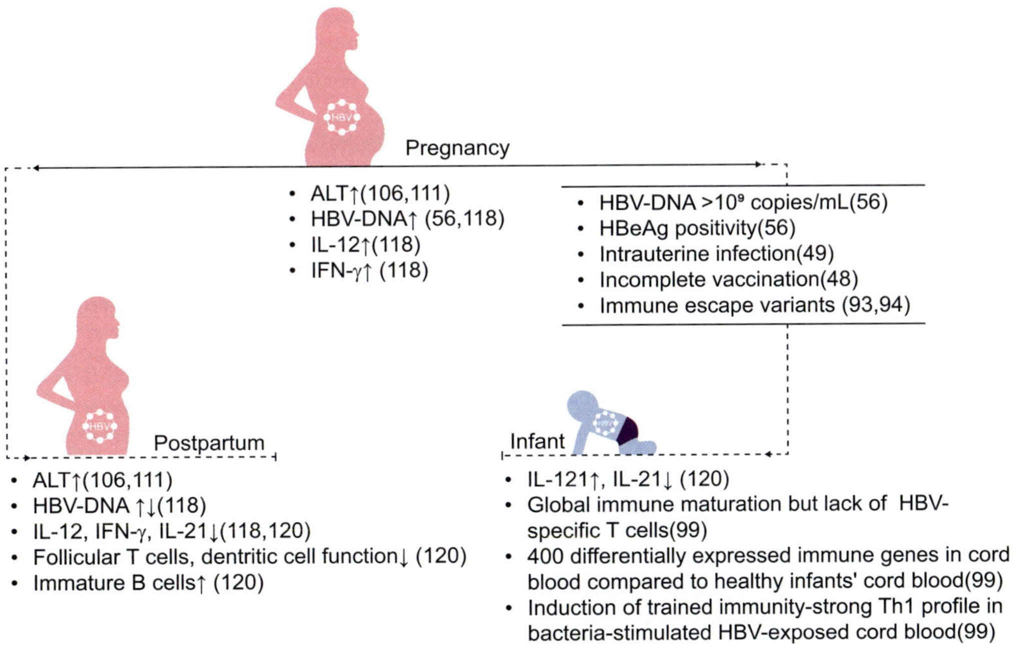


**FIG. 2**: Schematic representation of immunologic changes in the peripartum period in mothers with CHB and their infants.

*Source*: Joshi SS, Coffin CS. Hepatitis B and Pregnancy: Virologic and Immunologic Characteristics. Hepatol Commun. 2020;4(2):157-71.

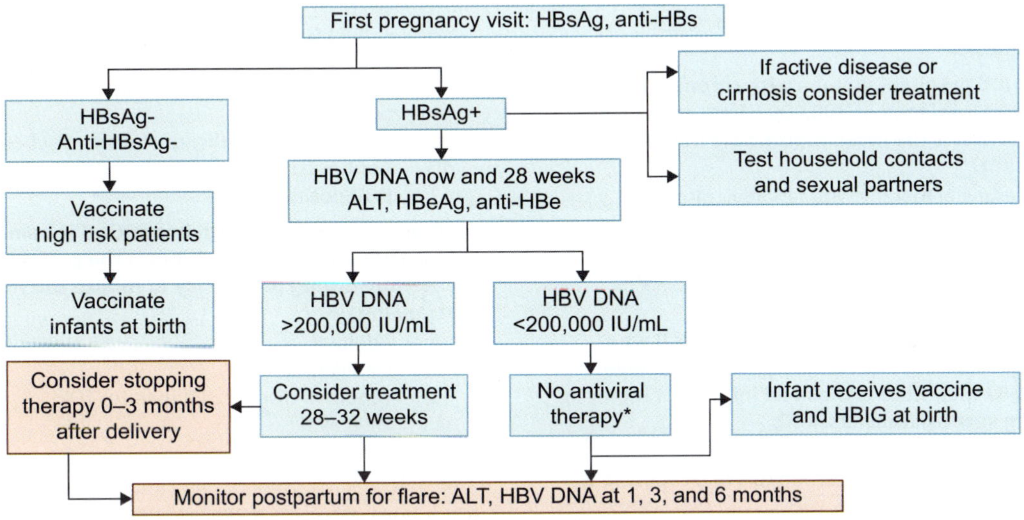


*Consider therapy if preterm labor or prior child with immunoprophylaxis failure.

**FLOWCHART 1**: Algorithm for hepatitis B virus during pregnancy.

*Source*: Ayoub WS, Cohen E. Hepatitis management in the pregnant patient: An Update. J Clin Transl Hepatol. 2016;4(3):241-7.

- Lamivudine (Category C in pregnancy) is an alternative but less preferred due to the potential for viral resistance.
- Entecavir is generally avoided in pregnancy due to safety concerns.

- *Follow-up*: Close monitoring for hepatitis B is crucial after delivery, especially for women who did not take antiviral medication during pregnancy or who stopped it early. This monitoring should continue for at least 6 months to watch for flares and changes in the virus. Long-term follow-up helps determine if future treatment is needed.
- *Postpartum antiviral therapy*: Based on liver function and HBV DNA levels, postpartum continuation of antiviral therapy may be considered. This is particularly relevant for those with elevated viral load and advanced liver disease.

## Prevention of Vertical Transmission

- *Newborn management*:
  - HBV vaccine: The baby should receive the first dose of the HBV vaccine within 12 hours of birth.
  - Hepatitis B immunoglobulin (HBIG): Administered within 12 hours after birth to reduce the risk of vertical transmission.
  - Follow-up testing for HBV at 9–12 months of age to determine whether the infant has contracted HBV.
- *Breastfeeding*: Safer if the infant receives the complete vaccine regimen (HBV vaccine) and HBIG.
- *Delivery considerations*:
  - Vaginal delivery is preferred unless there are other obstetric indications for a cesarean section.

## Points to Ponder

- *Universal screening*: Every pregnant woman should be tested for hepatitis B during her first prenatal visit. This identifies those who need closer monitoring and treatment to protect their babies.
- *Viral load matters*: High HBV DNA levels in the mother (above 200,000 IU/mL) increase the risk of transmission to the baby and require prompt action.
- *Anti-viral therapy*: Women who meet standard indications for HBV therapy should be treated. For women without standard indications but who have HBV DNA >200,000 IU/mL, antiviral therapy should be at 28 weeks to prevent mother-to-child transmission.
- *Protect the newborn*: Every baby born to a mother with hepatitis B should receive the hepatitis B vaccine and hepatitis B immune globulin (HBIG) within 12 hours of birth, ideally within 4 hours, for the best protection.
- *Breastfeeding*: Mothers with hepatitis B can breastfeed, especially if their baby receives timely vaccination and HBIG.
- *Monitoring*: Both mother and baby need continued monitoring and follow-up.
  - *The mother*: Regular liver function tests and HBV DNA level checks throughout the pregnancy and after delivery.
  - *The baby*: HBsAg and anti-HBs testing after completing the vaccination series.

## MULTIPLE CHOICE QUESTIONS

1. **Which of the following is the most appropriate initial step in the management of a pregnant woman with chronic hepatitis B (HBV)?**
   A. Immediate initiation of antiviral therapy
   B. Referral for a liver transplant evaluation
   C. Screening for hepatitis B virus (HBV) markers, including HBsAg and HBV DNA
   D. Routine cesarean delivery to prevent vertical transmission
2. **A 30-year-old pregnant woman with chronic hepatitis B (HBV) has a viral load of 300,000 IU/mL at 28 weeks' gestation. What is the most appropriate next step in management?**
   A. Start antiviral therapy with tenofovir disoproxil fumarate (TDF)
   B. Start antiviral therapy with lamivudine
   C. Initiate hepatitis C testing and delay treatment
   D. Plan for cesarean delivery at 39 weeks
3. **In a pregnant woman with chronic hepatitis B who is positive for HBeAg and has a high HBV DNA level (>200,000 IU/mL), what is the most important factor in preventing vertical transmission?**
   A. Initiating antiviral therapy in the third trimester
   B. Performing a cesarean section to avoid exposure to blood
   C. Administering hepatitis B immunoglobulin (HBIG) to the mother after delivery
   D. Administering hepatitis B vaccine to the mother after delivery
4. **Which of the following is not a recommended intervention for preventing HBV transmission to the newborn?**
   A. Administration of hepatitis B immunoglobulin (HBIG) within 12 hours of birth
   B. Hepatitis B vaccination for the newborn within 12 hours of delivery
   C. Starting antiviral therapy for the newborn after birth
   D. Continued breastfeeding after the birth of an HBV-positive infant
5. **A pregnant woman with hepatitis B is being considered for antiviral treatment. What is the preferred antiviral therapy during pregnancy to reduce the risk of vertical transmission?**
   A. Adefovir
   B. Lamivudine
   C. Tenofovir disoproxil fumarate (TDF)
   D. Entecavir

### Answers

1. (C); 2. (A); 3. (A); 4. (C); 5. (C)

## SUGGESTED READINGS


1. Dionne-Odom J, Cozzi GD, Franco RA, et al. Treatment and prevention of viral hepatitis in pregnancy. Am J Obstet Gynecol. 2022;226(3):335-46.
2. Brown RS, McMahon BJ, Lok ASF, et al. Antiviral therapy in chronic hepatitis B viral infection during pregnancy: A systematic review and meta-analysis. Hepatology. 2015;63(1):319-33.
3. Liao YJ, Li SS. Hepatitis B in pregnancy and its management: An overview. World Journal of Hepatology. 2015;7(27):2969-76.
4. American College of Obstetricians and Gynecologists (ACOG). (2020). Management of Hepatitis B in Pregnancy. ACOG Committee Opinion No. 794.
5. Lin CL, Kao JH. Management of Hepatitis B Virus Infection in Pregnancy. Clinics in Liver Disease. 2015;19(3):497-510.
6. Pan CQ, Dai E, Mo Z, et al. Tenofovir and Hepatitis B Virus Transmission During Pregnancy: A Randomized Clinical Trial. JAMA. 2024:e2422952.
7. Joshi SS, Coffin CS. Hepatitis B and Pregnancy: Virologic and Immunologic Characteristics. Hepatol Commun. 2020;4(2):157-71

CHAPTER

43

# An Approach to a Case of a 35-year-old Female with Lymph Node TB Presenting with New Onset Lymph Node

*Onkar Awadhiya, Sagar Sangole, Bharatsing D Rathod, Rajashree Khot*

**CASE VIGNETTE**

A 35-year-old female presented with a history of low-grade fever, decreased appetite, weight loss, and night sweats for 2–3 months. Clinical examination was remarkable for bilateral cervical lymphadenopathy. Fine-needle aspiration cytology (FNAC) of the lymph nodes showed epithelioid granulomas and caseous material. However, the ZN stain (for any acid-fast bacilli) and Xpert MTB/RIF assay were negative. With a presumptive diagnosis of lymph node tuberculosis (TB), she was started empirically on antitubercular treatment (ATT). Gradually, the symptoms improved but 2 months later, she presented again with fever and the appearance of new swellings in the neck with a discharging sinus.

## PROVISIONAL DIAGNOSIS

In a young lady who was diagnosed with tubercular lymphadenitis and presenting with new onset lymphadenopathy despite ongoing ATT, one of the most important provisional diagnoses is drug-resistant tuberculosis. However, nonadherence to ATT has to be ruled out first.

## DIFFERENTIAL DIAGNOSIS

Differential diagnoses of this clinical scenario are represented in **Flowchart 1**.

- *Poor adherence*: Recent studies in India have identified several factors contributing to nonadherence to antitubercular treatment (ATT). A study from Ahmedabad, with 200 participants found that financial strain, travel time to healthcare centers, adverse drug reactions, and stigma about TB were significant factors affecting adherence. Patients receiving treatment from government facilities showed higher nonadherence rates (50%) compared to those treated privately (38%), with challenges like lack of family support and difficulty in swallowing pills contributing to missed doses.
- *Drug-resistant tuberculosis (DR-TB)*: DR-TB should always be suspected and ruled out in patients with inadequate response or progression despite good compliance with ATT. DR-TB is a disease of international concern. Global estimates indicate that about 0.5 million new cases of rifampicin-resistant TB (RR-TB) occurred in 2019 with 78% of them having confirmed multidrug-resistant TB (MDR-TB). The estimated number of MDR/RR-TB cases in India is 124,000 (9.1/lakh population).

  Simple definitions of resistance patterns are as follows:
  - *RR-TB*: When resistance to R is detected.
  - *Isoniazid-resistant TB (Hr-TB)*: When resistance to isoniazid and susceptibility to rifampicin has been confirmed.
  - *MDR-TB*: When resistance to both H and R with or without resistance to other first-line anti-TB drugs.
- *Paradoxical reaction*: A paradoxical reaction (PR) in patients with lymph node tuberculosis (LNTB) is defined as either the worsening of pre-existing tuberculous lesions or the appearance of new lesions in those who showed initial improvement with ATT. It can be mistaken for treatment failure or relapse. PR in LNTB has a prevalence ranging from 13.3 to 35.3%. It typically begins within the first month of treatment but can arise up to a year later. The new nodal enlargement may be on the same or a different site, ipsilateral or contralateral. It can be complicated by abscess and sinus formation. PR with increased frequency and severity has been found in HIV co-infected patients on antiretroviral treatment (ART), than both HIV-negative and ART naïve HIV patients.

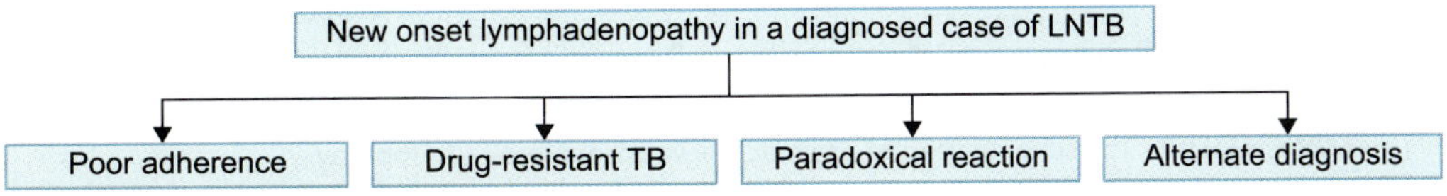


**FLOWCHART 1:** Differential diagnoses.

- *Alternate diagnosis*: When the primary cause of lymphadenopathy was an illness other than tuberculosis, the patient would not respond to ATT. A list of such etiologies includes the following:
  - *Infections*:
    - Bacterial: Brucellosis, Cat scratch disease, chancroid, lymphogranuloma venereum (LGV), syphilis, nontubercular mycobacteria (NTM), etc.
    - Viral: Infectious mononucleosis (Epstein–Barr virus), HIV, adenovirus, cytomegalovirus, etc.
    - Fungal: Coccidioidomycosis, cryptococcosis, histoplasmosis; helminthic, toxoplasmosis.
  - *Malignancy*: Lymphoma, leukemia, Kaposi sarcoma, skin neoplasms, and metastases.
  - *Autoimmune disorders*: Systemic lupus erythematosus, dermatomyositis, rheumatoid arthritis, Sjögren syndrome, Still's disease.
  - *Miscellaneous conditions*: Sarcoidosis, silicosis, Castleman disease, histiocytosis, Kawasaki disease, Kikuchi lymphadenitis, Kimura disease.
  - *Medications*: Allopurinol, atenolol, captopril, hydralazine, penicillin, phenytoin, trimethoprim/sulfamethoxazole, etc.

## CLINICAL APPROACH

A systematic method should be used to approach this case, (as depicted in **Flowchart 2**).

## HISTORY

A detailed history should be taken. Compliance with the ATT should be enquired. History of medications other than ATT should be noted. Symptoms may hint at the alternate cause of lymphadenopathy. Fever, chills, sore throat, and weight loss suggest an infective cause. However, constitutional symptoms of fever, anorexia, and night sweats may indicate underlying malignancy as well. Arthralgias, joint stiffness, and skin rash point toward autoimmune conditions. Some symptoms may indicate nonsuperficial lymphadenopathy such as cough or wheezing (airway compression); dysphagia (esophageal compression); or swelling of the neck, face, or arms (superior vena cava compression).

Tobacco and alcohol use and ultraviolet radiation exposure increase the risk for neoplasm. History of close contact with a case of tuberculosis should be enquired. A history of high-risk sexual behavior (syphilis, HIV, chancroid, LGV), occupational history (silicosis), and animal exposure (Cat scratch disease, brucellosis) is important.

## PHYSICAL EXAMINATION

Physical examination can provide clues for the diagnosis. The site, size, texture (soft, firm, rubbery, or hard), tenderness, signs of inflammation, and discharging sinus at skin overlying the LN should be noted. Classifying lymphadenopathy as generalized or localized narrows the differential diagnoses. Pallor, icterus, hepatosplenomegaly, skin rash, and joint swelling/tenderness, ENT examination may guide the workup. Splenomegaly implies a systemic illness such as infectious mononucleosis, lymphoma, acute or chronic leukemia, SLE, sarcoidosis, Cat scratch disease, etc.

### Imaging

Chest X-ray may show pulmonary infiltrates and mediastinal lymphadenopathy (TB, histoplasmosis, sarcoidosis, etc.). Ultrasonography, computed tomography, or magnetic resonance imaging may help characterize lymphadenopathy. These modalities may reveal hepatosplenomegaly or solid visceral tumors as well. If malignancy is suspected, a positron emission tomography (PET) scan should be performed.

### Biopsy

Fine-needle aspiration cytology (FNAC) is a quick, minimally invasive, and safe technique to evaluate patients with lymphadenopathy. Specimens should be sent for cytology, Xpert MTB/RIF test; microscopy and culture for *M.tb* with drug susceptibility testing.

Excisional biopsy should be done when FNAC is inconclusive or malignancy is suspected. Histopathology may show caseating (e.g., TB) or noncaseating (e.g., sarcoidosis) granulomas; histiocyte nuclear breakdown (karyorrhexis) with multiple necrotic foci and an absence of neutrophils and eosinophils (Kikuchi disease).

### Other Tests

Lab investigations are guided by history and physical examinations. CBC, LFT, KFT, peripheral smear, throat swab, ESR, CRP, rheumatoid factor, antineutrophilic (ANA)/anti-dsDNA antibodies, anti-HIV antibodies, VDRL, serum angiotensin-converting enzyme (ACE) levels, bone marrow aspiration and biopsy, immunohistochemistry, etc., may be used as indicated.

### Drug Susceptibility Testing

FNAC or the biopsy specimen should be sent for resistance testing in case of ATT failure. Rapid molecular diagnostic methods [Xpert MTB/RIF-cartridge-based nucleic acid amplification test (CBNAAT), Xpert MTB/XDR] are used for drug resistance testing.

Growth-based drug susceptibility testing is done by phenotypic tests wherein culture can be done on solid (Löwenstein–Jensen media) or liquid media (*Mycobacterium* growth indicator tube/MGIT system) and subsequently tested for drug susceptibility.

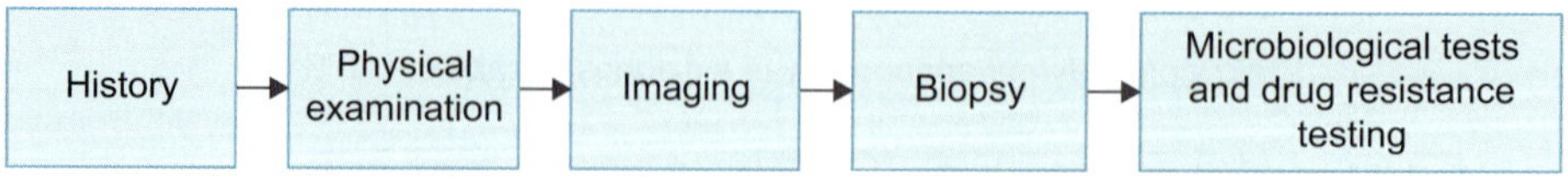


**FLOWCHART 2**: The scheme used to approach new onset lymphadenopathy.

## PATHOPHYSIOLOGY

In this section, we will discuss the pathophysiology of DR-TB and PR. A discussion on the pathophysiology of alternate diagnoses is beyond the scope of this chapter.

- *Drug-resistant TB*: The resistance is caused by a genetic mutation that makes a drug ineffective against the mutant mycobacterium. Significant mutations include the *rpoB* gene for rifampicin resistance; the *KatG* gene and the InhA promoter region mutation for isoniazid [and ethionamide (Eto)] resistance, and gyrA and gyrB mutations for fluoroquinolone resistance.

  An inadequate treatment regimen, improper supply of the drug, lack of resources, and premature termination of the treatment allow drug-resistant mutants to become the dominant strain.
- *Paradoxical reaction*: The exact mechanism of PR is not well understood. An immune response to *M. tuberculosis* after initiation of ATT and release of mycobacterial antigens has been implicated in the pathogenesis of PR. This hypothesis is supported by the fact that the biopsy or culture of nodes involved in PR typically shows granuloma formation, with or without positive AFB stains but negative culture results. A similar phenomenon of exaggerated immune reaction, known as immune reconstitution inflammatory syndrome (IRIS) has been seen in HIV/AIDS patients treated with ART.

## TREATMENT AND PREVENTION

- *Adherence*: Strengthening TB diagnostic and treatment services, adequate drug supply, nutritional and psychological support, and prompt identification and treatment of common adverse effects of ATT may improve compliance.
- *DR-TB*: Compared to the treatment for drug-susceptible TB (DS-TB), DR-TB regimens require a longer course, higher pill burden, and higher toxicity profile. Treatment follows a pretreatment evaluation to identify potential risk factors. Drugs are grouped into three groups **(Table 1)** and a combination of these is used to treat DR-TB. Previously, injectable drugs were used but nowadays, we are shifting toward all oral regimens. The DST results (H-mono/poly vs. M/XDR-TB), history of previous treatment, and adverse drug reactions are considered for the regimen selection. **Flowchart 3** depicts common regimens for DR-TB.

  BPaL regimen (6–9 months) for MDR-TB composed of bedaquiline, pretomanid, and linezolid may be used under operational research conditions in selected MDR-TB patients.
- *Paradoxical reaction*: There are no consensus guidelines for managing PR, and the approach should be based on the level of discomfort to the patient. Options include observation, aspiration, surgical excision, or a trial of nonsteroidal anti-inflammatory agents or corticosteroids. Steroids have been considered to reduce immune response in PR, but their use is controversial. Infliximab (anti-TNF-α inhibitor) has also been used in this setting. ATT should not be withheld.
- *Alternate diagnosis*: In conditions where the patient was presumptively diagnosed with tuberculosis, but the final diagnosis was a different disease, the ATT should be withheld. Treatment depends on the underlying cause of the lymphadenopathy. For example, corticosteroids for sarcoidosis, antiretroviral therapy (ART) for HIV/AIDS, disease-modifying drugs and immunosuppressants for autoimmune conditions (RA, SLE), symptomatic treatment + antivirals for infectious mononucleosis, and NSAIDs/steroids for Kikuchi disease are used. For the treatment of Hodgkins and non-Hodgkins lymphoma appropriate chemotherapeutic regimens (CHOP, R-CHOP, ABVD) are used as per the histological type, and stage of the disease.

Treatment options for NTM include macrolide antibiotics with ethambutol and rifamycin. Surgical intervention such as valve replacement or joint debridement may be needed.

**TABLE 1: Groups of drugs for the treatment of DR-TB.**

| Groups and steps | Medicine | Abbreviation |
|---|---|---|
| Group A | • Levofloxacin<br>• Moxifloxacin<br>• Bedaquiline<br>• Linezolid | • Lfx<br>• Mfx<br>• Bdq<br>• Lzd |
| Group B | • Clofazimine<br>• Cycloserine<br>• Terizidone | • Cfz<br>• Cs<br>• Trd |
| Group C | • Ethambutol<br>• Delamanid<br>• Pyrazinamide<br>• Imipenem-cilastatin<br>• Meropenem<br>• Amikacin (or Strepto-mycin)<br>• Ethionamide or prothionamide<br>• p-aminosalicylic acid | • E<br>• Dlm<br>• Z<br>• Ipm-Cln<br>• Mpm<br>• Am (or S)<br>• Eto or Pto<br>• PAS |

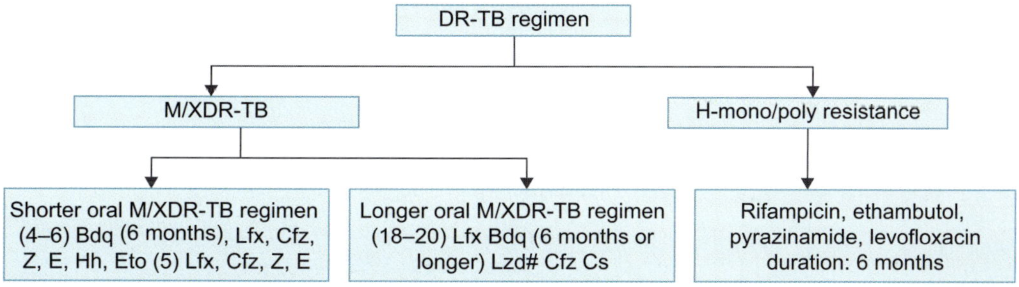


**FLOWCHART 3**: DR-TB regimen (numbers in parenthesis include duration in months).

## Points to Ponder

- Poor adherence is a significant cause of treatment (ATT) failure and should always be ruled out at the outset.
- A detailed history and physical examination help identify the alternative diagnosis, in case of no response to ATT or disease progression.
- Ruling out drug-resistant TB in such cases is important as the treatment (regimen and duration) and prognosis are different than those for DS-TB.
- Paradoxical reaction is an immunologically mediated phenomenon that usually mimics treatment failure (during the initial treatment period) or relapse (after completion).

## MULTIPLE CHOICE QUESTIONS

1. **Which gene mutation is most commonly associated with rifampicin resistance in *Mycobacterium tuberculosis*?**
   A. *katG*
   B. *gyrA*
   C. *inhA*
   D. *rpoB*
2. **Which feature distinguishes Kikuchi–Fujimoto disease from tuberculous lymphadenitis in lymph node biopsy?**
   A. Caseous necrosis
   B. Noncaseating granulomas
   C. Karyorrhexis with necrosis
   D. Langhans giant cells
3. **Which of the following findings is seen in a relapse of tuberculosis but not in case of paradoxical reaction?**
   A. Positive AFB
   B. New onset lymphadenopathy
   C. Positive CBNAAT
   D. Positive *M.tb* culture
4. **The recommended duration of treatment for a shorter bedaquiline-containing regimen is:**
   A. 4–6 months
   B. 6–9 months
   C. 9–11 months
   D. 12–15 months
5. **Which of the following is a cause of generalized lymphadenopathy?**
   A. HIV
   B. SLE
   C. Allopurinol
   D. All of the above

### Answers

1. (D); 2. (C); 3. (D); 4. (C); 5. (D)

## SUGGESTED READINGS


1. Subbaraman R, Thomas BE, Kumar JV, et al. Understanding Nonadherence to Tuberculosis Medications in India Using Urine Drug Metabolite Testing: A Cohort Study. Open Forum Infect Dis. 2021;8(6):ofab190.
2. WHO. Global Tuberculosis Report 2020 [Internet]. 2020. https://apps.who.int/iris/ bitstream/handle/10665/336069/9789240013131-eng.pdf. [Accessed 16 March 2021].
3. Carvalho ACC, De Iaco G, SaleriN, et al. Paradoxical reaction during tuberculosis treatment in HIV-seronegative patients. Clin Infect Dis. 2006;42:893-5.
4. Kumar RD, Kant S, Gupta VB, et al. Paradoxical reaction in peripheral lymph node tuberculosis: a review for its prevalence, clinical characteristics, and possible treatment. Monaldi Arch Chest Dis. 2023.
5. PMDT – Central Tuberculosis Division. Available from: https://tbcindia.mohfw.gov.in/pmdt/
6. Fontanilla JM, Barnes A, von Reyn CF, et al. Current diagnosis and management of peripheral tuberculous lymphadenitis. Clin Infect Dis. 2011;53(6):555-62.

# CHAPTER 44

# A Case-based Approach to a Case of Tuberculosis with Diabetes Mellitus

*Sirshendu Pal*

**CASE VIGNETTE**

A 45-year-old female from rural background who was suffering from diabetes came to OPD with cough and hemoptysis for 3 weeks. She had fever in the evenings. There was a history of weight loss. Family history of diabetes was present. There was no past history of tuberculosis. Physical examination revealed coarse crepitations in mid and lower zones of both lungs. Chest X-rays showed multilobe infiltrates. In blood reports ESR was 60 mm and HbA1c was 8.6%. Urinary albumin creatinine ratio was 303 mg/g. Sputum was sent for gram stain and culture sensitivity on the first day. Sputum was also sent for ZN stain and CBNAAT for tuberculosis which clinched the diagnosis.

## PROVISIONAL DIAGNOSIS

Pulmonary tuberculosis in a 45-year-old female with poorly controlled diabetes mellitus presenting with chronic cough, hemoptysis, evening fever, weight loss, and bilateral lung infiltrates.

## DIFFERENTIAL DIAGNOSES

The differentials in this patient of type 2 diabetes mellitus would include (a) Pulmonary tuberculosis (b) Bilateral pneumonia (c) Bronchiectasis (d) Interstitial lung disease (e) Congestive cardiac failure (f) Pulmonary edema in CKD.

### Epidemiological Evidence

A number of epidemiological studies have shown that diabetes increases risk of tuberculosis 3 times while tuberculosis increases risk of diabetes 2 times. Patients with diabetes are also mora likely to have latent TB infection which can reactivate and lead to active TB. The double burden of diabetes and tuberculosis is especially evident in low and middle income countries.

## CLINICAL APPROACH

### Symptoms and Signs

Diabetes patients with TB frequently have atypical symptoms compared to nondiabetic TB patients. Classic TB symptoms such as fever, cough, night sweats and weight loss are less common in diabetic individuals. However, hemoptysis is more common. Further, diabetes may delay or mask TB symptom recognition. Features of weight loss and fatigue may be thought to be due to diabetes rather than TB leading to diagnosis and treatment delays.

### Radiology

Chest radiographs of TB patients with diabetes often show atypical findings such as lower zone involvement, diffuse infiltrates, multiple or larger cavities and bilateral affection.

### Microbiology

TB along with DM patients have a greater bacterial load leading to higher sputum smear and culture positivity. This increased microbial burden causes severe disease with higher transmission risk. There may be delayed sputum smear and culture conversion pointing to slower therapeutic response.

### Complications

TB patients with diabetes have increased risk of developing extrapulmonary TB, including pleural TB, TB meningitis and lymphadenitis. The impaired immune response predisposes to spread of *Mycobacterium tuberculosis* beyond the lungs. Diabetes with TB patients are more susceptible to complications such as emphysema, bronchiectasis and respiratory failure. Further renal impairment, liver disease and cardiovascular disease can worsen the clinical course of TB.

## PATHOPHYSIOLOGY

### Effects of Diabetes on Tuberculosis

Diabetes impairs both innate and acquired immune responses, making patients prone to infections including TB. Hyperglycemia can impair the function of immune cells such as T cells and macrophages which are vital for controlling *Mycobacterium tuberculosis* infection. Diabetes is associated is associated with a higher risk of TB treatment failure due to the ineffective clearance of the mycobacteria by the impaired immune response. There is also increased chance of TB relapse which is attributed to factors such as poor glycemic control and persistent bacillary load which may not be cleared during the standard treatment course.

Chronic hyperglycemia leads to glycosylation of proteins and lipids, causing production of advanced glycation end products. AGEs promote a proinflammatory state and alters immune responses, facilitating the progression and persistence of TB infection.

Patients with diabetes frequently have nutritional deficiencies and other comorbidities that can impair their immune system. Chronic kidney disease, obesity or malnutrition which are common in patients with diabetes, further enhances the risk of tuberculosis.

### Effects of Tuberculosis on Diabetes

Active TB is a state of profound physiological stress that can increase blood glucose levels. The infection starts as an acute phase reaction, elevating the synthesis of stress hormones such as adrenaline, cortisol and glucagon which are known to produce hyperglycemia. TB infection stimulates the release of proinflammatory cytokines (e.g., IL-1, IL-6, TNF-α) which can alter insulin signaling and bigger insulin resistance, causing increased blood glucose levels.

*Mycobacterium tuberculosis* can directly añect the pancreas leading to inflammation and damage to pancreatic islet cells. This may hamper insulin secretions and promote hyperglycemia. Evidence suggests that TB infection may stimulate autoimmune responses that target pancreatic beta cells, as seen in type 1 diabetes, causing decreased insulin synthesis.

Tuberculosis frequently causes malnutrition and weight loss, which can in the early stages mask hyperglycemia but later result in abnormal glucose metabolism once nutritional status improves. The fat loss and muscle wasting associated with TB may influence insulin sensitivity. Recovery from tuberculosis leads to weight gain which can unmask or increase underlying insulin resistance.

## TREATMENT AND PREVENTION

### Management of Tuberculosis with Diabetes

Treatment of TB in patients with diabetes requires an integrated approach that addresses bath diabetes and tuberculosis. This includes regular sputum tests, regular monitoring of blood glucose levels, liver function tests, adjusting diabetes medication as needed and most importantly providing adequate and proper nutritional support. Frequent monitoring is required to ensure effective treatment response and to promptly identify and manage any adverse drug reactions or complications. Patient education to stress the importance of compliance to bath anti-TB and diabetes medication is essential. Patients should be alerted on potential drug interactions and the need for tight glycemic control.

Utilizing a multidisciplinary healthcare team, including infectious disease specialists or internists, dieticians and endocrinologists can optimize the treatment of coexisting diabetes and tuberculosis. Diabetes mellitus and tuberculosis mutually affect the treatment response causing delayed sputum conversion, higher rates of treatment failure, relapse and higher incidence of adverse drug reactions . These may require extending the duration of TB therapy if there is delayed sputum conversion or adjusting doses on the basis of basis of pharmacokinetic and pharmacodynamic data.

Diabetes medications may interact with anti-TB drugs. These interactions may influence drug efficiency and increase the chances of side effects. Newly diagnosed TB patients with diabetes are given the usual regimen. However, in previously treated tuberculosis patients injection. Streptomycin should be added to the regimen for the initial 8 weeks. DNI-TB in patients with morbid chronic kidney disease may need up to 50% dose reduction for ethambutol and pyrazinamide in patients with creatinine clearance less than 10 mL/min. In acute hepatitis TB treatment should be deferred until acute hepatitis has resolved. INH monotherapy is to be used and multidrug therapy avoided in patients coaffected with hepatitis B and C virus infections. If ATD induced hepatitis develops all hepatotoxic drugs to be stopped. TB treatment should be restarted after normalization of transaminases. Treatment should be started with lower doses of INH (50 mg) and rifampicin (150 mg) and up titrated every three or1our days to the recommended therapeutic doses. In patients with HIV, TB treatment must be started first followed by anti-retroviral therapy.

Metformin remains the oral hypoglycemic of choice and sulphonyl urea derivatives may be used as add on. But, sulphonyl urea have 30–80% lower efficacy with rifampicin. Alpha glucosidase inhibitors should be used only for mild post meal elevation, while thiazolidinediones, DPP-4 inhibitors and SGLT-2 inhibitors are used only selectively. Metformin should be avoided in patients with eGFR<g0ML/min/1.73 $m^2$. moulin should be used in patients with active tuberculosis in (1) HbA1c >9 w or FPG > 200 mg/dL (2) Ketonuria and/or hyperosmolar coma (3) on Mo. oral. medications but not reaching targets (4) significant catabolism (5) significant liver or renal dysfunction. vitamin A supplementation improves immune cell responses while vitamin D supplementation may improve TB outcomes. Cessation of smoking and alcohol and mild-to-moderate physical activity are a must.

Tuberculosis and diabetes have a complicated intricate relationship which poses a formidable challenge to the world health scenario. Diabetes hugely increases the risk of TB and complicates it with atypical clinical features leading to delayed diagnosis and also results in poorer outcomes. Similarly, TB can promote hyperglycemia leading to diabetes. Thus, each exacerbates the other, the mechanisms of which should be understood to implement integrated management strategies to reduce the burden of both these dreaded diseases. Comprehensive public health policies may be formulated to attain this objective and improve the quality of life in the poor and middle income countries.

## Points to Ponder

- *Tuberculosis in diabetes*: Patients with poorly controlled diabetes (HbA1c 8.6%) have a higher susceptibility to tuberculosis, which can present with atypical symptoms and more severe lung involvement.
- *Role of sputum testing*: Sending sputum for ZN stain and CBNAAT is critical in diagnosing tuberculosis, especially in regions with high TB prevalence and cases presenting with hemoptysis and chronic cough.
- *Importance of chest X-ray*: Multilobar infiltrates on chest X-ray in a patient with fever, hemoptysis, and weight loss should raise suspicion for pulmonary tuberculosis, especially in endemic areas.
- *Diabetes and secondary complications*: The presence of albuminuria (urinary albumin creatinine ratio of 303 mg/g) indicates diabetic nephropathy, which further complicates management and requires close monitoring.
- *Holistic management*: Along with antitubercular therapy, optimizing diabetes control and addressing nutritional and socioeconomic factors are essential to improving treatment outcomes.

## MULTIPLE CHOICE QUESTIONS

**1. Why does diabetes increase the risk of tuberculosis. Choose the incorrect response.**

A. Decreased cytokines
B Impaired humoral immunity
C. Pulmonary microangiopathy
D. Impaired cellular immunity

**2. In patients with diabetes which tubercular symptom is more common?**

A. Night sweats
B. Hemoptysis
C. Cough
D. Weight loss

**3. Treatment of TB in patients with diabetes who had previously been treated for TB should include in intensive phase.**

A. Levofloxacin
B. Inj. Kanamycin
C. Ethionamide
D. Inj. Streptomycin

**4. Sleep disturbance may occur with which ATD?**

A. Rifampicin
B. Pyrazinamide
C. INH
D. Ethambutol

**5. In DM-TB patients coaffected with chronic hepatitis B and C virus infection which therapy is to be used?**

A. Ethambutol
B. Levofloxacin
C. INH
D. Multidrug therapy

### Answers

1. (B); 2. (B); 3. (D); 4. (C); 5. (C)

## SUGGESTED READINGS


1. Restrepo BI. Diabetes and tuberculosis. Microbial Spectr. 2016;4(6):10.
2. Kant S, Lata H, Natu SM, et al. Diabetes mellitus with pulmonary tuberculosis: a double trouble. J Indian Med Assoc. 2013:111(3):187-91.
3. World Health Organization, Global Tuberculosis Report 2020. Geneva: World Health Organization: 2020. Available from: http// www who in. l/publications/i/item/Q7g9P4g0J3131.
4. International Diabetes Federation. IDF Diabetes Atlas, 9th edition. Brussels, Belgium: International Diabetes Federation. 2019.
5. Lin Y, Harris AO, Kumar AM, et al. Management of diabetes mellitus-tuberculosis: a guide to the essential practice. Paris: International Union Against Tuberculosis and Lung Disease; 2018.
6. Workneh MH, Bjune GA, Yimer SA. Prevalence and associated factors of tuberculosis and diabetes mellitus comorbidity: a systematic review. PLoS One. 2017;12(1):26.
7. Singh A, Prasad R, Balasubramanian V, et al. Prevalence of diabetes mellitus among tuberculosis patients in India: a systematic review and meta-analysis. Indian J Tuberc. 2019;66(4):528-34.
8. Marupuru S, Senapati P, Pathadka S, et al. Prevalence of diabetes mellitus among tuberculosis patients in India: a systematic review and meta-analysis. Indian J Tuberc. 2017;64(3):140-50.

CHAPTER 45

# An Approach to a Case of Dual Infection of Dengue and Malaria

*Kirandeep Kour, Rohit Singh, Ritu, Pratap Sharma, Taranpreet Kour*

**CASE VIGNETTE**

A 28-year-old male from a dengue- and malaria-endemic region presents with complaints of high-grade intermittent fever for 5 days, associated with chills, rigors, severe headache, muscle aches, and joint pain. Initially diagnosed with a viral fever, he was advised symptomatic treatment. However, he returned 2 days later due to worsening symptoms and a new erythematous rash. On examination, his vital signs include a temperature of 39.5°C, pulse rate of 110 beats/min, and blood pressure of 100/60 mm Hg. He shows mild hepatomegaly and positive tourniquet test results, along with a thrombocytopenia (platelet count 75,000/mm$^3$). This case highlights an initial non-specific presentation, evolving into a more complex dual infection that requires careful diagnostic and management strategies.

## PROVISIONAL DIAGNOSIS

Given the combination of symptoms—fever with chills (suggestive of malaria), myalgia and rash (suggestive of dengue), and thrombocytopenia—the provisional diagnosis is dual infection with dengue and malaria.

This case requires an open-ended approach in terms of early diagnosis and symptom-based management, considering each infection's characteristic signs:

- Malaria typically presents with cyclical fever, chills, and rigors, especially in regions where it's endemic.
- Dengue often features high fever, body aches, a distinctive rash, and thrombocytopenia.

An immediate differential diagnosis to rule out other febrile illnesses should be prioritized.

## DIFFERENTIAL DIAGNOSIS

With overlapping symptoms, other tropical and febrile diseases should be considered.

- *Leptospirosis:* Symptoms like fever, myalgia, and rash could overlap with dengue, but leptospirosis often involves kidney and liver damage, evident in symptoms like jaundice and conjunctival suffusion.
- *Typhoid fever*: High fever and abdominal symptoms are hallmarks of typhoid, but the fever is usually continuous rather than cyclical, and rash or thrombocytopenia is less common.
- *Chikungunya:* Although it can present with fever, rash, and severe joint pain, chikungunya usually lacks cyclical fever and thrombocytopenia.
- *Viral hepatitis*: Jaundice, elevated liver enzymes, and nausea are common, but it doesn't typically include cyclical fever or rash.
- *Bacterial sepsis*: A possibility when high fever and systemic symptoms are present, but sepsis usually involves organ dysfunction and lacks a specific fever pattern.

Clinicians should consider these possibilities and utilize lab and imaging tests to distinguish among these differentials.

## CLINICAL APPROACH

The approach involves a methodical assessment to confirm the dual infection and evaluate disease severity.

### History and Physical Examination

- *History:* Take a detailed travel history to assess potential exposure to vectors. Document fever characteristics, time of onset, pattern (cyclical or continuous), and associated symptoms like headache, rash, or bleeding.
- *Physical examination*: A full physical exam is necessary to identify organ involvement (liver and spleen enlargement), rash distribution, and bleeding signs. Perform a tourniquet test to assess capillary fragility, indicative of dengue.

### Laboratory Investigations

- *CBC:* Evaluate for anemia (suggesting malaria) and thrombocytopenia (suggesting dengue). Leukopenia is common in dengue.
- *Liver and renal function tests*: Elevation in liver enzymes supports dengue, while kidney function testing is vital to detect malaria-related complications.
- *Coagulation profile*: Coagulopathy or increased bleeding time may indicate severe dengue.
- *Dengue-specific tests*: NS1 antigen test is preferred in the early phase of dengue; serology (IgM and IgG) is useful in later stages. PCR for dengue is definitive but less widely available.

- *Malaria-specific tests*: A thick and thin blood smear is the gold standard for malaria detection, allowing parasite count and species identification. RDTs are useful for initial diagnosis, but confirmatory smear is preferred in endemic areas.

### Imaging

- *Ultrasound*: Detect hepatosplenomegaly or gallbladder wall thickening, which suggests dengue. Ascites or pleural effusion may also be seen in severe dengue.

The key characteristics of malaria, dengue, and concurrent infections are outlined in **Table 1** below.

## PATHOPHYSIOLOGY

Pathophysiology helps to explain the mechanisms and complications seen in dual infection.

### Dengue Virus Pathophysiology

- *Immune response*: Dengue virus infects monocytes and macrophages, triggering cytokine release and systemic inflammation, leading to capillary leak syndrome, bleeding, and hypovolemic shock.
- *Platelet dysfunction*: The virus suppresses bone marrow function and directly damages platelets, leading to thrombocytopenia and increased bleeding risk.

### Malaria Parasite Pathophysiology

- *Red blood cell invasion*: Plasmodium parasites multiply within RBCs, causing their destruction and leading to anemia. In *P. falciparum* malaria, sequestration in capillaries can lead to cerebral and multiorgan complications.
- *Immune evasion*: Malaria modulates immune response, which may exacerbate systemic inflammation in coinfection.

### Co-infection Pathophysiology

Co-infection intensifies immune activation, causing severe thrombocytopenia, vascular leak, and an increased risk of severe anemia. The overlapping inflammation and immune dysfunction demand close monitoring for rapid clinical changes.

## TREATMENT AND PREVENTION

Management should be targeted, with attention to supportive care, disease-specific therapy, and preventative measures.

### Supportive Care

- *Fever control*: Use paracetamol for fever and discomfort, but avoid NSAIDs due to bleeding risks associated with dengue.
- *Hydration:* IV fluids are critical in dengue to prevent hypovolemia. Balance carefully to avoid fluid overload, particularly in the critical phase.
- *Frequent monitoring*: Daily monitoring of vitals, platelet counts, hematocrit, and renal and liver function is essential to assess disease progression.

### Disease-specific Treatment

- *Malaria treatment*: Administer artemisinin-based combination therapy (ACT) according to regional guidelines, considering resistance patterns. ACT is highly effective and reduces parasite load quickly.
- *Dengue treatment:* Primarily supportive with careful fluid management. Patients with severe dengue may require platelet transfusions or blood products if bleeding is significant.

### Complications Management

- *Hemorrhage:* Platelet transfusion may be needed if platelet counts fall below 10,000/mm$^3$ or if there is active bleeding.
- *Organ dysfunction*: Multiorgan involvement, such as liver and renal impairment, requires ICU-level support and close monitoring.

### Prevention

Educate on the importance of vector control through insecticide-treated bed nets, especially in endemic areas.

Use of personal protective measures, including repellents, and community awareness on reducing mosquito breeding sites.

**TABLE 1: Key characteristics for malaria, dengue, and concurrent infections.**

| Characteristics | Malaria infection | Dengue infection | Concurrent infection |
|---|---|---|---|
| Mode of transmission | Mosquito-borne (*Anopheles*) | Mosquito-borne (*Aedes*) | Mosquito-borne (*Anopheles* + *Aedes*) |
| Fever | Acute febrile illness (chronic in some cases) | Acute febrile illness | Acute febrile illness |
| Myalgia | Detectable | Common | Common |
| Shock | Possible | Possible | Possible |
| Blood parasite | Positive | Negative | Positive |
| Atypical lymphocytosis | Usually negative | Usually positive | Usually positive |
| Hemoconcentration | Usually negative | Usually positive | Usually positive |
| Thrombocytopenia | Usually negative | Usually positive | Usually positive |
| Bleeding | Rare | Possible | Possible |
| Hemolysis | Possible | Rare | Rare |
| Tourniquet test | Usually negative | Usually positive | Usually positive |
| Treatment | Antimalarial drug | Fluid therapy | Antimalarial drug with fluid therapy |

## Points to Ponder

- *Consider endemic infections*: In regions where dengue and malaria are common, always consider these infections in cases of high-grade fever, even if the initial presentation is non-specific.
- *Monitor for symptom progression*: Worsening symptoms and the appearance of new signs like a rash can indicate a shift from a simple viral fever to a more serious condition, necessitating reevaluation.
- *Use specific diagnostic tests*: Positive tourniquet test, thrombocytopenia, and mild hepatomegaly suggest possible dengue. Confirmatory tests for both dengue and malaria are essential in endemic regions.
- *Focus on vital signs and organ involvement*: Persistent high fever, elevated pulse, and borderline blood pressure require careful monitoring. Check for complications like organ enlargement (hepatomegaly) and bleeding tendencies.
- *Adjust treatment based on evolution*: Initial symptomatic treatment may not suffice as the illness evolves. Dual infections necessitate tailored management, including antimalarial drugs and supportive care for dengue.

## MULTIPLE CHOICE QUESTIONS

**1. What clinical feature is a classic indicator of dengue?**
A. Cyclical fever
B. Jaundice
C. Thrombocytopenia with rash
D. Diarrhea

**2. Which test is essential for initial confirmation of malaria?**
A. Chest X-ray
B. Peripheral blood smear
C. Urinalysis
D. Coagulation profile

**3. What is the primary reason NSAIDs are avoided in dengue?**
A. Risk of gastrointestinal upset
B. Risk of bleeding complications
C. Ineffectiveness in reducing fever
D. Risk of renal impairment

**4. In dengue, what does a positive tourniquet test indicate?**
A. Dengue-specific antibody presence
B. Hypovolemia
C. Capillary fragility and potential for bleeding
D. Coagulation abnormalities

**5. Which intervention is effective in preventing both dengue and malaria?**
A. Antibiotics
B. Use of insecticide-treated bed nets
C. Vaccination
D. Avoiding crowded areas

### Answers

1. (C); 2. (B); 3. (B); 4. (C); 5. (B)

## SUGGESTED READINGS

1. Sharma SK, et al. Dengue and malaria co-infection: Clinical implications and challenges. J Trop Dis. 2023;18(3):123-34.
2. Gupta R, et al. Diagnostic approaches in febrile illnesses: Differentiating dengue from malaria. Int J Clin Pract. 2022;34(1):12-9.
3. Kumar A, et al. Severe dengue and malaria: A review of critical care strategies. Crit Care Med. 2021;29(5):320-8.
4. Singh V, et al. Clinical management of dengue and malaria co-infections. J Trop Med. 2020;15(7):245-53.
5. Joshi D, et al. Immunopathogenesis of dual infections: Dengue and malaria. Infect Dis Rev. 2022;36(4):567-74.
6. Anand K, et al. Approach to thrombocytopenia in tropical infections. Hematology Today. 2019;21(2):147-52.
7. Srivastava K, et al. Managing complications of dual mosquito-borne infections. Int J Trop Dis. 2019;17(3):85-92.
8. Patel L, et al. Vector control strategies in endemic regions: Evidence-based approaches. Global Health J. 2021;23(8):331-7.

CHAPTER 46

# An Approach to a Case of a Patient with Falling CD4 Counts

*Dipanjan Bandyopadhyay, Swarnadip Hazra, Rahul K Adhikary*

## CASE VIGNETTE

A 37-year-old male truck driver attends the ART center with the following CD4 counts over the past 2 years, as presented in **Table 1** below.

**TABLE 1: Patient's CD4 counts over the past 2 years.**

| Date | 03.2022 | 09.2022 | 03.2023 | 09.2023 | 03.2024 | 06.2024 | 09.2024 |
|---|---|---|---|---|---|---|---|
| CD4 count | 488 | 512 | 566 | 522 | 307 | 92 | 64 |

He has been on HAART since July, 2019 when he was started on ZLE (zidovudine, lamivudine, and efavirenz) regimen. He was well thereafter with progressive increase in CD4 counts and good weight gain, but was detected to have normochromic normocytic anemia (Hb 8.4 mg/dL) unresponsive to hematinics in 2021. His zidovudine was substituted with tenofovir and he continued this TLE regimen till mid 2022, when the new national guidelines necessitated his change from TLE to TLD regimen (tenofovir 300 mg OD, lamivudine 300 mg OD, and dolutegravir 50 mg OD).

## PROVISIONAL DIAGNOSIS

Treatment failure on HAART.

## DIFFERENTIAL DIAGNOSIS

A fall in CD4 counts raises the suspicion of treatment failure. However, inter-current illnesses and periods of physical trauma can temporarily reduce CD4 counts. Once such factors are ruled out, treatment failure needs to be considered.

## CLINICAL APPROACH

Treatment failure may be described as detailed in **Table 2**.

Identifying the cause of failure is important before deciding to modify the ART regimen. The following factors need to be assessed:

- *Treatment adherence*: A detailed assessment of adherence needs to be made. The reasons for non-adherence need to be explored. Unless these reasons are identified, a patient will find it difficult to adhere to the second-line regimen.
- *Drug–drug interactions*: Assessing whether the patient is concomitantly taking medications that interfere with ARV activity is important. For example, many patients may not reveal that they take herbal treatments along with the prescribed ART regimen. Common drugs like PPIs reduce serum levels of certain ARVs.

**TABLE 2: Treatment failure on HAART.**

| Failure | Definition | Comments |
|---|---|---|
| Virological failure | Plasma viral load ≥1,000 copies/mL | An individual must be taking ART for at least 6 months before it can be determined that a regimen has failed |
| Immunological failure | • CD4 count at 250 cells/mm$^3$ following clinical failure<br>• Persistent CD4 cell count below 100 cells/mm$^3$ | Concomitant or recent infection may cause a transient decline in the CD4 cell count. Some experts consider persistent CD4 counts of below 50 cells/mm$^3$ after 12 months of ART to be more appropriate |
| Clinical failure | New or recurrent clinical event indicating severe immunodeficiency (WHO clinical stage 4 condition) after 6 months of effective treatment | • The condition must be differentiated from IRIS<br>• Some WHO clinical stage 4 conditions (lymph node TB, uncomplicated TB pleural disease, esophageal candidiasis, recurrent bacterial pneumonia) may not indicate treatment failure<br>• For adults, certain WHO clinical stage 3 conditions (pulmonary TB and severe bacterial infections) may also indicate treatment failure |

Certain OIs and occult malignancies may lead to decline in the CD4 count, which may revert after treating those conditions.

Generally, causes of failure can be identified through history-taking and focused discussion with patient; however, in some cases these might not be obvious. Distinguishing among the causes of virological failure is important because the approaches to subsequent therapy may differ depending on the cause. Once failure is confirmed, steps should be taken to improve virological outcomes.

## PATHOPHYSIOLOGY

CD4 counts tend to rise on effective HAART. This increase is usually 50–100 cells/mm$^3$ within 6–12 months of ART initiation in ARV-naïve patients, who are taking ART with >95% adherence. Immunological response is defined as an increase of >50 CD4 cells/mm$^3$ at 6 months of ART. Transient fall in CD4 counts may occur with opportunistic infections, concomitant acute illnesses, or periods of physiological stress, and tend to reverse following cessation of this event. However, a persistent fall in CD4 count, despite adequate adherence of >95%, merits virological testing for the confirmation of treatment failure.

## TREATMENT AND PREVENTION

A case of immunological failure while on ART needs to be addressed with adherence counseling followed by virological testing and regimen switching **(Table 3)**.

For ART, a high level of sustained adherence is necessary to (1) suppress viral replication and improve immunological and clinical outcomes; (2) decrease the risk of developing ARV drug resistance; and (3) reduce the risk of transmitting HIV. Studies indicate that >95% of adherence is required for optimal viral load suppression. Lesser degree of adherence is often associated with virological failure. The checklist for ART adherence counseling encompasses issues like probable opportunistic infections (4S screening for cough, fever, weight loss, night sweats), social and psychological factors contributing to compromised adherence and support systems which might strengthen compliance.

There are a number of ways to measure adherence like self-reporting by patient, pill count, home visit, patient diary, etc. Pill count is the most used method to assess adherence. In each follow-up visit, the patient should be asked to bring the pill box with the unconsumed remaining pills.

The following formula is used to calculate the adherence:

- [Total number of pills the patient has actually taken/Total number of pills should have taken in that period] × 100
- This is [(Number of pills given to the client – Number of pills balance in the bottle)/Number of pills the client should have taken] × 100

**Example 1**

- Tenofovir + lamivudine + boosted atazanavir (TL+ATV/r) regimen
- Tablet TL once a day plus tablet ATV/r once a day;
- Patient received 30 tablets each and returns on 32nd day;
- Pill box shows remaining tablets TL: Nil; ATV/r: 1
- TL adherence = (30–0) / 32 × 100 = 30 / 32 × 100 = 94%
- ATV/r adherence = (30–1) / 32 × 100 = 29 / 32 × 100 = 91%
- Whenever a combination of two separate drugs is given, calculation has to be done for individual tablet and the drug with lower adherence has to be considered for reporting "overall adherence".

**Example 2**

- *ALD regimen*: Tablet AL (one tablet once a day) + dolutegravir (one tablet once a day)
- Patient received 30 tablets each and returns on 28th day
- Number of pill balance AL 5; dolutegravir 5
- *Adherence calculation*: (30–5)/(25) × 100 = 25 / 28 × 100 = 89%

**TABLE 3: Adherence counseling.**

| Counseling session | Counseling issues to be handled |
|---|---|
| Session 1 (just after receiving the test results indicating suspected treatment failure) | • Review patient understands of viral load<br>• Discuss possible reasons for high viral load<br>• Assess possible barriers to adherence<br>• Discuss patient's support systems<br>• Support patient in developing an adherence plan that addresses the identified issues<br>• Check the patient treatment adherence |
| Session 2 (15 days or 1 month—as deemed fit by the counselor at ART center after session-1) | • Review patient adherence between first and second sessions and discuss any emerging issues or gaps<br>• Follow-up on any referral services that the patient undertook<br>• Support patient in modifying the adherence plan to tackle the identified issues |
| Session 3 (15 days or 1 month as deemed fit by the counselor at ART centre after session-2) | • Review patient adherence between second and third sessions and discuss any emerging issues or gaps<br>• Support patient in modifying the adherence plan to tackle the identified issues<br>• *Decide next course of action based on adherence*: If adherence is good, plan a repeat plasma viral load test post 3 months of good adherence. If adherence is not adequate, plan further sessions with the patient before repeating plasma viral load test |
| Session after "repeat" plasma viral load test | • Discuss results of the repeat plasma viral load test<br>• Decide next steps based on repeat plasma viral load test results:<br>○ If plasma viral load count <1,000 copies/mL, appreciate the patient for his/her success and suggest continuation of current regimen; repeat plasma viral load as per the scheduled frequency of the patient. Next viral load test to be done after 12 months of the last viral load test in PLHIV on first line ART and after 6 months of the last viral load test in PLHIV on second line ART<br>○ If plasma viral load count ≥1,000 copies/mL, prepare the patient for a change in regimen |

Three step-up adherence counseling sessions are advocated before the viral load testing is performed.

Any change of ARVs prescribed should be carefully distinguished between substituting a drug within a given regimen and switching an entire ART regimen:

- *Substitution*: Substitution refers to replacement of ARV drug(s) in a virally suppressed PLHIV due to adverse effects of drug, drug–drug interactions or programme policy. This does not indicate change of regimen due to treatment failure. Any substitution after 6 months should be preceded by viral load testing. This helps to understand to whether a single drug substitution is enough (if plasma viral load <1,000 copies/mL) or whether the patient must be checked for treatment failure (if plasma viral load ≥1,000 copies/mL).
- *Switch*: Treatment failure refers to the loss of antiviral efficacy (plasma viral load ≥1,000 copies/mL) to the current regimen. When the regimen is changed because of ARV treatment failure, it is referred as the switch of the entire regimen.

It is important to make appropriate pre-work-up and timely referral to the State AIDS Clinical Expert Panel (SACEP) for evaluation of such patients. Once the patient has undergone viral load test and been evaluated by SACEP, one of the following possible decisions will be conveyed to the referring ART centre:

- Switch to "prescribed" second-line or third-line ART
- Continue current ART, reinforce adherence and re-evaluate.
- Evaluate for HIV-2.

The second line can be initiated at the ART center while for third line, initiation will be done at CoE/ART Plus Center. The objective of the second- and third-line ART is to prolong the survival of the PLHIV as much as possible with complete suppression of viral replication. This requires regular monitoring with viral load every 6 months for all patients on second/third-line ART.

Current recommendation for second-line ART is based on the following:

- *A new class of ARV*:
  - An integrase strand transfer inhibitor (INSTI) dolutegravir (DTG), if first line was NNRTI based
  - A ritonavir-boosted PI (atazanavir/ritonavir or lopinavir/ritonavir), if first line was INSTI based
- Supported by at least one new and unused NRTI (zidovudine or tenofovir)
- Continued lamivudine administration ensures reduced viral fitness.

*Steps in initiating second-line ART*:

- Define treatment failure by virological testing; see if adherence to treatment is adequate.
- Decide on NRTI component of the second-line regimen **(Table 4)**.
  - If zidovudine (AZT) is used in first line, NRTI choice in second line is tenofovir (TDF).
  - If TDF/ABC is used in first line, NRTI choice could be AZT, unless contraindicated by Hb < 9 g/dL.
  - Continuing lamivudine reduces viral fitness and must be part of second-line ART

**TABLE 4: Second-line ART regimens for PLHIV failing on first-line ART.**

| Failing first line ART regimen | | Second-line ART regimen |
|---|---|---|
| Tenofovir/Abacavir containing | INSTI-based first-line ART (DTG) | ***Hb ≥9 g/dL:***<br>• Zidovudine 300 mg + lamivudine 150 mg (FDC)–BD + atazanavir 300 mg + ritonavir 100 mg (FDC)–OD<br>***Hb <9 g/dL or past h/o zidovudine induced anemia:***<br>• Dolutegravir 50 mg BD + atazanavir 300 mg + ritonavir 100 mg (FDC)–OD + existing NRTI backbone* |
| Zidovudine containing | INSTI-based first-line ART (DTG) | Tenofovir (300 mg) + lamivudine (300 mg) (FDC)–OD + atazanavir (300 mg) + ritonavir (100 mg) (FDC)–OD |
| Zidovudine containing | NNRTI/PI based first line ART | • Tenofovir (300 mg) + lamivudine (300 mg) + dolutegravir (50 mg) – (FDC)<br>• If patient has contraindication to TDF, abacavir (600 mg) + lamivudine (300 mg) – OD + dolutegravir (50 mg) |
| Tenofovir/Abacavir containing | NNRTI based first line ART | *Hb ≥9 g/dL:*<br>• Zidovudine 300 mg + lamivudine 150 mg (FDC)–BD + dolutegravir 50 mg–OD Hb<br>*Hb <9 g/dL or past h/o zidovudine induced anemia:*<br>• Atazanavir 300 mg + ritonavir 100 mg (FDC)–OD + dolutegravir 50 mg–OD+ existing NRTI backbone* |
| | Boosted PI based first line ART | *Hb ≥9 g/dL:*<br>• Zidovudine 300 mg + lamivudine 150 mg (FDC)–BD + dolutegravir 50 mg OD<br>*Hb <9 g/dL or past h/o zidovudine induced anemia:*<br>• Darunavir 600 mg BD + ritonavir 100 mg BD + dolutegravir 50 mg–OD + existing NRTI backbone* |
| Multi NRTI exposed | NNRTI based first line ART | ATV/Ritonavir 300/100 mg (FDC)–OD + dolutegravir 50 mg–OD + existing NRTI backbone* |
| Multi NRTI exposed | PI-based first-line ART | Darunavir 600 mg–BD + ritonavir 100 mg–BD + dolutegravir 50 mg–OD + existing NRTI backbone |

*A combination of antiretroviral drugs that is used to treat HIV-1.

- *Decide on the other component*:
  - If patient had NNRTI in first line, INSTI (dolutegravir) will be preferred.
  - For patient who had INSTI in first line, give boosted PI (ATV/r) in combination. Use LPV/r in case of pregnant women or HIV-2.
- Patient education and agreement on treatment plan including follow-up and monitoring

The patient under discussion had good adherence. His plasma viral load testing detected 320,000 viral copies/mL. He was referred to SACEP and switched to the second line ART as follows:

- Present regimen TLD (INSTI based, with tenofovir and lamivudine as NRTI backbone)
- Switch to PI based with ATV/r (boosted atazanavir) and substitute tenofovir with alternative NRTI, keeping Lamivudine for reduced viral fitness.
- Patient has history of zidovudine induced anemia, hence zidovudine cannot be used. Accordingly, this patient will be switched to higher dose INSTI with dolutegravir 50 mg BD + atazanavir 300 mg–ritonavir 100 mg (FDC)–OD+ existing NRTI backbone (see **Table 3**)

## Points to Ponder

- A falling CD4 count is not essentially treatment failure. However, once intercurrent illnesses and poor adherence are ruled out, and virological testing documents treatment failure, a switch to second line HAART is essential.
- Designing a second line HAART regimen incorporates an idea of rational ARV combinations with particular attention to resistance issues and adverse drug events.

## MULTIPLE CHOICE QUESTIONS

**1. Switch is the change.**
   A. From ZLE to TLE due to Hb < 9 g/dL
   B. From ZLE to TLD due to falling CD4 counts
   C. TLD to ZLD due to rising creatinine
   D. ZLE to ZLN due to neuropsychiatric manifestations

**2. Annual increment in CD4 on effective initial HAART is:**
   A. 25–50 cells/year
   B. 50 –100 cells/year
   C. 100–200 cells/year
   D. 200–500 cells/year

**3. Patient presenting with TB meningitis on HAART for 3 years has:**
   A. Clinical failure
   B. Immunological failure
   C. Viorological failure
   D. IRIS

**4. Tenofovir intolerance is characterized by:**
   A. Anemia
   B. Pancytopenia
   C. Nephrotoxicity
   D. Drug rash

**5. Patient failing on TLD regimen with normal CBC will be shifted to:**
   A. TLE
   B. TLA/r
   C. ZLE
   D. ZLA/r

### Answers

1. (B); 2. (B); 3. (A); 4. (C); 5. (D)

## SUGGESTED READINGS


1. Patel P, Mouton CP. Management of HIV-related anemia in patients on antiretroviral therapy. Journal of Clinical Infectious Diseases. 2021;72(5):845-50.
2. Ghosh S, Kumar V. Evolving role of Tenofovir in the management of HIV/AIDS: A review. International Journal of HIV/AIDS. 2020;12(4):112-9.
3. Brown AE, Doi T. Impact of switching antiretroviral regimens: A review of current guidelines and clinical outcomes. HIV Therapy. 2022;13(3):161-73.
4. Smith MI, Jones LR. Anemia in HIV-infected individuals: A review of pathogenesis, diagnosis, and management. Journal of Acquired Immune Deficiency Syndromes. 2020;85(1):1-9.
5. World Health Organization. Updated HIV treatment guidelines: Emphasis on newer regimens. World Health Organization Technical Report Series. 2022;10(2):55-63.
6. Choudhary S, Saxena R. Role of Dolutegravir in the management of HIV in resource-limited settings. AIDS Research and Therapy. 2021;18(1):34-40.

CHAPTER 47

# An Approach to a Case of Metabolic Encephalopathy

*Krishna Padarabinda Tripathy, Deepthi Vemula*

## CASE VIGNETTE

A 65-year-old male with a history of hypertension, type 2 diabetes mellitus (T2DM), and stage 4 chronic kidney disease (CKD) was brought to the emergency department due to acute onset unusual behavior and altered sensorium. He had nausea and vomiting for several days with reduced food intake. There was no history of seizures or fever. On examination, the patient was stuporous with a GCS of E3V4M5. His pulse was 90 beats/min, blood pressure was 180/90 mm Hg, respiratory rate was 18 breaths/min, and temperature was 99.6°F, oxygen saturation was 96% on room air. He exhibited signs of mild dehydration, including dry mucous membranes. On CNS examination, there was no focal neurological deficit, exhibited asterixis and generalized hyperreflexia, bilateral plantar extensor responses and no neck stiffness. Given the subacute onset of presentation without focal neurological deficit, absence of fever and neck stiffness in an elderly male with diabetes mellitus (DM), hypertension and underlying CKD, the most probable diagnosis is metabolic encephalopathy. However, other possibilities such as cerebrovascular accident (CVA) and meningoencephalitis need to be ruled out.

A comprehensive diagnostic workup was undertaken. Laboratory tests revealed blood sugar of 136 mg/dL, elevated blood urea of (80 mg/dL), and creatinine (3.2 mg/dL), serum sodium of 108 mmol/L, and serum potassium of 5.8 mmol/L. Arterial blood gas analysis indicated metabolic acidosis with a pH of 7.32 and bicarbonate level of 18 mmol/L, $PaO_2$ of 92 mm Hg $PaCO_2$ of 32 mm Hg. Blood cultures were negative.

Neuroimaging showed no acute infarction, hemorrhage, or meningeal enhancement. Cerebrospinal fluid (CSF) analysis showed normal opening pressure, glucose and protein levels, no pleocytosis, and negative gram stain and cultures.

These findings, along with the laboratory results and imaging, pointed conclusively toward metabolic encephalopathy, attributed to the patient's CKD, which led to the accumulation of metabolic toxins compounded by dehydration and electrolyte imbalances, culminating in significant neurological disturbance. Patient was managed with hypertonic saline and renal replacement therapy and improved subsequently.

## PROVISIONAL DIAGNOSIS

Metabolic encephalopathy secondary to advanced CKD with severe hyponatremia and metabolic acidosis.

## DIFFERENTIAL DIAGNOSIS

Clinically, it is difficult to differentiate metabolic encephalopathy from other clinical conditions. The following differential diagnoses should be considered:

- Infectious encephalopathy (viral or bacterial)
- Structural brain lesions (tumor, abscess, hematoma)
- Vascular encephalopathy (strokes, transient ischemic attack, aneurysm)
- Neurodegenerative disorders (Alzheimer's disease, Parkinson's disease)
- Autoimmune encephalopathy
- Seizure disorders
- Psychiatric conditions (severe depression, schizophrenia)

However, a thorough history, general and neurological examination, along with imaging, CSF analysis, and EEG, will help differentiating these conditions.

## CLINICAL APPROACH (FLOWCHART 1)

### General Examination

Once the patient is stabilized, performing a comprehensive general examination in cases of altered sensorium requires skill and precision. Key areas to focus on include vital signs, skin condition, dehydration, flapping tremors, breathing patterns, unusual breath odor, checking for the loss of secondary sexual characteristics as in case of thyroid disorders. A detailed CNS examination, emphasizing focal neurological deficits and the presence of nuchal rigidity, can aid in differentiating from conditions that mimic similar symptoms.

Preservation of pupillary function is characteristic in metabolic encephalopathy due to intact brainstem reflexes. Horizontal

Suspected case of acute brain injury or with altered sensorium

↓

Evaluation and management of Airway, Breathing, Circulation

↓

History, medical records, general examination, CNS examination

↓

Preliminary investigations: Blood sugar, electrolytes, ABG, RFT, LFT

**Indications of CSF study:**
- Suspected infection
- Autoimmune encephalitis
- Meningeal irritation
- Subarachnoid hemorrhage
- Elevated intracranial pressure
- Neurodegenerative diseases with atypical presentation

**Indications of neuroimaging:**
- Suspected structural brain lesions
- Sudden onset of symptoms
- Focal neurological deficits
- Persistent or worsening symptoms despite treatment
- History of head trauma

**Indications of EEG:**
- Seizure activity
- Persistent or unexplained coma
- Monitoring for subclinical seizures
- Assessment of encephalopathy severity

**FLOWCHART 1:** Clinical approach to a case of metabolic encephalopathy.

gaze nystagmus is common in Wernicke's encephalopathy, with severe cases showing complete ophthalmoplegia. Mental status examination may reveal decreased arousal, disorientation, cognitive deficits, attention difficulties, hallucinations, sensory misperceptions, impaired memory, and disorganized thinking.

Motor examination findings often include generalized weakness, tremors, myoclonus, postural instability, and asterixis. Additional signs such as paratonia, brisk reflexes, and extensor plantar responses might be present. Classic findings like Chvostek's and Trousseau's signs indicate hypocalcemia.

### Screening Investigations

Routine tests include CBC, ESR, CRP, ABG, blood sugar, electrolytes (sodium, calcium, magnesium), LFT, and RFT. Specific tests involve serum ammonia, osmolarity, lactate, vitamin levels (D, B12, B1), CSF analysis, toxic screening, and hormone assessments (thyroid function, PTH, cortisol).

### Pathophysiology

Disruption of the blood–brain barrier can lead to significant changes in neurotransmitter levels and metabolic processes, contributing to metabolic encephalopathy through several mechanisms. Hypoxia and ischemia cause ATP depletion, cellular dysfunction, and neuronal injury due to reduced oxygen and nutrient delivery. Systemic diseases such as hepatic, renal, and endocrine disorders exacerbate these effects by disrupting neurotransmitter balance and causing imbalances in electrolytes and toxins. Toxins, including heavy metals and pesticides, further impair neuronal function, leading to oxidative stress and neuroinflammation.

## TREATMENT AND PREVENTION

- In an acute critical care setting, management begins with airway protection and hemodynamic stability, followed by prompt correction of potentially reversible metabolic abnormalities such as hypoglycemia, severe dehydration, hypo-osmolarity, and electrolyte imbalances.
- Sepsis, as a significant cause of altered sensorium, should be promptly evaluated, and broad-spectrum antibiotics should be initiated.
- Suspected toxins or drugs should be withdrawn, and thiamine supplementation should be administered immediately in cases of alcohol use disorder.
- If severe organ dysfunction, such as hepatic or uremic encephalopathy, is suspected, management should include renal replacement therapy like hemodialysis and appropriate treatment for hepatic encephalopathy.
- In unresponsive cases, evaluation for autoimmune encephalitis and paraneoplastic syndrome should be considered, with treatment focusing on managing the primary tumor and administering steroid therapy.

### Points to Ponder

- Metabolic encephalopathy and acute brain syndrome are closely related differential diagnoses.
- The presence of focal or sudden neurological deficits a nuchal rigidity suggests stroke and meningoencephalitis respectively.
- A thorough review of medical records and a detailed examination are essential.
- Metabolic encephalopathy is common in elderly people with degenerative brain disease, sepsis, and organ dysfunction
- The treatment should prioritize the prompt correction of electrolyte imbalances, the removal of toxins, and the management of organ dysfunction.

## MULTIPLE CHOICE QUESTIONS

1. **What is the most likely diagnosis for this patient?**
   A. Cerebrovascular accident
   B. Meningoencephalitis
   C. Metabolic encephalopathy
   D. Hypertensive encephalopathy
2. **Which electrolyte imbalance is most likely contributing to the patient's altered sensorium?**
   A. Hyperkalemia
   B. Hyponatremia
   C. Hypocalcemia
   D. Hypermagnesemia
3. **What clinical sign observed in this patient is characteristic of metabolic encephalopathy?**
   A. Focal neurological deficit
   B. Neck stiffness
   C. Asterixis
   D. Seizures
4. **What investigation was most useful in ruling out meningoencephalitis in this patient?**
   A. Blood culture
   B. CSF analysis
   C. Neuroimaging
   D. Serum lactate
5. **What was the primary management strategy for this patient's condition?**
   A. High-dose corticosteroids
   B. Broad-spectrum antibiotics
   C. Hypertonic saline and renal replacement therapy
   D. Anti-hypertensive therapy

### Answers

1. (C); 2. (B); 3. (C); 4. (B); 5. (C)

## SUGGESTED READINGS


1. Supanc V, Vargek-Solter V, Demarin V. Metabolic Encephalopathies. Acta Clin Croat. 2003;42(4):42.
2. Mohney L, Lindberg, RH. (2023). 'Metabolic Encephalopathies.' In StatPearls. Treasure Island, (FL): StatPearls. Available at https://www.ncbi.nlm.nih.gov/books/NBK564371/ (Last accessed: 1 December 2024).
3. Bathla G, Hegde AN. MRI and CT appearances in metabolic encephalopathies due to systemic diseases in adults. Clin Radiol. 2013;68(6):545-54.
4. Jeon SJ, Choi SS, Kim HY, et al. Acute Acquired Metabolic Encephalopathy Based on Diffusion MRI. Korean J Radiol. 2021;22(12):2034-51.
5. Rayi A, Mandalaneni K. (2023). 'Encephalopathic EEG Patterns.' In StatPearls. Treasure Island, (FL): StatPearls. Available at https://www.ncbi.nlm.nih.gov/books/NBK564371/ (Last accessed: 1 December, 2024).

# CHAPTER 48

# An Approach to a Case of Hypocalcemia

*Sumit Chatterjee, Paramita Bhattacharya*

**CASE VIGNETTE**

A 45-year-old woman presents to the emergency department with complaints of muscle cramps, tingling sensations around her mouth, and in her fingertips. She reports these symptoms have been escalating over the past week. Her medical history includes a thyroidectomy performed 6 months ago for thyroid cancer. On examination, she exhibits a positive Chvostek's sign. Laboratory tests reveal a serum calcium level of 7.0 mg/dL (normal range: 8.5–10.5 mg/dL) and a low parathyroid hormone (PTH) level. Her clinical presentation and laboratory findings strongly suggest hypocalcemia, likely secondary to hypoparathyroidism.

## PROVISIONAL DIAGNOSIS

Hypocalcemia is secondary to post-thyroidectomy hypoparathyroidism.

### Differential Diagnosis

Hypocalcemia has a broad differential diagnosis **(Fig. 1)**. Key conditions to consider include:

- *Hypoparathyroidism*:
  - *Postsurgical*: Following thyroidectomy or parathyroidectomy
  - *Autoimmune*: Autoimmune destruction of parathyroid glands
  - *Genetic disorders*: Such as DiGeorge syndrome, caused by congenital absence of parathyroid glands
- *Vitamin D deficiency*:
  - *Nutritional deficiency*: Inadequate dietary intake or lack of sunlight exposure.
  - *Malabsorption syndrome*: Conditions like celiac disease or Crohn's disease impairing vitamin D absorption
  - *Chronic liver or kidney disease*: Affecting the conversion of vitamin D to its active form
- *Chronic kidney disease (CKD)*:
  - *Impaired synthesis*: Decreased conversion of 25-hydroxyvitamin D to 1,25-dihydroxyvitamin D
  - *Phosphate retention*: Leading to secondary hyperparathyroidism
- *Hypomagnesemia*:
  - *Impaired PTH function*: Hypomagnesemia can inhibit PTH secretion and action. The causes include chronic alcoholism, malnutrition, and medications such as proton pump inhibitors

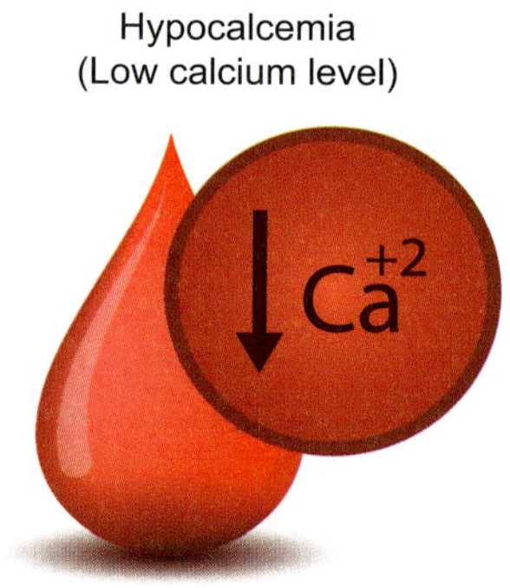


**FIG. 1:** Hypocalcemia.

- *Acute pancreatitis*:
  - *Saponification:* Calcium is deposited in necrotic fat tissue of the pancreas
- *Medications*:
  - *Bisphosphonates:* Used in osteoporosis, they can induce hypocalcemia
  - *Chemotherapeutic agents*: Such as cisplatin, which can reduce calcium levels

### Parathyroid Hormone (PTH) Resistance

*Pseudohypoparathyroidism (PHP):* These patients have clinical and biochemical features consistent with hypoparathyroidism but have neither a hypercalcemic nor phosphaturic response to exogenous parathyroid extract. Hypocalcemia is due to impaired mobilization of calcium from bone, reduced intestinal absorption of calcium, and increased urinary losses. In PHP1, there is usually an autosomal dominant inheritance of the mutation. Patients affected by PHP type IA (PHP1A) develop symptoms and signs of hypocalcemia in association with distinctive skeletal and developmental defects, referred to as Albright's hereditary osteodystrophy (AHO). The hypocalcemia is due to a deficient PTH response in the proximal renal tubules, probably leading to insufficient 1,25(OH)2 D production and thus impaired intestinal calcium absorption. Furthermore, PTH resistance in this portion of the kidney impairs urinary phosphate excretion, thus leading to elevated serum phosphate levels. Patients affected by PHP type 1B (PHP1B) also present with hypocalcemia and hyperphosphatemia but less frequently with obvious AHO features. If the mutation is passed down from the father, that allele is silenced in the proximal tubules of the kidney (through imprinting). The normal sequence from the maternal allele is expressed, and the biochemical and mineral abnormalities are absent. Only the AHO phenotype is present in such an individual. This is called pseudopseudohypoparathyroidism (PPHP).

## Clinical Approach

### History and Physical Examination

- *Detailed medical history*:
  - Recent surgeries, particularly thyroid or parathyroid surgeries
  - Dietary habits, including calcium and vitamin D intake
  - History of gastrointestinal disorders, kidney disease, or malnutrition
  - Medication history, including supplements and drugs that affect calcium metabolism
  - Family history
- *Symptoms review*:
  - *Neuromuscular*: Muscle cramps, tetany, paresthesias, and seizures
  - *Cardiovascular*: Palpitations, prolonged QT interval on ECG
  - *Dermatologic*: Dry skin, brittle nails, hair loss
- *Physical examination*:
  - *Neurological signs*: Look for Chvostek's sign (facial twitching) and Trousseau's sign (carpopedal spasm)
  - *Cardiac examination:* Assess for arrhythmia, check the ECG for QT prolongation
  - *Dermatological examination:* Evaluate skin texture and hair quality
  - *AHO features*: Short stature, round facies, brachydactyly, obesity, and subcutaneous calcifications
  - Features of hypothyroidism, hypogonadism, and mental retardation

### Laboratory Tests

1. *Serum calcium levels*: Measure total serum calcium and correct for albumin levels. Ionized calcium is the most accurate measure of biologically active calcium
2. *Parathyroid hormone*: Low PTH levels suggest hypoparathyroidism. Elevated PTH levels are indicative of secondary hyperparathyroidism
3. *Vitamin D levels*: Measure 25-hydroxyvitamin D to assess for deficiency.
4. *Magnesium levels*: Check serum magnesium levels, as hypomagnesemia can exacerbate hypocalcemia
5. *Phosphate levels*: Elevated phosphate levels are often seen in CKD and hypoparathyroidism.

### Imaging and Additional Tests

- *Electrocardiogram*: To identify prolonged QT intervals or other arrhythmias
- *Bone density scans/bone mineral density (BMD)*: Useful for assessing bone mineral density in chronic cases
- *Renal function tests*: To evaluate for CKD

## Pathophysiology

Surgical removal or damage to the parathyroid glands during thyroidectomy leads to reduced PTH secretion. PTH deficiency impairs calcium homeostasis by decreasing calcium resorption from bones, reducing renal calcium reabsorption, and lowering intestinal calcium absorption due to decreased activation of vitamin D, resulting in hypocalcemia.

## Treatment and Prevention

### Acute Hypocalcemia

- *Intravenous calcium administration*:
  - *Calcium gluconate*: Preferred for its safety profile, it is administered intravenously under cardiac monitoring
  - *Calcium chloride*: More potent but should be given via central venous access due to local irritation risks
- *Monitoring*:
  - Continuous ECG monitoring during IV calcium administration to detect arrhythmias
  - Regular serum calcium levels to guide ongoing treatment

### Chronic Hypocalcemia

- *Oral Calcium supplements*: *Calcium carbonate or calcium citrate*: For maintenance therapy, with doses adjusted based on serum calcium levels
- *Vitamin D supplementation*:
  - *Calcitriol*: The active form of vitamin D, used for faster action in patients with impaired conversion
  - *Ergocalciferol or cholecalciferol*: For long-term maintenance therapy.
- *Magnesium supplementation*: Essential if hypomagnesemia is present. Magnesium sulfate is commonly used

### Specific Treatments

- *Hypoparathyroidism*:
  - Lifelong calcium and active vitamin D supplementation
  - Recombinant PTH (e.g., Natpara) may be considered for patients with severe hypocalcemia and inadequate response to conventional therapy
- *Vitamin D deficiency*: High-dose vitamin D therapy initially, followed by maintenance dosing to restore normal levels
- *Chronic kidney disease*:
  - Manage phosphate levels with dietary restrictions and phosphate binders
  - Use active vitamin D analogs (e.g., calcitriol) to mitigate secondary hyperparathyroidism

## Points to Ponder

- *Early recognition and intervention*: Prompt diagnosis and treatment of hypocalcemia are crucial to prevent severe complications such as seizures, tetany, and cardiac arrhythmias. Early intervention can significantly improve patient outcomes.
- *Importance of monitoring:* Regular monitoring of serum calcium, vitamin D, and magnesium levels is vital, especially in patients at high risk, such as those with CKD or post-thyroidectomy. Adjusting treatment based on these levels helps maintain optimal calcium balance.
- *Patient education:* Educate patients on the importance of medication adherence, dietary calcium and vitamin D intake, and recognizing symptoms of hypocalcemia. Providing clear guidelines can enhance patient compliance and reduce the risk of recurrent hypocalcemia.
- *Interdisciplinary collaboration:* Effective management of hypocalcemia often requires a multidisciplinary approach involving endocrinologists, nephrologists, cardiologists, and primary care providers. This collaboration ensures comprehensive care and addresses all aspects of the patient's condition.

## MULTIPLE CHOICE QUESTIONS

1. **What is the most likely cause of the patient's hypocalcemia?**
   A. Vitamin D deficiency
   B. Chronic kidney disease
   C. Post-thyroidectomy hypoparathyroidism
   D. Malabsorption syndrome
2. **Which clinical sign is most indicative of hypocalcemia in this patient?**
   A. Trousseau's sign
   B. Positive Chvostek's sign
   C. Muscle weakness
   D. Hyperreflexia
3. **What is the primary hormone responsible for regulating serum calcium levels that is deficient in this patient?**
   A. Calcitonin
   B. Parathyroid hormone
   C. Vitamin D
   D. Aldosterone
4. **What is the immediate treatment for this patient's symptomatic hypocalcemia?**
   A. Oral calcium supplements
   B. Intravenous calcium gluconate
   C. Vitamin D analogs
   D. Bisphosphonates
5. **Which long-term treatment is most appropriate to prevent the recurrence of hypocalcemia in this patient?**
   A. Calcitonin therapy
   B. Vitamin D supplementation and oral calcium
   C. Diuretics to promote calcium retention
   D. Dietary calcium intake adjustment

### Answers

1. (C); 2. (B); 3. (B); 4. (B); 5. (B)

## SUGGESTED READINGS

1. Bilezikian JP, Brandi ML, Cusano NE, et al. Management of Hypocalcemia. Endocr Rev. 2016;37(5):489-8.
2. Cooper MS, Gittoes NJL. Diagnosis and Management of Hypocalcaemia. BMJ. 2008;336(7656):1298-302.
3. Peacock M. Calcium Metabolism in Health and Disease. Clin J Am Soc Nephrol. 2010;5(S1).
4. Shoback D. Clinical Practice. Hypoparathyroidism. N Engl J Med. 2008;359(4):391-403.
5. Turner JJ, Finch JL. Diagnosis and Management of Hypocalcaemia. Best Pract Res Clin Endocrinol Metab. 2017;31(3):359-70.

CHAPTER

49

# An Approach to a Case of Raised Prolactin

*Silima Subhasnigdha Tarenia, Niladri Das, Rana Bhattacharjee*

**CASE VIGNETTE**

A 38-year-old woman was brought to the emergency room by her relatives in a drowsy state, presenting with a history of headache, vomiting, and visual disturbances. She was resuscitated, and neuroimaging (CT and MRI) revealed a hemorrhage within a pituitary tumor, consistent with pituitary apoplexy. Her medical history revealed that she had been asymptomatic 6 months earlier when she consulted a local gynecologist for irregular menstrual cycles and galactorrhea. At that time, she was found to have elevated prolactin levels (112 ng/mL) and was started on cabergoline 0.25 mg twice weekly. Recent evaluation revealed secondary hypothyroidism, low cortisol levels, and low prolactin, indicating pituitary dysfunction. She underwent surgical decompression of the tumor and was started on hormone replacement therapy.

## PROVISIONAL DIAGNOSIS

Pituitary apoplexy in a nonfunctioning pituitary adenoma.

## DIFFERENTIAL DIAGNOSIS

- Cerebrovascular accident
- Encephalitis
- Subarachnoid hemorrhage

## CLINICAL APPROACH

When evaluating hyperprolactinemia, it is crucial to exclude common causes such as lactation, pregnancy, untreated primary hypothyroidism, renal failure, hepatic failure, and pharmacological factors. In drug-induced hyperprolactinemia, if the clinical situation allows, the offending drug should be withdrawn for at least 3 days, and serum prolactin levels retested. If hyperprolactinemia persists after drug withdrawal, or if the drug cannot be discontinued, a pituitary MRI should be performed to investigate pituitary-related causes like prolactinoma or a nonfunctioning pituitary tumor with stalk compression. Serum prolactin levels generally correlate with the size of the prolactinoma.

In microadenomas (maximum diameter <10 mm), serum prolactin levels are typically <200 ng/mL, whereas macroadenomas (maximum diameter >10 mm) are usually associated with levels >200 ng/mL. However, some macroadenomas may present with serum prolactin levels below 200 ng/mL. In patients with prolactin-secreting macroadenomas and very high serum prolactin levels, falsely low values can occur when measured using older two-site immunometric assays due to the high-dose hook effect. Serum prolactin measurement with serial dilutions should be performed if this is suspected.

In cases of cystic prolactinoma, where > 50% of the tumor volume is cystic, serum prolactin levels may be < 200 ng/mL. It is important to differentiate cystic prolactinomas from other cystic sellar lesions, such as Rathke's cleft cyst, craniopharyngioma, and arachnoid cyst, to ensure appropriate therapeutic intervention.

Another entity, macroprolactinemia, should be considered when high serum prolactin levels are observed with no or minimal symptoms of hyperprolactinemia. Large prolactin molecules (macroprolactin) with low biological activity lead to falsely elevated serum prolactin levels, resulting in minimal or no symptoms. Polyethylene glycol (PEG) precipitation or chromatography separates macroprolactin from monomeric prolactin, while chromatography is more definitive, is an expensive and time-consuming method for confirming macroprolactin.

## PATHOPHYSIOLOGY (FIG. 1)

Prolactin is secreted by lactotrophs in the anterior pituitary gland. Unlike other anterior pituitary hormones, prolactin is primarily under tonic inhibitory control by dopamine, which acts through D2 receptors on lactotrophs. Additionally, prolactin regulates its

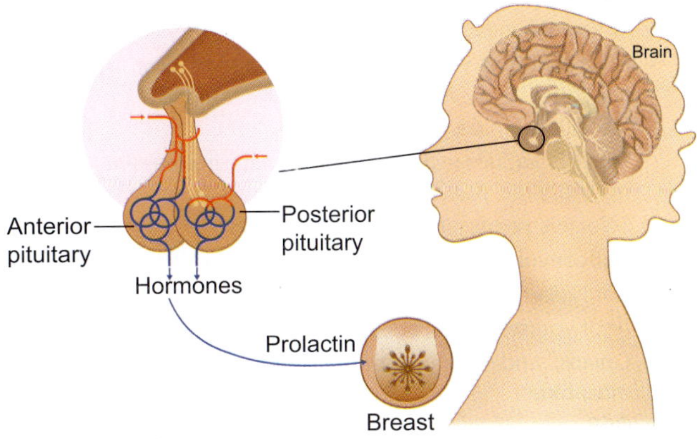


**FIG. 1:** Hyperprolactinemia.

own secretion via short-loop negative feedback by stimulating tuberoinfundibular dopamine (TIDA) cells. Thyrotropin-releasing hormone (TRH), vasoactive intestinal peptide (VIP), endothelial growth factor, serotonin, estrogen, and oxytocin also function as prolactin-releasing factors.

## CAUSES OF HYPERPROLACTINEMIA (BOX 1)

Pathological causes of hyperprolactinemia include prolactinoma, acromegaly, and nonfunctional sellar or parasellar tumors. In the last situation, hyperprolactinemia typically results from stalk compression or disruption of vascular connections between the pituitary and hypothalamus, with serum prolactin levels generally not exceeding 100 ng/mL. In contrast, prolactinomas are characterized by significantly elevated prolactin levels, often above 100 ng/mL, with levels exceeding 200 ng/mL strongly indicative of prolactinoma.

Drug-induced hyperprolactinemia commonly occurs with neuroleptics and atypical antipsychotics due to their D2 receptor-blocking effects. Among these, risperidone has a potent prolactin-stimulating effect, whereas drugs like olanzapine and clozapine have minimal effects. In drug-induced hyperprolactinemia, serum prolactin levels usually do not exceed 200 ng/mL, except in cases involving risperidone **(Box 1)**.

**BOX 1: Causes of hyperprolactinemia.**

*Physiologic*:
- Pregnancy
- Nipple stimulation
- Sleep
- Stress
- Sexual intercourse
- Exercise

*Pathological*:
- *Pituitary causes*:
  - Prolactinoma
  - Hypophysitis
  - Acromegaly
  - Plurihormonal adenoma
- *Hypothalamic pituitary stalk damage*:
  - Suprasellar, parasellar mass
  - Craniopharyngioma
  - Germinoma
  - Rathke's cleft cyst
  - Brain irradiation
  - Head injury
  - Sellar surgery
  - Pituitary/hypothalamic metastases
- *Systemic illness*:
  - Chronic renal failure
  - Chronic liver disease
  - Polycystic ovary syndrome
  - Seizures
  - Chest wall injury

*Pharmacologic*:
- *Typical antipsychotics*:
  - Phenothiazines: Chlorpromazine, perphenazine
  - Butyrophenones: Haloperidol, droperidol
  - Thioxanthenes: Flupenthixol, clopenthixol
  - Atypical antipsychotics: Clozapine, risperidone, olanzapine, sulpiride
  - Metoclopramide, domperidone
  - Tricyclic antidepressants: Amitriptyline, imipramine, nortriptyline, doxepin
  - Selective serotonin reuptake inhibitors
  - Anticonvulsants: Phenytoin
  - Antihistaminics: H2-blockers
  - Antihypertensives: Labetalol, reserpine, verapamil
  - Opiates and opiate antagonist: Methadone, apomorohine, morphine
  - OCP

## CLINICAL APPROACH

Symptoms of hyperprolactinemia arise both from elevated prolactin levels and from tumor mass effects in pituitary-related causes. Elevated prolactin can cause menstrual irregularities and galactorrhea. At the same time, tumor-related mass effects may lead to headaches, visual field defects, reduced visual acuity, and symptoms of deficiencies in other pituitary hormones.

In females, hyperprolactinemia typically presents with menstrual irregularities like oligomenorrhea, amenorrhea, infertility, low libido, and galactorrhea. Approximately 50% of women with hyperprolactinemia experience galactorrhea. Very few males have galactorrhea, as male mammary tissue is less sensitive to the lactogenic effects of elevated prolactin. Men commonly present with infertility, oligospermia, reduced libido, erectile dysfunction, and tumor mass effects. Symptoms of tumor expansion include headaches, visual defects, external ophthalmoplegia, or symptoms of secondary adrenal or thyroid failure.

In prepubertal or peripubertal children, hyperprolactinemia may present with delayed or arrested puberty, headaches, visual field defects, or growth arrest.

## TREATMENT AND PREVENTION

Before starting treatment, the cause of hyperprolactinemia must be ascertained.

In cases of drug-induced hyperprolactinemia, treatment is necessary if the patient develops hypogonadism or troublesome galactorrhea. If possible, antipsychotics causing hyperprolactinemia can be replaced with alternatives such as olanzapine or risperidone, which has minimal prolactin-elevating effects.

In nonfunctional pituitary macroadenoma with stalk compression (like in our patient), surgical excision of the SOL is needed. For prolactinoma, medical treatment with dopamine agonists is the preferred therapy. Cabergoline, a long-acting dopamine agonist, is the most commonly used medication. Cabergoline is usually started at a dose of 0.25 mg once or twice weekly and adjusted based on tolerance and response. Patients are advised to start with small doses taken with food at bedtime.

Approximately 15% of patients fail to normalize prolactin levels or achieve significant tumor reduction with optimal cabergoline doses, indicating resistance. In such cases, surgery or radiotherapy may be necessary. Initial side effects of dopamine agonists, such as nausea, vomiting, and gastrointestinal discomfort, often subside after dose adjustment. Rare side effects include nasal stuffiness, depression, digital vasospasm, somnolence, postural hypotension, and impulse control disorders. Patients experiencing intolerable side effects may benefit from intravaginal bromocriptine to mitigate gastrointestinal symptoms.

Medical therapy can be withdrawn after at least 2 years of treatment in absence of any visible tumor mass on MRI with normalization of serum prolactin level. Transsphenoidal surgery is considered for patients resistant to maximally tolerable medical therapy. Pituitary apoplexy with compressive features also warrants surgery.

Surgical resection of microprolactinomas and well-circumscribed macroprolactinomas (Knosp grade 0 and 1) by an experienced neurosurgeon may be considered as first-line. For adenomas with a lower likelihood of surgical remission (Knosp grade ≥ 2), medical therapy remains the preferred initial approach.

Radiotherapy is generally reserved for aggressive or malignant prolactinomas, especially after medical surgical failure, though its maximal effects take time to manifest. Temozolomide, an alkylating agent, may be used in cases of malignant prolactinoma.

## Points to Ponder

- Hyperprolactinemia involves a broad range of etiologies—always establish diagnosis before starting treatment.
- Careful history-taking and clinical assessment help in narrowing down differentials.
- Medications are the most common causes of pathological raised prolactin.
- Mildly elevated prolactin can occur due to large sellar or parasellar masses with stalk compression.
- Interpretation of prolactin reports should be done carefully keeping macroprolactin and hook-effect in mind.
- Treatment goals of hyperprolactinemia include restoration and maintenance of gonadal function, relieving distressing galactorrhea and prevention of osteoporosis.
- Dopamine agonists are first-line of treatment for most prolactinomas, where treatment is indicated.

## MULTIPLE CHOICE QUESTIONS

1. **Which of the following drugs is least associated with hyperprolactinemia?**
   A. Aripiprazole
   B. Amisulpride
   C. Domperidone
   D. Risperidone
2. **A 22-year-old unmarried female was referred for a prolactin level of 96 ng/mL. History reveals that her menstrual cycles were cyclic and predictable. There was no galactorrhea. She has not taken any incriminating drugs in the last 1 month. What to do next?**
   A. Prolactin in dilution
   B. LH/FSH
   C. PEG precipitation
   D. MRI-HP AREA
3. **In a case of hyperprolactinemia due to primary hypothyroidism, all of the following are true, except:**
   A. Prolactin levels are usually < 100 ng/mL
   B. Appropriate treatment normalizes prolactin
   C. Prolactin levels are always > 200 ng/mL
   D. There is lactotroph hyperplasia due to increased TRH drive
4. **All of the following are true about prolactinoma, except:**
   A. They are the most common pituitary tumor
   B. Macroprolactinomas are more common in men
   C. Surgical modality is the treatment of choice
   D. Women may present with galactorrhea, oligomenorrhea and infertility
5. **All of the following are true, except:**
   A. TRH acts as a prolactin releasing factor
   B. Estrogen inhibits prolactin
   C. Prolactin levels may be raised in CKD
   D. Prolactin can inhibit gonadotrophs

### Answers

1. (A); 2. (C); 3. (C); 4. (C); 5. (B)

## SUGGESTED READINGS


1. Liu JW, Ben-Jonathan N. Prolactin-releasing activity of neurohypophysial hormones: structure-function relationship. Endocrinology. 1994;134(1):114-8.
2. Bernard V, Lamothe S, Beau I, et al. Autocrine actions of prolactin contribute to the regulation of lactotroph function in vivo. FASEB J. 2018;32(9):4791-7.
3. Karavitaki N, Thanabalasingham G, Shore HCA, et al. Do the limits of serum prolactin in disconnection hyperprolactinaemia need re-definition? A study of 226 patients with histologically verified non-functioning pituitary macroadenoma. Clin Endocrinol (Oxf). 2006;65(4):524-9.
4. Ajmal A, Joffe H, Nachtigall LB. Psychotropic-induced hyperprolactinemia: a clinical review. Psychosomatics. 2014;55(1):29-36.
5. Frieze TW, Mong DP, Koops MK. "Hook effect" in prolactinomas: case report and review of literature. Endocr Pract. 2002;8:296-303.
6. Glezer A, Bronstein MD. Hyperprolactinemia. [Updated 2022 Jan 5]. In: Feingold KR, Anawalt B, Blackman MR, et al., editors. Endotext [Internet]. South Dartmouth (MA): MDText.com, Inc.; 2000.
7. Muhtaroglu S, Keti DB, Hacıoglu A. Macroprolactin: an overlooked reason of hyperprolactinemia. Journal of Laboratory Medicine. 2019;43(3):163-8.
8. Melmed S, Auchus RJ, Goldfine AB, et al., editors. Williams Textbook of Endocrinology. 14th ed. Philadelphia: Elsevier; 2020.
9. Melmed S, Casanueva FF, Hoffman AR, et al. Diagnosis and treatment of hyperprolactinemia: an Endocrine Society clinical practice guideline. J Clin Endocrinol Metab. 2011;96(2):273-88.
10. Petersenn S, Fleseriu M, Casanueva FF, et al. Diagnosis and management of prolactin-secreting pituitary adenomas: a Pituitary Society international Consensus Statement. Nat Rev Endocrinol. 2023;19(12):722-40.

CHAPTER 50

# An Approach to a Case of Asymptomatic Hypercreatininemia

*Raj Datta*

**CASE VIGNETTE**

A 65-year-old gentleman who has a 20-year history of diabetes mellitus and a 10-year history of hypertension visits the outpatient department for consultation about his laboratory reports in which the serum creatinine is outside the reference range. He was previously treated for diabetic retinopathy and is otherwise well with no physical complaints. The patient's blood pressure measured in the office is 142/88 mm Hg, weight is 72 kg, most recent blood glycosylated hemoglobin (HbA1c) measurement was 8.2%, and most recent low-density lipoprotein (LDL) cholesterol level was 145 mg/dL. The patient's current regimen for blood pressure control includes amlodipine 5 mg/day and atenolol, 25 mg/day; and for blood glucose control he uses glipizide at 5 mg/day. The patient has no known history of heart disease or congestive heart failure. Result of a serum creatinine test obtained just before this visit is 1.6 mg/dL, which is the same result as that obtained 3 months earlier. The reference ranges for serum creatinine are 0.7–1.3 mg/dL in men and 0.6–1.1 mg/dL in women. The patient has persistently elevated serum creatinine over the past 3 months, with an estimated glomerular filtration rate (eGFR) of 48 mL/min/1.73 $m^2$, indicating stage 3 chronic kidney disease (CKD). Investigations reveal proteinuria and a high albumin-to-creatinine ratio, suggesting diabetic nephropathy. Management includes optimal blood pressure and glucose control, with medications like losartan to reduce proteinuria. The patient was also prescribed rosuvastatin and advised on lifestyle changes. Follow-up showed a reduction in proteinuria, and a nephrology consultation was recommended.

## PROVISIONAL DIAGNOSIS

Stage 3 chronic kidney disease due to diabetic nephropathy.

## DIFFERENTIAL DIAGNOSIS

Rise in serum creatinine can be due to (1) Increased production, (2) Decreased excretion, (3) Interference with laboratory assay.

## PATHOPHYSIOLOGY

Diabetic nephropathy occurs due to prolonged hyperglycemia leading to glomerular hyperfiltration, endothelial dysfunction, and accumulation of extracellular matrix, which results in glomerular injury, fibrosis, and progressive decline in renal function.

First, it is essential to understand a bit about creatinine synthesis and metabolism **(Fig. 1)**. Creatinine is a byproduct of creatine and creatine phosphate in muscles, produced based on muscle mass. It is synthesized in the liver and kidneys from amino acids and plays a role in ATP production. Serum creatinine can temporarily increase due to factors like a large meat meal, rhabdomyolysis, or creatine supplement intake.

Creatinine is primarily excreted by the kidneys through glomerular filtration **(Fig. 2)** and tubular secretion. Diseases that reduce glomerular filtration rate can lead to elevated serum creatinine levels. Certain drugs can inhibit tubular secretion of creatinine, causing a reversible rise in serum creatinine without affecting the glomerular filtration rate (eGFR). Examples of such drugs include trimethoprim, dronedarone, dolutegravir, cimetidine, PARP inhibitors like olaparib, and tyrosine kinase inhibitors like imatinib.

Serum creatinine is often measured using the alkaline picrate method (Jaffe reaction), which can be interfered with by substances like acetoacetate and glucose. Many labs now prefer an enzymatic method, which offers more accuracy by converting creatinine to creatine and further processing it.

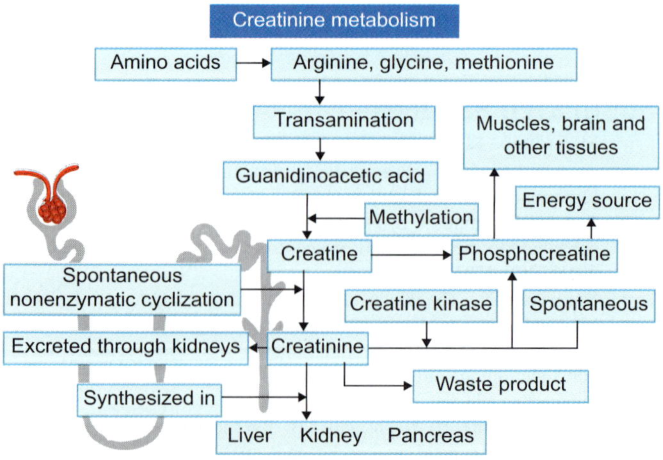


**FIG. 1:** Creatinine synthesis and metabolism.

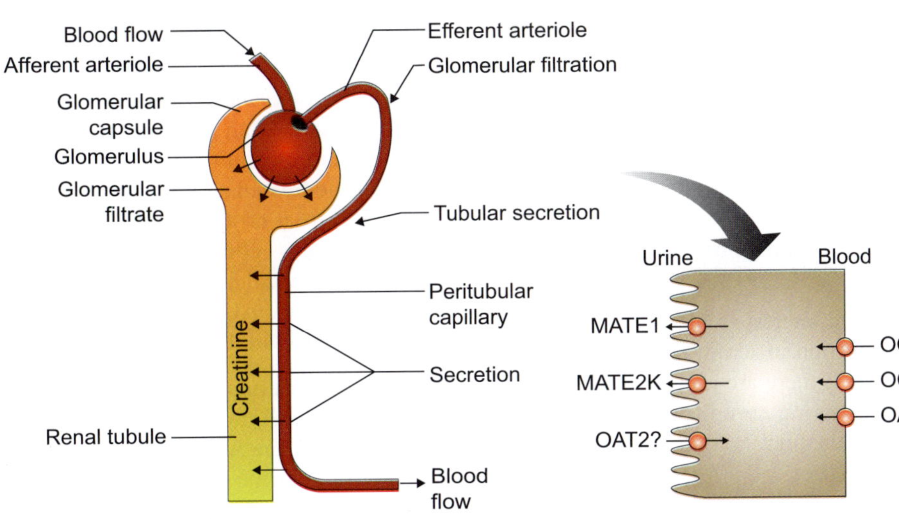


**FIG. 2:** Creatinine excretion.

*Source*: 10.1124/dmd.115.067694 at ASPET Journals on March 4, 2016 dmd.aspetjournals.org.

## CLINICAL APPROACH

A thorough history searching for risk factors for CKD is warranted. A review of medications as well as prior serum creatinine and urinalysis reports should be sought for if available. Risk factors for acute or subacute kidney injury should be searched for as well. Physical examination **(Box 1)** should include vitals and search for renovascular or polycystic kidney disease, microvascular complications like neuropathy if diabetic, any signs of autoimmune disease like rash or purpura or scleroderma, and assessment of volume status (*Note*: Pallor cannot reliably differentiate between acute kidney injury and chronic kidney disease). Based on history, clinical examination and review of medications and previous laboratory reports, it should be determined whether the patient can be categorised into (1) known chronic kidney disease, (2) acute kidney injury or acute kidney disease (3) seemingly well patient without risk factors for kidney disease. The definitions (KDIGO) for these are given below:

1. *Chronic kidney disease* ***(Table 1)***: Presence of kidney damage (evidenced by structural abnormalities detected on imaging or functional abnormalities like abnormal urine sediment or urinary albumin excretion >30 mg/day) or decreased kidney function (eGFR < 60 mL/min) for 3 or more months.
2. *Acute kidney injury (AKI)* ***(Table 2)***: Rise in serum creatinine >0.3 mg/dL within 48 hours or more than 50% increase in serum creatinine which is known or presumed to have occurred within the prior 7 days or decrease in urine output <0.5 mL/kg/hr for > 6 hours.
3. *Acute kidney disease (AKD)*: AKI or GFR < 60 mL/min/1.73 $m^2$ for < 3 months, or decrease in GFR by >35% or increase in serum creatinine by > 50% for < 3 months.

**BOX 1: Targeted physical examination.**

- Signs of volume depletion
- Signs of volume overload
- Presence of retinopathy on fundoscopy
- Abdominal bruit
- Enlarged kidneys
- Peripheral neuropathy
- Rash
- Palpable purpura
- Skin thickening and skin hardness
- Signs of liver disease

**TABLE 1: Risk factors for CKD.**

| | |
|---|---|
| Diabetes | Known renal anatomical abnormalities or obstruction |
| Hypertension | Recurrent, complicated urinary tract infections or kidney stones |
| Cardiovascular, cerebrovascular or peripheral vascular disease | Family history of genetically transmitted kidney disease like polycystic kidney disease, Alport's syndrome, sickle cell disease |
| Prior acute kidney injury | Cancer treated with chemotherapy/immunotherapy/radiotherapy |
| Obesity | Prior urologic/pelvic surgery, known or suspected pelvic/retroperitoneal malignancy |
| Heart failure | Exposure to nephrotoxins or toxic environmental exposures like lead, lithium, analgesic, toxin containing herbal medicine |
| Autoimmune disease | Agricultural work in hot climate or other geographical environmental exposures, e.g., schistosomiasis |

## TREATMENT AND PREVENTION

- *Seemingly well patient without risk factors for kidney disease*: The creatinine elevation may be due to some easily remediable cause (e.g., hypovolemia) or it may be transient. Reviewing and addressing medications that may

| TABLE 2: Risk factors for AKI. | |
|---|---|
| Volume depletion | Recent cardiac or major non-cardiac surgery |
| Known chronic disease (kidney/liver/heart) | Critical illness |
| Nephrotoxin exposure like drugs or contrast | Cancer |
| Sepsis | Burns or trauma |

increase serum creatinine or interfere with creatinine assay is required. A transient elevation in serum creatinine does not require further evaluation if there are no worrisome clinical features. A persistent or rising serum creatinine requires further monitoring and evaluation.

- *Known chronic kidney disease*:
  - *Stable serum creatinine elevation:*
    - If the cause of CKD is unknown, it has to be evaluated with relevant tests like urinalysis, urine ACR, and other tests as appropriate.
    - The stage of CKD has to be determined based on eGFR and degree of albuminuria.
    - Risk factors and comorbid conditions like diabetes, hypertension, obstructive uropathy, complications of CKD need to be addressed, and reversible causes/complications need to be treated.
    - Medication doses should be adjusted based on eGFR.
  - *Unstable serum creatinine:*
    - Steady progression (slowly rising serum creatinine over months or years) —risk factors and underlying disease have to be addressed. Nephrology consultation has to be taken as well.
    - Abrupt rise in serum creatinine (days to weeks) — needs to be evaluated for acute or subacute kidney injury (in the setting of CKD).
- *Acute or subacute kidney injury*:
  - If there is an obvious, remedial cause for increase in serum creatinine like hypovolemia, the reason needs to be addressed.
  - If there is no apparent remedial reason, further evaluation includes complete hemogram, serum electrolytes, glucose, calcium, phosphate, uric acid, urinalysis along with urine ACR, and ultrasound imaging.
  - Results will dictate further evaluation.

**When to consult nephrology?**

- eGFR < 30 mL/min/1.73 m$^2$
- Persistent urine ACR >300 mg/g
- Abnormal urine microscopy (cellular casts, nonoliguric hematuria, sterile pyuria)
- Personal history of autoimmune disease
- Large cystic kidneys by imaging or examination
- Known history of multiple myeloma or monoclonal gammopathy
- Evidence of rapidly progressive renal dysfunction (reduction in eGFR by >5 mL/min/1.73 m$^2$/year)
- Recurrent extensive nephrolithiasis
- Resistant hypertension
- Pregnancy
- Young patients with unclear cause of CKD who may need a kidney biopsy
- Confirmed or presumed hereditary disease
- Patients with single kidney and eGFR <60 mL/min/1.73 m$^2$
- Difficult to manage laboratory abnormalities, e.g., anemia, metabolic acidosis, hyperkalemia

## Points to Ponder

- Even a slightly elevated serum creatinine level can indicate presence of clinically significant kidney disease, despite being asymptomatic. Therefore, estimated glomerular filtration rate, instead of absolute serum creatinine level, should be used to evaluate kidney function.
- Creatinine elevation may be due to increased production, decreased excretion or interference with laboratory assay. Certain drugs may interfere with assay as well without causing actual reduction in glomerular filtration rate.
- Reviewing past records is helpful if available, to check for duration of renal dysfunction and to categorise patients on this basis.
- Patients with any degree of chronic kidney disease should have their blood pressure, blood glucose level, and blood cholesterol level managed aggressively to help reduce or prevent the progression of kidney disease as well as to reduce risk of cardiovascular events.
- Nephrology consultation is essential when indicated.

## MULTIPLE CHOICE QUESTIONS

1. **Which of the following is the most likely cause of the patient's elevated serum creatinine?**
   A. Acute glomerulonephritis
   B. Diabetic nephropathy
   C. Hypertensive nephropathy
   D. Renal artery stenosis
2. **What is the most appropriate next step in managing this patient's diabetic nephropathy?**
   A. Start insulin therapy
   B. Increase the dose of glipizide
   C. Start angiotensin-converting enzyme (ACE) inhibitors
   D. Increase amlodipine dosage
3. **Which of the following is the target blood pressure for a patient with chronic kidney disease?**
   A. ≤140/90 mm Hg
   B. ≤130/80 mm Hg
   C. ≤120/80 mm Hg
   D. ≤150/90 mm Hg
4. **Which medication is most commonly used to reduce proteinuria in patients with diabetic nephropathy?**
   A. Furosemide
   B. Losartan
   C. Metformin
   D. Amlodipine

5. **What is the recommended HbA1c target for diabetic patients with chronic kidney disease?**
   A. ≤8%
   B. ≤7%
   C. ≤6%
   D. ≤9%

## Answers

1. (B); 2. (C); 3. (B); 4. (B); 5. (B)

## SUGGESTED READINGS


1. Johnson RJ, O'Hare LC. Diabetic Nephropathy: Diagnosis and Treatment. Lancet Diabetes Endocrinol. 2018;6(2):91-104.
2. Stevens MA, Levey JS. Chronic Kidney Disease: Evaluation and Management. N Engl J Med. 374(8):769-81.
3. Perazella MA. Kidney Disease and Hypertension: A Guide to Managing Patients with CKD. Am J Kidney Diseases. 2017;69(2):267-75.
4. Parikh RMJ, Tuttle MK. Kidney Disease and Diabetes: A Pathophysiological Approach. Diabetes Care. 2020;43(5):1056-65.
5. Collins SJ, Kasiske DL. Managing Diabetic Nephropathy in Clinical Practice. Kidney Int., 2019;96(1):21-8.

CHAPTER

51

# A Case-based Approach to Renal Tubular Acidosis

*Sayan Kar, Boudhayan Das Munshi, Dipesh Kumar Dhoot, Saikat Mondal*

**CASE VIGNETTE**

Mr AS, a 44-year-old man presented with flaccid paralysis of all four limbs, and tetanic spasm of the hand. He had a history of a similar episode 1-year-ago that progressed to respiratory paralysis, needing assisted ventilation. The past episode was attributed to hypokalemia and hypocalcemia. He received treatment outside, under an empirical diagnosis of familial periodic paralysis (FPP), with oral potassium and calcium supplementation, with acetazolamide to combat muscle weakness. The patient was stringently taking the drugs. He was normotensive, with normal blood sugar and normal renal function (urea 11 mg/dL and creatinine 0.6 mg/dL). The present episode was also associated with persistent hypokalemia ($K^+$ 1.8 mmol/L) and hypocalcemia (6.4 mg/dL with albumin of 3.8 g/dL. ABG showed hyperchloremic metabolic acidosis (plasma $HCO_3$: 16, pH 7.21, Na: 138, Cl: 110, anion gap 12 mEq/L). Abdominal ultrasonography revealed bilateral nephrocalcinosis. Routine urinalysis showed pH-6.7, glycosuria and 2+ proteinuria by dipstick. Urinary potassium creatinine ratio was 6.77 and TTKG was 10 with a urine anion gap of 32 mEq/L. TSH, vitamin D, and PTH levels were normal. Beta-2 microglobulin was high and spot urinary ACR was normal. The patient was put on oral Shohl's solution (custom-made by the in-house biochemistry department providing 1 mEq/mL of alkali) at a dose of 10 mEq/kg body weight of $HCO_3^-$ for 2 weeks, restoring arterial $HCO_3^-$ level to 22 mEq/L. We then estimated the fractional excretion of $HCO_3^-$, which came out to be 24%. Tubular reabsorption of phosphate was determined to be 78%. These, along with the qualitative demonstration of glycosuria by Benedict's method, established a proximal tubular origin of acidosis as well.

## PROVISIONAL DIAGNOSIS

Case is a rare entity having features of both proximal as well as distal RTA and belongs to the rare category of type 3 RTA.

## DIFFERENTIAL DIAGNOSIS

- *Familial periodic paralysis (FPP)*: A genetic disorder causing recurrent episodes of hypokalemia and muscle weakness.
- *Proximal renal tubular acidosis (pRTA)*: Characterized by bicarbonate wasting, glycosuria, and nephrocalcinosis.
- *Hypokalemic periodic paralysis*: Can present with hypokalemia and muscle paralysis, often triggered by factors like stress or medication.

## CLINICAL APPROACH (FLOWCHARTS 1 AND 2)

*Step 1*: Confirm metabolic acidosis via arterial blood gas and assess compensation for chronic respiratory alkalosis.

*Step 2*: Calculate serum anion gap (AG) and correct for albumin.

$$AG = Na^+ - [(Cl^-) + (HCO_3^-)] \text{ [Normal: } 12 \pm 2 \text{ mEq/L]}$$

Corrected AG = AG + [2.5 × (4 – Albumin)].

*Step 3*: Measure urinary anion gap (UAG) and osmolal gap (UOG).

$$UAG = (UNa^+ + UK^+) - UCl^-$$

*Normal/RTA*: +30 to +50 mmol/L; Extrarenal causes: < −20 mmol/L

UOG = Measured urinary osmolality − Calculated osmolality

*Normal UOG*: 10–100 mOsmol/kg; Elevated (>100) indicates high $NH_4^+$.

*Step 4*: Measure urine pH and serum potassium. Fresh urine sample is preferable, and urine pH is best measured by electrode.

*Step 5*: Assess proximal tubular function in proximal RTA (Fanconi syndrome), which includes glycosuria, hypophosphatemia, and aminoaciduria.

*Step 6*: Additional testing for RTA types:

- *Type 1 (distal RTA)*: Urine pH > 5.5, urine ammonium low, diagnosis with ammonium chloride acidification test.
- *Type 2 (proximal RTA)*: Bicarbonate wasting, diagnosis by raising serum bicarbonate with sodium bicarbonate infusion. Urine pH > 7.5 and $FEHCO_3^-$ > 15–20%.
- *Type 3 (carbonic anhydrase II deficiency)*: Mixed RTA with both proximal and distal features, seen in the middle east and Mediterranean.
- *Type 4 (hyperkalemic RTA)*: Characterized by hyperkalemia, assess with plasma renin activity, aldosterone levels, and transtubular potassium gradient (TTKG). TTKG > 8 suggests mineralocorticoid deficiency.

## PATHOPHYSIOLOGY

The patient's symptoms suggest a combination of proximal renal tubular acidosis (pRTA) with hypokalemia and hypocalcemia.

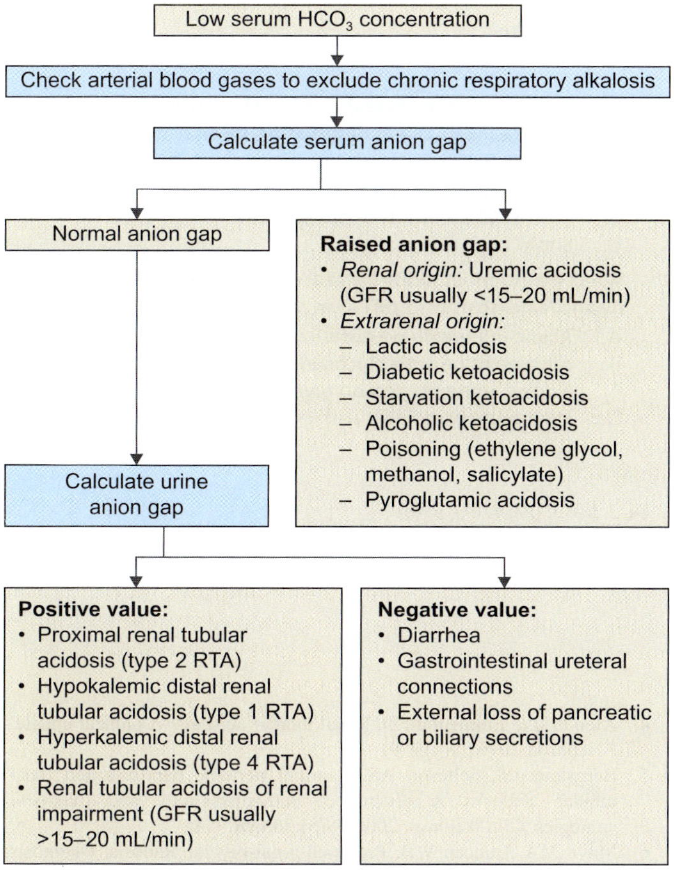


**FLOWCHART 1:** Approach to metabolic acidosis.

pRTA results from impaired bicarbonate reabsorption in the proximal tubule, leading to metabolic acidosis. Glycosuria and proteinuria, along with nephrocalcinosis, are indicative of tubular dysfunction. The hypokalemia is likely exacerbated by renal potassium wasting, as evidenced by the low urinary potassium levels. The elevated beta-2 microglobulin reflects tubular injury, while the normal PTH, vitamin D, and TSH help rule out other metabolic causes.

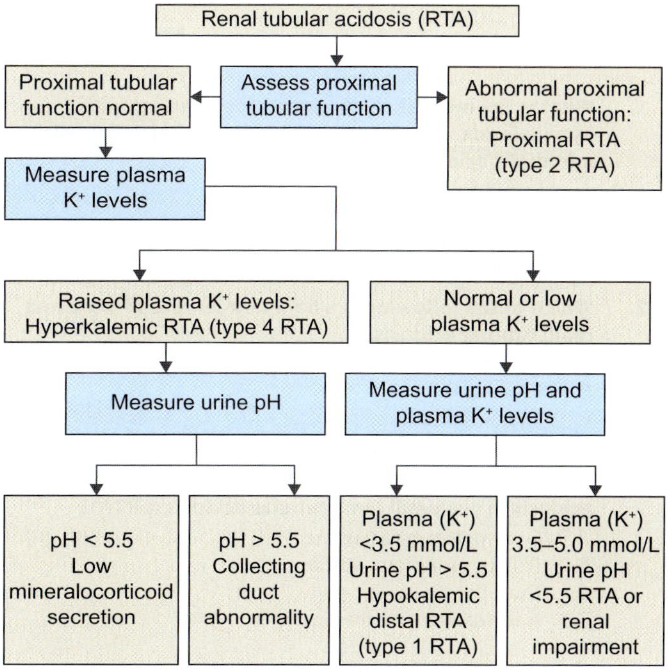


**FLOWCHART 2:** Approach to renal tubular acidosis.

## TREATMENT AND PREVENTION

### Treatment

- Shohl's solution (sodium bicarbonate) to correct metabolic acidosis.
- Potassium supplementation to address hypokalemia.
- Calcium supplementation to correct hypocalcemia.
- Monitor renal function and electrolytes regularly.

### Prevention

- Long-term alkali therapy to manage pRTA and prevent recurrent episodes of acidosis.
- Regular potassium and calcium monitoring to prevent imbalances.
- Avoidance of triggers that precipitate episodes of paralysis.

### Points to Ponder

- *Nephrocalcinosis in pRTA*: The deposition of calcium salts in the kidneys is often a result of chronic metabolic acidosis and renal tubular dysfunction, as seen in pRTA.
- *Fractional excretion of bicarbonate ($FEHCO_3$)*: This test helps assess the kidney's ability to reabsorb bicarbonate, with high values indicating proximal tubular dysfunction.
- *Importance of glycosuria in pRTA*: Glycosuria in the absence of hyperglycemia suggests proximal tubular dysfunction, commonly seen in conditions like pRTA.
- *Potassium wasting in pRTA*: Proximal tubular acidosis can lead to potassium wasting, contributing to hypokalemia, which may trigger episodes of muscle paralysis.
- *Management of pRTA*: Long-term treatment with alkali therapy, such as sodium bicarbonate, is crucial to correct metabolic acidosis and prevent complications such as bone disease and nephrocalcinosis.

## MULTIPLE CHOICE QUESTIONS

**1. What is the most likely diagnosis for a patient with hypokalemia, hypocalcemia, and nephrocalcinosis with metabolic acidosis?**
- A. Familial periodic paralysis
- B. Proximal renal tubular acidosis (pRTA)
- C. Hypokalemic periodic paralysis
- D. Distal renal tubular acidosis (dRTA)

**2. Which of the following is a hallmark feature of proximal renal tubular acidosis?**
- A. Hyperkalemia
- B. Glycosuria
- C. Hypokalemia
- D. Elevated urine pH

**3. What is the most common treatment for metabolic acidosis in proximal renal tubular acidosis (pRTA)?**
- A. Oral sodium bicarbonate
- B. Calcium supplementation
- C. Diuretics
- D. Antihypertensive medications

**4. Which test is used to assess the fractional excretion of bicarbonate ($FEHCO_3$) in diagnosing pRTA?**
- A. Urine potassium creatinine ratio
- B. Ammonium chloride test
- C. Fractional excretion of phosphate
- D. Shohl's solution test

**5. What would most likely be seen in a patient with nephrocalcinosis and pRTA on a urinalysis?**
- A. Acidic urine with no proteinuria
- B. Alkaline urine with glycosuria and proteinuria
- C. Normal urine pH and no glycosuria
- D. High urine osmolality with no glycosuria

### Answers

1. (B); 2. (B); 3. (A); 4. (A); 5. (B)

## SUGGESTED READINGS

1. Goswami RP, Mondal S, Karmakar PS, et al. Type 3 renal tubular acidosis. Indian J Nephrol. 2012;22:466-8.
2. Palmer BF, Kelepouris E, Clegg DJ. Renal Tubular Acidosis and Management Strategies: A Narrative Review. Adv Ther. 2021;38(2):949-68.
3. Emmett M, Palmer BF. Etiology and diagnosis of distal (type 1) and proximal (type 2) renal tubular acidosis. In: UpToDate, Connor RF (Ed), Wolters Kluwer. (Accessed on August 8, 2024)
4. Alon US, & Emmanouil D. Renal tubular acidosis: A clinical update. J Nephrol. 2016;29(1):1-9.
5. Bergstein JM, Johnson AS. Familial periodic paralysis and renal tubular acidosis: A review of pathophysiology and treatment strategies. Clin Nephrol. 2002;58(5):365-74.
6. Mayo MA, Duncan WB. Proximal renal tubular acidosis: Diagnosis and management. Am J Kidney Dis. 2019;73(6):819-26.

CHAPTER 52

# An Approach to a Case of Renal Failure on Antituberculosis Treatment

*Sabu Augustine, Visvesvaran Salitteeswaran*

**CASE VIGNETTE**

A 60-year-old male, diagnosed with isoniazid-resistant pulmonary tuberculosis, began treatment following the standard protocol. However, he developed acute kidney injury (AKI) and was diagnosed with rifampin-induced AKI. This case highlights the challenge of managing patients with isoniazid resistance, where rifampin remains the only first-line treatment option. In such situations, several approaches can be considered: Rifampin can be temporarily discontinued and reintroduced once renal function improves, potentially with a short course of steroids; alternatively, the patient may undergo rifampin desensitization before reintroduction when renal parameters stabilize. As another option, second-line drugs that are renal-safe, such as fluoroquinolones and linezolid, can be used to manage the condition.

## PROVISIONAL DIAGNOSIS

Rifampin-induced acute kidney injury (AKI) in a patient with isoniazid-resistant pulmonary tuberculosis.

## DIFFERENTIAL DIAGNOSIS

- Isoniazid-induced hepatotoxicity (less likely, as no liver dysfunction is reported).
- Fluoroquinolone-induced AKI (alternative TB treatment).
- Sepsis-related AKI (due to underlying infection or TB progression).

## PATHOPHYSIOLOGY

Rifampin-induced AKI is primarily caused by hypersensitivity reactions or nephrotoxicity, resulting in tubular damage and impaired renal function. Immune-mediated mechanisms may play a role, particularly in patients with pre-existing renal impairment or those on multiple medications. Rifampin (R), pyrazinamide (Z), and isoniazid (H) are mainly excreted via the biliary route, while streptomycin (S) and other aminoglycosides are excreted exclusively by the kidneys. Ethambutol (E) is predominantly excreted through the kidneys. Although both isoniazid and ethambutol have been linked to AKI, rifampin is the most frequently implicated anti-TB drug in causing AKI, as reported in most studies. Renal injury from anti-tuberculosis treatment (ATT) is more common in the elderly, primarily due to comorbid conditions, and recovery tends to be slower compared to younger patients.

## CLINICAL APPROACH

- *Initial management*: Discontinue rifampin and assess renal function (creatinine, electrolytes, urine output).
- *Treatment options* **(Table 1)**: Consider steroid therapy or rifampin desensitization once AKI improves.
- *Alternative drugs*: Use second-line TB medications such as fluoroquinolones or linezolid that are less nephrotoxic.
- *Monitor renal function*: Regularly assess renal parameters and reintroduce rifampin cautiously when renal function normalizes.

## PHARMACOKINETICS AND MODIFICATION REQUIREMENT OF ATT

Refer to **Table 1**.

## TREATMENT AND PREVENTION

In the management of isoniazid-resistant pulmonary tuberculosis with rifampin-induced AKI, treatment involves careful monitoring and adjustment of therapy. Rifampin may need to be temporarily discontinued until renal function improves, with the option of reintroducing it once the kidney injury resolves, potentially with the aid of a short course of steroids. Desensitization to rifampin is another strategy for reintroduction once renal parameters stabilize. Alternatively, second-line drugs such as fluoroquinolones and linezolid, which are renal-safe at all doses, can be used. Prevention includes early identification of drug resistance, close monitoring of renal function during treatment, and adjusting therapy to minimize renal toxicity while ensuring effective tuberculosis treatment.

**TABLE 1: Dosage adjustment of ATT according to established degree of renal function.**

| Antimycobacterial agent and normal dose | Established creatinine clearance (CrCL) | | | Intermittent hemodialysis (IHD) | Peritoneal dialysis (PD) | Comments and recommendations |
|---|---|---|---|---|---|---|
| | 30–60 mL/min | 10–29 mL/min | <10 mL/min | | | |
| Rifampicin 10 mg/kg/day up to 600 mg | No dose adjustment is required | | | | | It can be used safely in renal disease |
| Isoniazid 5 mg/kg/day up to 300 mg | | | | | | It can be used safely in renal disease |
| Pyrazinamide 25 mg/kg/day | No dose adjustment is required | 25–30 mg/kg q48h | 25–30 mg/kg 3 times/week | 25–30 mg/kg 3 times/week after dialysis sessions | No dose adjustment is required | It can be used safely in renal disease |
| Ethambutol 15 mg/kg/day | No dose adjustment is required | 15 mg/kg q48h | | 15 mg/kg 3 times/week after dialysis sessions | 15 mg/kg q48h | Avoid use unless essential in renal disease with CrCl <30 mL/min. The main route of clearance is renal |
| Levofloxacin 750-1,000 mg daily | 750–1,000 mg q48 h | 750–1,000 mg 3 times/week | | | Consult with a renal physician | Unlike moxifloxacin, levofloxacin is significantly eliminated by the kidneys; moxifloxacin may be preferred in significant renal impairment |
| Moxifloxacin 400 mg/day | No dose adjustment is required | | | | | |
| Bedaquiline 400 mg daily for 2 weeks; 200 mg thrice weekly thereafter | No dose adjustment is required | Use with caution and consider TDM | | | | No dose adjustment is recommended for mild to moderate renal impairment, but caution is recommended in more severe renal failure |
| Clofazimine 100 mg daily | No dose adjustment is required | | | | | It can be used safely in renal disease |
| Linezolid 600 mg/day | | | | | | It can be used with caution in renal disease |
| Streptomycin 15 mg/kg/day | 15 mg/kg individual doses with interval between doses adjusted to achieve undetectable plasma trough levels | | | | | It can be used with significant caution in renal disease. The main route of clearance is renal. Dose adjustment and therapeutic drug monitoring (TDM) are required. For hemodialysis patients, doses can be administered intravenously at the end of the dialysis session |
| Amikacin 15 mg/kg/day | | | | | | |
| Capreomycin 15 mg/kg/day | Capreomycin is no longer recommended for the treatment of drug-resistant tuberculosis. | | | | | |
| Prothionamide 15–20 mg/kg/day in divided doses | No dose adjustment is required | No dose adjustment is required | 250 mg q12h | | | It can be used in renal disease |
| Cycloserine 10–15 mg/kg/day in divided doses | 250 mg q12h | 250 mg q24h | 250 mg q24h | 250 mg q24h or 500 mg 3 times per week | 500 mg q48h or 3 times per week | Avoid if possible in renal disease. The main route of clearance is renal |
| Para-aminosalicylic acid (PAS) 8–12 g/day in divided doses | No dose adjustment required | 4g q12h | | | | Use with significant caution in renal disease. The main route of clearance is renal |
| Pretomanid 200 mg daily | There are no safety or efficacy data on use in patients with renal impairment or receiving renal replacement therapy. Use is not currently recommended | | | | | The main route of clearance of active drugs is extrarenal however, the pharmacokinetics of metabolites are not well understood currently |
| Delamanid 100 mg twice daily | No dose adjustment required with CrCl > 50 mL/min | There are no safety or efficacy data on use in patients with renal impairment or receiving renal replacement therapy. Use is not currently recommended | | | | |

## Points to Ponder

- *Rifampin-induced AKI*: Careful monitoring of renal function is essential when using rifampin, especially in patients with pre-existing conditions or drug resistance.
- *Managing isoniazid resistance*: In patients with isoniazid resistance, rifampin remains the primary first-line treatment, but its potential for nephrotoxicity requires close monitoring.
- *Renal-safe alternatives*: Second-line drugs like fluoroquinolones and linezolid can be effective and renal-safe alternatives when rifampin use is contraindicated.
- *Desensitization protocol*: Gradual reintroduction of rifampin through a desensitization protocol can be a viable option in patients with rifampin-induced AKI after renal recovery.
- *Steroid use in rifampin-induced AKI*: Short courses of steroids may help manage inflammatory responses in rifampin-induced AKI, aiding in renal recovery before reintroducing the drug.

## MULTIPLE CHOICE QUESTIONS

**1. What is the most likely cause of AKI in a patient with isoniazid-resistant pulmonary tuberculosis on rifampin?**

A. Acute tubular necrosis
B. Rifampin-induced AKI
C. Fluoroquinolone toxicity
D. Isoniazid toxicity

**2. Which of the following is an appropriate management option for rifampin-induced AKI in a patient with isoniazid-resistant tuberculosis?**

A. Continue rifampin without modification
B. Discontinue rifampin and start a second-line drug immediately
C. Temporarily stop rifampin and reintroduce once renal function improves
D. Switch to a different first-line drug

**3. Which second-line drug is renal-safe at all doses for managing tuberculosis in patients with rifampin-induced AKI?**

A. Isoniazid
B. Rifampin
C. Fluoroquinolones
D. Streptomycin

**4. What is the first step in managing a patient with rifampin-induced AKI and isoniazid resistance?**

A. Start a short course of steroids
B. Discontinue rifampin temporarily
C. Initiate dialysis
D. Increase the dose of rifampin

**5. How can the patient be desensitized to rifampin in the context of rifampin-induced AKI?**

A. By starting rifampin at a higher dose
B. Through gradual dose escalation after renal function improves
C. By using corticosteroids with rifampin
D. By switching to an alternative first-line drug

### Answers

1. (B); 2. (C); 3. (C); 4. (B); 5. (B)

## SUGGESTED READINGS


1. World Health Organization. Global Tuberculosis Report. Blood. 2015: 1–98 pp.
2. Nahid P, Dorman SE, Alipanah N, et al. Official American Thoracic Society/Centers for Disease Control and Prevention/Infectious Diseases Society of America Clinical Practice Guidelines: Treatment of Drug-Susceptible Tuberculosis. 2016;63:853-67.
3. Queensland Health. Treatment of tuberculosis in renal disease in adults. 2023;1-15.
4. Milburn H, Ashman N, Davies P, et al. Guidelines for the prevention and management of *Mycobacterium tuberculosis* infection and disease in adult patients with chronic kidney disease. Thorax. 2010;65(6): 559-70.
5. Kwon SH, Kim JH, Yang JO, et al. Erratum: Ethambutol-induced acute renal failure. Nephrol Dial Transplant. 2004;19(5):1335-6.
6. Trainin EB, Turin RD, Gomez-Leon G. Acute renal insufficiency complicating isoniazid therapy. Int J Pediatr Nephrol. 1981;2(1):53-4.
7. Kumar S, Mehta JA, Trivedi HL. Light-chain proteinuria and reversible renal failure in rifampin-treated patients with tuberculosis. Chest. 1976;70(4):564-5.
8. Chang CH, Chen YF, Wu VC, et al. Acute kidney injury due to anti-tuberculosis drugs: A five-year experience in an aging population. BMC Infect Dis. 2014;14:23.
9. Chen X. Chinese clinical practice guideline for acute kidney injury. National Medical Journal of China. 2023;103(42):3332-66.
10. Bedi RS. Management of Tuberculosis in Special Situations. Lung India. 2005;22(4):138-41.

CHAPTER 53

# An Approach to a Case of Post-renal Transplant Patient with Fever and Headache

*Sagar Khadanga*

**CASE VIGNETTE**

*Clinical presentation*: A 45-year-old male presents with fever (101°F) and headache for the past 3 days. He underwent a renal transplant 6 months ago and is on triple immunosuppressive therapy (tacrolimus, mycophenolate mofetil, and prednisone). There are no associated neurological deficits, seizures, or neck stiffness, but the patient complains of mild photophobia.

*Clinical concerns*: Given the patient's immunosuppressed state, the differential diagnosis includes:

*Infectious causes*: Opportunistic infections such as viral (CMV, HSV, or VZV), fungal (cryptococcal meningitis), bacterial (Listeria, nocardiosis), or parasitic (toxoplasmosis).

*Non-infectious causes*: Drug toxicity (e.g., tacrolimus-related neurotoxicity) or post-transplant lymphoproliferative disorder (PTLD).

## INITIAL EVALUATION

- *History*: Duration and progression of symptoms, compliance with immunosuppressants, recent exposures, and prophylactic regimens.
- *Examination*: Detailed neurological assessment for meningitis or focal deficits.
- *Investigations*:
  - *Blood tests*: CBC, renal function, CRP, and cultures.
  - *Serologies*: CMV, EBV, and toxoplasmosis.
  - *Lumbar puncture*: CSF analysis for cell count, glucose, protein, culture, and PCR for viral/fungal pathogens.
  - *Imaging*: MRI brain with contrast to evaluate for abscesses, meningoencephalitis, or PTLD.

## MANAGEMENT

- *Empiric therapy*: Initiate broad-spectrum antibiotics and antifungals (e.g., ceftriaxone + vancomycin + liposomal amphotericin B) while awaiting results. Adjust immunosuppressive therapy under infectious disease and nephrology guidance.
- *Specific treatment*: Tailored based on confirmed etiology, with close monitoring of graft function.

This approach highlights the complexity of managing infections and complications in postrenal transplant patients, emphasizing early and aggressive evaluation to prevent adverse outcomes.

## PROVISIONAL DIAGNOSIS

Opportunistic infection (e.g., cryptococcal meningitis or CMV encephalitis) in an immunosuppressed postrenal transplant patient presenting with fever and headache.

## DIFFERENTIAL DIAGNOSIS

- *Infectious causes*: Cryptococcal meningitis, CMV/EBV encephalitis, bacterial meningitis (e.g., Listeria), or nocardiosis.
- *Noninfectious causes*: Tacrolimus neurotoxicity, post-transplant lymphoproliferative disorder (PTLD), or metabolic disturbances.

## PATHOPHYSIOLOGY

Post-transplant immunosuppression reduces the host's immune defense, particularly T-cell-mediated immunity, predisposing the patient to opportunistic infections. Reactivation of latent infections or new infections with pathogens like *Cryptococcus* or CMV is common, leading to systemic or CNS involvement manifesting as fever and headache.

## CLINICAL APPROACH

- *History*: Focus on transplant timeline, immunosuppressant regimen, and infection prophylaxis.
- *Examination*: Assess for signs of meningitis, focal deficits, or systemic involvement.
- *Investigations*:
  - *Blood*: CBC, inflammatory markers, cultures, and serologies for opportunistic infections.
  - *CSF analysis*: Evaluate for infectious pathogens.
  - *Imaging*: MRI brain for structural abnormalities.

## TREATMENT AND PREVENTION

Management involves hospitalization and initiation of empiric therapy, including antibiotics (e.g., ceftriaxone, vancomycin), antifungals (liposomal amphotericin B), or antivirals (ganciclovir) based on the most likely etiology. Immunosuppressants may be adjusted with nephrology consultation. Definitive therapy is tailored to identified pathogens, with close monitoring of graft function and patient response.

Prevention includes strict adherence to infection prophylaxis (e.g., cotrimoxazole for PCP, valganciclovir for CMV), regular monitoring of infection markers, and vaccination before transplantation. Education on early symptom recognition and regular follow-ups are crucial to minimize morbidity and mortality in post-transplant patients.

## Points to Ponder

- Fever and headache in a postrenal transplant patient require urgent evaluation due to the high risk of life-threatening opportunistic infections.
- *Cryptococcus neoformans* and CMV encephalitis are key pathogens to consider in post-transplant CNS infections.
- Early lumbar puncture and brain imaging are critical for diagnosing CNS involvement while ruling out contraindications for the procedure.
- Drug interactions between immunosuppressants and antimicrobial agents must be carefully managed.
- Prevention through infection prophylaxis and vaccination pretransplant significantly reduces morbidity.

## MULTIPLE CHOICE QUESTIONS

**1. Which of the following is the most common opportunistic fungal infection in postrenal transplant patients presenting with fever and headache?**
A. *Candida albicans*
B. *Cryptococcus neoformans*
C. *Aspergillus fumigatus*
D. *Histoplasma capsulatum*

**2. What is the most specific diagnostic test for cryptococcal meningitis?**
A. CSF gram stain
B. CSF India ink preparation
C. CSF cryptococcal antigen test
D. Serum galactomannan test

**3. Which immunosuppressant is most commonly associated with neurotoxicity?**
A. Tacrolimus
B. Mycophenolate mofetil
C. Cyclosporine
D. Prednisone

**4. What is the first-line empiric treatment for suspected bacterial meningitis in an immunosuppressed patient?**
A. Piperacillin-tazobactam
B. Ceftriaxone and vancomycin
C. Meropenem and linezolid
D. Ciprofloxacin and metronidazole

**5. What is the primary prophylactic drug for preventing *Pneumocystis jirovecii* pneumonia (PCP) in postrenal transplant patients?**
A. Cotrimoxazole
B. Dapsone
C. Azithromycin
D. Valganciclovir

### Answers

1. (B); 2. (C); 3. (A); 4. (B); 5. (A)

## SUGGESTED READINGS


1. Fishman JA. Infection in Solid-Organ Transplant Recipients. New England Journal of Medicine. 2007;357(25):2601-4.
2. Cohen J, Powderly WG, Opal SM. Infectious Diseases. 4th Edition, Elsevier, 2016.
3. Perfect JR, Dismukes WE, Pappas PG et al. Clinical Practice Guidelines for the Management of Cryptococcal Disease. Clinical Infectious Diseases: 2010 update by the infectious diseases society of America. Clin Infect Dis. 2010;50(3):291-322.
4. Abbo LM, Grossi PA. Surgical site infections: Guidelines from the American Society of Transplantation Infectious Diseases Community of Practice. Clinical Transplantation [Internet]. 2019;33(9).
5. Kumar D, Humar A. Opportunistic Infections in Transplantation. Infectious Disease Clinics of North America. 2010;24(2):461-76.
6. Singh N, Paterson DL. Approach to Fever and Infections in Solid-Organ Transplant Recipients. Clinical Microbiology Reviews. 2005;18(1):71-108.
7. Alangaden GJ. Infectious Complications of Renal Transplantation. Critical Care Clinics. 2019;35(1):185-207.

CHAPTER 54

# An Approach to a Case of Asymptomatic Renal Cyst

*Puranjoy Chakrabarty, Arunangshu Banerjee*

**CASE VIGNETTE**

Mr Kumar, 58-year-old software engineer working in a MNC visited his local physician in a perplexed state. He informed that he was having a chronic backache for last few months especially toward the evening. His friends and office colleagues have warned him that his symptoms might be due to kidney ailments and so he went through a whole-body checkup including ultrasound of abdomen. Ultrasound had reported fatty liver and a simple cyst in the right kidney. After examination and going through his reports, Mr Kumar was assured by his physician of the benign nature of his cyst and only asked to follow a healthy lifestyle and proper hydration.

## PROVISIONAL DIAGNOSIS

- Simple renal cyst (asymptomatic)
- Fatty liver
- Mechanical backpain

## DIFFERENTIAL DIAGNOSIS

- Complex renal cyst
- Acquired cystic renal disease

## CLINICAL APPROACH

Renal cysts are a common finding often detected incidentally during abdominal imaging for other causes. Majority of them are simple renal cysts which are acquired and their prevalence increases with age reaching up to 50% above 50 years of age as reported in some autopsy series. They are thin walled completely fluid-filled renal mass of epithelial origin; are usually asymptomatic and do not warrant any further investigation other than surveillance based on their grade. Apart from simple renal cysts, other inherited causes constitute a spectrum of renal cystic disorders which can be classified for easier understanding and approach.

### Etiological Classification of Renal Cysts

- *Autosomal dominant polycystic kidney disease (ADPKD)*:
  - Classic ADPKD of adults and older children
  - ADPKD in infants (in the spectrum of glomerulocystic disease)
  - Classic ADPKD associated with, tuberous sclerosis (''contiguous gene syndrome'': *ADPKD-TSC/TSC2-PKD1)*
- *Autosomal recessive polycystic kidney disease (ARPKD)*:
  - Classic ARPKD of newborn and young infants
  - ARPKD and congenital hepatic fibrosis in older children and adults
- Unilateral renal cystic disease (URCD) or localized or segmental cystic disease of the kidney
- Solitary and multiple renal simple cysts
- *Dysplastic kidney*:
  - Multicystic dysplastic kidney
  - Hypoplastic dysplastic kidney
- Pluricystic kidney of multiple malformations syndromes (e.g., diffuse cystic dysplasia of the kidney)
- Juvenile nephronophthisis (JNPHP) and medullary cystic kidney disease (MCKD)
- Medullary sponge kidney
- Glomerulocystic kidney disease (GCKD)
- Multilocular renal cyst–cystic nephroma (MLC–CN) and congeners
- *Renal cysts in hereditary syndromes*:
  - Tuberous sclerosis (TSC)
  - Von Hippel–Lindau syndrome (VHL)
- Renal lymphangioma/peripyelic-pericalyceal lymphangiectasis
- Acquired renal cystic disease
- Renal cell carcinoma with cystic change
- Pseudocystic change of the kidney

## SIMPLE RENAL CYST

Majority of the cysts encountered in clinical practice are like the one mentioned in the case vignette. A cyst is termed simple when the following criteria are met as per radiological consensus and reporting on ultrasound:

- Anechoic
- Homogenous content
- Posterior enhancement
- Imperceptible wall

On computed tomography, these cysts are classified according to Morton Bosniak classification system **(Table 1)** when they meet the following criteria:

- Water attenuation (– to +15 HU)
- Homogenous
- *Post contrast*:
  - o Homogenous
  - o <+10 HU increase in attenuation
- Imperceptible wall

Management depends on the grade of the cyst and change if any over time.

## POLYCYSTIC KIDNEY DISEASE

Among the inherited etiologies, polycystic kidney diseases are relatively common. Autosomal dominant polycystic kidney disease is a disease associated with bilateral renal cysts which enlarge in size and distort the architecture of the kidneys with increasing age. *PKD1* and *PKD2* genes have been implicated; other complex associations are also found as in childhood onset or rapidly progressing phenotypes. For example, "contiguous gene syndrome" as in *PKD1* and *TSC* gene. End-stage renal disease is encountered in sixth or seventh decades. Asynchronous or unilateral or asymmetrical ADPKD has also been described. Family history, intracranial aneurysm, hepatic cysts and slow progression to ESRD are its characteristics.

Autosomal recessive polycystic disease is associated with *PKHD1* gene mutation and has a neonatal or early childhood presentation. Associated Potters sequence, hepatic fibrosis and ESRD in childhood differentiates it from ADPKD.

## ACQUIRED RENAL CYSTIC DISEASE

Bilateral renal cysts encountered in patients undergoing dialysis probably due to accumulation of growth factors. 40–90% of dialysis patients have this condition depending on the duration of dialysis. Increased propensity for papillary tumors and other renal cell carcinomas warrants strict vigilance.

## GENETIC SYNDROMES

Commonly encountered in neonates and early childhood, this spectrum includes varied diseases with genetic mutations and variable cortico-medullary renal cysts. Hyperuricemia is a common finding. Common implicated genes include *NPHP1, NPHP2, FHJN,* and *UMOD*. Diseases included are:

- Juvenile nephronophthisis
- Medullary cystic kidney disease
- Familial hyperuricemic juvenile nephropathy

Among others that need mention include medullary sponge kidneys (MSK) which is a nongenetically transmitted disease involving papillary duct ectasia which take the "bouquet of flower" appearance. Nephrolithiasis with staghorn calculi is the major clinical presentation.

## GLOMERULOCYSTIC KIDNEY DISEASE (GCKD)

This group of diseases is characterized by Bowman's space and proximal convoluted tubule dilation resulting in renal cortical cysts. Infantile type is associated with ADPKD while sporadic type is found in older individuals. Familial GCKD occurs due to HNF-1β mutation and present with smaller kidneys.

Glomerulocystic kidneys on the other hand represent kidneys in the background of complex inheritable malformation syndromes like tuberous sclerosis, oral-*facial* -digital syndrome–type I, brachymesomelia renal syndrome, trisomy 13, short-rib-polydactyly syndrome–Majewski type and Saldino-Noonan type.

## PATHOPHYSIOLOGY

Various intrinsic mechanism work in an orchestrated fashion to lead to renal cyst formation. The most accepted theory is cyst formation starts at the level of distal tubules as simple outpouchings of tubular epithelium. Among inherited diseases, autosomal dominant polycystic kidney disease provides a model to understand the molecular mechanism of cyst formation. *PKD1* and *PKD2* genes encode polycystin-1 and polycystin-2 proteins which play an important role in calcium mediated intracellular signaling pathways. Elevated levels of cAMP can lead to excess Cl-driven fluid secretion which leads to dilation of the tubules and subsequent cyst formation. Other theories like loss planar cell polarity assist in cyst expansion.

## TREATMENT AND PREVENTION

Simple renal cysts are treated as per their grades where IIF onwards surveillance is needed at 3, 6, 9, and 12 months and annually therafter. Symptomatic simple cysts (pain, hemorrhage, recurrent infections or uncontrolled hypertension) may be treated by image guided aspiration (with or without sclerotic agents) or surgical excision (open/laparoscopic/robotic). Ethanol sclerotherapy is more popular although recurrence and complications like extravasation or bleeding are sometimes encountered.

**TABLE 1: Bosniak classification of renal cysts.**

| Stage | Cyst wall | Septa | Calcification | Enhancement |
|---|---|---|---|---|
| I | Hairline thin | No | No | No |
| II | Minimal regular thickening | Few, hairline septa | Smooth, hairline thin | No |
| IIF* | Minimal regular thickening | Multiple, minimal smooth thickening | Thick, nodular | No |
| III | Irregular thickening | Measurably, thick irregular | Thick, nodular, irregular | Yes |
| IV | Gross irregular thickening | Irregular gross thickening | Thich, nodular, irregular | Yes, tissue and cyst |

*F: follow-up.

Treatment for ADPKD has advanced with robust trials like TEMPO and REPRISE showing evidences for efficacy of tolvaptan in slowing renal disease progression in selective patients.

Renal cell carcinoma is increasingly encountered in patients with renal cysts. Vigilance for the same is essential through image based follow-up documenting any sudden increase in size or character of cyst. Clinically red flag signs like hematuria, weight loss and pain should prompt a re-evaluation with necessary imaging.

## Points to Ponder

- Renal cysts are common and majority are simple renal cysts which needs only surveillance rarely.
- Inherited causes include syndromes and disorders which need identification and management.
- PCKD is common, genetic and slowly progressive renal disease which now can be managed with disease modifying agents like tolvaptan.
- Symptomatic renal cysts may need surgical interventions.
- Vigilance for renal cell carcinoma is warranted in background of complex cysts and genetic syndromes.

## MULTIPLE CHOICE QUESTIONS

**1. True about renal cyst is:**

A. All renal cysts should be evaluated with CT scan
B. Renal cysts may be associated with hypertension
C. Polycystic kidney disease is always autosomal dominant
D. Renal cysts never lead to malignancies

**2. All may be associated with renal cyst except:**

A. Cortical tuber
B. Hematuria
C. Weight loss
D. Ovarian cyst

**3. ADPKD least associated with:**

A. Hepatic cysts
B. Thunderclap headache
C. Primary biliary cirrhosis
D. Hypertension

**4. Smoking is associated with all except:**

A. Alzheimer's disease
B. Renal cyst
C. SCC
D. Coronary artery disease

**5. Pathophysiology of renal cyst generation includes:**

A. Cyclic AMP
B. Chloride channels
C. PKD1 and 2 genes
D. All of the above

### Answers

1. (B); 2. (D); 3. (C); 4. (A); 5. (D)

## SUGGESTED READINGS


1. Ferro F, Vezzali N, Comploj E, et al. Pediatric cystic diseases of the kidney. J Ultrasound. 2019;22(3):381-93.
2. Chin HJ, Ro H, Lee HJ, et al. The clinical significances of simple renal cyst: is it related to hypertension or renal dysfunction? Kidney Int 2006;70:1468-73.
3. Bisceglia M, Galliani CA, Senger C, et al. Renal cystic diseases: a review. Adv Anat Pathol. 2006;13(1):26-56.
4. Satariano M, Ghose S, Raina R. The Pathophysiology of Inherited Renal Cystic Diseases. Genes. 2024;15(1):91.
5. Hélénon O, Crosnier A, Verkarre V, et al. Simple and complex renal cysts in adults: Classification system for renal cystic masses. Diagnostic and Interventional Imaging. 2018;99(4):189-218.
6. Skolarikos A, Laguna MP, De La Rosette JJ. Conservative and radiological management of simple renal cysts: a comprehensive review. BJU International. 2012;110(2):170-8.
7. Eknoyan G. A clinical view of simple and complex renal cysts. J Am Soc Nephrol. 2009;20:1874-6.
8. Terada N, Arai Y, Kinukawa N, et al. The 10-year natural history of simple renal cysts . Urology. 2008;71:7-12.
9. Okeke AA, Mitchelmore AE, Keeley FX Jr, et al. A comparison of aspiration and sclerotherapy with laparoscopic de-roofing in the management of symptomatic simple renal cysts. BJU Int. 2003;92: 610-3.

CHAPTER 55

# A Case-based Approach to Secondary Myopathies

*Siddharth Singh, Anand Dev, Abhay Kumar, Santosh Kumar Nayan, Santosh Kumar Swain*

**CASE VIGNETTE**

Sunita Devi (name changed), a 60-year-old female farmer from rural Bihar, has a history of poorly controlled type 2 diabetes for over 20 years, along with hypothyroidism for 10 years as well as primary hyperparathyroidism for past three years. Her medical history also includes hypertension, hyperlipidemia, chronic kidney disease, and obesity (BMI 35). Limited healthcare access and irregular medication adherence have exacerbated her condition.

Sunita presented to the Indira Gandhi Institute of Medical Sciences (IGIMS) in Patna with a one-year history of worsening muscle weakness, particularly in her thighs and shoulders, making it difficult to climb stairs or rise from a seated position. She reported severe fatigue, muscle cramps, intermittent pain, unintentional weight loss, and persistent dry skin.

On physical examination, she exhibited proximal muscle weakness (3/5), visible atrophy in her thighs, diminished deep tendon reflexes, mild peripheral neuropathy with reduced sensation in her feet, and dry skin with generalized oedema. Her medication regimen included metformin, levothyroxine, amlodipine, atorvastatin, and losartan.

## CLINICAL FINDINGS AND INVESTIGATIONS

- *Lab values:*
  - Fasting blood glucose 220 mg/dL, HbA1c 9.8%
  - Creatine kinase 600 IU/L
  - TSH 25 (elevated), low Free T4
  - Serum calcium 11.5 mg/dL, PTH 120 pg/mL (elevated), vitamin D 15 ng/mL
  - Elevated AST and ALT, normal electrolytes, negative autoimmune panel
- *Imaging and biopsy:*
  - MRI of thighs showed increased signal intensity in T2-weighted images.
  - DEXA scan indicated Osteopenia.
  - Muscle biopsy revealed muscle fiber necrosis, increased connective tissue, inflammatory cell infiltration, and muscle fiber regeneration with atrophy.

## PROVISIONAL DIAGNOSIS

Proximal myopathy, secondary to poorly controlled diabetes and hypothyroidism, compounded by chronic kidney disease and primary hyperparathyroidism.

## DIFFERENTIAL DIAGNOSIS

- Diabetic myopathy
- Hypothyroid myopathy
- Hyper parathyroid myopathy
- Chronic kidney disease-related myopathy
- Inflammatory myopathies (e.g., polymyositis)
- Drug-induced myopathy (e.g., statins)

## CLINICAL APPROACH

Approaching a case of secondary myopathy requires a thorough understanding of the complex interplay between systemic diseases and muscle pathology. This involves a comprehensive evaluation process that integrates clinical insights with advanced diagnostic tools to accurately diagnose and effectively manage the underlying conditions contributing to muscle dysfunction (**Flowchart 1**).

- *Laboratory test:* As per our differential diagnosis
- *Electromyography (EMG):* Short duration and decreased amplitude of action potential
- *Muscle biopsy:* Reveals muscle fiber necrosis, increased connective tissue, inflammatory cell infiltration, and muscle fiber regeneration with atrophy.
- *Imaging (MRI):* An MRI of the thighs reveals increased signal intensity on T2-weighted images, indicating muscle inflammation and edema, along with fatty infiltration and muscle atrophy.

## PATHOPHYSIOLOGY

Secondary myopathies arise as a result of systemic diseases, metabolic derangements, or hormonal imbalances rather than the primary muscle pathology. Key mechanism includes:

- *Endocrine disorders:* Conditions like hypothyroidism, hyperthyroidism, and Cushing's syndrome disrupt normal muscle metabolism. Hypothyroidism leads to impaired protein synthesis and accumulation of glycosaminoglycans, resulting in muscle weakness and myalgia.

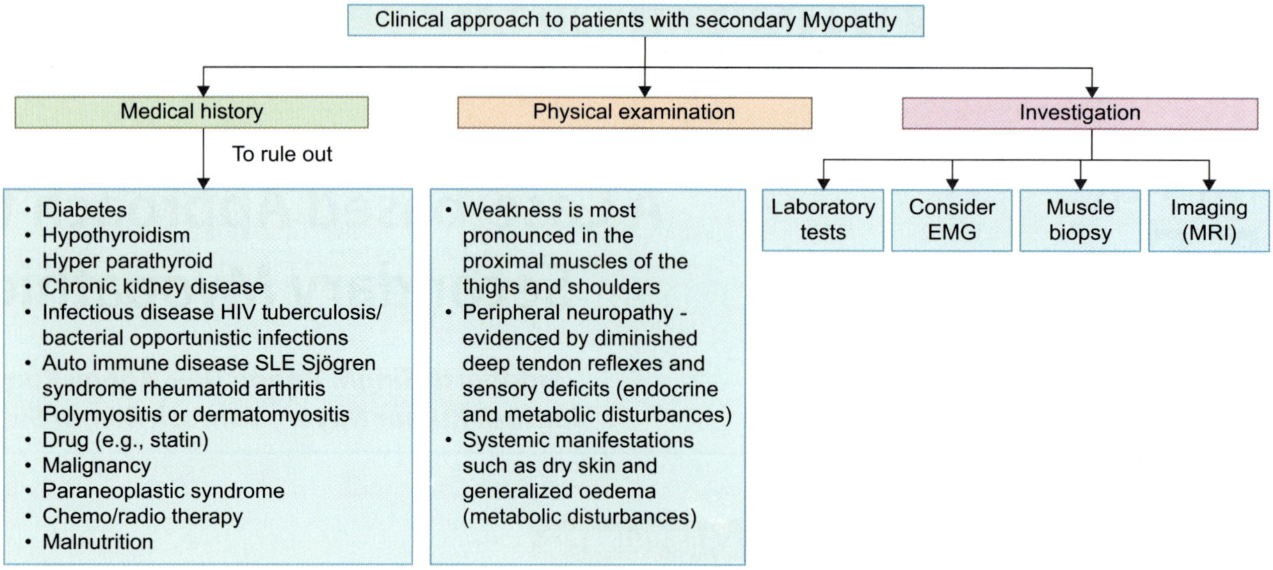


**FLOWCHART 1:** Showing the clinical approach to patients with secondary myopathy.

- *Metabolic disorders:* Poorly controlled diabetes can result in diabetic myopathy through microvascular damage, chronic inflammation, and oxidative stress. This contributes to muscular atrophy and reduced strength.
- *Electrolyte imbalances:* Abnormal levels of calcium, potassium, or magnesium, often seen in chronic kidney disease or hyperparathyroidism, impair neuromuscular transmission and muscle function.
- *Chronic inflammatory states:* Conditions like rheumatoid arthritis or systemic lupus erythematosus cause muscle inflammation, mitochondrial dysfunction, and atrophy.
- *Medications:* Long-term use of corticosteroids or statins can lead to steroid-induced or statin-associated myopathy, characterized by muscle weakness, and myonecrosis.

These factors combine to impair muscle structure and function, further resulting in weakness, atrophy, and associated symptoms.

## TREATMENT AND PREVENTION

- *Improving glycemic control:* Initiated Insulin glargine 20 units subcutaneously at bedtime and Insulin lispro 10 units before each meal. Continued metformin 500 mg twice daily, and added liraglutide 0.6 mg daily, titrating up as tolerated.
- *Managing thyroid dysfunction:* Levothyroxine was increased to 75 mcg daily based on the TSH levels.
- *Treating Hyperparathyroidism:* Parathyroidectomy was considered; initiated calcitriol 0.25 mcg daily and calcium carbonate 500 mg twice daily.
- *Comprehensive management:* Addressed chronic kidney disease and its complications, physical therapy, nutritional support, pain management, and bone health with calcium 1,000 mg daily, vitamin D 1,000 IU daily, and bisphosphonates (alendronate 70 mg weekly).

### Points to Ponder

- *Interconnectedness of endocrine disorders*: Understanding the physiological interactions between diabetes, hypothyroidism, and hyperparathyroidism is crucial, as these conditions collectively impact muscle metabolism, leading to significant muscle weakness.
- *Role of hormonal imbalances in myopathy*: Elevated blood glucose and calcium levels, along with the altered thyroid function, can exacerbate muscle protein catabolism and impair muscle repair mechanisms, highlighting the need for targeted endocrine management.
- Understanding the link between systemic diseases and muscle pathology is crucial for accurate diagnosis and treatment.
- Clinicians must adopt a holistic, patient-centered approach to manage secondary myopathies effectively.

## MULTIPLE CHOICE QUESTIONS

1. **What is the most likely cause of Sunita's proximal muscle weakness and muscle cramps?**
   A. Hypothyroidism
   B. Hyperlipidemia
   C. Hyperparathyroidism-induced hypercalcemia
   D. Chronic kidney disease-related mineral imbalance
2. **Which of the following symptoms in Sunita is most consistent with chronic hypothyroidism?**
   A. Muscle cramps
   B. Dry skin and generalized edema
   C. Peripheral neuropathy
   D. Weight loss
3. **What could be a contributing factor to Sunita's peripheral neuropathy?**
   A. Diabetes mellitus
   B. Primary hyperparathyroidism
   C. Obesity
   D. Hypothyroidism
4. **Which investigation would be the most useful to evaluate Sunita's proximal muscle weakness?**
   A. Serum calcium and parathyroid hormone levels
   B. Nerve conduction studies
   C. Serum creatine kinase levels
   D. Thyroid function tests
5. **What lifestyle modification should be prioritized for Sunita's management?**
   A. Weight loss and dietary adjustments
   B. Intensive physical therapy
   C. Reduction in statin dosage
   D. Increased fluid intake

### Answers

1. (D); 2. (B); 3. (A); 4. (C); 5. (A)

## SUGGESTED READINGS

1. Adams RD, Victor M, Ropper AH, et al. Principles of Neurology. Neuropsychiatry, Neuropsychology & Behavioral Neurology. 1997;10(3):220.
2. Engel A, Franzini-Armstrong C. Myology: Basic and Clinical. McGraw-Hill Medical Publishing; 2004.
3. Loscalzo J, Fauci AS, Kasper DL, et al. Harrison's Principles of Internal Medicine, Twenty-First Edition (Vol. 1 & Vol. 2). McGraw Hill Professional; 2022.
4. Lazarou IN, Guerne PA. Classification, diagnosis, and management of idiopathic inflammatory myopathies. J Rheumatol. 2013;40(5):550-64.
5. Dalakas, MC. Inflammatory Muscle Diseases. N Engl J Med. 2006;355(9):917-27.
6. Barohn RJ. Approach to the patient with muscle disease: A six-step plan. Cleveland Clinic Journal of Medicine, 2003;70(5):409-22.
7. Dimachkie MM, Barohn RJ. Idiopathic inflammatory myopathies. Neurologic Clinics. 2024;32(3):595-628.
8. Feltkamp TE, Kirkpatrick P, & Myones BL. Secondary myopathies. Current Opinion in Rheumatology 2001;13(6):521-25.
9. Bohan A, Peter JB. Polymyositis and dermatomyositis (first of two parts). N Engl J Med. 1970;292(7):344-7.
10. Silliman CC, Peterson PK. Bacterial infections in HIV-infected patients. Infectious Disease Clinics of North America 1993;7(2):373-92.

CHAPTER 56

# An Approach to a Case of Atypical Parkinsonism

*S Sreenivas*

**CASE VIGNETTE**

A 70-year-old man Mr X presents with Gait difficulty and a tendency to fall backwards. Mr X also complaints of difficulty walking downstairs. On examination patient has a characteristic expression of surprise and has an inability to stop clapping after being asked to clap threetimes. What is the diagnosis?

## PROVISIONAL DIAGNOSIS

The diagnosis is progressive supranuclear palsy.

Explanation of symptoms and signs **(Fig. 1)**:

- The frequent backward falls is because of increased extensor tone and postural instability.
- Difficulty walking downstairs is because of the combination of retrocollis and impaired downgaze.
- Characteristic expression of surprise (PROCERUS SIGN) is due to facial dystonia.
- Inability to stop clapping after three times (APPLAUSE SIGN) is a nonspecific sign of frontal lobe dysfunction.

## DIFFERENTIAL DIAGNOSES

The differential diagnosis of Parkinson's disease (PD) are:

- Idiopathic PD
- Parkinsonian syndromes
- Progressive supranuclear palsy
- Multisystem atrophy (MSA)
- MSA-parkinsonian (striatonigral degeneration)
- MSA-cerebellar (olivopontocerebellar degeneration, sporadic form)
- MSA-autonomic (Shy–Drager syndrome)
- Diffuse Lewy body disease

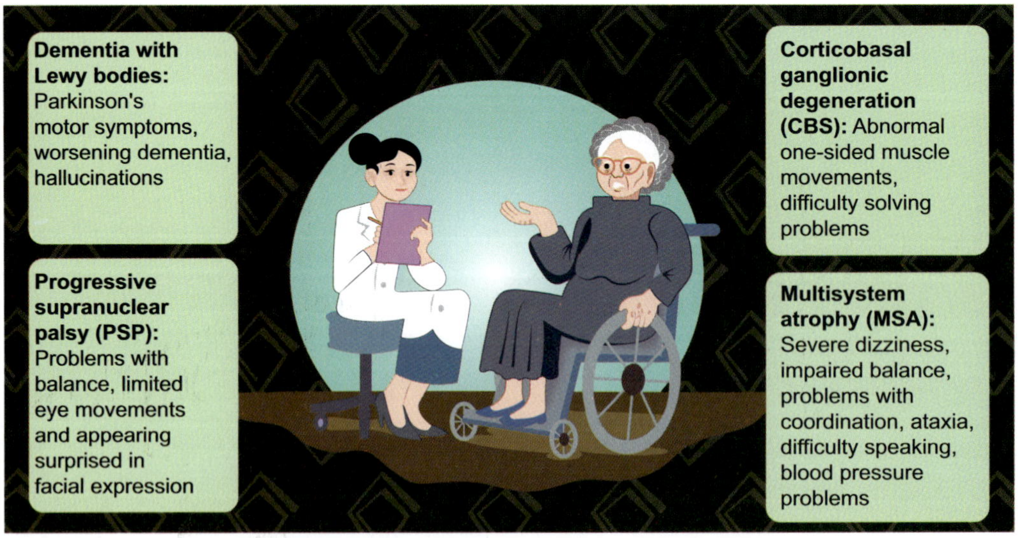


**FIG. 1:** Types and symptoms of atypical Parkinson's disease.
*Source*: ©Verywell/Ellen Lindner.

- Corticobasal degeneration
- Drug-induced parkinsonism
- Dopa-responsive dystonia
- Other non-Parkinson's akinetic-rigid syndromes
- Huntington's disease (rigid or juvenile form)
- Wilson's disease
- Essential tremor.

## CLINICAL APPROACH

Clinical features suggesting an atypical Parkinsonism are as follows in **Table 1**.

## PATHOPHYSIOLOGY (FIG. 2)

Atypical Parkinsonism encompasses several neurodegenerative disorders that share some symptoms with Parkinson's disease

**TABLE 1: Signs and symptoms with possible alternate diagnoses for atypical Parkinsonism.**

| Symptoms/Signs | Alternative diagnosis to consider |
|---|---|
| ***History*** | |
| Early speech and gait impairment (lack of tremor, lack of motor asymmetry, early falls) | Atypical parkinsonism |
| Exposure to neuroleptics | Drug-induced parkinsonism |
| Onset prior to age 40 years | Genetic form of PD, Wilson's disease, DRD |
| Liver disease | Wilson's disease, non-Wilsonian hepatolenticular degeneration |
| Early hallucinations and dementia with later development of PD features | Dementia with Lewy bodies |
| Diplopia, impaired vertical gaze | PSP |
| Poor or no response to an adequate trial of levodopa | Atypical or secondary parkinsonism |
| ***Physical examination*** | |
| Dementia as first or early feature | Dementia with Lewy bodies |
| Prominent orthostatic hypotension | MSAP |
| Prominent cerebellar signs | MSAC |
| Slow saccades with impaired downgaze | PSP |
| High-frequency (6–10 Hz) symmetric postural tremor with a prominent kinetic component | Essential tremor |

(DRD: dopa-responsive dystonia; MSAC: multiple system atrophy–cerebellar type; MSAP: multiple system atrophy–Parkinson's type; PD: Parkinson's disease; PSP: progressive supranuclear palsy)

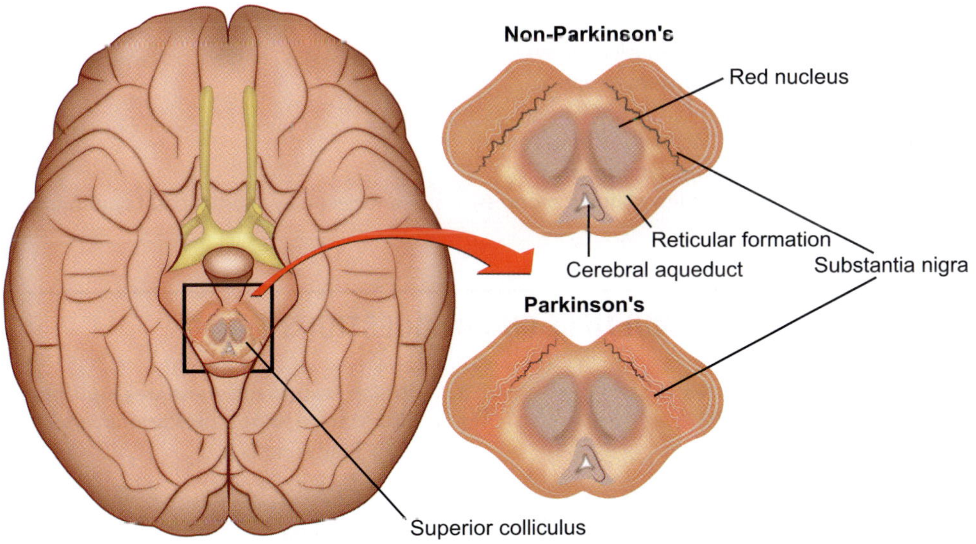


**FIG. 2:** Pathophysiology: Atypical Parkinsonism.

*Source*: © Medical gallery of Blausen Medical 2014. WikiJournal of Medicine 1 (2), 2014.

(PD) but have distinct clinical features, faster progression, and poorer response to dopaminergic therapy. These include:

- *Progressive supranuclear palsy (PSP)*: Characterized by tau protein accumulation, which leads to neuronal damage in brainstem structures, basal ganglia, and the frontal cortex, resulting in postural instability, supranuclear gaze palsy, and cognitive decline.
- *Multiple system atrophy (MSA)*: Involves glial cytoplasmic inclusions and neuronal loss affecting various systems, including the cerebellum, basal ganglia, and autonomic systems, leading to parkinsonism, cerebellar ataxia, and autonomic dysfunction.
- *Corticobasal degeneration (CBD)*: Exhibits asymmetric cortical atrophy and tau protein deposition, manifesting as parkinsonism, alien limb syndrome, and cognitive dysfunction.

## TREATMENT AND PREVENTION

*Dementia with Lewy bodies (DLB)*: Involves the widespread presence of Lewy bodies (alpha-synuclein inclusions) in the cortex, leading to parkinsonism with early cognitive decline and visual hallucinations.

### Treatment

Refer to **Flowchart 1**.

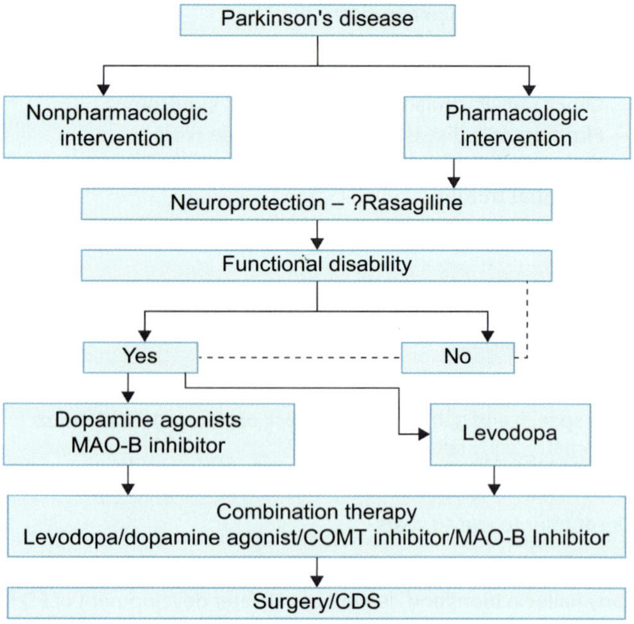


**FLOWCHART 1:** Parkinson's disease management.

*Note*: Nonpharmacologic intervention-Exercise is generally recommended for all PD patients as it increases enkephalins, endorphins and dopamine.

(CDS: continuous dopaminergic stimulation; COMT: catechol-O-methyltransferase; MAO-B: monoamine oxidase type B)

### Points to Ponder

- Clinically PD is characterized by tetrad of TRAP—T: Tremor; R: Rigidity; A: Akinesia; P: Postural disturbances.
- Features predictive of atypical parkinsonism:
  - Rapid disease progression.
  - Early gait instability, falls.
  - Absence or paucity of tremor.
  - Irregular jerky tremor, myoclonus.
  - Poor or absent response to levodopa.
- Additional features of atypical parkinsonism:
  - Abnormal eye movements (Progressive supranuclear palsy).
  - Pyramidal tract/cerebellar signs (Multiple system atrophy).
  - Dysautonomia (Multiple system atrophy).
  - Severe dysarthria, dysphonia or stridor (Multiple system atrophy).
  - Apraxia, alien limb, myoclonus (Corticobasal syndrome).
  - Early prominent dementia (Dementia with lewy bodies, progressive supranuclear palsy/corticobasal syndrome).

## MULTIPLE CHOICE QUESTIONS

**1. Which of the following is a hallmark feature of progressive supranuclear palsy (PSP)?**
A. Resting tremor
B. Supranuclear gaze palsy
C. Bradykinesia
D. Hypokinetic dysarthria

**2. Atypical parkinsonism is characterized by all of the following except:**
A. Rapid disease progression
B. Absence or paucity of tremor
C. Strong response to levodopa
D. Early gait instability and falls

**3. Which feature differentiates multiple system atrophy (MSA) from idiopathic Parkinson's disease?**
A. Bradykinesia
B. Autonomic dysfunction
C. Rest tremor
D. Akinesia

**4. Which of the following is not a common feature of corticobasal degeneration (CBD)?**
A. Alien limb phenomenon
B. Apraxia
C. Supranuclear palsy
D. Cognitive decline

5. **Which protein accumulation is primarily implicated in progressive supranuclear palsy (PSP)?**
   A. Alpha-synuclein
   B. Tau protein
   C. Amyloid plaques
   D. Beta-amyloid

## Answers

1. (B); 2. (C); 3. (B); 4. (C); 5. (B)

## SUGGESTED READINGS


1. Williams DR, Lees AJ. Progressive supranuclear palsy: clinicopathological concepts and diagnostic challenges. The Lancet Neurology. 2009;8(3):270-9.
2. Wenning GK, Stankovic I, Vignatelli L, et al. The Movement Disorder Society Criteria for the diagnosis of multiple system atrophy. Movement Disorders [Internet]. 2022 Apr 21;37(6):1131-48.
3. Goedert M, Spillantini MG, Del Tredici K, et al. 100 years of Lewy pathology. Nature Reviews Neurology. 2012;9(1):13-24.
4. Stankovic I, Wenning GK. Neuropsychiatric manifestations in atypical parkinsonian syndromes. In: Neuropsychiatric symptoms of neurological disease. 2014. pp. 141-70.
5. Armstrong MJ, Litvan I, Lang AE, et al. Criteria for the diagnosis of corticobasal degeneration. Neurology. 2013;80(5):496-503
6. Papp MI, Kahn JE, Lantos PL. Glial cytoplasmic inclusions in the CNS of patients with multiple system atrophy (striatonigral degeneration, olivopontocerebellar atrophy and Shy-Drager syndrome). Journal of the Neurological Sciences. 1989;94(1–3):79-100.

CHAPTER
57

# An Approach to a Case of Subarachnoid Hemorrhage from a Physician's Perspective

*Pavithra Ravi, Mugundhan Krishnan*

## CASE VIGNETTE

A 55-year-old man with a history of type 2 diabetes presented to the emergency department after developing a sudden severe headache in the posterior neck and radiating to the top of his head. He had no other neurologic symptoms. The patient had no history of alcohol or tobacco use. He took metformin daily for diabetes. On examination, his blood pressure was 155/88 mm Hg, heart rate was 81 bpm, respiratory rate was 22 breaths/min, and oxygen saturation was 98% on room air. He was conscious and oriented. Cranial nerves, spinomotor examination and sensation were all intact. His laboratory values were within normal limits except for glucose of 296 mg/dL. Plain CT brain was taken which showed acute subarachnoid hemorrhage (SAH) in the premedullary, prepontine, and perimesencephalic cisterns and further extended into the suprasellar, sylvian, and the quadrigeminal cisterns. MRI brain with MRA and MRV showed no other abnormalities except SAH. CT angiography was performed but in which no cerebrovascular abnormalities were detected. Especially, no intracranial aneurysm or vertebral artery dissection was seen **(Fig. 1)**.

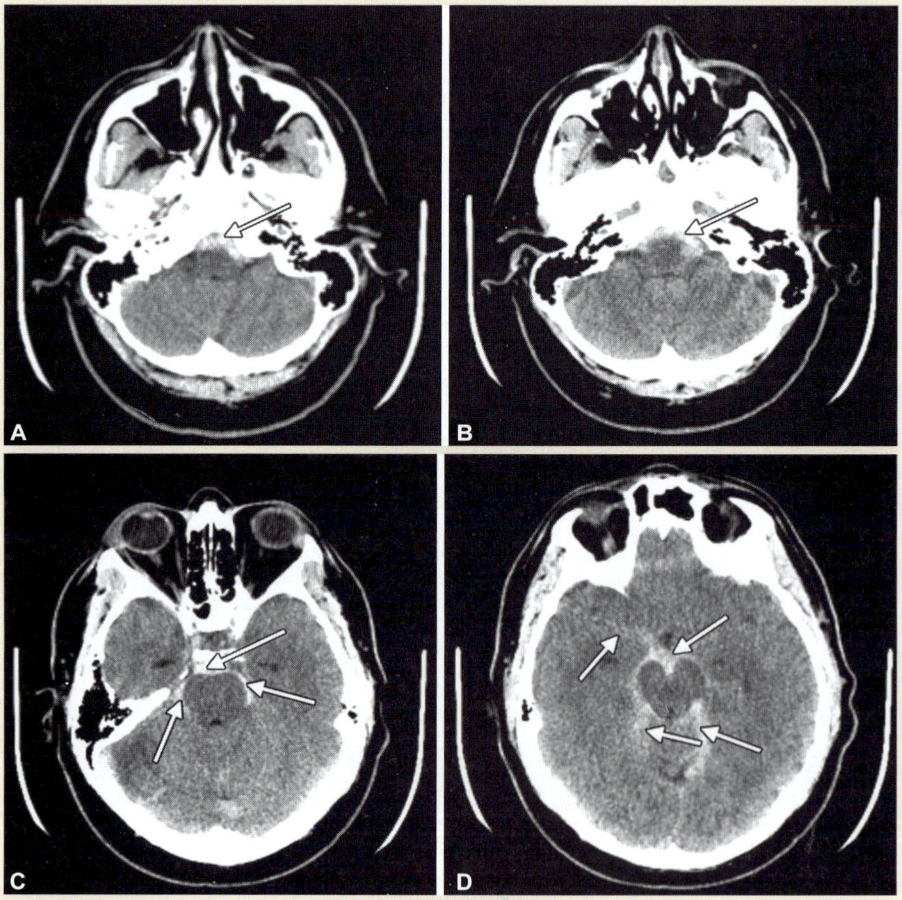


**FIGS. 1A TO D:** (A) SAH in premedullary cistern. (B) SAH in prepontine cistern. (C) SAH in perimesencephalic cistern. (D) SAH extending anteriorly suprasellar and sylvian cisterns and posteriorly, the quadrigeminal cistern.

The patient was admitted and started on nimodipine 60 mg orally every 4 hours for prevention of delayed cerebral ischemia. The patient remained in the critical care unit under close monitoring for the next 7 days. He remained neurologically intact except for headache and neck pain treated with oral paracetamol. IV antihypertensives given intermittently for hypertension control and blood sugars were managed with insulin. He has been evaluated for vasculitis and it was unremarkable.

He underwent DSA after 1 week of SAH, but no abnormalities detected. Since, no cerebral aneurysm or other vascular abnormalities were found, and blood pressure controlled to a SBP less than 140 mm Hg and the patient remained stable, he was discharged with oral antihypertensives.

## PROVISIONAL DIAGNOSIS

### The Ottawa Subarachnoid Hemorrhage Rule

Investigate if one or more high-risk variables present:
- Age ≥40 years
- Neck pain or stiffness
- Witnessed loss of consciousness
- Onset during exertion
- Thunderclap headache (reaching maximum intensity within 1 minute of onset)
- Limited neck flexion on examination

## DIFFERENTIAL DIAGNOSIS

- SAH secondary to occult trauma
- Blood dyscrasias and sickle cell disease
- Non visualized AV malformation or an unseen small aneurysm
- Thrombosis of a ruptured aneurysm
- Dural/spinal AV malformation
- CVT
- Intracranial arterial dissections
- Cerebral amyloid angiopathy
- Cocaine abuse
- Pituitary apoplexy
- Vasculitis (PAN and Wegener's granulomatosis)

This patient had atypical CT features for a possible underlying aneurysmal source for the bleed. Although most non-aneurysmal SAHs have a benign clinical course, in atypical cases, patients can develop delayed cerebral vasospasm, delayed hydrocephalus, or even rebleeding from an occult cerebral aneurysm not visualized on the initial imaging. We must closely monitor these patients for these rare complications for several days and to perform a second DSA to confirm the absence of cerebral vascular malformation.

Perimesencephalic SAH is considered a non-aneurysmal benign variant of primary SAH for which prognosis is excellent. Unlike aneurysmal SAH, perimesencephalic SAH affects men more often than women. Approximately 10% of perimesencephalic SAHs are due to rupture of posterior circulation aneurysm.

## CLINICAL APPROACH

### Symptoms

- Severe headache usually with vomiting – most common symptom (97%), the classic description is "the worst headache of my life", sudden in onset (paroxysmal). This may go off and the patient may not seek medical attention (known as sentinel headache or warning headache, occur in 30–60% of patients presenting with SAH).
- DDs for severe, acute paroxysmal headache includes: SAH, crash migraine, RCVS, airplane headache, benign orgasmic cephalgia
- Neck pain (meningism us)
- Photophobia
- Loss of consciousness
- Focal cranial nerve deficits (third CN palsy causing diplopia/ptosis)
- Low back pain due to irritation of lumbar roots (by dependant blood)

### Signs

- Nuchal rigidity
- Positive Kernig's sign
- Positive Brudzinski sign
- Hypertension
- Oculomotor palsy
- Hemiparesis
- Obtundation or coma (due to raised ICP, hydrocephalus, delayed ischemia, seizure, reduced cerebral blood flow)
- Ocular hemorrhage (sub hyaloid/preretinal hemorrhage, intraretinal hemorrhage, vitreous hemorrhage/Terson syndrome)

### Evaluation

*Non-contrast high-resolution CT brain* **(Figs. 2 and 3)**: It will detect SAH in ≥ 95% if done within 48 hours. For subtle SAH, occipital horns of lateral ventricles and dependant portion of Sylvian fissures have to be seen in CT brain.

It is also used to assess – ventricular size, hematoma, infarct, and amount of blood in cisterns and fissures which is important for prognostication for vasospasm.

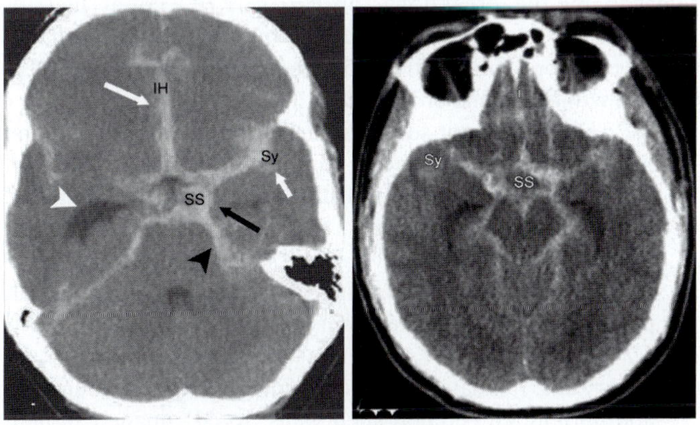


**FIG. 2:** Non-contrast high-resolution CT brain.
(I/IH: interhemispheric fissure; Sy: Sylvian fissure; SS: suprasellar cistern)

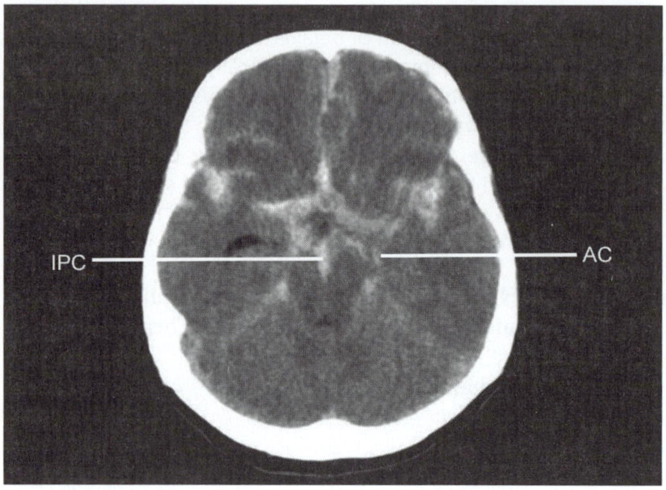


**FIG. 3:** High-resolution non-contrast CT scan of the brain.

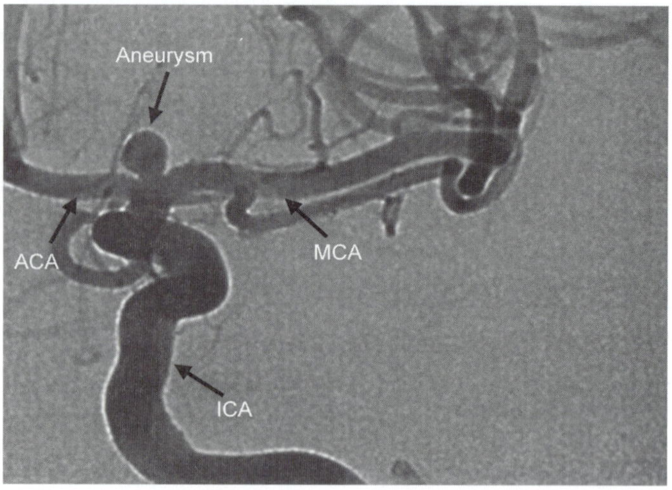


**FIG. 4:** CT angiography showing ICA aneurysm.

CT can predict aneurysm location based on pattern of blood in 78% cases:

- Blood in anterior interhemispheric fissure with or without blood in lateral ventricles or within the gyrus rectus – suggest Acom aneurysm
- Blood predominantly in Sylvian fissure – PCOM or MCA aneurysm on that side
- Blood predominantly in prepontine or peduncular cistern suggests a basilar apex or SCA aneurysm
- Blood in third and fourth ventricle – suggests lower posterior fossa source – PICA aneurysm or VA dissection
- Blood primarily in third ventricle – a basilar apex aneurysm

## Lumbar Puncture

It is the most sensitive test for SAH. However, false positives can occur due to traumatic tap.

*Caution*: lowering the CSF pressure may precipitate rebleeding by increasing the transmural pressure. Therefore, only small amount of CSF is to be removed and small ≤ 20 G spinal needle to be used.

Findings in SAH: elevated opening pressure, non-clotting bloody fluid that does not clear with sequential tubes, xanthochromia of CSF supernatant after centrifugation due to heme pigments released by the breakdown of RBCs. RBC count usually >100,000 RBCs/mm$^3$ (compare RBC count in first to last tube – should not drop significantly). CSF protein will be elevated. CSF glucose will be normal or reduced.

- *MRI brain*: It is not sensitive for SAH within 24–48 hours. But it is better for subacute to remote SAH, >10–20 days. FLAIR MRI is the most sensitive study for detecting blood in the subarachnoid space.
- *Magnetic resonance angiography (MRA)*: It is 87% sensitive and 92% specific for detecting intracranial aneurysms with poorer sensitivity for aneurysms <3 mm diameter.
- *CT angiography (CTA)*: It is useful for detecting 97% of aneurysms. It is safe and effective imaging study for ruptured and unruptured cerebral aneurysms. Its 3D image can help differentiate adherent vessels from those arising from the aneurysm. It is also useful for evaluation of vasospasm **(Figs. 4 and 5)**.

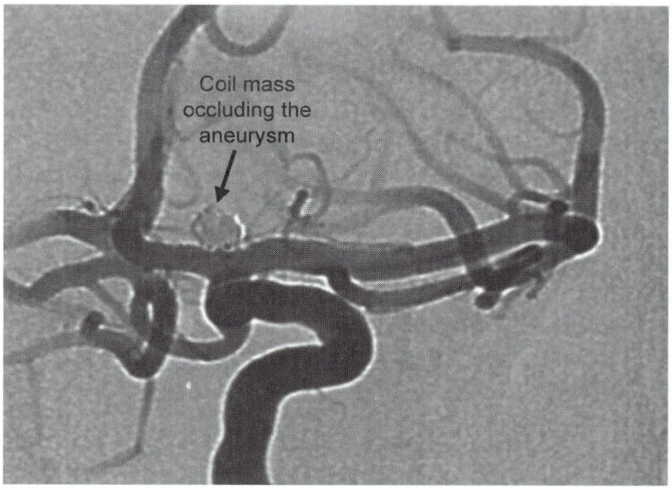


**FIG. 5:** CT angiography showing coiling done for ICA aneurysm.

*Catheter angiogram*: Digital subtraction angiography (DSA) is the gold standard for evaluation of cerebral aneurysms. It demonstrates source in 80–85% cases and the remainder are called "SAH of unknown etiology". It also shows vasospasm and assess primary feeding arteries, and collateral flow.

*Transcranial doppler:* TCD ultrasound is used for monitoring of cerebral artery flow velocity. It is used as a low-risk non-invasive tool to monitor for the presence of cerebral vasospasm following acute SAH. TCD is used to detect vasospasm particularly in the proximal segments of the middle cerebral artery (MCA) and internal carotid artery (ICA). It is less reliable in detecting vasospasm in the anterior cerebral artery (ACA) branches and posterior circulation arteries. When using TCD to monitor cerebral vasospasm, results must be interpreted with clinical correlation, and negative TCD studies do not rule out the presence of vasospasm or the risk for symptomatic delayed cerebral ischemia.

Diagnostic algorithm for evaluating a patient with SAH is given in **Flowchart 1**.

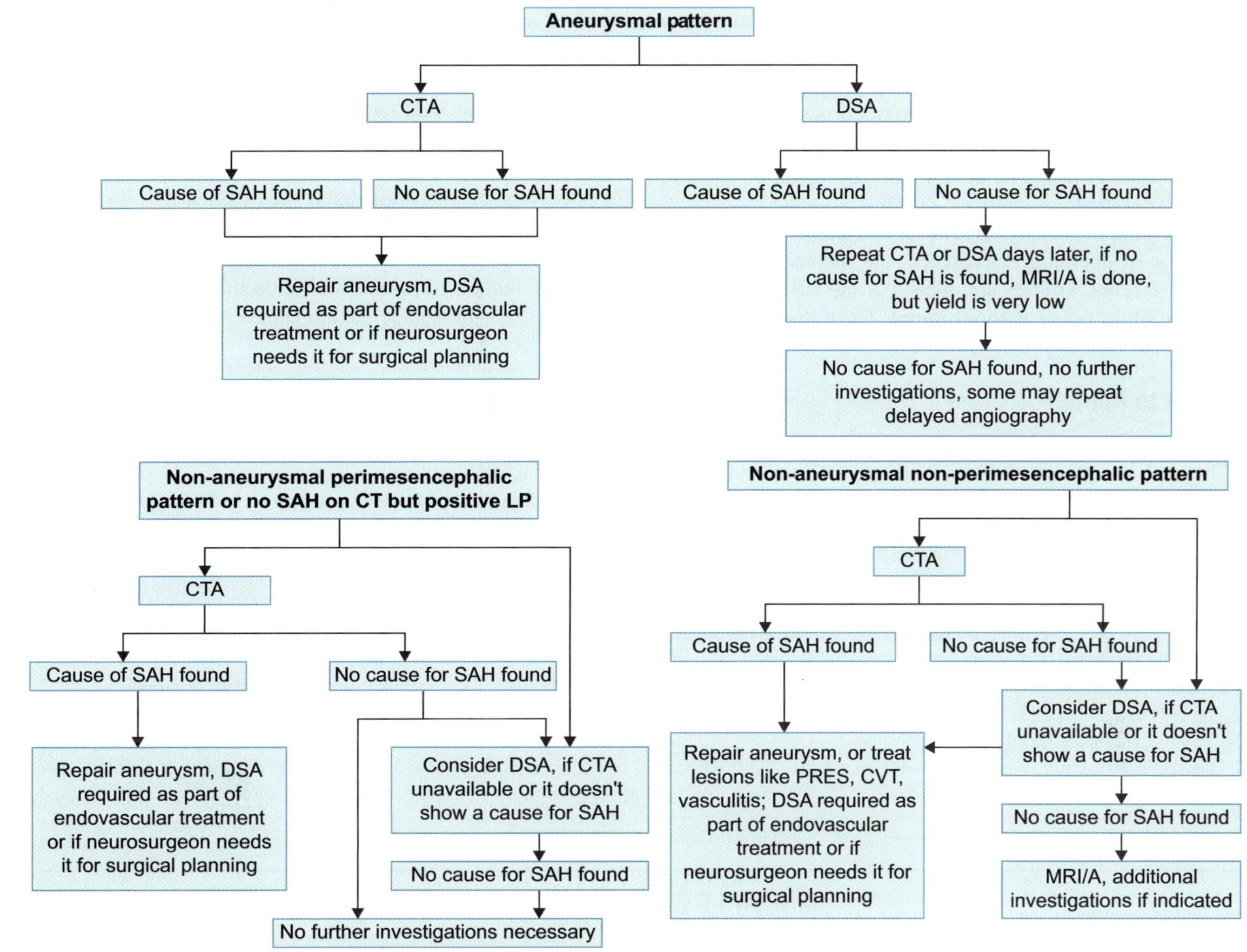


**FLOWCHART 1:** Algorithm for investigating a patient with SAH.

*Source*: Adapted from Chou SH. Subarachnoid Hemorrhage. Continuum (Minneap Minn). 2021;27(5):1201-45.

## PATHOPHYSIOLOGY

Subarachnoid hemorrhage (SAH) occurs when blood enters the subarachnoid space, typically due to rupture of a cerebral aneurysm or trauma. This leads to increased intracranial pressure, reduced cerebral perfusion, and irritation of the meninges. The breakdown products of blood in the cerebrospinal fluid can trigger vasospasm, potentially causing delayed cerebral ischemia. Additionally, the release of inflammatory mediators and disruption of the blood-brain barrier contribute to neurological deficits and complications.

## TREATMENT AND PREVENTION

### Management before Securing Aneurysm

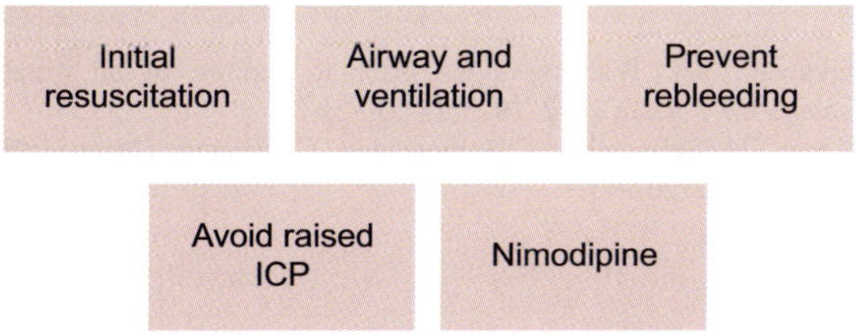


*BP control*: Mean arterial blood pressure of <110 mm Hg is recommended. Short-acting easily titratable agents such as IV calcium-channel blockers (nicardipine, clevidipine) are used. IV nitrates should be avoided as they have the propensity to raise ICP.

To maintain systolic BP below 160 mm Hg and if more than this, anti-hypertensives can be used.

*Antifibrinolytics*: They are used to prevent rebleeding. They are not routinely used but may be considered in whom the aneurysm treatment cannot proceed immediately. Aminocaproic acid was given in a dose of 24 g/day IV for 3 days, followed by oral administration for 3 weeks or until surgery.

*Hyponatremia*: It is the most common electrolyte disturbance in patients with aneurysmal SAH (30–50% cases). Etiology could be cerebral salt wasting more than SIADH. Due to multitude of factors contributing to hyponatremia, it is not treated with fluid restriction, but with free water restriction and mildly hypertonic fluids. Vasopressin receptor agonists are also used.

*Seizures*: It occurs in 20% of patients, especially with intraparenchymal bleeding. However, data are lacking for routine antiseizure medications and routine prophylaxis is not recommended.

*Management of aneurysm*: Definitive treatment on early securement of aneurysm is within 72 hours, or ideally within 24 hours of diagnosis. Obliteration of aneurysm is essential to prevent rebleeding. It can be done by neurosurgical clipping or endovascular coiling.

Surgical clipping of a ruptured aneurysm requires craniotomy. With the use of operating microscope, the subarachnoid spaces around the cerebral arteries are opened at the base of the skull to mobilize brain tissue without injury. Once the aneurysm is reached, a titanium clip is placed across the neck of the aneurysm to mechanically close the sac at its neck while preserving blood flow through the adjacent normal arteries.

Endovascular treatment for the ruptured aneurysm involves navigating a catheter under fluoroscopic guidance from an entry point, typically the femoral artery in the groin up to the parent artery of aneurysm. A microcatheter is then passed into the aneurysm sac and metal coils are placed into the aneurysm lumen through the microcatheter. This process arrests the intra-aneurysmal blood flow and induces thrombus formation, thereby occluding the aneurysm and eliminating the immediate risk of rerupture.

## Points to Ponder

- Timely recognition and correct diagnosis of SAH is associated with better outcomes.
- The most common cause of spontaneous SAH is a ruptured cerebral aneurysm (85%).
- Approximately 10–15% of patients with SAH do not have an identifiable bleeding source; of these, approximately 38% have non-aneurysmal perimesencephalic SAH, which is a benign variant of SAH with excellent prognosis.
- Hyperacute life-threatening complications are acute cardiopulmonary failure, acute hydrocephalus, diffuse cerebral edema, and aneurysm rebleeding.
- Timely insertion of an external ventricular drain for acute symptomatic hydrocephalus is lifesaving.
- Early brain injury following SAH occurs at the time of aneurysm rupture when sudden rise in ICP causes transient global cerebral ischemia and brain damage by intracranial hematoma.
- Delayed cerebral ischemia develops 3–21 days following aneurysm rupture and it is the strongest predictor of poor outcome.
- The only drug with Class I evidence for decreasing the risk of poor outcome in SAH is nimodipine. It is to be started within 96 hours of the initial bleed and continued for 21 days.
- The 'Triple H therapy' is associated with increased cardiopulmonary complications. It is not recommended in modern neurocritical care for SAH.

## MULTIPLE CHOICE QUESTIONS

1. **What is the most likely cause of this patient's acute subarachnoid hemorrhage (SAH)?**
   A. Intracranial aneurysm
   B. Arteriovenous malformation
   C. Non-aneurysmal perimesencephalic SAH
   D. Hypertensive crisis
2. **Which medication was started to prevent delayed cerebral ischemia in this patient?**
   A. Paracetamol
   B. Nimodipine
   C. IV antihypertensives
   D. Insulin
3. **What imaging technique is considered definitive for detecting aneurysmal causes of SAH?**
   A. Plain CT brain
   B. MRI brain
   C. CT angiography
   D. Digital Subtraction Angiography (DSA)
4. **Which of the following is true about the patient's clinical course?**
   A. He developed neurological deficits during hospitalization.
   B. Hypertension was uncontrolled during his stay.
   C. He remained neurologically intact except for headache and neck pain.
   D. Cerebral vasculitis was confirmed as the cause of SAH.
5. **What was the recommended blood pressure target for this patient during hospitalization?**
   A. SBP < 160 mm Hg
   B. SBP < 140 mm Hg
   C. SBP < 130 mm Hg
   D. SBP < 120 mm Hg

### Answers

1. (C); 2. (B); 3. (D); 4. (C); 5. (B)

## SUGGESTED READINGS

1. Lawton MT, Vates GE. Subarachnoid Hemorrhage. N Engl J Med. 2017;377(3):257-66.
2. Thilak S, Brown P, Whitehouse T, et al. Diagnosis and management of subarachnoid haemorrhage. Nat Commun. 2024;15(1):1850.
3. Jovin T, Caplan LR. Subarachnoid hemorrhage, aneurysms, and vascular malformations. In: Caplan LR, ed. Caplan's Stroke: A Clinical Approach. Cambridge University Press. 2016:439-76.
4. Okawara SH. Warning signs prior to rupture of an intracranial aneurysm. J Neurosurg. 1973;38(5):575-80.
5. Chou SH. Subarachnoid Hemorrhage. Continuum (Minneap Minn). 2021;27(5):1201-45.

CHAPTER 58

# An Approach to a Case of Hyperkinetic Movement Disorders from a Physician's Perspective

*Jaydeep Majumdar, Bhaskar Ghosh*

## CASE VIGNETTE

A 68-year-old hypertensive and diabetic female with a history of poor glycemic control presented with involuntary, irregular, non-repetitive, dance like movements of the left upper limb and left lower limb for 2 days, which she noticed after attending a reception party of one of her relatives. She denied any history of weakness of limbs, slurring of speech or difficulty in deglutition. Detailed enquiry regarding drug history only revealed that she was on antihypertensive and antidiabetic medication for last 20 years but often skipped her routine antidiabetic medication for last 6 months. General and neurological examination findings were unremarkable except the choreiform movement of left extremities. Laboratory investigations showed random blood sugar 624 mg/dL, glycated hemoglobin (HbA1c) 12.6%, serum osmolality 330 mOsmol/L, urine sugar 4+, urine ketones-absent. Otherwise, routine laboratory parameters were within normal range. Non-contrast MRI brain revealed altered signal intensity over right caudate nucleus and right putamen region which appeared hyperintense on T1-weighted image and hypointense on T2-weighted image. She was diagnosed with non-ketotic hyperglycemic chorea. The treatment strategy included urgent control of hyperglycemia, correction of hydration status and symptomatic treatment for chorea. The patient symptomatically improved gradually over the next 7 days with complete resolution of involuntary movements.

## PROVISIONAL DIAGNOSIS

Non-ketotic hyperglycemic hemichorea-hemiballismus (NKH-HH) syndrome.

## DIFFERENTIAL DIAGNOSIS

- Stroke (ischemic or hemorrhagic) involving the basal ganglia
- Wilson's disease
- Sydenham's chorea
- Hyperthyroidism-related chorea
- Drug-induced dyskinesias

## CLINICAL APPROACH

Common hyperkinetic movement disorders include tremor, chorea, tics, myoclonus, dystonia, athetosis and ballismus **(Fig. 1)**. Due to variable, complex, overlapping and often bizarre presentation of these movement disorders, correct diagnosis can become problematic and challenging for the attending physician.

- Detailed history taking, including drug history, phenomenology identification, pattern recognition of movement disorder, thorough systemic and neurological examinations and finally, identification of the etiology are essential to arrive at a correct diagnosis. Hyperkinetic movement disorders are frequently encountered in routine practice of physicians.
- Detailed history, especially the drug history, which is often overlooked, to be emphasized upon. Analysis of phenomenology, pattern recognition of the movement disorders, thorough neurological and systemic examination and ultimate search for an etiology remain the cornerstone for arriving at a correct diagnosis.
- An appropriate clinical context would also warrant the physician to exclude functional hyperkinetic movement disorders.
- A correct etiological diagnosis, arrived through a stepwise and structured approach, helps to formulate a treatment strategy for these hyperkinetic movement disorders.

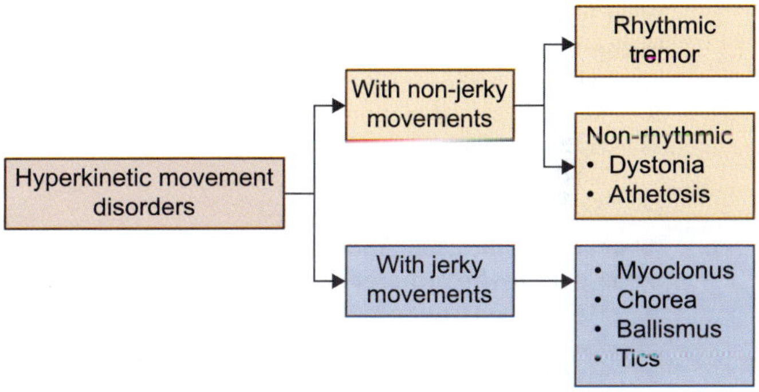


**FIG. 1:** Spectrum of hyperkinetic movement disorders.

### Pathophysiology

Non-ketotic hyperglycemic chorea occurs due to metabolic derangement from poorly controlled diabetes. Hyperglycemia leads to a hyperosmolar state, disrupting basal ganglia neurotransmitter regulation, particularly in the striatum (caudate and putamen). This results in impaired GABAergic inhibition, excessive glutamatergic activity, and abnormal neuronal firing, manifesting as choreiform or ballistic movements. MRI findings of hyperintensities in the basal ganglia (T1-weighted) reflect metabolic injury or gliosis.

## Treatment

- *Glycemic control*: Immediate correction of hyperglycemia using insulin therapy
- *Hydration*: Correcting dehydration with intravenous fluids
- *Symptomatic management*: Dopamine depletor (e.g., tetrabenazine, deutetrabenazine), receptor blockers (e.g., haloperidol) or benzodiazepines for severe chorea
- *Monitoring and supportive care*: Close monitoring of electrolytes, renal function, and neurological status

## Prevention

- Maintain strict glycemic control with regular monitoring of blood glucose and HbA1c
- Adhere to antidiabetic medications consistently
- Educate the patient about recognizing early symptoms of hyperglycemia
- Regular follow-ups with healthcare providers to manage chronic conditions like diabetes and hypertension

## Points to Ponder

- *Hyperglycemia and movement disorders*: Non-ketotic hyperglycemic chorea (NKHC) is a rare manifestation of poorly controlled diabetes, highlighting hyperglycemia as a potential cause.
- *Critical role of history*: Medication nonadherence and overlooked drug history are key contributors to complex clinical presentations.
- *Diagnostic imaging*: MRI findings of basal ganglia hyperintensities provide definitive clues for NKHC diagnosis.
- *Stepwise approach*: Combining history, clinical examination, and imaging ensures accurate differentiation between organic and functional movement disorders.
- *Effective management*: Timely glucose control, hydration, and symptomatic care can reverse NKHC, preventing complications and recurrence.

## MULTIPLE CHOICE QUESTIONS

**1. Which region of the brain is most commonly affected in non-ketotic hyperglycemic hemichorea?**

A. Frontal lobe
B. Basal ganglia
C. Cerebellum
D. Occipital lobe

**2. What is the primary cause of the involuntary movements in non-ketotic hyperglycemic chorea?**

A. Ischemia in the motor cortex
B. Metabolic dysfunction of the basal ganglia due to hyperglycemia
C. Dehydration-related neuronal damage
D. Excessive dopamine production

**3. What is the typical MRI finding in non-ketotic hyperglycemic hemichorea?**

A. Hypointensity on T1-weighted images and hyperintensity on T2-weighted images
B. Hyperintensity on T1-weighted images and hypointensity on T2-weighted images
C. Diffuse brain edema on T2-weighted images
D. Normal MRI findings

**4. Which of the following is the most important initial step in the management of non-ketotic hyperglycemic chorea?**

A. Administer antipsychotic medication
B. Perform emergency MRI
C. Correct hyperglycemia with insulin therapy
D. Start anticoagulation therapy

**5. Which of the following is a key preventive measure for non-ketotic hyperglycemic hemichorea?**

A. Avoiding high-protein diets
B. Maintaining strict glycemic control
C. Regular screening for basal ganglia abnormalities
D. Use of prophylactic dopamine receptor blockers

### Answers

1. (B); 2. (B); 3. (B); 4. (C); 5. (B)

## SUGGESTED READINGS

1. Deuschl G, Bain P, Brin M. Consensus statement of the Movement Disorder Society on Tremor. Ad Hoc Scientific Committee. Mov Disord.1998;13:2-23.
2. Stimming EF, Bega D, Chorea. Continuum (Minneap Minn). 2022; 28(5):1379-408.
3. Abdo WF, van de Warrenburg BPC, Burn DJ, et al. The clinical approach to movement disorders. Nat Rev Neurol. 2010;6:29-37.
4. Kojovic M, Cordivari C, Bhatia K. Myoclonic disorders: a practical approach for diagnosis and treatment. Ther. Adv Neurol Disord. 2011;4 (1):47-62.
5. Batla A. Dystonia: A review. Neurol India. 2018;66:S48-S58.
6. Kumar D, Srivastava A, Faruq M, et al. Spinocerebellar ataxia type 12: an update. Ann Mov Disord. 2019;2:48-57.

CHAPTER
59

# An Approach to a Case of Different Types of Tremors

*Shafat Iqbal Bhati*

## CASE VIGNETTE

A 72-year-old man sought a neurology evaluation for a bilateral hand tremor, which he had experienced since high school. The tremor was initially modest, infrequent, and did not interfere with daily functioning. His mother, grandmother, maternal uncle, and cousin all suffered identical tremors. The accountant's tremor became annoying in his fifties when it interfered with writing, typing, and computer use. He struggled to pour himself coffee at home and to use the tools in the garage and garden. He found it hard to eat soup with a spoon and spaghetti with a fork, so he avoided going out to eat with friends. He noticed improvement in his tremors with a glass of wine. He received propranolol 160 mg daily, which provided some relief. He received primidone as an additional drug to treat his tremors. He tolerated the medications without experiencing dizziness, nausea, or gait instability. Despite on treatment, the patient's problems persisted that prompted him an early retirement. Examination revealed a moderately significant arm tremor affecting the metacarpophalangeal and wrist joints when he stretched his arms forward. The tremor was also observed during writing, drawing spirals, and doing the finger-nose-finger movement. The tremor was not present while his arm was resting. He considered deep brain stimulation (DBS) surgery to control his symptoms.

## PROVISIONAL DIAGNOSIS

Essential tremor (ET) with functional impairment and poor response to pharmacological treatment.

## DIFFERENTIAL DIAGNOSIS

The various conditions that can be considered in patients who present tremors are as follows:

- Essential tremors
- Physiologic tremors
- Parkinson disease tremors
- Dystonic tremors
- Drug-induced tremors (drugs such as amiodarone, atorvastatin, caffeine carbamazepine, theophylline, thyroid hormones, TCA, and valproic acid)
- *Tremors associated with genetic disorders*: Fragile X associated tremors/Ataxia syndrome, Wilson disease tremors
- Holmes tremors
- Functional tremors
- Psychogenic tremors

## CLINICAL APPROACH

Tremors are diagnosed through a clinical history and physical examination. While tremor syndromes can overlap and vary, the fundamental aspects of the tremor often serve as a major diagnostic clue. Its approach can be explained by **Flowcharts 1 and 2 and Table 1** as follows.

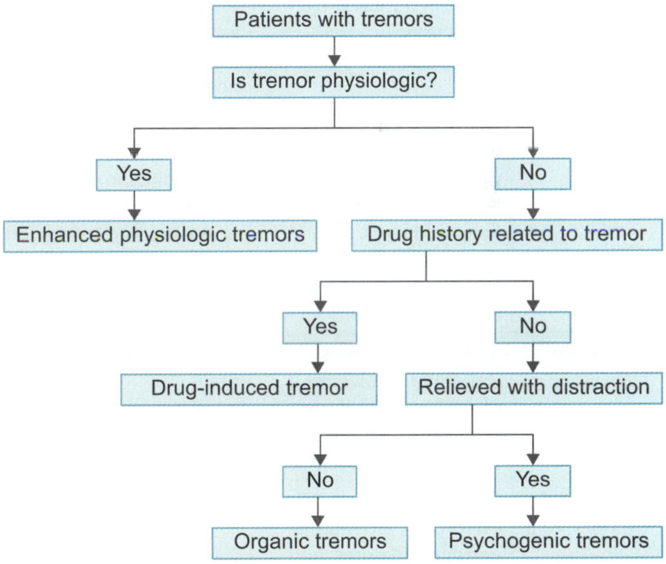


**FLOWCHART 1:** How to approach a patient clinically with tremors?

While clinical diagnosis is still the primary method for tremors, several imaging modalities can aid in distinguishing between various causes. Non-contrast MRI brain and CT scan head can rule out the secondary etiologies of tremors, such as multiple sclerosis, space occupying mass lesions, or cerebrovascular accident, especially when the history and

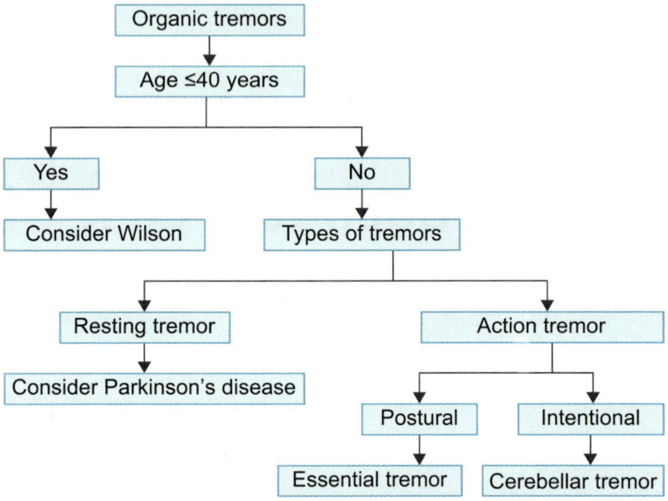


**FLOWCHART 2:** Clinical approach to organic tremors.

**TABLE 1: Characteristics of common tremor disorders.**

| Tremors | Clinical features | Diagnostic tests |
|---|---|---|
| Essential tremors | Postural tremors; symmetrical; affects hands/wrists, lower extremities, head, or voice; family history; improves with minor amounts of alcohol consumption | There is no specific test, although a complete blood count, thyroid function test, and serum biochemical profile can rule out other diseases |
| Enhanced physiologic tremors | Postural tremors with modest amplitude and usage of aggravating medicines | History of caffeine usage or anxiety; liver function testing, glucose (to look for hypoglycemia), and thyroid-stimulating hormone |
| Parkinsonian tremors | Asymmetrical rest tremor that affects the distal extremities, becomes less noticeable with voluntary movement, stiffness and bradykinesia, and postural instability | For atypical presentations, use single-photon emission computed tomography or positron emission tomography, rest no specific test |
| Cerebellar tremors | Intentional tremors; ipsilateral involvement of the lesion; abnormal finger-to-nose and heel-to-shin test; imbalance | CT scan head or MRI brain |
| Psychogenic tremors | Sudden onset, remission on its own, alterations in tremor features, and extinction by distraction | Clinical history |

physical examination points toward a structural lesion or in case of parkinsonism with atypical features or refractory to levodopa.

## PATHOPHYSIOLOGY

Essential tremor is primarily attributed to dysfunction in the cerebellothalamocortical circuit, particularly involving the cerebellum and its connections with the thalamus. Abnormal oscillatory activity in this pathway leads to rhythmic, involuntary movements characteristic of the disorder. ET is associated with:

- *Cerebellar dysfunction*: Purkinje cell loss or structural abnormalities in the cerebellum contribute to impaired motor coordination
- *Thalamic hyperactivity*: Increased oscillations in the ventral intermediate nucleus (VIM) of the thalamus amplify tremor signals
- *Neurotransmitter imbalance*: Altered GABAergic and glutamatergic signaling disrupts inhibitory mechanisms, facilitating tremor.
- *Genetic factors*: Mutations in genes such as LINGO1 have been linked to familial ET

In cases of functional impairment and poor pharmacological response, the pathophysiology may reflect more extensive cerebellar degeneration or advanced neural circuit disruption.

## Treatment and Prevention

Principles of management for different types of tremors involves considering various factors such as the underlying cause, severity, impact on daily life, and individual patient characteristics. Here's a general approach for different types of tremors.

- Identify the type and cause of tremor as explained above.
- *Assessment and diagnosis*: Detailed medical history and physical examination. Consider imaging (e.g., MRI) or neurophysiological studies if needed
- General principles of management: *Lifestyle modifications*: Avoid triggers (e.g., caffeine), stress reduction techniques, adequate rest
  - *Physical and occupational therapy*: Exercises to improve coordination and reduce tremor severity.
  - *Speech therapy*: For tremors affecting speech.
- *Specific management approaches*:
  - *Essential tremor*:
    - Medication: Beta blockers (e.g., propranolol) or anticonvulsants (e.g., primidone).
    - Surgical Options: DBS for severe cases resistant to medication.
- *Parkinsonian tremor*:
    - Levodopa: Often effective, but careful titration is needed to manage motor fluctuations.
    - DBS: Particularly effective for tremor-dominant Parkinson's disease.
  - *Dystonic tremor*:
    - Botulinum toxin injections: Targeting dystonic muscles.
    - Medication adjustments: Anticholinergics or muscle relaxants may help
  - *Drug-induced tremor*:
    - Medication review: Adjust or discontinue offending medications.
    - Alternative treatments: Depending on the underlying condition.
  - *Physiologic tremor*:
    - Identify and manage triggers: Address underlying causes (e.g., anxiety, stimulants)
- *Multidisciplinary approach*:
  - Collaboration between neurologists, physical therapists, occupational therapists, and speech therapists for comprehensive care

  - Regular follow-up and adjustment of treatment plans based on patient response
- *Patient-centered care*:
  - Tailor treatment plans based on individual patient goals, preferences, and severity of tremors
  - Provide ongoing support and education to patients and caregivers

By following these principles, healthcare providers can effectively manage different types of tremors, improve patient outcomes, and enhance quality of life. Each patient's management plan should be personalized based on their specific needs and clinical presentation.

## Points to Ponder

- *Identification and classification*: Differentiate among various types of tremors according to their attributes such as frequency, amplitude and causes. Correct identification is useful for guiding the treatment approach.
- *Etiology and pathophysiology*: Appreciate the reasons and mechanism underlying each type of tremor. This insight plays a critical role in care delivery.
- *Tailoring treatment approaches*: Develop personalized intervention plans depending on the kind of tremor. Possible pharmaceutical interventions (e.g., beta-blockers for essential trembling or dopamine agonists for Parkinson's ones), physiotherapy options and sometimes surgical procedures (such as deep brain stimulation) should be taken into consideration.
- *Monitorig and adjustements*: Keep track of patient's response to therapy regularly and change it accordingly where necessary. Tremors may progress with time that might require adjustments in medication, intensity of therapy or even revaluation of initial diagnosis made earlier.

## MULTIPLE CHOICE QUESTIONS

**1. What is the most likely diagnosis for the patient's condition?**
A. Parkinson's disease
B. Dystonia
C. Essential tremor (ET)
D. Multiple sclerosis

**2. Which of the following features supports the diagnosis of essential tremors?**
A. Tremor present at rest
B. Family history of similar tremors
C. No response to propranolol
D. Gait instability observed during examination

**3. What is a known temporary alleviating factor for ET in this patient?**
A. Caffeine intake
B. Consumption of alcohol
C. Resting the hands
D. Stress reduction

**4. Which of the following treatment options has the patient already tried?**
A. Levodopa
B. Deep brain stimulation
C. Propranolol and primidone
D. Botulinum toxin injections

**5. What surgical option is the patient considering due to persistent symptoms?**
A. Thalamotomy
B. Deep brain stimulation
C. Vagal nerve stimulation
D. Carotid endarterectomy

### Answers

1. (C); 2. (B); 3. (B); 4. (C); 5. (B)

## SUGGESTED READINGS

1. Wippold FJ II, Brown DC, Broderick DF, et al. (2015). Expert Panel on Neurologic Imaging. American College of Radiology Appropriateness Criteria: Dementia and movement disorders. [online] https://acsearch.acr.org/docs/69360/Narrative/.[Last accessed December, 2024].
2. Crawford P, Zimmerman EE. Differentiation and diagnosis of tremor. Am Fam Physician. 2011;83(6):697-702.
3. Crawford P, Zimmerman EE. Tremor: Sorting Through the Differential Diagnosis. Am Fam Physician. 2018;97(3):180-6.

CHAPTER

60

# An Approach to a Case of Myelopathy

*Mrinal Kanti Roy, Debaleena Mukherjee*

**CASE VIGNETTE**

A 30-year-old male presented with acute onset, progressive symmetric weakness of bilateral lower limbs, along with numbness and tingling paresthesias up to his umbilicus for the past 2 weeks. He reported a girdle-like sensation around his umbilicus. This was associated with painful urinary retention requiring catheterization and decreased perianal sensation. After 4 days, he also developed acute onset painful, diminution of vision in both eyes along with color desaturation. Examination revealed bilateral optic neuritis. He had decreased tone and power (MRC grade 1) of both lower limbs along with absent deep tendon reflexes. Sensory examination showed a sensory level at D10 with all modalities impaired below it. A clinical diagnosis of acute dorsal myelopathy with bilateral optic neuritis was made. Investigations confirmed a long-segment myelitis and bilateral optic neuritis on MRI spine, brain and orbit. Aquaporin-4 antibody positivity confirmed NMO-spectrum disorder.

## PROVISIONAL DIAGNOSIS

Neuromyelitis optica spectrum disorder (NMOSD) with acute longitudinally extensive transverse myelitis (LETM) and bilateral optic neuritis.

## DIFFERENTIAL DIAGNOSIS

With respect to disease onset, myelopathies are classified as hyperacute (<6 hours from onset to nadir), acute (6–48 hours), subacute (2–21 days) or chronic (>21 days). The course may be monophasic, relapsing/remitting or progressive.

Etiologically, myelopathies have long been classified as compressive and noncompressive myelopathies **(Table 1)**.

While the terminologies compressive and noncompressive myelopathies have been used traditionally, the newer approach as inflammatory and noninflammatory myelopathies leads to a more comprehensive etiological search.

## CLINICAL APPROACH

Diagnosis of myelopathies requires comprehensive history taking and step-wise detailed neurological evaluation along with appropriate neuroimaging and laboratory assessment.

### Step 1: When to Suspect Spinal Cord Lesion?

Myelopathies should be suspected whenever a patient presents with a combination of motor, sensory and sphincter abnormalities, especially if a sensory level or a girdle like sensation on the trunk is reported.

#### *Clinical Cues*

*Motor*: Weakness patterns range from quadriparesis to paraparesis and even monoparesis. In the acute stages, tone is often flaccid (spinal shock stage), as is common in complete cord involvement. In chronic stages, upper motor neuron (UMN) features (spasticity, hyperreflexia, pyramidal weakness) are observed below the level of lesion along with extensor plantar response, while segmental lower motor neuron (LMN) involvement (wasting and fasciculations) are noted at the level of lesion. In case of longitudinally extensive lesions (involving > 3 vertebral segments), involving the anterior horn cells, chronic flaccid weakness occurs.

*Sensory*: This results from involvement of the spinothalamic tracts (carries pain, temperature sensations and crude touch) and posterior column (carries fine touch, vibration, joint position and vibration sense) and spinocerebellar tracts (unconscious proprioception).

*Complaints include*:

- Negative symptoms (numbness, unsteadiness worsening in the dark or with eye closure suggestive of sensory ataxia)
- Positive symptoms [paresthesias, burning sensation, plaster cast sensation, band such as sensation, Lhermitte's sign (electrical pain and tingling elicited down the spine with neck flexion)]

Identifying a sensory level with loss of modalities below it, helps in localizing symptoms to the spinal cord. While a history of girdle like sensation and a sensory level is easier to identify in dorsal myelopathies, it is often not reported in case of cervical. False localizing thoracic sensory levels are often noted in cervical compressive myelopathies as the leg fibers are more superficial in the ascending tracts and prone to compression. Lhermitte sign is frequently associated with both inflammatory and noninflammatory cervical myelopathies resulting from posterior column involvement. Central cord lesions classically

| TABLE 1: Etiologies of compressive and noncompressive myelopathies. | |
|---|---|
| **Compressive myelopathies** | |
| Degenerative | Spondylotic myelopathy |
| Traumatic | Bone lesion, disc herniation, epidural hemorrhage |
| Infective | Abscess |
| Tumors | Intramedullary, intradural extramedullary, extradural extramedullary |
| Vascular | Spinal arterio-venous fistulas, arteriovenous malformations |
| Syrinx | |
| **Noncompressive myelopathies** | |
| Infective | • *Viral*: HSV, VZV, CMV, EBV, adenovirus, enterovirus, cox sackie virus, HHV-6, HIV, HTLV-1<br>• *Bacterial*: *Mycobacterium tuberculosis*, *Staphylococcus aureus*, *Streptococcus*, *Brucella*<br>• *Spirochetes*: Syphilis and Lymes<br>• *Fungal*: *Cryptococcus*, *Aspergillus* |
| Demyelination | • *Primary demyelination*: Multiple sclerosis, MOGAD, NMOSD, ADEM, GFAP astrocytopathy<br>• *Secondary demyelination*: SLE Sjögren's syndrome, sarcoidosis |
| Immune-mediated | *Autoimmune/connective tissue disorders*: SLE, Sjögren's syndrome, sarcoid, Behçet's disease paraneoplastic |
| Vascular | • CNS vasculitis (primary/secondary)<br>• Spinal artery thrombosis |
| Metabolic | Vitamin B12 deficiency, vitamin E deficiency, copper deficiency |
| Degenerative/Genetic | Friedreich's ataxia, SCA, HSP, PLS, hexosaminidase deficiency, adrenomyeloneuropathy |
| Toxin | Lathyrism, organophosphorus |
| Idiopathic | |

present with suspended sensory loss spinal tract crossed findings (e.g., ipsilateral pyramidal signs, posterior column involvement and contralateral spinothalamic findings) as seen in hemicord syndromes and dissociated sensory loss (involvement of pain and temperature with sparing of vibration and proprioception) are other clues for spinal cord localization.

*Autonomic dysfunction*: In the acute stages, the bladder often remains in a state of shock (detrusor hyporeflexia/areflexia) causing urinary retention. In the chronic stages, detrusor hyperreflexia and detrusor sphincter dyssynergia (DSD) are noted. Detrusor hyperreflexia causes urinary urgency, frequency and urge incontinence, while DSD manifests as a urinary hesitancy, sense of incomplete evacuation and retention. Fluctuations in blood pressure and heart rate further indicate autonomic dysreflexia.

Once spinal cord lesion if suspected, further localization is done as follows in **Table 2**.

## Step 2: Anatomical Localization

1. **Longitudinal localization—at what level does the lesion lie?**

- *Motor*: LMN features at level of lesion, UMN features below
- *Sensory*: Girdle like sensation at level of lesion, sensory loss below
- *Reflexes*: Loss of deep tendon reflexes at level of lesion, exaggerated below when beyond shock stage
- *Local features*: Pain, tenderness and deformity
- *Additional clues for each level*:
  - o *Foramen magnum syndrome*: Down beat nystagmus, cerebellar ataxia, lower cranial nerve palsies, suboccipital neck pain and papilledema are pointers. Pattern of weakness can be cruciate (crossed weakness of contralateral upper limb and ipsilateral lower limb) or Elsberg phenomenon (progression of weakness in a U-shaped manner starting with one upper limb followed by ipsilateral lower limb then contralateral lower limb and finally the contralateral upper limb)
  - o *High cervical cord lesion*: Quadriparesis with diaphragmatic weakness, Lhermitte's sign and Balaclava helmet pattern (loss of pain and temperature over lateral face with sparing of central face) are observed. Horner's syndrome may occur. Though lower cervical segments are responsible for wasting and weakness of small muscles of hand, this feature is often observed in high cervical cord lesions. Considered to be a false localizing sign, it is hypothesized that arterial watershed zone or venous congestion are the possible explanations. Myelopathic hand is a deformity characterized by inability to adduct and extend the little finger, which suggests spinal cord lesion above C6.
  - o *Lower cervical and thoracic cord lesion*: Typically characterized by LMN features at level of lesion and UMN features below. Inverted supinator reflex (absent supinator as well as biceps with presence of finger flexion) and inverted triceps reflex (elbow flexion instead of extension) localizes lesion at the C5-C6 and C7 levels respectively. Lesion above D6 results in mass reflex or autonomic dysreflexia. Lesion above D10 levels causes upwards contraction of the umbilicus on trunk flexion (Beevor's sign)
  - o *Conus medullaris lesion*: Characterized by early, flaccid bladder involvement with bilateral saddle sensory loss and lumbosacral pattern LMN weakness.

**TABLE 2: Patterns of spinal cord involvement and their respective etiologies.**

| Pattern | | Etiology |
|---|---|---|
| Complete spinal cord involvement | Involvement of all tracts of the spinal cord | • Spinal cord trauma<br>• Hematomyelia<br>• NMOSD<br>• Paraneoplastic necrotizing myelopathy **(Table 3)**<br>• Late radiation myelitis |
| Brown–Séquard syndrome/Hemispinal cord syndrome | Ipsilateral corticospinal, ipsilateral posterior column, contralateral spinothalamic tract and autonomic fibers | • Multiple sclerosis<br>• Cord compression<br>• Penetrating trauma<br>• Varicella zoster virus |
| Posterior cord syndrome | Posterior columns with or without dorsal roots | • Tabes dorsalis<br>• Early cervical spondylotic myelopathy<br>• Multiple sclerosis<br>• Vitamin B12/Copper deficiency<br>• Radiation myelopathy<br>• Chemotherapy toxicity<br>• Paraneoplastic sensory neuronopathy |
| Posterolateral cord syndrome | Posterior column and lateral cortico-spinal tracts | • Vitamin B12 and copper deficiencies<br>• Cervical spondylotic myelopathy<br>• HIV myelopathy<br>• HTLV-1 associated myelopathy<br>• Paraneoplastic myelopathy<br>• Hereditary spastic paraparesis<br>• AMN |
| Central cord syndrome | Crossing of spinothalamic tracts, corticospinal tract and autonomic tracts | • Syringomyelia<br>• Intramedullary tumor<br>• Hyperextension injury<br>• NMOSD |
| Anterior cord syndrome | Anterior horns, corticospinal tract, spinothalamic tracts and autonomic tracts | • Anterior spinal artery infracts<br>• Polio, WNV<br>• Disc herniation<br>• Multiple sclerosis<br>• SMA |
| Anterior horn syndrome | Selective damage to anterior horn cells only | • *Infection*: WNV, JE, polio<br>• Kennedy disease<br>• Monomelic/Bimelic amyotrophy<br>• Paraneoplastic |
| Anterior horn cell + corticospinal tract | Anterior horn cell and corticospinal tract only | • Cervical myeloradiculopathy<br>• Amyotrophic lateral sclerosis |
| Conus involvement | Spinal segments S1–S5, but classic conus medullaris can extend upto L2 | • Lumbar disc<br>• Metastasis<br>• Abscess<br>• CMV infection<br>• MOGAD |

**TABLE 3: Clinical clues for compressive versus noncompressive myelopathy.**

| | Compressive | Noncompressive |
|---|---|---|
| Pattern of involvement | Non-selective, sequential | Selective tract involvement |
| Sensory level | Clear, LMN signs above UMN signs | +/– |
| Radicular pain | +++ | – |
| Funicular pain | – | + |
| Local pain | ++ | – |
| Bony deformity and tenderness | ++ | – |

2. **Cross-sectional localization—which tracts are involved? (Table 2)**
3. **Is the lesion compressive or noncompressive? (Table 3)**
4. **If compressive, is it extramedullary or intramedullary (Table 4)?**
5. **If extramedullary, is it intradural or extradural?**

Intradural lesions are more associated with radicular pain. In extradural lesions, features acquire quicker symmetry than in intradural lesions owing to the small extradural space. Furthermore, they are associated with local deformity and tenderness.

## TREATMENT AND PREVENTION

A comprehensive history and neurological examination are indispensable for clinical localization and understanding the extent of disease involvement. Further diagnostic tests are required for confirmation of clinical diagnosis and etiological evaluation. Magnetic resonance imaging (MRI) of the spinal cord is essential to differentiate compressive from noncompressive pathologies **(Table 5, Figs. 1 and 2)**. Other advanced imaging modalities include digital substraction angiography in suspected cases of vascular myelopathies. **Flowchart 1** provides a diagnostic algorithm for evaluation of different etiologies. It is imperative to promptly identify the treatable options to avoid devastating sequelae. In cases of infective myelitis treatment is tailored as per infective agent along with additional role of steroids and intravenous immunoglobulin (IVIg) depending on the causative organism. Amongst the demyelinating pathologies, Multiple sclerosis is treated using short course steroids and disease modifying therapies. Non-MS demyelination are largely treated with intravenous methylprednisolone/IVIg/plasmapheresis in the acute phases followed by steroids and steroid sparing immunomodulators. Metabolic myelopathies require supplementation of the deficiencies (vitamin B12/vitamin E). Treatment of genetic etiologies are entirely supportive, though adrenal insufficiency must be investigated and addressed in adrenomyeloneuropathy. Treatment of spinal cord ischemia and strokes is limited with focus on use of augmented perfusion pressure (induced hypertension) and reducing external cord pressure. Vascular malformations are treated via open surgical repairs or endovascular procedures.

**TABLE 4: Clinical clues for extramedullary intradural versus extradural involvement.**

| | **Intramedullary** | **Extramedullary** |
|---|---|---|
| Onset | Symmetric | Asymmetric |
| Sphincter involvement | Early and common | Late |
| Radicular pain | Uncommon | Common |
| Funicular pain | Common | Uncommon |
| Sensory deficit | • Dissociation present<br>• Suspended sensory loss<br>• Initial sacral sparing | No dissociation |
| Pattern of progression of sensory involvement | Descending loss | Ascending loss |
| Lhermitte symptoms | Uncommon | Common |
| UMN signs | Late and mild | Prominent and early |
| LMN signs | Diffuse and prominent | At segmental level |
| Trophic signs | More marked | Not marked |
| Brown–Séquard | Less common | Common |

**TABLE 5: Salient features of magnetic resonance imaging of the spine of commonly encountered myelopathies.**

| | |
|---|---|
| Spondylotic myelopathy | • Spinal canal stenosis, spondylolisthesis, disc herniations, osteophyte formation, ossification of posterior longitudinal ligament, ligamentum flavum hypertrophy and calcification<br>• Initial stages, edema is present at compression site with progression to myelomalacia. "Pancake sign" is observed in T1 weighted contrast as focal, thin transverse band of cord enhancement, affecting peripheral white matter tracts, at the focus of spinal stenosis. Owl's eye sign (hyperintensity of the anterior horns) is also noted in compressive myelopathies |
| Spinal epidural lipomatosis | In T1 weighted MRI, compression of the thecal sac causes a polygonal deformation of dural sac (Y sign) |
| Multiple sclerosis | Longitudinally multiple, short segment (<2 vertebral segments) and cross-sectionally small and peripheral lesions. Occasionally, it can be long segment |
| NMOSD | Longitudinally extensive (involving > 3 vertebral segments) lesions often extending upto medulla and cross-sectionally involves central gray matter. Cord expansion and bright spotty lesions are noted |
| MOGAD | Longitudinally extensive or segmental lesions often involving conus, cross-sectionally involves central gray matter (H sign) |
| Immune mediated | *Long segment hyperintensity*: Neurosarcoid particularly has dorsal cord, leptomeningeal involvement and crescentic posterior and lateral subpial enhancement called trident sign |

*Continued*

*Continued*

| | |
|---|---|
| Viral myelitis | Classically involves the anterior horn cells showing T2 hyperintensity—Owl's eye sign/snake eye sign. HIV characterized by symmetric nonenhancing symmetric T2 hyperintensity of posterior columns (Vacuolar myelopathy) |
| Syphilitic myelitis | Flip flop sign, candle guttering sign |
| Vascular | • Anterior spinal artery infarct, T2 hyperintensity of anterior horn cells—Owl's eye appearance. DWI should be asked when clinical suspicion is high<br>• Dural AVF, causes T2 hyperintensity in cord and cord expansion due to venous congestion and dilated perimedullary veins are seen as multiple flow voids on the surface |
| Metabolic | Vitamin B12 deficiency causes inverted V sign or inverted Rabbit ear signs—T2 hyperintensity of the posterior columns |

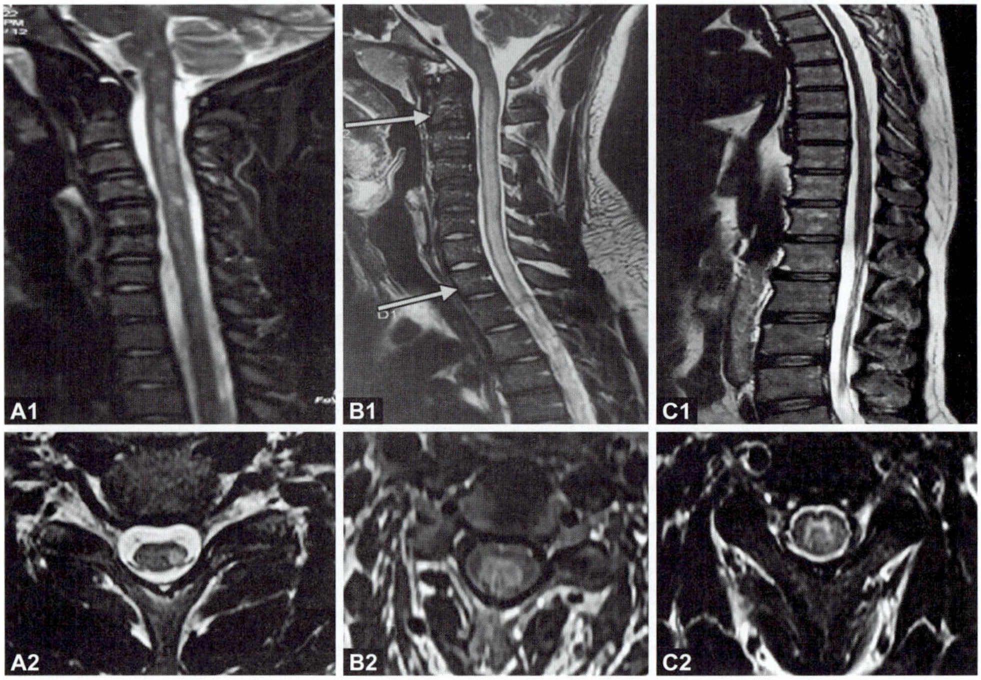


**FIGS. 1A TO C:** Magnetic resonance imaging of spine (T2 weighted images) showing: (A1) Sagittal view of spine in MS showing multiple small discrete lesions, (A2) axial section of spine showing small and peripherally located lesion (B1) Sagittal view of spine in NMOSD showing longitudinally extensive myelitis involving cervico-dorsal cord, (B2) axial section of spine showing central and large T2 hyperintense lesion, (C1) Sagittal view of spine in MOGAD showing longitudinally extensive myelitis extending up to conus, (C2) axial section of spine showing central and large T2 hyperintense lesion with H shaped pattern.

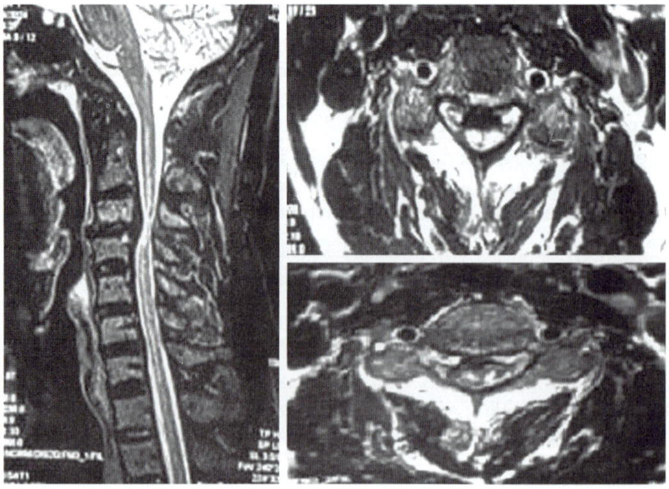

**FIG. 2:** Sagittal and axial views of cervical spine showing compressive myelopathy at C3-C4 with signal changes in cord and hyperintensity of anterior horn cells, Owl's eye appearance.

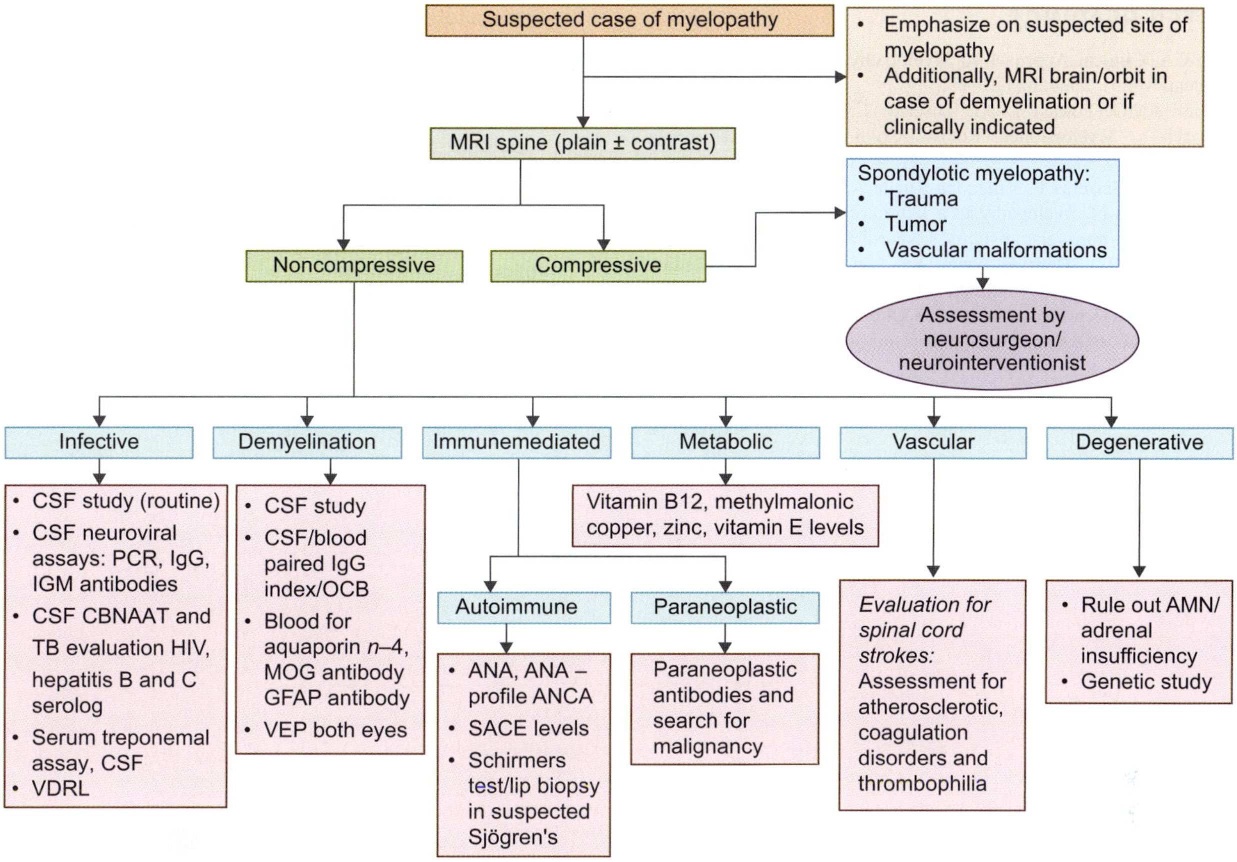


**FLOWCHART 1:** Algorithm for diagnostic approach in myelopathies.

## Points to Ponder

- Comprehensive history taking and neurological examination play a key role in narrowing down the differentials and guiding diagnostic imaging.
- Clinical localization is crucial to determine the part that needs to be scanned to avoid missing the diagnosis.
- Further importance lies in differentiation of compressive versus noncompressive etiologies with emphasis on search for immune- mediated and vascular etiologies for precision therapy.
- Prompt recognition of reversible etiologies can avoid devastating consequences.

## MULTIPLE CHOICE QUESTIONS

**1. What is the most likely diagnosis for a patient presenting with acute progressive weakness of bilateral lower limbs, sensory loss, and optic neuritis?**

A. Multiple sclerosis
B. Neuromyelitis optica spectrum disorder (NMOSD)
C. Guillain–Barré syndrome
D. Transverse myelitis

**2. Which antibody is commonly associated with NMOSD?**

A. Anti-aquaporin-4 antibody
B. Anti-MOG antibody
C. Anti-myelin basic protein antibody
D. Anti-NMDA receptor antibody

**3. Which of the following symptoms is NOT typically associated with NMOSD?**

A. Acute optic neuritis
B. Longitudinally extensive transverse myelitis
C. Progressive upper limb weakness
D. Girdle sensation around the umbilicus

**4. What Is the most common initial presentation in a patient with NMOSD?**

A. Visual disturbances
B. Gait abnormalities
C. Painful urinary retention
D. Sensory loss below the umbilicus

**5. Which MRI finding is characteristic of NMOSD?**

A. Longitudinally extensive transverse myelitis
B. Demyelination of the basal ganglia
C. Multiple white matter lesions in the brain
D. Confluent periventricular lesions

## Answers

1. (A); 2. (A); 3. (C); 4. (A); 5. (A)

## SUGGESTED READINGS

1. Pardo CA. Clinical Approach to Myelopathy Diagnosis. Continuum (Minneap Minn). 2024;30(1):14-52.
2. Sanchez AMG, Posada LMG, Toscano CAO et al. Diagnostic Approach to Myelopathies. Revista Colombiana De Radiología. 2011;22(3):3231-51.
3. Murphy OC, Barreras P, Villabona-Rueda A, et al. Identification of specific causes of myelopathy in a large cohort of patients initially diagnosed with transverse myelitis. J Neurol Sci 2022;442:120425.
4. Ray BK. (2022). Bedside Neurology. Jaypee Brothers Medical Publishers Pvt Limited. [Online]. http://books.google.ie/books?id=407IEAAAQBAJ&printsec=frontcover&dq=bed+side+neurology++BK+ray&hl=&cd=1&source=gbs_api=frontcover&dq=bedside+neurology+clinical+approach&hl=&cd=1&source=gbs_api. [Last accessed December, 2024].
5. Campbell WW, DeJong RN. (2005). DeJong's the Neurologic Examination. Lippincott Williams & Wilkins. [Online]. http://books.google.ie/books?id=CvgxUpZ7ZfUC&pg=PP8&dq=dejong&hl=&cd=1&source=gbs_api [Last accessed December, 2024].
6. Khadilkar SV, & Singh G. (2023). IAN Textbook of Neurology. Jaypee Brothers Medical Publishers Pvt Limited. [Online]. http://books.google.ie/books?id=48OjzwEACAAJ&dq=IAN+textbook+of+neurology&hl=&cd=1&source=gbs_api [Last accessed December, 2024].
7. Jadhav AP. Vascular Myelopathies. Continuum (Minneap Minn). 2024;30(1):160-79.

CHAPTER

61

# An Approach to a Case of New-onset Seizure

*Aradhya Sekhar Bagchi*

**CASE VIGNETTE**

A 24-year-old man, cab driver by profession, presented with history of a paroxysmal episode at night—semiology: There was no history of aura; tonic posturing of all limbs for 5–10 seconds, followed by clonic movements of both upper limbs lasting for 30–60 seconds. There was tongue bite in the left lateral margin, with no incontinence. Postictal drowsiness lasted for 30 minutes. The event was seen and described by the patient's wife who woke up during the episode. There was no family history of epilepsy, and no prior history of neurological disease/brain injury. Patient was not an alcoholic. Neurological examination was essentially normal. He presented to the outpatient department 3 days after the event, for opinion on further management. Examination and routine blood tests (CBC, CMP, LFT, RFT, electrolytes including calcium and magnesium) were normal. MRI brain (epilepsy protocol) and EEG (awake and sleep) were also normal. Given the nocturnal event with unwitnessed onset, the risk of recurrence was >60%, so antiseizure medication (ASM) was initiated after discussing risks and benefits. He was started on Levetiracetam 1 g/day (20 mg/kg/day) and advised to strictly avoid driving and consider a career change. Tapering was discussed as an option after 2–3 years of seizure freedom, with a risk of recurrence. Rejoining as a driver was advised only after at least 10 years of seizure freedom.

## PROVISIONAL DIAGNOSIS

Generalized tonic–clonic seizure (GTCS) likely idiopathic epilepsy.

## DIFFERENTIAL DIAGNOSES

Based on the patient's history, in all probability he had a seizure. The semiology that has been described is of GTCS, of unknown onset (as onset was not witnessed by his wife). However, any such paroxysmal episode can have quite a few differentials **(Table 1)**

The commonest differentials for seizure are syncope and psychogenic nonepileptic seizure (PNES).

- *Syncope*: It is a close mimic of seizure, however, can be reliably differentiated with history alone **(Table 2)**. The closest differential of seizure is a convulsive syncope, in which the patient lands in orthostatic position after syncopal attack, causing transient hypoxemia to the brain which in turn leads to a convulsion. Characteristics of a seizure include the presence of an aura, cyanosis, unconsciousness, motor manifestations lasting >30 seconds, postictal confusion, muscle soreness, and sleepiness. In contrast, a syncopal episode is to be suspected if the event was provoked by acute pain or anxiety or occurred immediately after arising from recumbent or sitting position. In patients with suspected postural hypotension, an autonomic function test/tilt table test may be needed to rule out syncopal attack.
- *Psychogenic nonepileptic seizure*: It is a conversion reaction precipitated by underlying psychological distress. Certain behaviors, such as side-to-side head turning, asymmetric

**TABLE 1: Differential diagnoses of seizure.**

| Observation | Seizure |
|---|---|
| Metabolic disturbances | • Alcoholic blackouts<br>• Delirium tremens<br>• Hypoglycemia<br>• Hypoxia<br>• Psychoactive drugs (e.g., hallucinogens) |
| Sleep disorders | • Narcolepsy/Cataplexy<br>• Benign sleep myoclonus<br>• Psychogenic seizure |
| Psychological disorders | • Hyperventilation<br>• Panic attack |
| Transient ischemic attack (TIA) | • Basilar artery TIA<br>• Tics |
| Movement disorders | • Nonepileptic myoclonus<br>• Paroxysmal choreoathetosis |
| Migraine | • Confusional migraine<br>• Basilar migraine<br>• Breath-holding spells<br>• Migraine with recurrent abdominal pain and cyclic vomiting |
| Special considerations in children | • Benign paroxysmal vertigo<br>• Apnea<br>• Night terrors<br>• Sleepwalking |

**TABLE 2: Clinical indicators to differentiate seizure from syncope.**

| Observation | Seizure | Syncope |
|---|---|---|
| Onset | Sudden | More gradual |
| Duration | Minutes | Seconds |
| Jerks | Frequent | Rare |
| Headache | Frequent (after) | Occasional (before) |
| Postevent confusion | Frequent | Rare |
| Incontinence | Frequent | Rare |
| Eye deviation | Horizontal | Usually absent |
| Tongue biting | Frequent | Rare |
| Prodrome | Aura | Dizziness, nausea, sweating |

and large-amplitude shaking movements of the limbs, pelvic thrusting are more commonly associated with psychogenic rather than epileptic seizures. The best means to diagnose this would be a video recording of the event, and if that is also not conclusive, a video EEG.

## CLINICAL APPROACH

### History

The first step in any patient presenting with a paroxysmal episode is a thorough history, preferably eyewitness accounts regarding the semiology of the event. It has to be ascertained from history whether the episode is a true seizure or more likely to be a seizure mimic.

Once history points toward a diagnosis of seizure, history of precipitating factors should be sought, particularly history of alcohol, drug and psychoactive medication use; history of comorbid conditions which may precipitate electrolyte imbalance like chronic kidney disease, diabetes mellitus, or other endocrine disturbances. Family history of epilepsy, and history of prior events, which may not be seizure but just aura like déjà vu, sudden feeling of fear, bad smell or taste, and brief language difficulties should also be sought for, as the presence of the such episodes in the recent or remote past might indicate that it is not a new-onset, rather recurrent seizures, fulfilling a diagnosis of epilepsy.

### Examination

Soon after history, a thorough general and systemic, including neurologic examination, should be done to look for potential 'provoking' sources of seizure. The following signs should be looked for:

- Infection-cutaneous or systemic
- Malignancy lymphadenopathy should be extensively searched. Breast examination is compulsory in female patients
- Signs of alcohol use or drug intoxication
- Neurocutaneous disorders, like neurofibromatosis or tuberous sclerosis
- Chronic liver disease/chronic kidney disease/congestive heart failure
- Organomegaly in storage disorders and lymphoreticular malignancies
- Signs of head trauma-recent or remote

**BOX 1: Baseline investigations to look for "provoking" causes of seizure.**

*Baseline investigations in any patient presenting with seizure*:

- Random blood sugar
- Electrolytes: sodium, potassium, calcium, magnesium
- Complete blood count
- Renal function tests, liver function tests
- Arterial blood gas
- Pregnancy test

**BOX 2: Risk factors associated with a seizure recurrence rate of ≥60% after a first unprovoked seizure.**

*Factors associated with seizure recurrence risk*:

- Prior brain injury
- Abnormal neuroimaging
- Focal or generalized epileptiform discharges on EEG
- Nocturnal seizure

### Investigations

About 25–30% of all seizure cases will be provoked/acute symptomatic seizure. The most common provoking factors are electrolyte disturbances, most notably hypoglycemia and hyponatremia, with other factors being hypocalcemia and hypomagnesemia **(Box 1)**. Pregnancy test should be done in all females of reproductive age group. Provoked seizures have a low risk of recurrence, if the provoking factor is addressed. Prophylactic antiepileptics may be given for a period of 3–6 months, and may be gradually withdrawn after this period if there are no other factors which might predispose to a higher risk of recurrence **(Box 2)**.

If no obvious provoking factor is found, patient is to be subjected to other investigations:

- *EEG*: Has a sensitivity of 17% in picking up epileptiform discharges, further sensitivity may be increased by performing the EEG within the first 24 hours, doing a 60-minute record, and three serial routine EEGs. If these too fail to detect IEDs, a sleep deprived EEG may be performed within 7 days of the episode. EEG is also necessary if a patient presents with persistent altered sensorium after a single episode of seizure, to rule out nonconvulsive status epilepticus.
- *Neuroimaging*: MRI is preferred over CT, unless there is any contraindication to MRI.
  - 3-Tesla MRI is preferable to 1.5.
  - Axial and coronal ≤ 3 mm T2/FLAIR cuts are needed.
  - MPRAGE and SWI/GRE sequences to look for hemosiderin/calcification are also needed in the protocol. Contrast studies may be needed in patients above 50 years of age due to higher likelihood of metastatic or primary brain neoplasms in this age.
  - CT may be preferred in the acute setting if patient is restless and MRI facility is not available.
- *Lumbar puncture (LP)*: It may be considered in an acute presentation of seizure, if:
  - Patient has fever

- Patient has severe headache
- Patient is immunocompromised has history of malignancy
- Patient is in persistent altered mental state after seizure

## Treatment

If MRI shows structural brain lesion/EEG shows presence of focal IEDs/generalized epilepsy, antiepileptic drugs need to be started (discussed in the following section). Definitive treatment of the underlying condition, if any such is detected on MRI or LP (e.g., arterial or venous stroke/neuroinfection/trauma/tumor) should be initiated.

## PATHOPHYSIOLOGY

The case suggests a GTCS, likely due to abnormal synchronous neuronal discharges across the bilateral cerebral cortex. The tonic phase (posturing of limbs) results from sustained muscle contraction due to increased excitatory activity, while the clonic phase (rhythmic jerking) follows as inhibitory mechanisms intermittently counteract the excitatory bursts. The post-ictal drowsiness reflects temporary neuronal exhaustion and recovery. Despite normal imaging and EEG, the risk of recurrence remains high due to underlying neuronal hyperexcitability, necessitating antiseizure medication (ASM) therapy.

## TREATMENT AND PREVENTION

*First episode of provoked seizure*:

1. **Should we treat?**
*Ans*: Treatment should be directed at removing the provoking factor. Prophylactic ASMs are usually not needed, unless there is a recurrence. However, may be given after deciding on a case-to-case basis.

2. **How long should we treat?**
*Ans*: If at all ASMs are given, they are to be given for a short duration of 3–6 months after deciding on a case-to-case basis.

*First episode of unprovoked seizure*:

1. **Should we treat?**
*Ans*: If any of the risk factors for a recurrence risk of 60% or more (**Table 2**) are present, ASMs are to be initiated.

2. **How long should we treat?**
*Ans*: If structural lesion is not present on neuroimaging, and if it is not an epilepsy syndrome, then for a minimum of 2–3 years: thereafter tapering may be tried based on an assessment of the risks and benefits to the patient. If any of the aforementioned two are present, treatment is to be given lifelong.

**What should be the drug(s) of choice?**
*Ans*: For GTCS semiology, 1st line drugs are Valproate, and Lamotrigine. For focal seizures, 1st line drugs are Lamotrigine, Levetiracetam and Carbamazepine/Oxcarbazepine. However, in view of minimal adverse effects, levetiracetam may be used in both. Other drugs that may be used are enumerated in **Table 3**.

*Anti-seizure medications in pregnancy*: Levetiracetam and lamotrigine are the two commonly used drugs in pregnancy due to their established safety profile. Other drugs, particularly valproate may be avoided due to risk of neural tube defects. Folic acid supplementation (0.4 mg/day) is necessary along with all ASMs in pregnancy.

**TABLE 3: List of first line and alternative drugs used in focal and generalized seizures.**

| | Focal seizures | Generalized tonic–clonic seizures |
|---|---|---|
| First line | • Lamotrigine<br>• Carbamazepine<br>• Oxcarbazepine<br>• Levetiracetam<br>• Phenytoin | • Valproate<br>• Lamotrigine<br>• Topiramate |
| Alternatives | • Topiramate<br>• Zonisamide<br>• Valproate<br>• Lacosamide<br>• Phenobarbital<br>• Clobazam<br>• Perampanel | • Levetiracetam<br>• Zonisamide<br>• Phenytoin<br>• Phenobarbital |

### Points to Ponder

- All paroxysmal events are not seizures. Meticulous history (with review of video of event if available) should be taken to rule out mimics.
- A single seizure does not warrant a diagnosis of epilepsy, unless associated with specific risk factors that confer a risk of recurrence more than 60%.
- 25–30% of the seizures are provoked. Provoking etiology may be worked up by means of lab investigations and urine drug and toxin screen. Mere correction of the provoking factor may lead to a very low risk of recurrence, and antiepileptic even if initiated may be given for a short period of time.
- In a first episode of unprovoked seizure, neuroimaging and electroencephalography have to be done: Antiepileptics are to be started if the expected risk of recurrence is more than 60%.
- In a first episode of unprovoked seizure, with expected risk of recurrence less than 60% after neuroimaging and electroencephalography, there needs to be an extensive discussion with the patient regarding initiation of antiseizure medication, with due consideration being given to socioeconomic, psychosocial and cultural factors.

## MULTIPLE CHOICE QUESTIONS

1. **What is the most likely diagnosis for the described episode in this patient?**
   A. Psychogenic nonepileptic seizure (PNES)
   B. Generalized tonic–clonic seizure
   C. Focal seizure with secondary generalization
   D. Transient ischemic attack
2. **Which feature of the semiology strongly supports the diagnosis of a seizure?**
   A. Absence of an aura
   B. Tonic posturing and clonic movements
   C. Absence of urinary incontinence
   D. Postictal drowsiness lasting 30 minutes
3. **The presence of a tongue bite in the left lateral margin suggests:**
   A. Focal seizure origin
   B. Syncope
   C. Generalized tonic–clonic seizure
   D. Psychogenic seizure
4. **Which of the following features makes PNES less likely?**
   A. History described by the patient's wife
   B. Tonic–clonic movements lasting 30–60 seconds
   C. Absence of urinary incontinence
   D. Presence of tongue bite
5. **What would be the most appropriate next step in the management of this patient?**
   A. Reassurance and discharge without further workup
   B. EEG and brain imaging (MRI)
   C. Initiate antiepileptic drugs immediately
   D. Refer to psychiatry for PNES evaluation

### Answers

1. (B); 2. (D); 3. (C); 4. (D); 5. (B)

## SUGGESTED READINGS

1. Hauser WA, Annegers JF, Kurland LT. Incidence of epilepsy and unprovoked seizures in Rochester, Minnesota: 1935-1984. Epilepsia. 1993;34(3):453-68.
2. Fisher RS, Acevedo C, Arzimanoglou A, et al. ILAE official report: a practical clinical definition of epilepsy. Epilepsia. 2014;55(4):475-82.
3. Sridharan R, Murthy BN. Prevalence and pattern of epilepsy in India. Epilepsia 1999;40:6316.
4. Sandeep P, Cherian A, Iype T, et al. Clinical profile of patients with nascent alcohol related seizures. Ann Indian Acad Neurol. 2013;16(4):530-3.
5. Saygi S, Katz A, Marks DA. Frontal lobe partial seizures and psychogenic seizures: comparison of clinical and ictal characteristics. Neurology. 1992;42(7):1274-7.
6. Bouma HK, Labos C, Gore GC, et al. The diagnostic accuracy of routine electroencephalopgraphy after a first unprovoked seizure. Eur J Neurol. 2016;23:455-63.
7. Burkholder DB, Britton JW, Rajasekaran V, et al. Routine vs extended outpatient EEG for the detection of interictal epileptiform discharges. Neurology. 2016;86:1524-30.
8. Geut I, Weenink S, Knottnerus ILH, et al. Detecting interictal discharges in first seizure patients: ambulatory EEG or EEG after sleep deprivation? Seizure. 2017;51:52-4.
9. Baldin E, Hauser WA, Bucchalter JR, et al. Yield of epileptiform electroencephalogram abnormalities in incident unprovoked seizures: a population-based study. Epilepsia. 2014;55:1389-98.
10. Wellmer J, Quesada CM, Rothe L, et al. Proposal for a magnetic resonance imaging protocol for the detection of epileptogenic lesions at early outpatient stages. Epilepsia. 2013;54:1977-87.
11. Knake S, Triantafyllou C, Wald LL, et al. 3T phased array MRI improves the presurgical evaluation in focal epilepsies: a prospective study. Neurology. 2005;65:1026-31.
12. Phal PM, Usmanov A, Nesbit GM, et al. Qualitative comparison of 3-T and 1.5-T MRI in the evaluation of epilepsy. AJR Am J Roentgenol. 2008;191:890-5.
13. Chen T, Si Y, Chen D, et al. The value of 24-hour video-EEG in evaluating recurrence risk following a first unprovoked seizure: a prospective study. Seizure. 2016;40:46-51.

CHAPTER 62

# An Approach to a Case of Lower Back Pain

*Joydeep Mukherjee*

## CASE VIGNETTE

Lower back pain (LBP) is one of the most common symptoms in medicine and neurology clinics. There are numerous causes behind it. We must look closer at the problem to solve it efficiently. A 24-year-old athlete male with LBP for 1 week with radiation to lower limb with lower limb weakness → MRI showed disk prolapse at L4/5 level → Surgical decompression by microdiscectomy and patient improved.

A 52-year-old farmer male with LBP for 3 months along with leg pain without any limb weakness → MRI showed ligamentum flavum hypertrophy and obliteration of subarachnoid space at the level of L3, L4, and L5 → physical therapy, analgesics, gabapentin, muscle relaxants relieved him slowly.

A 65-year-old retired-police male with LBP for 2 months with significant weight loss and occasional fever → MRI showed epidural abscess → surgical decompression done → epidural fluid culture showed tuberculosis → bed rest, antitubercular medicines, and symptomatic therapy let him recover.

A 66-year-old housewife with LBP for 6 months with occasional leg pain → MRI lumbosacral spine showed vertebral fracture with M band in serum protein electrophoresis → multiple myeloma referred to hematologist for treatment.

A 52-year-old shop-owner male with LBP for 2 months with stooped posture → other clinical features suggested parkinsonism → MRI brain normal with MRI lumbosacral spine showed degenerative pine disease → Levodopa therapy and analgesics helped him to recover.

A 70-year-old housewife with LBP for 1 year → MRI and bone scan showed osteoporotic vertebral fracture → treated with analgesics, calcium vitamin D, later vertebroplasty.

A 20-year-old female with fever and LBP for two weeks with abdominal heaviness and lower urinary tract symptoms → MRI lumbosacral spine unremarkable → CT abdomen showed free fluid in pelvis → urine examination suggestive of infection → antibiotics and analgesics relieved her.

A 16-year-old school student with LBP for 1 year with morning stiffness, past history of redness in eyes and blood in stool → MRI sacroiliac joint showed inflammation in bilateral sacroiliac joints → anti-inflammatory therapy improved him.

## PROVISIONAL DIAGNOSIS

*Pain-sensitive structures of the back* **(Fig. 1):**

- Vertebra or pelvis
- Facet joints
- Dura mater
- Paraspinal muscles
- Lumbosacral nerve roots
- Lumbosacral plexus
- Peripheral nerves
- Blood vessels

Apart from these, there is referred pain from intra-abdominal organs.

## DIFFERENTIAL DIAGNOSES

- *A 24-year-old athlete male*: Provisional diagnosis—Lumbar disk prolapse (L4/5). Differential diagnosis—lumbar radiculopathy due to spinal stenosis.
- *A 52-year-old farmer male*: Provisional diagnosis—lumbar spinal stenosis with ligamentum flavum hypertrophy. Differential diagnosis—degenerative disk disease.
- *A 65-year-old retired police male*: Provisional diagnosis—tuberculous epidural abscess. Differential diagnosis—spinal malignancy (e.g., metastasis).
- *A 66-year-old housewife*: Provisional diagnosis—multiple myeloma with vertebral fracture. Differential diagnosis—osteoporotic vertebral compression fracture.
- *A 52-year-old shop-owner male*: Provisional diagnosis—degenerative spine disease with parkinsonism. Differential diagnosis—lumbar spondylosis.
- *A 70-year-old housewife*: Provisional diagnosis—osteoporotic vertebral fracture. Differential diagnosis—metastatic vertebral lesion.
- *A 20-year-old female*: Provisional diagnosis—lower urinary tract infection (UTI) with pelvic free fluid. Differential diagnosis—pelvic inflammatory disease (PID).

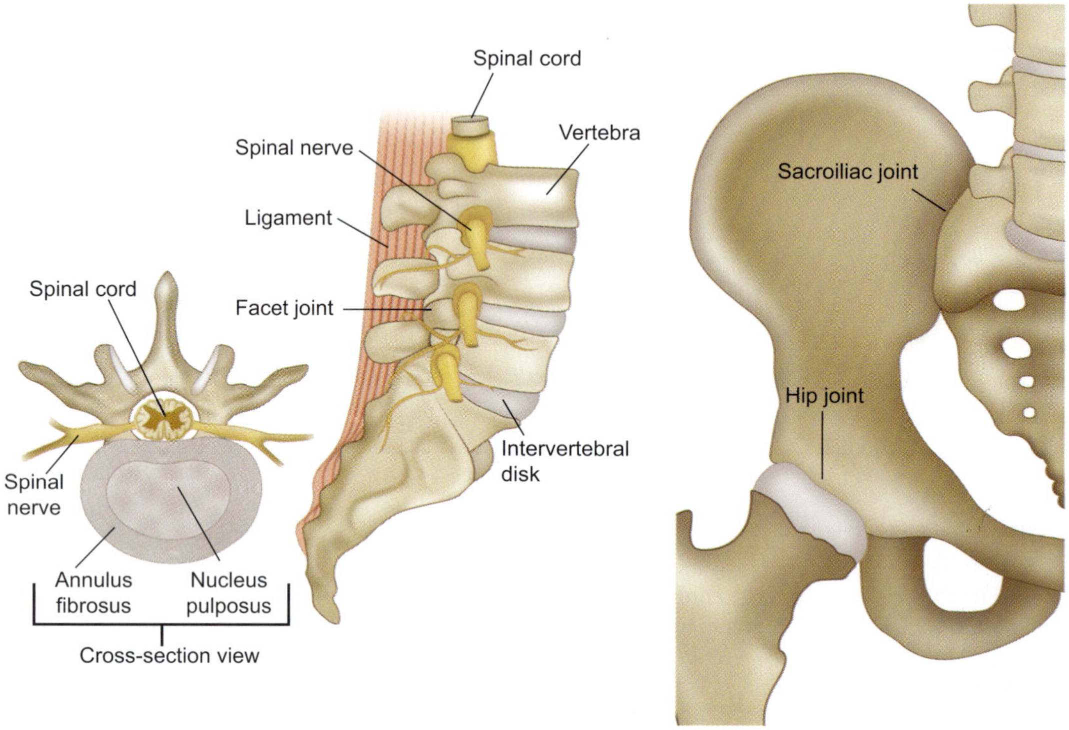


**FIG. 1:** Pain-sensitive structures related to lower back pain.

- *A 16-year-old school student*: Provisional diagnosis—ankylosing spondylitis with sacroiliitis. Differential diagnosis—juvenile idiopathic arthritis.

## PATHOPHYSIOLOGY

- *Mechanical pain (may be due to lumber spondylosis, vertebral or disk destruction or inflammation, sacroiliac joint inflammation, facet joint inflammation)*: In all cases, movement exacerbates pain. SI joint pain lateral to the lower spine. Facet pain is unilateral or bilateral paraspinal pain. It occurs due to paraspinal muscle and ligament strain/tear, bony and connective tissue pain. It is a dull aching pain without any radicular component.
- *Neuropathic pain (radiculopathy, plexopathy, mononeuropathy, polyneuropathy)*: The spinal stenosis pain remains in the lower back, buttocks, and legs with an increment while standing, walking, and back extension. Radiculopathy patients have back pain radiating to the leg following a dermatome and increasing with coughing or straining. The sensory-motor loss follows a root distribution in radiculopathy. Plexopathy cases have back and leg pain with dysesthesia, burning, or electric-shock-like sensation.
- *Non-neurological pain (mostly referred pain) (urolithiasis, abdominal aortic aneurysm, endometriosis, enlarged ovarian mass, pelvic inflammatory disease, etc.)*: Ovarian origin pain remains in the hip and lower back with bowel disturbance in advanced cases. Uterine-origin pain remains in the pelvis but occasionally goes to the back and legs. Urolithiasis pain radiates from the upper or mid-back laterally to the groin. Pain from the retroperitoneal structures remains in the back bilateral to the spine along with a neuropathic component in case of plexus or nerve involvement.
- Patients may have either one type of pain or a combination.

## CLINICAL APPROACH

- *Lumber spine stenosis*: Late middle-aged and older adults. Disk disease, bony hypertrophy, ligamentum flavum thickening cause direct pressure on cauda equina and nerve roots. Vascular supply compromise due to lumbar spine extension during standing (bulging ligamentum flavum) causes nerve root ischemia, leading to severe pain and weakness. Leg pain is exacerbated by standing, walking, and relieved by sitting. The prone position lying down worsens the pain by spinal extension. MRI of the lumber spine shows obliteration of subarachnoid space at the level of the lesion. Leg weakness or sphincter problem leads to surgical decompression. Otherwise, physical therapy and medication will help.
- *Cauda equina syndrome*: Direct compression of nerve roots below the termination of the spinal cord in degenerative bony disease, lumbar disk disease, abscess, hematoma, tumor, or acute trauma. Conus medullaris syndrome occurs due to damage to the terminal spinal cord at a bit higher level than cauda equina syndrome. Back pain, leg pain, weakness, and cramps of leg muscles are common. Sensory loss, neuropathic pain, and sphincter disturbances also occur. The latter syndrome is more rapidly progressive, and more symmetrical, with earlier back pain, and sphincter problems than the former one. MRI of the lumbosacral spine with contrast is required. Treatment is according to the etiology and severity of the disease.
- *Lumbosacral radiculopathy*: Infringement of neural foramen by a herniated disk (young patients), or osteophytes (older patients). They have back pain radiating down the leg following the nerve root. MRI of the lumbosacral spine is diagnostic. NCV may show the F or H wave delay. EMG can differentiate between radiculopathy and peripheral neuropathy by showing the denervation in muscles in either

distribution. Anti-inflammatory and muscle relaxants help in mild disease. Surgical decompression is needed in motor or sphincter deficit patients.

- *Arachnoiditis*: Inflammation of the arachnoid surrounding the spinal cord due to injury surgery, chronic compression, intrathecal chemotherapy/contrast agents, infection, or neoplasm. Patients have back and leg pain along with a suggestive history. MRI shows clumped nerve roots ardent to each other and dura. CSF is necessary. Treatment is symptomatic. Prevention is the best method and is achieved by avoiding injury and administering steroids with the intrathecal agent.
- *Plexopathy*: Plexopathy is caused by lumbosacral plexus involvement due to abscess, hematoma, or neoplasm. Patients may have back pain with leg motor and sensory symptoms. CT abdomen is necessary along with an MRI lumbosacral plexus with contrast.
- *Acute inflammatory demyelinating polyradiculoneuropathy*: Back pain may be present before the motor and sensory deficits in the limbs. MRI may show an enhancement in the lumbosacral nerve roots. NCV and CSF will aid in the diagnosis.
- *Piriformis syndrome*: Piriformis muscle compresses the sciatic nerve or superior gluteal branch. Patients have pain in the buttock, radiating to the leg, and exacerbating during hip flexion and adduction (prolonged sitting and climbing stairs). Treatment is by anti-inflammatory agents and local injection of steroids.
- *Meralgia paresthetica*: Lateral femoral cutaneous nerve dysfunction due to compression by inguinal ligament in cases of obesity, pregnancy, and diabetes. There is pain and sensory loss over the lateral thigh. Conservative management by weight loss, neuropathic medicines, and nerve block.
- *Femoral neuropathy*: Femoral nerve gets injury in pelvis or below the inguinal ligament resulting in weakness in the psoas ± quadriceps (stronger) and sensory loss over anterior thigh and medial calf. Adductors are spared due to supply by the obturator nerve (despite same root—differentiate L234 radiculopathy from femoral neuropathy). Physical therapy, weight loss, avoiding hip flexion usually resolve it.
- *Peroneal neuropathy*: Peroneal neuropathy occurs in the prolonged bed rest, knee hyperflexion, cross-legged sitting, ballet dancers, leg casting leading to compression at the fibular neck. They have foot drop.
- *Herpes zoster*: Rash and neuropathic pain occurs in a single nerve distribution following the reactivation of varicella zoster virus. Treatment by antiviral and neuropathic medicines, especially carbamazepine.
- *Claudication of leg arteries*: Walking and other activities increases the ischemia of iliac arteries, and the terminal branches causes pain, weakness, and vascular changes in the lower limbs. There is no back pain or pain increment on spinal extension. Ultrasonography doppler or invasive angiography are the diagnostic modality. Medical therapy (cilostazol, statin, and other) and angioplasty are the treatments.
- *Sacroiliitis*: Pain is isolated to back and paraspinal region in ankylosing spondylitis, psoriasis, autoimmune arthritis, degenerative, infective, or destructive process.
- *Hip joint pathology*: Pain in the groin with increment with movement, occasionally with history of long-term steroid or trauma makes us suspicious about ipsilateral hip joint pathology. Patrick test is positive with pain over anterior part of groin.
- *Facet joint pain syndrome*: Paraspinal pain is exacerbated by extension or ipsilateral bending. Repetitive strenuous activity, excessive weight, and abnormal posture predisposes to the degenerative process leading to pain.
- *Lumber spine compression*: Compression of the vertebral bodies due to acute trauma, osteoporosis, infection, or tumor leads to low back pain without a radicular component. Radicular pain may be present in case of collapsed vertebra compression the nerve root. Pain is exacerbated by movement of spine (bending or twisting). MRI or bone scan differentiates it from tumor or degeneration. Treatment is by bed rest, bracing, analgesics, and surgery (vertebroplasty for unstable lesion, spinal/neural compression). Corticosteroid and radiation therapy for malignant vertebral collapse.
- *Spinal tumor*: Patients might have dull aching low back pain, radicular pain, sensory and motor loss according to the location of the tumor in spine. MRI with contrast is diagnostic.
- *Lumber diskitis*: Lower back pain and markedly restricted spine flexion without any radicular component occur due to inflammation of the intervertebral disks from infections (most common *Staphylococcus aureus* and mycobacteria). MRI shows changes in the endplates of adjacent vertebra. High ESR, CRP with elevated tracer uptake in the infected disks in the bone-scan are present. Organism is identified with biopsy. Treatment is by bed rest and antibiotics. But rarely diskectomy with fusion of the adjacent vertebra is required.
- *Spinal epidural abscess*: Bacterial infection of the epidural space leads to fever back pain, and neurologic deficits. MRI and blood/tissue culture clinches the diagnosis. Empiric treatments, aspiration, and open surgery are the treatment options.
- *Lumber spine osteomyelitis*: Lower back pain is associated with systemic inflammatory signs, tender vertebra, tight paraspinal muscles, decreased back movement. MRI shows local tissue oedema. The commonest organism is *Staphylococcus aureus*. Treatment is by bed rest, antibiotics ± surgical debridement.

*Some tips and tricks in clinical approach*:

- Middle-age, anemia, renal failure → myeloma
- Cachectic appearance → malignancy, tuberculosis
- Generalized rashes → meningitis
- Bruises → trauma
- Distended bladder → myelopathy, prostate carcinoma
- Stiff back → ankylosis spondylitis
- Stooping forward posture, slowness, rigidity, imbalance, tremor → parkinsonism
- Exaggerated lumber lordosis, difficulty in bending forward → Stiff-person syndrome
- Multiple lymphadenopathy → tuberculosis, lymphoma, malignancy
- Abnormal limb or back posture, may increase after activity or diurnal variation → dystonia
- Straight leg raising test below 60° → lumber disk herniation
- Patrick/FABER test or figure-of-4 test → patient lies supine. The testing lower limb hip is abducted, externally rotated, and leg flexed. Then the leg is placed on the other knee (figure of 4). The testing knee is pressed downwards after fixating the opposite anterior superior iliac spine. If there is pain on the (a) same side anteriorly over pelvis → hip joint

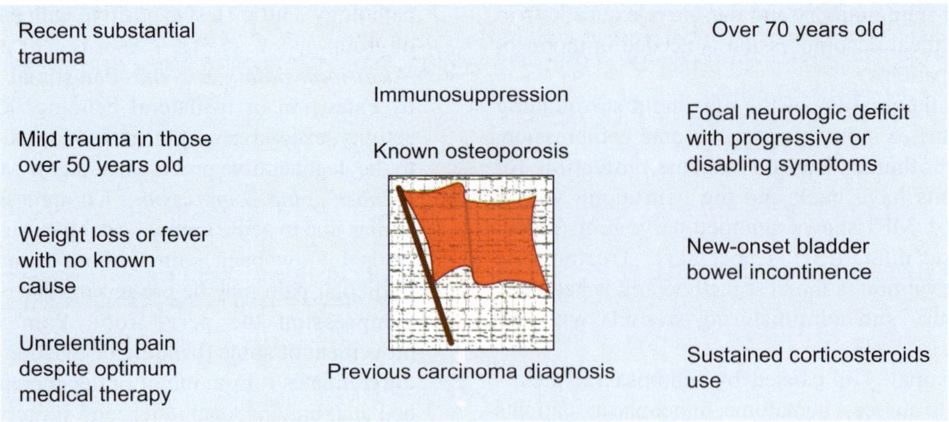


**FIG. 2:** Red flags for low back pain when urgent neuroimaging is required.

pathology; (b) same/opposite side posteriorly over pelvis → sacroiliac joint pathology; (c) same side back of thigh → nerve root pathology.

- *Brisk lower limb deep tendon reflexes or extensor planter response*: Possible corticospinal tract involvement at the level of brain or cervical/dorsal cord.

2. *When to do imaging*: We should not do routine imaging in case of low back pain. If we get a red flag sign **(Fig. 2)**, then only we go for an MRI of the concerned area (MRI of lumbosacral spine or sacroiliac joint or lumbosacral plexus or hip joint).

## TREATMENT AND PREVENTION

- *MRI lumbosacral spine ± contrast*: Lower back pain with red flag signs **(Fig. 2)**
- *MRI sacroiliac joint/hip joint ± contrast*: Suspected pathology in respective joints
- *MRI dorsal spine ± contrast*: If brisk deep tendon reflex in lower limbs, paraspinal tenderness at dorsal level, Lhermitte's sign
- *MRI cervical spine ± contrast*: If brisk deep tendon reflex in lower limbs, wasting or fasciculation in the upper limbs, Lhermitte's sign
- *MRI brain*: Parkinsonism, dystonia
- *Nerve conduction study*: Plexopathy, acute demyelinating polyradiculoneuropathy
- *Electromyography*: Radiculopathy
- *Cerebrospinal fluid*: Acute demyelinating polyradiculoneuropathy, meningitis, tuberculosis, malignancy
- *Serum protein electrophoresis*: Lower back pain, middle to advanced age, polyradiculoneuropathy
- *Whole body PET scan*: Suspecting malignancy
- *CT abdomen*: Suspecting pelvic pathology, plexopathy

### Points to Ponder

- ❑ *Disks prolapse:* Common in young adults with acute lower back pain radiating to limbs; MRI confirms the diagnosis.
- ❑ *Tuberculosis of spine:* Consider in chronic back pain with systemic symptoms (fever, weight loss) and epidural abscess.
- ❑ *Multiple myeloma:* Suspect in older adults with vertebral fractures and M band on serum electrophoresis.
- ❑ *Ankylosing spondylitis:* Look for morning stiffness, sacroiliitis, and systemic features (uveitis, GI symptoms) in young patients.
- ❑ *Osteoporotic fractures:* Common in elderly; managed with calcium, vitamin D, and vertebroplasty when indicated.

## MULTIPLE CHOICE QUESTIONS

**1. In a 24-year-old athlete with lower back pain radiating to the lower limb and limb weakness, which MRI finding is most likely?**
   A. Ligamentum flavum hypertrophy
   B. Epidural abscess
   C. Disk prolapse at L4/5 level
   D. Vertebral fracture

**2. A 65-year-old male with lower back pain, weight loss, fever, and an epidural abscess is most likely suffering from:**
   A. Osteoporotic vertebral fracture
   B. Tuberculosis of the spine
   C. Lumbar disk prolapse
   D. Multiple myeloma

**3. What is the most likely diagnosis in a 16-year-old with lower back pain, morning stiffness, and MRI showing bilateral sacroiliac joint inflammation?**
   A. Juvenile idiopathic arthritis
   B. Ankylosing spondylitis
   C. Degenerative spine disease
   D. Spinal epidural abscess

**4. In a 66-year-old woman with lower back pain and vertebral fracture, which test result suggests multiple myeloma?**
   A. MRI showing ligamentum flavum hypertrophy
   B. Epidural fluid culture positive for tuberculosis
   C. Serum protein electrophoresis showing M band
   D. Bone scan showing osteoporotic changes

5. **What is the most appropriate treatment for a 70-year-old housewife with osteoporotic vertebral fracture?**
   A. Antitubercular therapy
   B. Surgical decompression
   C. Calcium, vitamin D, and vertebroplasty
   D. Anti-inflammatory therapy

## Answers

1. (C); 2. (B); 3. (B); 4. (C); 5. (C)

## SUGGESTED READINGS


1. Allegri M, Montella S, Salici F, et al. Mechanisms of low back pain: a guide for diagnosis and therapy. F1000 Research. 2016;5:F1000 Faculty Rev-1530.
2. Misulis KE, Murray EL. Lower back and lower limb pain, In: Daroff RB, Jankovic J, Mazziotta JC, Pomeroy SL (Eds). Bradley's Neurology in Clinical Practice. 7th edition. Philadelphia, Elsevier. 2016. p. 332-41.

CHAPTER 63

# An Approach to a Case of Neurological Manifestations of Systemic Disease

*Pradeep K Maheshwari, Akhilesh Kumar Singh, Ruhani Ahuja*

**CASE VIGNETTE**

A 40-year- old lady presented with cognitive dysfunction in the form of decreased self care, memory impairment and generalized weakness for 6 months. Further, history revealed that patient was having amenorrhea for about 7 years after last child birth. Physical examination revealed pallor, alopecia, dry coarse skin, hypotension and hung up reflexes. Mental status examination revealed disorientation to time and place, impaired attention, calculation and memory. On the basis of these manifestations patient was diagnosed clinically as Sheehan's syndrome. Her laboratory work up revealed anemia (hemoglobin-8.4 g%), hyperkalemia (serum potassium-5.4 mEq/L), decreased level of thyroid stimulating hormone (TSH)-0.3 mIU/L, free thyroxine 4 (fT4) -0.13 ng/dL and cortisol-0.16 µg/dL at 8.00 AM. Magnetic resonance imaging (MRI) of brain demonstrated partial empty sella turcica. Hence, we want to emphasize that an endocrinopathy may present with neurological manifestation. It is very important to understand neurological aspects of systemic diseases as it enables timely diagnosis and treatment and thus creating holistic treatment plan for better prognosis.

## PROVISIONAL DIAGNOSIS

Sheehan's syndrome (postpartum pituitary insufficiency).

## DIFFERENTIAL DIAGNOSIS

- Pituitary adenoma with hypopituitarism
- Lymphocytic hypophysitis
- Empty sella syndrome (primary or secondary)
- Chronic adrenal insufficiency (Addison's disease)
- Hypothyroidism due to other causes (e.g., autoimmune thyroiditis).

## CLINICAL APPROACH

Approaching to a case of neurological manifestations of systemic diseases, involves a systematic and comprehensive approach to diagnose and manage the patient.

### Detailed Medical History

Initially, a detailed medical history is essential, focusing on the chief complaints, including the onset, duration and progression of neurological symptoms. It's important to review the patient's past medical history for systemic diseases such as diabetes, hypertension, autoimmune diseases, thyroid illness, chronic liver disease (CLD), chronic kidney disease (CKD), malignancy or infections, etc. As many diseases have genetic predisposition, family history should be taken carefully. Social, occupational and travel history provide information regarding exposure to toxins and unusual infections.

### Thorough Physical Examination

A thorough physical examination starting with vital signs and general examination, clinicians should look for signs of systemic disease such as (malar rash, oral ulcers, polyarthritis—systemic lupus erythematosus), (symmetric small joint polyarthritis—rheumatoid arthritis), (palpable purpura—small vessel vasculitis), (coarse dry skin, alopecia, bradycardia, hung up reflexes—hypothyroidism), (hyperpigmentation on palmer crease and dorsum of foot suggestive of Addison's disease), (obesity, moon facies, buffalo hump, purple skin striae, hirsutism—Cushing's syndrome), (lymphadenopathy—malignancy and infection), (hepatosplenomegaly—hematological disorder and infection), (irregularly irregular pulse—atrial fibrillation leading to thromboembolic stroke), (asymmetrical or absent pulses and stroke—Takayasu arteritis), (headache, hemianopia—pituitary adenoma), (headache, diminution of vision, polymyalgia rheumatica, anemia in elderly patient—giant cell arteritis).

### Investigations

Accordingly we will plan relevant blood investigation, cerebrospinal fluid analysis (CSF), imaging studies (chest X-ray, ultrasonography, computed tomography scan, MRI of brain and spinal cord), nerve conduction studies, etc., depending upon suspected systemic disease.

## PATHOPHYSIOLOGY

Sheehan's syndrome occurs due to ischemic necrosis of the pituitary gland following severe postpartum hemorrhage.

Excessive blood loss leads to hypovolemic shock, causing reduced blood flow to the already enlarged pituitary gland during pregnancy, making it vulnerable to ischemia. This results in partial or complete destruction of the pituitary tissue, leading to panhypopituitarism with deficiencies in anterior pituitary hormones (e.g., TSH, ACTH, LH, FSH, GH, and prolactin). The resulting hormonal deficits manifest as hypothyroidism, adrenal insufficiency, amenorrhea, and other systemic symptoms **(Fig. 1)**.

## Management and Prevention

Assessment of neurological manifestation in systemic disease is crucial for several reasons as it helps in early detection and diagnosis, comprehensive patient management, preventing complications, research and understanding and prognostic significance.

Management of these cases requires multidisciplinary approach including neurologist, rheumatologist, endocrinologist, internist, etc., depending upon nature of systemic illnesses and primarily focus on treating the underlying systemic diseases and providing symptomatic treatment for neurological manifestation additionally, supportive care have to be provided to these patients to prevent in hospital complications. Rehabilitation including physiotherapist, speech therapist, occupational therapist, etc., helps patients to recover from after effects of disease and to improve quality of life.

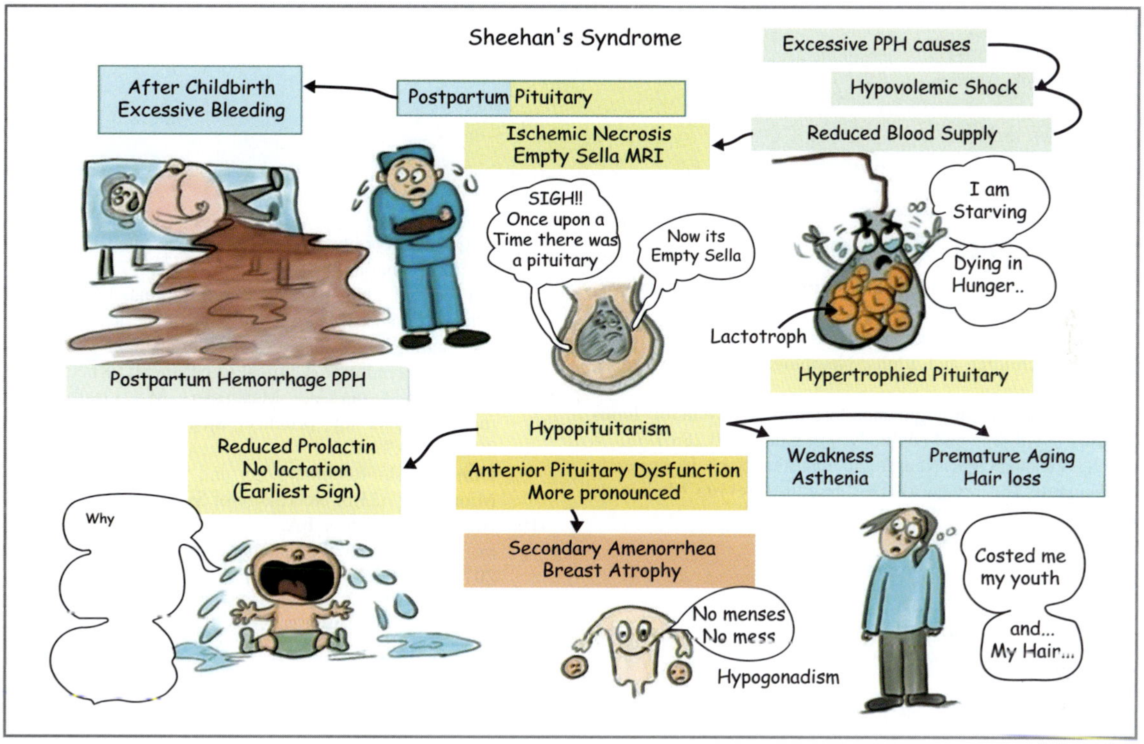


**FIG. 1:** Sheehan's syndrome (postpartum hypopituitarism).
*Source*: © 2024 Creative Med Dose.

### Points to Ponder

- As management of these cases consists of interdisciplinary approach, it is very important to timely find out underlying systemic disease with neurological manifestation.
- Interdisciplinary approach ensures treatment plans to address all facets of disease and improving overall outcome of patients.
- Educating patients about potential complication, encouraging them to adopt preventive measures and to follow-up regularly are vital for effective management.

## MULTIPLE CHOICE QUESTIONS

1. **What is the most likely diagnosis for a postpartum woman presenting with amenorrhea, cognitive dysfunction, and generalized weakness?**
   A. Addison's disease
   B. Sheehan's syndrome
   C. Pituitary adenoma
   D. Hypothyroidism
2. **Which hormonal abnormality is typically seen in Sheehan's syndrome?**
   A. Elevated TSH and cortisol
   B. Decreased TSH and cortisol
   C. Elevated free T4 and cortisol
   D. Decreased potassium and hemoglobin
3. **What MRI finding is characteristic of Sheehan's syndrome?**
   A. Pituitary adenoma
   B. Normal sella turcica
   C. Partial empty sella turcica
   D. Brainstem lesion
4. **Which physical examination finding supports a diagnosis of hypothyroidism in this case?**
   A. Hypertension
   B. Alopecia and dry coarse skin
   C. Hyperreflexia
   D. Tachycardia
5. **What is the likely cause of hyperkalemia in this patient?**
   A. Chronic kidney disease
   B. Adrenal insufficiency due to cortisol deficiency
   C. Excess potassium intake
   D. Hyperaldosteronism

### Answers

1. (B); 2. (B); 3. (C); 4. (B); 5. (B)

## SUGGESTED READINGS


1. Aminoff MJ. The neurological manifestations of systemic disease. Lancet Neurol. 2007;6(4):331-40.
2. Muscal E, Brey RL. Neurologic manifestations of systemic lupus erythematosus in children and adults. Neurologic Clinics [Internet]. 2009;28(1):61-73.
3. Muscal E, Brey RL. Neurologic manifestations of systemic lupus erythematosus in children and adults. Neurol Clin. 2010;28:61-73.
4. Massardo L, Vásquez MJ. Neurologic manifestations in systemic lupus erythematosus: a review of the literature. Revista Medica de Chile. [2015)
5. DeQuattro K, Imboden JB. Neurologic Manifestations of Rheumatoid Arthritis. Rheum Dis Clin North Am. 2017;43:561-71.
6. CA, et al. Neurologic manifestations of rheumatoid arthritis. Rheumatic Disease Clinics of North America. 2009.
7. La Paglia RTM, et al. Neurological manifestations of primary Sjögren's syndrome. Clinical Experimental Rheumatology. 2019.
8. Perzyńska-Mazan J, Maślińska M, Gasik R. Neurological manifestations of primary Sjögren's syndrome. Reumatologia. 2018;56(2):99-105.
9. Dimberg EL. Rheumatology and Neurology. Continuum (Minneap Minn). 2017;23(3, Neurology of Systemic Disease):691-721.
10. Amaral TN, Peres FA, Lapa AT, et al. Neurologic involvement in scleroderma: a systematic review. Semin Arthritis Rheum. 2013;43(3):335-47.

CHAPTER
64

# A Case-based Approach to Cerebral Salt-Wasting Syndrome

*Narmada Prasad Patel, Pooja Baradia*

**CASE VIGNETTE**

A 17-month-old female child was brought to the emergency with alleged history of fall from 20 feet building. She was bleeding from right ear with swelling of right side of head. On examination, weight was 7.5 kg, pulse rate 110/min, respiratory rate 32/min, $SpO_2$ 98%, blood pressure 90/60 mm Hg. Glasgow Coma Scale (GCS): 10/15, sluggishly reacting unequal pupils, increased tone, and extensor planters. She was started on intravenous fluids, phenytoin, dexamethasone, and antibiotics. CT head showed fracture of skull bone with subdural hematoma, extradural hematoma, subarachnoid hemorrhage and contusion. On day 3, she had multiple episodes of seizures which were controlled with antiepileptics. On day 10, child had polyuria (9 mL/kg/hr) with hyponatremia (128 mEq/L). Blood urea was 22 mg/dL and creatinine were 0.6 mg/dL. Possibility of SIADH and CSW was considered. Urine osmolality and urine sodium were 400 mOsmol/L and 146 mEq/L, respectively, serum osmolality was 265 mOsmol/L. Serum uric acid was 3.5 mg/dL. Uric acid (24.8%) and sodium (4.16%) fractional excretion were increased. normal saline was given. Patient still had hyponatremia, 3% NaCl infusion was started. Polyuria (reached up to 15 mL/kg/hr) was not controlled despite saline infusion. On day 13 she was started on oral fludrocortisone 0.1 mg/day, in two divided doses which increased to 0.2 mg/day after 2 days. Urine output improved gradually and polyuria subsided. Fludrocortisone was tapered and stopped on day 20. On discharge, her sensorium was normal, had normal urine output and no seizures.

## PROVISIONAL DIAGNOSIS

Traumatic brain injury (TBI) with skull fracture, intracranial hemorrhages, and cerebral salt-wasting syndrome (CSW).

## DIFFERENTIAL DIAGNOSIS

- CSW
- SIADH

Hyponatremia secondary to head trauma is generally considered SIADH. Both SIADH and CSW have hyponatremia, increased urinary sodium excretion and high urinary osmolality. However, SIADH is a volume expanded state whereas CSW is a volume depleted state. In CSW, the fluid balance is net negative. If there are any postural blood pressure abnormalities, tachycardia, or poor skin turgor, the clinical history and assessment results may be useful. Regretfully, there are times when this distinction is not clinically discernible. In a study by Chung et al., the clinical assessment of the ECFV status in 58 patients without edema and hyponatremia was investigated; only 47% of patients with hypovolemia and 48% of patients with euvolemia were accurately diagnosed.

The period of time between an injury and the onset of CSW might range from days to weeks. Elevated levels of BNP may support CSW but may not be present in all patients. It has been shown that the natriuretic peptides decrease intramedullary collecting-duct sodium absorption as well as direct tubular sodium resorption. Additionally, it is thought that they directly suppress the release of renin and aldosterone from the adrenal gland and juxtaglomerular cells, respectively. To detect brain pathology any new deficit should be assessed by neurological examination, CSF examination or electroencephalogram. Other known causes of renal sodium loss should be excluded.

To differentiate between the two uric acid level can be measured. Initially both conditions have low serum uric acid level and high fractional excretion of uric acid. In SIADH sodium reabsorption in proximal tubule is decreased leading to less uric acid absorption and increased loss in urine. Whereas in CSW exact mechanism is not known. There is impaired urate transport in proximal tubules. The differentiation can be made by the observation that Fe uric acid continues to be high even after correction of hyponatremia in CSW.

## CLINICAL APPROACH

The etiology is not completely understood. Hyponatremia develops quickly in the first 2 weeks following SAH. There is natriuresis and volume depletion with SAH, so patients become hyponatremic and hypovolemic. Brain natriuretic peptide (BNP) and atrial natriuretic peptide have a role in producing salt-wasting syndrome. Following an injury, they are released, and a breached blood-brain barrier allows them to enter the systemic circulation. BNP inhibits sodium reabsorption and reduces renin release via acting on the collecting ducts of renal tubules. It clears over the course of 1–2 weeks in the setting of SAH.

## Causes of CSW

- Subarachnoid hemorrhage
- Head trauma
- Intracranial neoplasm
- Metastatic neoplasm
- Infections or carcinomatous meningitis
- Encephalitis
- Central nervous system surgery

Cerebral salt-wasting syndrome is characterized by hyponatremia, inappropriate natriuresis, with hypovolemia. The disorders associated with CSW may include subarachnoid hemorrhage (SAH), traumatic brain injury, encephalitis and meningitis. It has to be differentiated from SIADH because cerebral salt-wasting will respond to aggressive fluid and Na-Cl repletion whereas in SIADH fluid is restricted. CSW resolves within weeks to months after onset. Comparison between CSW and SIADH is listed in **Table 1**.

Wijdicks et al. discovered that 17 out of 134 individuals who had subarachnoid hemorrhage had SIADH in a retrospective analysis. These 15 patients deteriorated after fluid restriction and thus might have had CSW. In case 1, there was no evidence of actual cerebral injury. In a study by Askar et al., they reported patients who presented with CSW without evidence of cerebrovascular injury or brain edema. It suggests that in patients with neurological disorders, even in absence of injury, hyponatremia secondary to CSW can occur. In children there are limited case reports and case series. Children with CSW usually have low blood pressure and shock due to polyuria, increased urinary sodium loss, and contraction of extracellular fluid.

## PATHOPHYSIOLOGY

In traumatic brain injury (TBI), damage to the brain, particularly to the hypothalamus or pituitary gland, disrupts sodium and fluid balance. Cerebral salt-wasting syndrome (CSW) occurs due to increased release of natriuretic peptides, which cause renal loss of sodium and water. This leads to hyponatremia, polyuria, and hypovolemia. Unlike SIADH, where fluid retention occurs, CSW involves a primary renal sodium loss despite normal adrenal and renal function. The resulting hyponatremia and polyuria require careful sodium and volume replacement, as seen in this case **(Fig. 1)**.

## TREATMENT AND PREVENTION

First treatment strategy is directed at underlying brain pathology. Second, patient must be volume repleted.

**TABLE 1: Comparison of CSW and SIADH.**

| Parameters | Cerebral salt-wasting (CSW) | Syndrome of inappropriate ADH secretion (SIADH) |
|---|---|---|
| Cerebral injury | Usually, evident | May be present |
| Volume status | Hypovolemic/ Dehydrated | Euvolemic/ Hypervolemic |
| Blood pressure | Decreased | Normal |
| Hematocrit | Increased | Normal |
| Central venous pressure | Decreased | Normal/Increased |
| Serum sodium | Decreased | Decreased |
| Plasma osmolality | Decreased | Decreased |
| Urine volume | Increased | Normal/Decreased |
| Urine sodium | Increased | Increased/Normal |
| Urine osmolality | Increased | Increased |
| Urinary sodium concentration | Increased | Increased |
| Fractional excretion of uric acid | High | |
| Remains high even after correction of sodium | High | |
| Brain natriuretic peptide (BNP) | Normal/Increased | Normal |
| Treatment | Salt and water repletion with fludrocortisone | Salt intake and free water restriction |

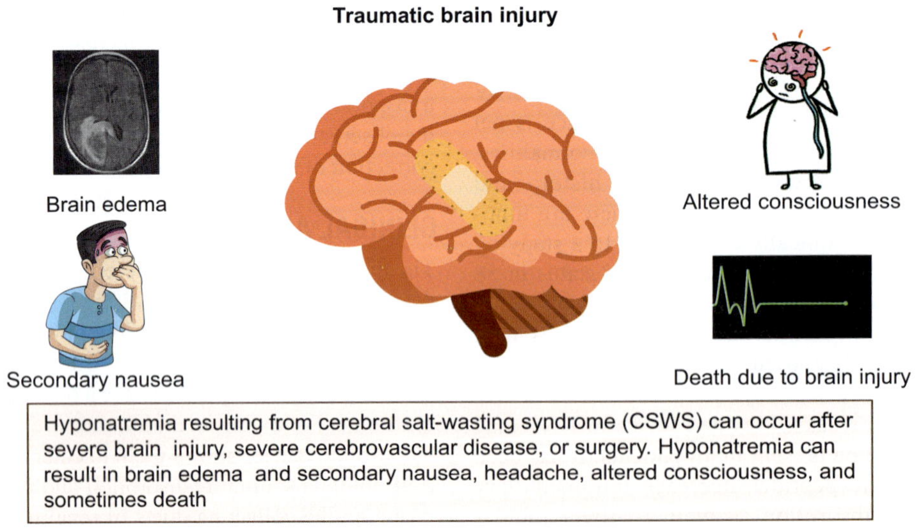


**FIG. 1:** Hyponatremia resulting from cerebral salt-wasting syndrome (CSWS) post brain injury.

The way that SIADH and CSW react to fluid therapy is another significant distinction between the two. Free water restriction is the recommended treatment for SIADH when increasing fluid intake will worsen the hyponatremia. However, CSW is a sodium-wasting and volume-depleted state that needs isotonic solutions to replenish lost fluid. Excessive natriuresis, sometimes associated with hyponatremia, requires a substantial intake of salt and water to facilitate intravascular volume expansion. The sodium and water intake required for hypervolemia can be effectively decreased while simultaneously avoiding hyponatremia by fludrocortisone-induced natriuresis inhibition.

Early correction of hyponatremia is important to prevent complications. For mild-to-moderate hyponatremia normal saline can be administered. For moderate-to-severe case hypertonic saline may be required. There is the risk of central pontine myelinolysis if the hyponatremia is corrected too quickly, specially for long-standing hyponatremia. It is recommended that no more than 10 mEq/L/24 hours or 1 mEq/L every 2 hours of sodium should be corrected. Fludrocortisone can be used for treatment. It reabsorbs sodium and water from distal tubule, expanding the extracellular fluid volume. The underlying pathophysiology linked to CSW and the clinical history of the hyponatremia determine how long therapy should last. Once underlying pathology has been corrected, CSW resolves within 3–4 weeks.

### Points to Ponder

- Cerebral salt-wasting syndrome is not a rare occurrence, it can be managed and can lead to better patient outcomes.
- Care for such patients must be coordinated between multiple specialties like primary care provider, neurologist, neurosurgeon, nephrologist. Patient's neurological assessment should be done regularly.
- Differentiating CSW from SIADH and other etiologies of hyponatremia is important when treating patients with brain injuries. Obtaining a favorable outcome depends on a prompt and accurate diagnosis, as the two illnesses require distinct treatments.
- There is also need for a diagnostic criterion for CSW for better understanding and prompt diagnosis.

## MULTIPLE CHOICE QUESTIONS

1. **What is the most likely cause of persistent hyponatremia and polyuria in this child with traumatic brain injury?**
   A. Syndrome of inappropriate antidiuretic hormone (SIADH)
   B. Diabetes insipidus
   C. Cerebral salt-wasting syndrome (CSW)
   D. Acute kidney injury
2. **Which laboratory finding is characteristic of cerebral salt-wasting syndrome (CSW)?**
   A. Low urine sodium and high serum osmolality
   B. High urine sodium and low serum osmolality
   C. Low urine osmolality and hypernatremia
   D. Low serum osmolality and normal urine output
3. **What treatment helped resolve polyuria in this child?**
   A. Normal saline infusion
   B. 3% sodium chloride infusion
   C. Oral fludrocortisone
   D. Phenytoin therapy
4. **What distinguishes CSW from SIADH in hyponatremic states?**
   A. CSW is associated with fluid retention, while SIADH involves hypovolemia
   B. CSW causes hypovolemia, while SIADH involves fluid retention
   C. CSW causes hypernatremia, while SIADH causes hyponatremia
   D. CSW involves normal renal function, while SIADH involves renal failure
5. **Which clinical feature suggests significant brain injury in this case?**
   A. GCS of 10/15 with unequal pupils
   B. Hyponatremia and low serum osmolality
   C. Polyuria of 9 mL/kg/hr
   D. Normal blood pressure and $SpO_2$

### Answers

1. (C); 2. (B); 3. (C); 4. (B); 5. (A)

## SUGGESTED READINGS

1. Tenny S, Thorell W. Cerebral Salt Wasting Syndrome. [Updated 2023 Aug 28]. In: StatPearls [Internet]. Treasure Island (FL): StatPearls Publishing; 2024 Jan-. Available from: https://www.ncbi.nlm.nih.gov/books/NBK534855/
2. Younas H, Tarif N, Baig I, et al. [Internet]. [cited 2024 Jul 21]. Available from: https://www.jcpsp.pk/archive/2015/Jan2015/18.pdf
3. Momi J, Tang CM, Abcar AC, et al. Hyponatremia-what is cerebral salt wasting? Perm J. 2010;14(2):62-5.
4. Askar A, Tarif N. Cerebral salt wasting in a patient with head trauma: management with saline hydration and fludrocortisone. Saudi J Kidney Dis Transpl. 2007;18:95-8.
5. Chaudhary N, Pathak S, Gupta MM, et al. Cerebral salt wasting syndrome following head injury in a child managed successfully with fludrocortisone. Case Rep Pediatr. 2016;2016:6937465.

CHAPTER 65

# A Case-based Approach to New-onset Seizure

*Man Mohan Mehndiratta, Abhishek Dixit, Nishant Tomar*

**CASE VIGNETTE**

A 76-year-old female with no previous history of cognitive impairment presented with complaints of intermittent forgetfulness for two weeks. Episodic memory disturbances increased over time. She experienced a seizure characterized by tonic posturing of the right followed by left upper limb with right facial deviation and loss of consciousness for 3 to 5 minutes.

## PROVISIONAL DIAGNOSIS

Seizure with possible underlying paraneoplastic limbic encephalitis or acute symptomatic focal epilepsy.

## DIFFERENTIAL DIAGNOSIS

- Neuroinfection (e.g., viral encephalitis such as herpes encephalitis)
- Metabolic derangements
- Seizures in the elderly (multifactorial)
- Autoimmune encephalitis

## CLINICAL APPROACH

The 2017 Classification of Epilepsies by the International League Against Epilepsy (ILAE) **(Fig. 1)**.

The clinical approach relied on a thorough history, routine investigations including complete blood count and serum electrolytes, neuroimaging (MRI brain with contrast), and lumbar puncture for CSF analysis.

*Investigations revealed*:

- Hyponatremia (Serum sodium: 122 mEq/L)
- MRI brain showed asymmetrical FLAIR hyperintensities in medial temporal lobes
- *CSF analysis*: No cells, protein 69 mg/dL, sugar 78 mg/dL, biofire panel negative for herpes
- Autoimmune encephalitis antibody panel positive for LGI1 antibody

This finding **(Fig. 2)** is suggestive of autoimmune encephalitis, particularly LGI1 antibody-associated encephalitis,

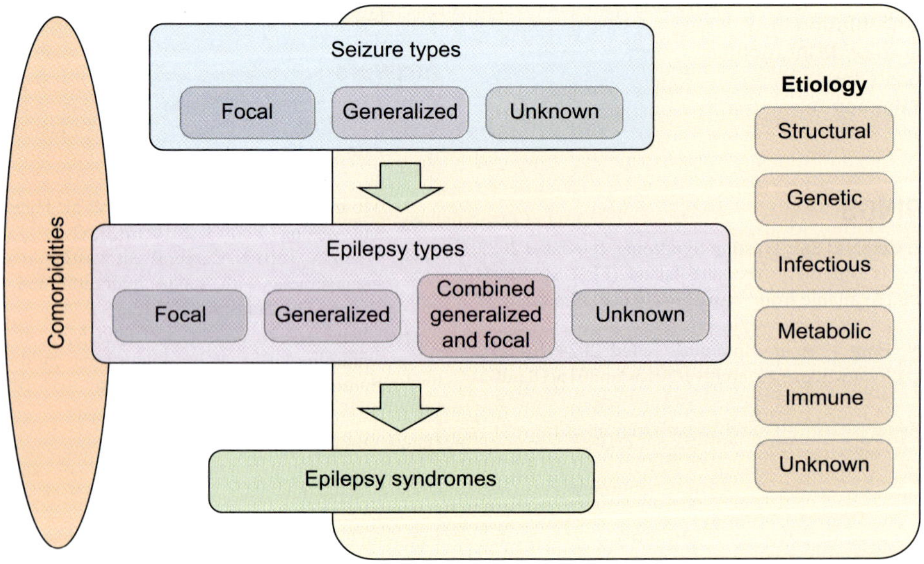


**FIG. 1:** The ILAE 2017 Classification of the Epilepsies, showing the hierarchical approach from seizure type to epilepsy type to epilepsy syndrome. This classification guides the clinical approach and management of epilepsy.

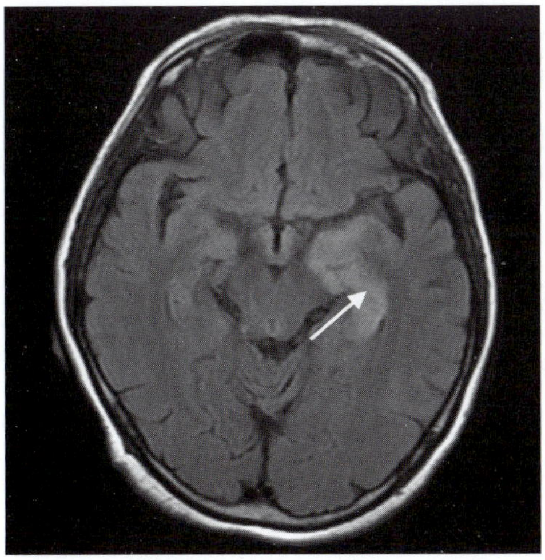

**FIG. 2:** T2-weighted FLAIR MRI image showing asymmetrical hyperintensities in the medial temporal lobes (arrow).

as opposed to the more symmetrical involvement typically seen in herpes encephalitis.

Laboratory report showing positive results for LGI1 antibodies in the autoimmune encephalitis panel **(Table 1)**.

This finding **(Table 1)** confirms the diagnosis of LGI1 antibody-associated autoimmune encephalitis.

## PATHOPHYSIOLOGY

In autoimmune encephalitis, autoantibodies (such as LGI1 antibodies) target neural synaptic proteins, leading to inflammation and dysfunction in the brain, particularly in regions controlling

**TABLE 1: Autoimmune encephalitis antibody panel results.**

| **Autoimmune encephalitis panel (BLK)** ***Immunofluorescence*** | |
|---|---|
| **Sample type** | **Serum** |
| Titre | 1:10 |
| NMDA (antiglutamate receptor against NR1) | Negative |
| AMPA (antiglutamate) Glu-R1 | Negative |
| AMPA (antiglutamate) Glu-R2 | Negative |
| GABA-B receptor antibody | Negative |
| LGI-1 antibody (VGKC type) | Positive |
| CASPR2 antibody (VGKC type) | Negative |

memory and movement. This results in cognitive impairment, seizures, and neurological deficits. The inflammatory response disrupts normal neuronal activity, causing focal seizures, including Faciobrachial dystonic seizures, and other associated symptoms like memory disturbances.

## TREATMENT AND PREVENTION

Management of autoimmune encephalitis involves acute treatment and maintenance therapy:

- *Acute phase*: IV antiepileptics, immunotherapy with intravenous immunoglobulin (2 g/day for 5 days), and supportive treatment
- *Maintenance phase*: Low-dose steroids
- *Prevention*: Early recognition and treatment of underlying causes, such as autoimmune or vascular conditions, can help prevent seizures and cognitive decline.

### Points to Ponder

- Hyponatremia with memory disturbances and Faciobrachial seizures may suggest LGI1 antibody-associated autoimmune encephalitis.
- Asymmetrical FLAIR hyperintensities in medial temporal lobes on MRI help differentiate autoimmune encephalitis from herpes encephalitis.
- New-onset seizures in adults require thorough evaluation for causes like autoimmune or infectious encephalitis.
- Initial normal MRI or CSF does not rule out conditions like autoimmune encephalitis or early tuberculous meningitis.
- Early diagnosis with tools like FDG-PET and timely treatment can significantly improve outcomes.

## MULTIPLE CHOICE QUESTIONS

1. **What is the most likely cause of intermittent forgetfulness and seizures in an elderly patient?**
   A. Alzheimer's disease
   B. Autoimmune encephalitis
   C. Stroke
   D. Meningitis
2. **Which clinical feature in this case strongly suggests focal seizure onset?**
   A. Intermittent forgetfulness
   B. Loss of consciousness for 3–5 minutes
   C. Tonic posturing of right and left upper limbs
   D. Right facial deviation
3. **Which diagnostic tool is most helpful to identify autoimmune encephalitis?**
   A. EEG
   B. MRI brain with FLAIR sequences
   C. CSF analysis
   D. FDG-PET
4. **What antibody is commonly associated with Faciobrachial dystonic seizures?**
   A. NMDA receptor antibody
   B. LGI1 antibody
   C. GAD65 antibody
   D. CASPR2 antibody

5. **What is the most appropriate initial treatment for autoimmune encephalitis?**
   A. Antiepileptic drugs alone
   B. Intravenous immunotherapy (steroids, IVIG)
   C. Antibiotics
   D. Antiviral therapy

## Answers

1. (B); 2. (C); 3. (B); 4. (B); 5. (B)

## SUGGESTED READINGS

1. Hauser WA, Annegers JF, Elveback LR. Mortality in patients with epilepsy. Epilepsia. 1980;21:399-412.
2. Fisher RS, Acevedo C, Arzimanoglou A, et al. ILAE official report: a practical clinical definition of epilepsy. Epilepsia. 2014;55:475-82.
3. Scheffer IE, Berkovic S, Capovilla G, et al. ILAE classification of the epilepsies: Position paper of the ILAE Commission for Classification and Terminology. Epilepsia. 2017;58:512-21.
4. Mehndiratta MM, Aggarwal V. Neurological disorders in India: past, present, and next steps. Lancet Glob Health. 2021;9(8):e1043-4.
5. Vegda M, Mehndiratta M. GAD-65-Associated Limbic Encephalitis — Early Diagnosis and Course of Disease, Treated with IV Methylprednisolone. Ann Indian Acad Neurol. 2023;26(5):785-7.

CHAPTER

66

# An Approach to a Case of Reversible Dementias

*U Meenakshisundaram, Shrivarthan R, Priyanka B, Sreesha S*

## CASE VIGNETTE

A 70-year-old gentleman was brought for evaluation of a gradually progressing neurological disorder that had been causing memory disturbances for the past three months. He had also been experiencing difficulty with his walking and was responding slowly to questions from his family. Initial examination by an ENT specialist revealed a need for wax removal and significant hearing loss, for which a hearing-aid was provided. His memory improved after this, which his family attributed to his enhanced understanding. Subsequent eye checkup revealed the need for spectacles. However, his condition worsened, and he began experiencing urinary incontinence. After consulting a urologist, a neurological opinion was sought. The patient had no other previous comorbidities. Examination revealed bilateral parkinsonian features in the form of bradykinesia and significant psychomotor slowing. Magnetic gait with marked difficulty clearing the feet off the ground was noted. Cranial MRI **(Figs. 1A to C)** studies revealed features consistent with normal pressure hydrocephalus. After counseling, a ventriculoperitoneal shunt was placed, leading to significant improvement in gait and memory.

Normal pressure hydrocephalus is a potential cause of reversible dementia in the elderly. The classic triad of symptoms includes ataxia, urinary disturbances, and memory problems. Patients typically have a short, broad-based gait with slow movements and feet glued to the ground, known as "magnetic gait". Following imaging studies, a CSF tap test is performed where a large volume lumbar puncture (40–50 cc) is done. Comparing gait and memory before and after the CSF tap test can help identify patients who may benefit from a diversion procedure (14).

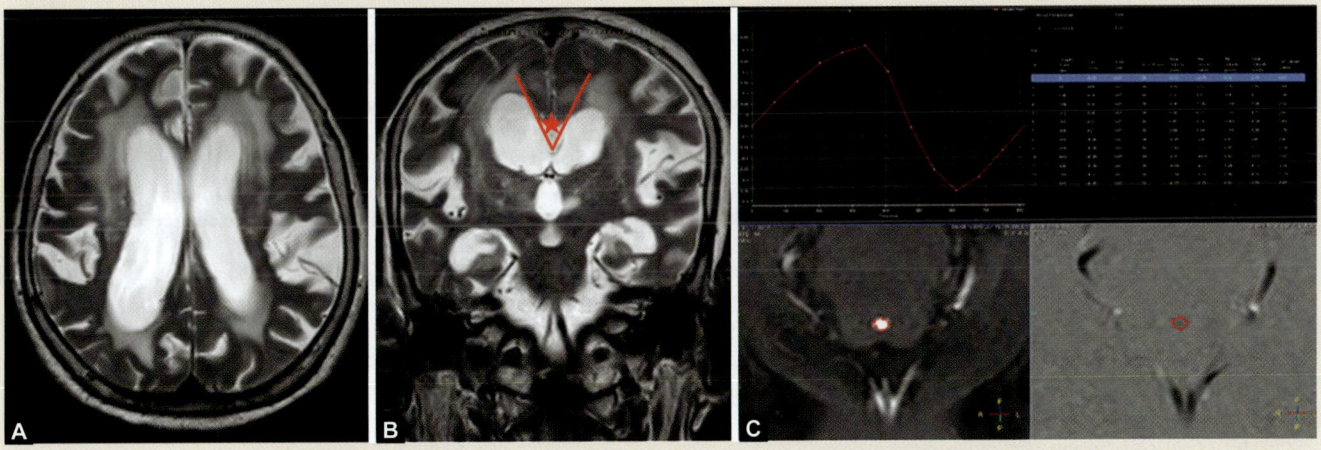


**FIGS. 1A TO C:** Cranial MRI in a patient with normal pressure hydrocephalus that shows hydrocephalus as demonstrated by increased Evan's index (A), decrease in callosal angle a finding typically seen in NPH (B), and CSF flow study showing features consistent with hyperdynamic CSF circulation (C).

## PROVISIONAL DIAGNOSIS

Normal pressure hydrocephalus (NPH).

## DIFFERENTIAL DIAGNOSIS

- Parkinson's disease
- Alzheimer's disease
- Vascular dementia
- Chronic subdural hematoma
- Vitamin B12 deficiency

## CLINICAL APPROACH

The clinical evaluation should focus on symptoms of gait disturbances, cognitive decline, and urinary incontinence, which are hallmark features of NPH. MRI findings consistent with ventriculomegaly without significant cortical atrophy confirm the diagnosis. Management typically includes ventriculoperitoneal shunting, which can result in significant symptom improvement. Differential diagnosis should consider other neurodegenerative or vascular causes of similar symptoms, and a thorough workup with neuroimaging and clinical assessment is essential.

## PATHOPHYSIOLOGY

NPH is characterized by accumulation of cerebrospinal fluid (CSF) in the ventricles, leading to ventricular enlargement without a corresponding increase in intracranial pressure. The enlarged ventricles exert pressure on surrounding brain structures, particularly the frontal lobes and periventricular white matter, resulting in gait disturbances, cognitive impairment, and urinary incontinence. The exact cause of impaired CSF absorption is unclear but may involve dysfunction of the arachnoid villi or venous outflow obstruction, leading to altered CSF dynamics and brain compression.

## TREATMENT AND PREVENTION

The primary treatment for normal pressure hydrocephalus (NPH) is the placement of a ventriculoperitoneal (VP) shunt, which diverts excess cerebrospinal fluid (CSF) from the ventricles to the peritoneal cavity, relieving pressure on the brain and improving symptoms, particularly gait and cognitive function.

There are no known preventive measures for NPH, as it typically occurs due to age-related changes or secondary causes like head trauma or infections. Early diagnosis and intervention with a VP shunt can significantly improve outcomes and prevent further neurological deterioration. Regular monitoring and management of underlying conditions can also help mitigate progression.

### Points to Ponder

- The mnemonic dementias enables one to remember the potentially reversible etiologies of dementia.
- Considering the irreversibility of the majority of dementias, an astute clinical physician should always be vigilant to evaluate for the potentially reversible causes of the syndrome, thus providing a platform for treating and ameliorating these conditions and improving cognitive functions, functional status, and quality of life.
- Careful consideration of the risks and benefits of any medication prescribed to elderly individuals is essential to avoid this situation.
- Drug-induced dementia is potentially the most reversible form of dementia, so clinicians should be diligent in identifying this cause, particularly in elderly patients on multiple medications.
- Clinicians can utilize tools like the Beers criteria developed by the American Geriatrics Society or the STOPP/START criteria developed by the European Geriatrics Society to identify medications associated with higher risk of inducing cognitive dysfunction in the elderly.

## MULTIPLE CHOICE QUESTIONS

**1. Which clinical feature is most indicative of normal pressure hydrocephalus (NPH)?**
  A. Bradykinesia and tremors
  B. Gait disturbances, cognitive decline, and urinary incontinence
  C. Short-term memory loss and personality changes
  D. Progressive paralysis and visual disturbances

**2. What is the primary treatment for normal pressure hydrocephalus (NPH)?**
  A. Levodopa therapy
  B. Ventriculoperitoneal (VP) shunt placement
  C. Anticholinergic drugs
  D. Cognitive behavioral therapy

**3. Which of the following is a characteristic MRI finding in normal pressure hydrocephalus (NPH)?**
  A. Cortical atrophy with enlarged ventricles
  B. Periventricular white matter lesions
  C. Enlarged ventricles without significant cortical atrophy
  D. Brainstem compression

**4. What symptoms did the patient initially improve after receiving a hearing aid?**
  A. Cognitive function
  B. Memory disturbance
  C. Gait disturbance
  D. Urinary incontinence

**5. Which condition is not typically included in the differential diagnosis of normal pressure hydrocephalus (NPH)?**
  A. Parkinson's disease
  B. Alzheimer's disease
  C. Vascular dementia
  D. Peripheral neuropathy

### Answers

1. (B); 2. (B); 3. (C); 4. (B); 5. (D)

## SUGGESTED READINGS

1. American Psychiatric Association D, American Psychiatric Association D. Diagnostic and statistical manual of mental disorders: DSM-5. Vol. 5. American Psychiatric Association Washington, DC; 2013.
2. Day GS. Reversible Dementias. Contin Lifelong Learn Neurol. 2019;25(1):234.
3. Little MO. Reversible Dementias. Clin Geriatr Med. 2018;34(4): 537-62.
4. Brooks JO, Hoblyn JC. Neurocognitive costs and benefits of psychotropic medications in older adults. J Geriatr Psychiatry Neurol. 2007;20(4):199-214.
5. American Geriatrics Society 2015 updated Beers criteria for potentially inappropriate medication use in older adults. J Am Geriatr Soc. 2015;63(11):2227-46.
6. O'Mahony D, O'Sullivan D, Byrne S, et al. STOPP/START criteria for potentially inappropriate prescribing in older people: version 2. Age Ageing. 2015;44(2):213-8.
7. Tetsuka S. Depression and Dementia in Older Adults: A Neuropsychological Review. Aging Dis. 2021;12(8):1920-34.
8. Honig LS. Reversible Dementias. In: Hachinski V, (Ed). Treatable and Potentially Preventable Dementias [Internet]. Cambridge: Cambridge University Press; 2018 [cited 2024 Aug 18]. pp. 110-9. Available from: https://www.cambridge.org/core/books/treatable-and-potentially-preventable-dementias/reversible-dementias/8D184D6B47EF3010B00C4AA39021D2B1
9. Chung MC, Yu TM, Shu KH, et al. Hyponatremia and increased risk of dementia: A population-based retrospective cohort study. PLoS ONE. 2017;12(6):e0178977.
10. Tripathi M, Vibha D. Reversible dementias. Indian J Psychiatry. 2009;51(Suppl. 1):S52-5.

CHAPTER

67

# A Case-based Discussion on Psychogenic Nonepileptic Seizures

*Saikat Ghosh*

**CASE VIGNETTE**

A 35-year-old female with multiple comorbidities like diabetes, hypertension and depression attended hospital with a paroxysmal event. She was previously hospitalized for a suicidal attempt 5 years back. She was otherwise in her usual state of health until the last few days when she appeared quite perturbed with a feeling that her husband was cheating on her and might be contemplating divorce. She didn't have any past history of seizures. Few days after knowing about her husband's recent deeds, she was involved in a minor car accident but didn't sustain any head trauma and didn't lose consciousness. Later that day, she was talking to her mother over the phone with her daughter beside her watching TV. Just as she was discussing regarding the divorce, her daughter saw her fall over on the sofa, eyes rolling backwards before she 'shook all over'. She was almost unresponsive during the event which lasted approx. 10 minutes and was tired and sore all over the body following the ictus. She didn't appear too confused though and had clarity of thoughts and events. She was rushed to a nearby hospital where she was administered injection levetiracetam. Urgent noncontrast CT brain, ECG and electrolytes done were normal. Recurrent events kept occurring over the next week despite increasing doses of levetiracetam and even adding new antiseizure medications. EEG appeared abnormal at the onset due to temporal spikes which were ultimately found to be wicket spikes in subsequent EEG which is a normal variant. Adding antiseizure medication hardly offered relief and she was thence referred to a psychiatrist. She was put on antidepressants and after undergoing three sessions of psychological counselling, she is currently doing better now.

## PROVISIONAL DIAGNOSIS

The history of recurrent paroxysmal events with apparent loss of consciousness lasting almost 10 minutes without any postictal confusion not responding to incremental doses of antiseizure medications in a middle-aged female with depression and recent stressor heavily points toward a diagnosis of psychogenic nonepileptic seizure (PNES).

## DIFFERENTIAL DIAGNOSES

- Seizure
- Convulsive syncope
- Transient ischemic attacks
- Transient global amnesia
- Paroxysmal movement disorders
- Hypoglycemia
- Panic attacks
- Conversion reaction

## CLINICAL APPROACH (WHEN TO SUSPECT PNES?)

- Semiology inconsistent with epileptic seizures.
- High frequency of events (several, daily)
- Associated psychiatric diagnoses
- Attacks precipitated by triggers unusual for epilepsy (e.g., acute stress, pain, sounds, getting upset, etc.)
- Attacks in presence of audience/medical personnel.
- General demeanor, affect, low level of concern (la belle indifference), overdramatization.
- Failure to present with features like postictal confusion, incontinence, occurrence out of sleep, significant injury, and lateral tongue bites, etc.
- Complete resistance of episodes to antiseizure medications.

Psychogenic nonepileptic attacks (PNEA) are probably the most common reason for misdiagnosis of epilepsy in patients presenting to referral epilepsy centres and epilepsy monitoring units. Misdiagnosis of PNES as epilepsy is a major clinical problem and it represents a challenge in both diagnosis and management. Upto 20% of referrals for surgical treatment of apparently drug-resistant epilepsy have exclusively PNES as have upto 50% of patients entering ICUs for presumed drug resistant status epilepticus. PNES mostly affects women than men (4:1 ratio) in the age group 15–35 years. Video EEG monitoring is the gold standard for diagnosis of PNES. Induction or activation using a placebo has been used to demonstrate suggestibility associated with psychogenic etiologies. The diagnosis hinges on recording the typical event with a normal or unchanged ictal EEG **(Table 1)**. It has to be kept in mind, however that 1–2% of adult patients with abnormal interictal epileptiform discharges may not have clinical evidence of epilepsy.

**TABLE 1: Differences between psychogenic and epileptic seizures.**

| Attack feature | Psychogenic seizure | Epileptic seizure |
|---|---|---|
| Stereotypy of attack | Often variable | Stereotypical |
| Onset or progression | Gradual | More rapid |
| Duration | May be prolonged | Typically 1–2 minutes |
| Diurnal variation | Daytime | Nocturnal or daytime |
| Injury | Rare | Can occur with tonic–clonic seizures |
| Tongue biting | Rare (typically tip of tongue) | Can occur with tonic–clonic seizures (lateral tongue or inside of cheek) |
| Ictal eye closure | Common | Rare (eyes typically open) |
| Urinary incontinence | Rare | Frequent |
| Vocalization | May occur; variable (often crying, moaning) | Tonic–clonic seizures may have ictal cry at onset |
| Motor activity | Prolonged, uncoordinated; pelvic thrusting, back arching | Typically unilateral rhythmic jerking, dystonic posturing of a limb, or synchronous tonic–clonic activity |
| Prolonged loss of muscle tone | Common | Rare |
| Postictal confusion | Rare | Common (several minutes, often fatigued for hours desiring sleep) |
| Postictal headache | Rare | Common |
| Postictal crying | Common | Rare |
| Relation to medication changes | Unrelated | Usually related |
| Relation to menses in women | Uncommon | Occasionally increased |
| Triggers | Emotional disturbances | Sleep deprivation, illness, medication nonadherence |
| Frequency of attacks | More frequent, up to daily | Less frequent |
| Interictal EEG findings | Normal | Frequently abnormal |
| Reproduction of attack by suggestion | Sometimes | No |
| Ictal EEG findings | Normal | Abnormal |
| Presence of secondary gain | Common | Uncommon |
| Presence of others | Frequently | Variable |
| Psychiatric disturbance | Very common (though not always apparent) | Variable |

*Source*: Bradley and Daroff's Textbook of Neurology in Clinical Practice 8th edition.

## PATHOPHYSIOLOGY

The pathophysiology of PNES is unclear, but it is thought to be a network disorder that affects the brain's emotional regulation, sensorimotor processing and stress response. Some evidence suggests that PNES may be caused by:

- Abnormal brain structure in areas like amygdala, hippocampus, insula, prefrontal cortex as evidenced by functional neuroimaging studies.
- Altered brain connectivity in regions that are associated with memory, attention, emotion processing, sensory and motor functions.
- Dysfunction in arousal tolerance, cognitive-emotional information processing and volitional control.

## TREATMENT AND PREVENTION

The initial step to treat PNES is to first deliver the diagnosis to the patient, which may itself be effective in 15% of patients. Pithiatism (Greek word meaning "curable by persuasion") involves the art of delivering psychological information to the patient. It is both crucial and serves as a window of opportunity to effect remission as well as to gain the patient's needs to accept psychotherapy. Delivering information to both the patients and their relatives is integral to the ultimate treatment process along with tapering non-essential medications including antiseizure medications, which might otherwise produce unwanted adverse reactions. Timely referral to a psychiatrist is of paramount importance as far as a neurologist is concerned. However, many psychiatrists are uncomfortable to manage these set of patients when either patients or relatives or both continue to believe that at least some or all of the episodes are in fact epilepsy and insist on treatment with antiseizure medications. Another limitation is that some psychiatrists tend to be skeptical about the diagnosis of psychogenic symptoms even when PNES has been confirmed by video EEG monitoring. The role of the neurologist should not end when when the diagnosis of PNES is made. Patients should be explained that the symptoms are genuine, attacks are "real" and can be frightening or disabling. The predisposing, precipitating and the perpetuating factors should all be taken into account and a holistic approach needs to be initiated. Patients' reactions can include disbelief, denial and anger. Psychological approaches, such as cognitive behavioral treatment remain the cornerstone of treatment with some pharmacological support for coexisting depression and anxiety when necessary. Treatment may be long enough and effective only when patients consciously and unreservedly agree and accept the diagnosis and possible aftermath.

## Points to Ponder

- PNES are involuntary experimental and behavioral responses to psychological triggers that may clinically resemble epileptic seizures, but are not associated with detectable abnormal electrical activity in the brain.
- PNES most frequently start in late adolescence or early adulthood especially in females.
- The spectrum of psychiatric disorders that can generate PNES is broad and includes conversion, anxiety and dissociation.
- Approximately 10% of people with PNES have concurrent epilepsy that, as a rule precedes the onset of PNES. Also, people with PNES are 6 times more likely to report having witnessed someone in a seizure before experiencing their own first nonepileptic seizure than people with epilepsy prior to their seizure onset.
- Average time between onset of PNES to effective diagnosis may be delayed upto 7 years.
- Video EEG is the mainstay of diagnosis of PNES.
- PNES is mostly refractory to antiseizure medications.
- The management of PNES by neurologists alone is problematic. Although reassurance that epilepsy has been ruled out may temporarily help, PNES tend to recur as long as their psychiatric causes remain unsolved.

## MULTIPLE CHOICE QUESTIONS

**1. How common is it for normal adults to have an abnormal EEG despite not having epilepsy ?**

A. 2%
B. 5%
C. 10%
D. 20%

**2. How frequent is it for PNES to present as drug resistant status epilepticus in ICUs?**

A. 10%
B. 25%
C. 50%
D. 75%

**3. Which of the following clinical entity doesn't mimic a seizure?**

A. Hypoglycemia
B. PNES
C. Convulsive syncope
D. Tardive dyskinesia

**4. Which is the best modality to treat PNES?**

A. Electroconvulsive therapy
B. Surgery
C. Antiseizure medications
D. Psychotherapy and counselling

**5. Semiology of PNES includes all except:**

A. Pelvic thrusting
B. Opisthotonic posturing
C. Weeping
D. Lateral tongue bite

### Answers

1. (A); 2. (C); 3. (D); 4. (D); 5. (D)

## SUGGESTED READINGS


1. Brown RJ, Reuber M. Psychological and psychiatric aspects of psychogenic non-epileptic seizures: a systemic review. Clin Psychol Rev. 2016;45:157-82.
2. Baslet G, Dworetzky B, Perez DL, et al. Treatment of psychogenic nonepileptic seizures: updated review and findings from a mindfulness-based intervention case series. Clin EEG Neurosc. 2015;46(1):54-64.
3. Elger CE, Schmidt D. Modern management of epilepsy: A practical approach. Epilepsy Behav. 2008;12(4):501-39.
4. Chen DK, La France WC. Diagnosis and treatment of non-epileptic seizures. Continuum (Minneap Minn). 2016;22(1):116-31.
5. Hall-Patch L, Brown R, House A, et al. Acceptability and effectiveness of a strategy for the communication of the diagnosis of psychogenic nonepileptic seizures. Epilepsia. 2010;51(1):70-7.
6. Benbadis SR, Agrawal V, Tatum 4th WO. How many patients with psychogenic nonepileptic seizures also have epilepsy? Neurology. 2001;57:915-7.
7. Martin R, Bumeo JG, Prasad A, et al. Frequency of epilepsy in patients with psychogenic seizures monitored by video-EEG. Neurology. 2003;61(12):1791-2.
8. Goldstein LH, Robinson EJ. Characteristics of 698 patients with dissociative seizures. A UK multicentre study. Epilepsia. 2019; 60(11):2182-93.

CHAPTER 68

# An Approach to a Case of Deviation of Angle of Mouth to the Left Side

*Soumya Bhowmik*

**CASE VIGNETTE**

A 65-year-old gentleman with a history of hypertension and type 2 diabetes mellitus for 10 years presented to the emergency with sudden onset lower facial paresis of right side with deviation of the angle of his mouth to the left side, accompanied by right-sided hemiparesis.

## PROVISIONAL DIAGNOSIS

Given the sudden onset of right-sided upper motor neuron (UMN)-type facial paresis with accompanying right-sided corticospinal tract involvement, the provisional diagnosis is a cerebrovascular accident (CVA) in the left suprapontine cerebral hemisphere, affecting the contralateral corticobulbar tract between its origin in the precentral gyrus and the pontine facial motor nucleus. Understanding the neuroanatomy of the facial nerve and its supranuclear control is essential to precisely localize the lesion.

## DIFFERENTIAL DIAGNOSIS

Understanding the level of the lesion aids in distinguishing central from peripheral causes of facial paralysis, essential for accurate diagnosis and management.

In localizing unilateral facial paresis, facial nerve (cranial nerve VII) lesions can occur at various levels, each presenting with distinct clinical features.

- *Supranuclear lesions (central facial palsy)*: In cortical or corticobulbar tract lesions, facial paresis primarily affects the contralateral lower face, sparing the upper face due to dual (bilateral) cortical innervation. This type may include dissociation between voluntary and emotional facial movements, suggesting specific cortical pathway involvement.
- *Nuclear and fascicular lesions (pontine lesions)*: Lesions in the pons affect the entire ipsilateral face. May be associated with ipsilateral lateral gaze palsy (abducens nerve involvement) and contralateral hemiplegia, as seen in brainstem stroke syndromes like Millard–Gubler or Foville syndromes.
- *Posterior fossa lesions (cerebellopontine angle)*: Tumors here, such as acoustic neuromas, can affect multiple cranial nerves, leading to ipsilateral facial paralysis with hearing loss, tinnitus, and vertigo.
- *Temporal bone lesions*: Lesions within the temporal bone's facial canal lead to facial motor paralysis with additional symptoms based on the exact site. Proximal lesions near the geniculate ganglion affect taste, lacrimation, and hyperacusis, while more distal lesions primarily cause facial weakness without such disturbances.
- *Distal lesions beyond the stylomastoid foramen*: These lead to isolated facial muscle paralysis often caused by trauma, infection, or tumors affecting the nerve after it exits the skull.

## CLINICAL APPROACH

### History

A thorough history focuses on the onset, progression, and associated risk factors of unilateral facial paresis. Clinicians should inquire about hypertension, diabetes, recent infections, trauma, or other relevant medical conditions. A sudden onset with associated neurological deficits may suggest a vascular cause, while gradual progression raises suspicion for chronic inflammatory conditions. Recent upper respiratory infections or viral symptoms might point to Bell's palsy.

### Examination

The physical examination emphasizes distinguishing UMN from lower motor neuron (LMN) lesions. Involvement of the upper face, such as the inability to close the eye or move the forehead, is consistent with LMN lesions. Preserved upper face movement indicates an UMN lesion. Neurological examination for long tract signs, such as left-sided hemiparesis accompanying right-sided LMN facial palsy, suggests brainstem involvement in pons, potentially due to stroke or demyelination. Absence of these signs points toward alternative causes, including CPA tumors, jugular foramen syndrome, basal meningitis, or sarcoidosis. Bell's palsy is considered in an isolated LMN facial palsy without any identifiable secondary cause.

## Investigations

### Laboratory Investigations

Blood tests play a critical role in evaluating systemic conditions. Tests such as Lyme disease serology, angiotensin-converting enzyme (ACE) levels, and markers of infection or inflammation help identify underlying causes like sarcoidosis or infections. CSF studies, including analysis for elevated proteins, pleocytosis, or specific infectious agents like *Mycobacterium tuberculosis*, can confirm diagnoses like basal meningitis or Guillain–Barré syndrome.

### Imaging

MRI or CT scans are essential to detect brainstem strokes, CPA tumors, or structural lesions affecting the facial nerve. Gadolinium-enhanced MRI can provide detailed imaging of the facial nerve course and surrounding structures, aiding in the diagnosis of tumors, demyelination, or inflammatory changes. This structured approach helps to differentiate between central and peripheral causes and supports targeted treatment.

Here's a simplified flowchart **(Flowchart 1)** outlining the anatomical localization of unilateral facial paresis, tracing the pathway from the cortex to the facial nerve.

The below **Flowchart 1** organizes the differential diagnoses of unilateral facial palms based on the clinical findings, providing a systematic approach in evaluating facial nerve involvement at different anatomic levels.

## PATHOPHYSIOLOGY

Brief neuroanatomy of the facial nerve **(Fig. 1)**.

The facial nerve (cranial nerve VII) is a complex mixed nerve with motor, sensory, and parasympathetic components. It provides motor innervation to the facial muscles, taste sensation from the anterior two-thirds of the tongue, and parasympathetic supply to the lacrimal, submandibular, and sublingual glands.

The motor division originates in the caudal pons from the facial motor nucleus, which is organized into subnuclei: The dorsomedial group (innervating auricular and occipital muscles), intermediate group (frontalis and corrugator), ventromedial group (platysma), and lateral group (buccinator and buccolabial muscles). Additionally, the orbicularis oculi is controlled by neurons in the dorsolateral facial nucleus. Motor fibers course dorsally, loop around the abducens nucleus to form the genu of the facial nerve, and emerge laterally from the brainstem. Supranuclear control is mediated by the corticobulbar tract

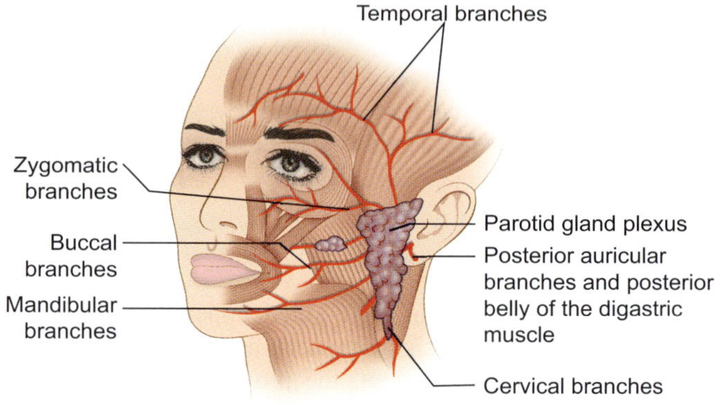


**FIG. 1:** Neuroanatomy of the facial nerve.

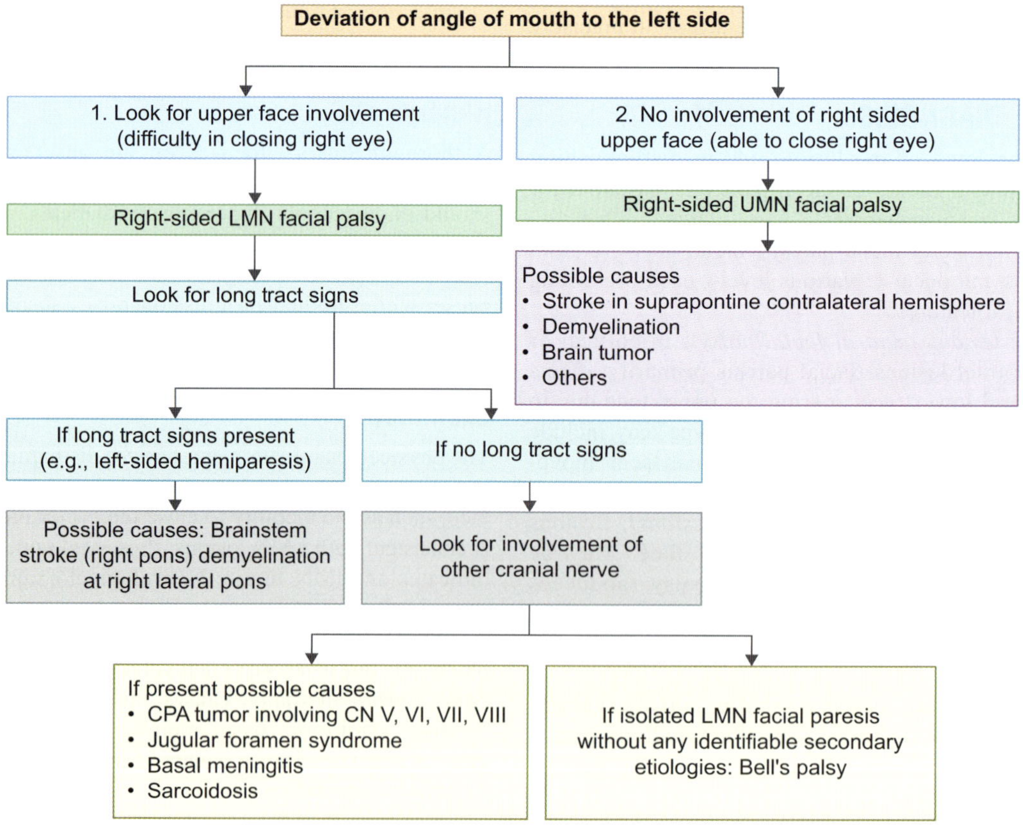


**FLOWCHART 1:** Clinical approach to unilateral facial paresis.

from the lower precentral gyrus, which crosses to innervate the facial nucleus contralaterally. The nerve's sensory and parasympathetic components, known as the nervus intermedius, carry taste sensation and secretomotor functions. Control over facial expressions is divided between voluntary movements, governed by corticobulbar fibers, and emotional expressions, which are regulated by the right hemisphere and basal ganglia pathways.

Upper motor neuron lesions typically cause weakness in the lower face due to bilateral cortical innervation of the upper face, while LMN lesions affect the entire side of the face, producing features such as flattening of the nasolabial fold, poor eyebrow elevation, weak eye closure, and Bell's phenomenon.

### Bilateral Facial (Bifacial) Paresis

Bilateral facial palsy is characterized by weakness or paralysis affecting both sides of the face. Infections like Lyme disease, HIV, and syphilis can lead to facial nerve involvement bilaterally, while autoimmune conditions such as Guillain–Barré syndrome (especially the Miller Fisher variant) and sarcoidosis (Heerfordt syndrome) are significant inflammatory causes. Neuromuscular conditions like myasthenia gravis and some muscular dystrophies can also manifest as bilateral facial weakness. In rare instances, brainstem lesions, multiple sclerosis, or bilateral Bell's palsy may be implicated. Understanding these etiologies is essential for clinicians to accurately diagnose and manage bifacial palsy, as treatment varies significantly depending on the underlying cause.

## TREATMENT AND PREVENTION

### Treatment of Possible Causes of Unilateral Facial Paresis

The treatment of unilateral facial paresis depends on the underlying etiology. For brainstem strokes, management focuses on reperfusion therapy in ischemic strokes and supportive care. Demyelinating conditions such as multiple sclerosis may require corticosteroids or disease-modifying therapies. CPA tumors, including schwannomas and meningiomas, often require surgical resection or radiotherapy. Infectious causes like basal meningitis in tuberculosis are treated with anti-tubercular therapy, while sarcoidosis may respond to corticosteroids. Bell's palsy, a diagnosis of exclusion, is typically treated with corticosteroids and antiviral agents if indicated. For UMN facial palsy, treatment targets the primary condition, such as anticoagulation or antiplatelets for strokes or specific disease-modifying therapies for demyelinating diseases. Early diagnosis and tailored therapy are essential for optimizing recovery.

### Points to Ponder

- *UMN versus LMN lesions*: UMN lesions usually spare the upper face; LMN lesions affect the entire side.
- *Associated signs*: Contralateral hemiparesis with facial palsy suggests brainstem involvement.
- *Differential diagnosis*: A structured approach helps identify causes at different lesion levels.
- *Imaging and tests*: MRI, CT, and specific lab tests aid in diagnosing structural and systemic causes.
- *Bell's palsy*: Considered when other secondary causes of LMN paresis are excluded.

## MULTIPLE CHOICE QUESTIONS

**1. A 70-year-old man with a history of hypertension and diabetes presents with right sided lower facial weakness and right-sided hemiparesis. His forehead movement is intact. What is the most likely location of the lesion?**

A. Right cerebellopontine angle
B. Right temporal bone
C. Left corticobulbar tract
D. Right pontine facial nucleus

**2. A 60-year-old man presents with right-sided facial paralysis affecting both upper and lower face muscles, right-sided horizontal gaze palsy, and left-sided hemiparesis. Which anatomical lesion is most consistent with this presentation?**

A. Left precentral gyrus affecting the corticospinal and corticobulbar tracts
B. Right lateral pons involving the facial nerve nucleus, abducens nucleus, and corticospinal tract
C. Right cerebellopontine angle affecting cranial nerves V, VII, and VIII
D. Midbrain tectum affecting the oculomotor nerve and red nucleus

**3. Which of the following findings is most characteristic of a lesion at the cerebellopontine angle?**

A. Ipsilateral facial paralysis, tinnitus, and vertigo
B. Contralateral lower facial weakness with preserved upper facial movement
C. Flattening of the nasolabial fold and widened palpebral fissure on one side
D. Isolated lower facial weakness with intact upper face and forehead movement

**4. All of the following are true about Bell's palsy, except:**

A. It is commonly associated with reactivation of the herpes simplex virus
B. Bell's palsy affects the upper and lower parts of the face on the same side
C. Steroid therapy is considered the first-line treatment in most cases
D. The absence of taste sensation on the posterior third of the tongue is a hallmark feature

5. **Which of the following conditions is most likely to cause bifacial (bilateral) facial palsy?**
   a. Millard–Gubler syndrome
   b. Temporal bone fracture
   c. Guillain–Barré syndrome
   d. Cerebrovascular accident in the precentral gyrus

## Answers

1. (C); 2. (B); 3. (A); 4. (D); 5. (C)

**1:** (C) Left corticobulbar tract
*Explanation*: Intact forehead movement and motor symptoms (right-sided hemiparesis) on the same side of lower facial paresis, indicate a central lesion, specifically in the contralateral corticobulbar tract, consistent with an UMN facial palsy.

**2:** (B) Right lateral pons involving the facial nerve nucleus, abducens nucleus, and corticospinal tract
*Explanation*: Foville Syndrome results from a lesion in the dorsal pons affecting the abducens nucleus (causing horizontal gaze palsy), the facial nerve nucleus (causing ipsilateral facial paralysis), and the corticospinal tract (leading to contralateral hemiparesis). This combination of symptoms matches a lesion in the right lateral pons.

**3:** (A) Ipsilateral facial paralysis, tinnitus, and vertigo
*Explanation*: Cerebellopontine angle lesions often affect multiple cranial nerves (e.g., CN VII, VIII), leading to ipsilateral facial weakness and auditory symptoms like tinnitus and vertigo.

**4:** (D) The absence of taste sensation on the posterior third of the tongue is a hallmark feature
*Explanation*: Bell's palsy is linked to herpes simplex virus reactivation and causes unilateral facial weakness affecting both upper and lower parts of the face. Steroid therapy is the first-line treatment. It impacts taste on the anterior two-thirds of the tongue, not the posterior third, which is innervated by the glossopharyngeal nerve.

**5:** (C) Guillain–Barré syndrome
*Explanation*: Guillain–Barré syndrome, particularly the Miller Fisher variant, is associated with bifacial palsy, whereas the other conditions typically cause unilateral facial involvement.

## SUGGESTED READINGS

1. Adour KK. Bell's palsy: The clinical management of facial paralysis. Oxford University Press, 1991.
2. Bae YJ, Kim JH, Choi BS, et al. Clinical anatomy of the facial nerve: An updated review of the extracranial and intracranial pathways. Neurographics. 2019;9(1):47-56.
3. House JW, Brackmann DE. Facial nerve grading system. Otolaryngol Head Neck Surg. 1985;93(2):146-7.
4. Eviston TJ, Croxson GR, Kennedy PG, et al. Bell's palsy: Aetiology, clinical features and multidisciplinary care. J Neurol Neurosurg Psychiatry. 2015;86(12):1356-61.
5. Rowland LP, Pedley TA. Merritt's Neurology. 14th ed. Wolters Kluwer Health; 2015.
6. Ellenbogen JR, Waqar M, Kitchen ND. Anatomy and clinical significance of the cerebellopontine angle. World Neurosurgery. 2014;82(5):64-8.
7. Kishore LT, Menon V. Central versus peripheral facial palsy: A comprehensive guide to clinical localization. Journal of Neurology & Neuroscience. 2018;9(4):1-10.
8. Preston DC, Shapiro BE. Electromyography and Neuromuscular Disorders: Clinical-Electrophysiologic Correlations. 4th ed. Elsevier, 2020.
9. Prasad S, Galetta S. Approach to a patient with facial nerve palsy. Continuum (Minneap Minn). 2008;14(2):131-42.
10. Baringer JR. Localization in Clinical Neurology. 7th ed. Wolters Kluwer, 2019.

CHAPTER 69

# An Approach to a Case of Progressive Muscle Weakness

*Biva Bhakat*

**CASE VIGNETTE**

A 52-year-old female without any known comorbidities presented with insidious onset, slowly progressive, proximal weakness of all four limbs for last 5 months along with difficulty in lifting head from the bed and turning over bed. But no complaint of distal weakness. It was associated with muscle pain in calf, thigh, arm, and forearm region. Also, difficulty in opening mouth with some clicking sound, difficulty in deglutition of food. No history of any sensory and bowel, bladder abnormalities. No history of anorexia, cough, weight loss, chest pain.

On examination—vital stable. Tone-normal, power—neck flexor-severe weak, neck extensor-normal, truncal weakness—present, Jaw opening weakness-present, shoulder 2/5, elbow 3/5, wrist 4/5, moderate weakness of small muscle of hand, hip flexor, extensor 0/5 knee 3+ ankle, EHL, FHL. Normal DTRs: All lost, plantar-bilateral no response. Sensory, cerebellar function—normal.

## PROVISIONAL DIAGNOSIS

Immune mediated necrotising myositis.

## DIFFERENTIAL DIAGNOSIS

*Systemic diseases*:

- *Rheumatological disorder*: Small/Large joint—polyarthritis
- *Metabolic diseases*: Insulin dependent or noninsulin dependent diabetes mellitus, thyroid disorders, primary or secondary adrenal insufficiency, hypokalemia, hyperkalemia hypocalcemia, etc.
- Moderate-to-severe anemia of any etiology
- Deconditioning due to some long-term illness
- Depression

*Neurological diseases*:

- Anterior horn cell diseases
- Polyradiculopathy
- Plexopathy
- Neuropathy
- Neuromuscular junction disorders
- Myopathies

*Causes of myopathies*:

- *Idiopathic Inflammatory myopathies*:
  - o Dermatomyositis
  - o Antisynthetase syndrome
  - o Immune-mediated necrotizing myopathy
  - o Overlap myositis
- *Toxin induced myopathies*: Alcohol, drugs like statins, etc.
- *Infectious myositis*: Viral (echo, coxsackie, adeno, influenza, HIV, COVID-19, etc.), mycoplasma, etc.
- *Metabolic myopathic disorder*: Carnitine palmitoyl transferase II deficiency, McArdle's disease
- *Rhabdomyolysis*: Neuroleptic malignant syndrome, post-status epilepticus/exercise, hypokalemia, para infectious

## CLINICAL APPROACH

The patient presented with B/L symmetrical proximal pure motor LMN quadriparesis without any atrophy, fasciculation, radicular pain, fatigability, or diurnal variation—so myopathy is the diagnostic consideration here.

Detailed clinical history and neurological examination are necessary to have a clear idea about the neuroaxis involved, the possible pathophysiology and to have differential diagnosis and plan investigation accordingly to confirm or reject the diagnostic possibility.

- *To differentiate true muscle weakness from mimics*: Proper history and examination will help to differentiate true muscle weakness from other conditions such as polyarthralgia, anemia, depression deconditioning, etc.

  While taking history one should focus on identifying how much the weakness is hampering the patient's daily activities and what are the activities involved, i.e., the degree of disabilities, e.g., a person suffering from proximal weakness is unable to carry out overhead activities like combing hair, reaching for overhead objects, standing from sitting posture, climbing upstairs, etc., person suffering from distal weakness usually complains of dexterity weakness like buttoning, unbuttoning, frequent tripping, slippage of *chappals* with awareness, etc. Associated neck weakness causes difficulty in lifting neck from pillow, truncal weakness causes difficulty in getting up from bed, orbital muscle weakness causes double vision (that patient may interpret as blurred vision), drooping of eyelids, etc., involvement of the bulbar muscles lead to nasal intonation of voice, nasal regurgitation of food, i.e., difficulty in swallowing, weakness of tongue or facial muscles lead to difficulty in manipulating food inside mouth or slurred speech. Weakness of the respiratory muscles lead to weak cough, exertional dyspnea, or orthopnea. Cardiomyopathy can also cause exertional dyspnea or orthopnea or palpitations.

- *Pattern of weakness*: The pattern recognition approach is the cornerstone for any neurological diagnosis. For example, the typical pattern for myopathies is bilaterally symmetrical and proximal weakness. Most of the myopathies, idiopathic Inflammatory myopathies, endocrine myopathies, periodic paralyses, toxic myopathies, congenital myopathies, muscular dystrophies all follow this pattern of involvement. However, both proximal and distal weakness are seen in late stages of muscular dystrophies. Only distal weakness seen in inclusion body myositis, myotonic dystrophy type-1, some distal myopathies like Udd, Welander, Markesbery–Griggs, Laing, Nonaka, and Miyoshi. Myopathies having asymmetric involvement are focal myositis, facioscapulohumeral dystrophy (FSHD), inclusion body myositis, oculo-bulbar weakness seen in oculopharyngeal muscular dystrophy (OPMD), thyroid orbitopathy, and mitochondrial myopathy. Facial muscle involved in FSHD, OPMD, myotonic dystrophy-1.
- *Age at symptom onset*: The age at which the patients begin to experience the symptoms can help the physician to narrow down the diagnostic possibilities. one must enquire even about the subtle symptoms as the patient might have ignored them for decades. History regarding the achievement of motor milestones, walking/running abilities in childhood, comparison with peers are helpful. Congenital myopathies, muscular dystrophies, myofibrillar myopathies begins early in the life whereas idiopathic inflammatory myopathies present in the fourth to sixth decade of life, but can occur in childhood also.
- *Family history*: A family tree should be crafted carefully to identify the inheritance pattern if any. For example, X-linked inheritance is found in Duchenne and Becker muscular dystrophy, maternal transmission seen in mitochondrial myopathies, autosomal dominant inheritance seen in LGMD-1, myotonic dystrophy I and II, FSHD, OPMD, autosomal recessive seen in LGMD-2, metabolic myopathies.
- *Any precipitating factor*: History regarding the antecedent respiratory or gastrointestinal infection (para infectious or post infectious myositis), drug history (e.g., statin, chemotherapeutic drugs, colchicine, amiodarone, hydroxychloroquine), long term intake of corticosteroids, toxin exposure (alcohol) should be asked for.
- *Onset and progression of weakness*: Muscle weakness can develop and progress in an acute (over hours to days), subacute (over weeks), chronic (over months) manner. For example, periodic paralyses, rhabdomyolysis can develop acutely, idiopathic inflammatory myopathies develop over weeks and the congenital or inherited myopathies have a chronic course.
  - *Other system involvement*: The presence of skin rash (dermatomyositis), mechanics hand (anti-synthetase syndrome—ASS), ILD (IIM, ASS), cataract (myotonic dystrophy-1), cognitive impairments (congenital myopathies, DMD, myotonic dystrophies etc) should be looked for.

## EXAMINATION

A carefully performed general survey is very much important as it can provide some important clues regarding the underlying disease. For example, any dysmorphic facies, skeletal abnormalities, joint contracture may indicate presence of congenital myopathies or muscular dystrophies. One should look for presence of skin rash because most of the cases of inflammatory myopathies shows characteristic skin lesions. Patients of dermatomyositis may show presence of gottron's sign (erythematous plaques over the metacarpophalangeal and interphalangeal joint), heliotrope sign (presence of violaceous skin lesions over periorbital region and upper eyelids), V sign (presence of erythematous skin rash over neck), shawl sign (presence of erythematous skin rash over back of neck and upper shoulder), holster's sign (erythematous skin rash over lateral thigh). Examination of the nails is to be done to look for nail bed telangiectasia, ragged appearance of cuticle, etc. Examination of the hand also shows skin thickening over palm with presence of calluses and cracks (mechanics hand) seen in anti-synthetase syndrome.

### Neurological Examination

Examination of muscles is very much important. The inspection and palpation should focus on identifying presence of any atrophy or hypertrophy in a patterned distribution and the consistency and presence of tenderness, e.g., presence of calf hypertrophy should suggest dystrophinopathies. Muscle tenderness may be present on cases of myositis (infectious or inflammatory). Power examination should be done to assess the MRC grading in the following muscle group-around neck (extensor and flexor), shoulder joint (abduction, external and internal rotation), elbow and wrist (flexion and extension), fingers flexors and extensors in the upper limb. In the lower limbs one should focus on muscles around hip joint (flexors, extensors, adductors, and abductors), knee (flexors, extensors), ankle (plantar flexors and dorsiflexors).

## INVESTIGATIONS

Specific investigations in a case of myopathies must include:

- *Electrophysiological examination*: A needle electromyogram (EMG) is very much helpful as it rules out mimics of myopathies such as motor neuron disorders or polyradiculopathies and determine the extent of muscle involvementand also assist in the selection of muscle for biopsy. EMG shows combination of spontaneous activity—fibrillations, positive waves, complex repetitive discharges or true myotonic discharges and early recruitment of small, short-duration, and polyphasic motor unit potentials.
- *Creatine kinase*: Creatine kinase moderate elevation (10–50 times) seen in dermatomyositis sand polymyositis, very high elevation (50 times) seen in immune mediated necrotizing myositis, rhabdomyolysis, mild elevation (<10 times) seen in inclusion body myositis. In long standing disease, creatine kinase level is usually normal.
- *Muscle MRI*: It is the imaging modality of choice for the diagnosis of IIM. It assists in distinguishing muscle edema from fat infiltration—muscle edema is characterized by high

T2 and STIR signal, and fat infiltration has abnormally high T1 signal. It also outline the pattern and extent of muscle involvement and help in selecting the optimal target for muscle biopsy and facilitate assessment of response to therapy.

- *Immunology*: The role of immunology is mainly in cases of inflammatory myopathies. With the recent advancements in the field of immunology, the yield of antibody testing in idiopathic inflammatory myopathies is now increased to about 65–70%. There are mainly two types of antibodies—myositis-specific antibodies (MSA) and myositis-associated antibodies (MAA). It has advanced the classification of idiopathic inflammatory myopathies and allows recognition of syndromes with distinct epidemiologic associations, extramuscular and histopathologic features, and prognosis.
  - Myositis-specific antibodies:
    - Dermatomyositis: Anti-NXP-2, anti-TIF1-γ, anti-MI-2, anti-MDA-5, anti-SAE
    - Anti-synthetase syndrome: Anti-aminoacyl tRNA synthetase antibodies, anti-jo-1 antibody, anti-PL-7, anti-PL-12, anti-OJ, anti-EJ, anti-KS, anti-Zo, and anti-HA
    - Immune-mediated necrotizing myopathy: Anti-SRP, anti–HMG-CoA reductase IgG, antimitochondrial M2 antibodies
  - Myositis-associated antibodies: Antibodies that are associated with myositis but are not specific for it. They can also be detected in numerous connective tissue diseases, e.g., anti-Ro52, anti-U1 RNP, anti-U2 RNP, anti-PM-Scl-75, anti-PM-Scl-100, anti-Ku.
- *Genetics*: Genetics are confirmatory diagnostic test for congenital myopathies, dystrophinopathies, and limb girdle muscular dystrophies and myotonic dystrophies.

## PATHOPHYSIOLOGY

The pathogenesis of polymyositis and dermatomyositis involves a complex interaction between genetic and environmental factors **(Fig. 1)**. Genetic predispositions, including HLA and non-HLA genes, combined with environmental triggers like infections, toxins, and UV light, create an "immunologic danger" that activates the immune system. This leads to an upregulation of MHC class I/II molecules, contributing to immune responses. Both innate (e.g., dendritic cells, macrophages, cytokines) and adaptive immunity (B cells, T cells) are involved, with regulatory factors like Tregs playing a role. Nonimmune factors such as ER stress, hypoxia, and altered metabolism also contribute, leading to muscle inflammation characteristic of myositis.

## TREATMENT AND PREVENTION

In this chapter, the treatment of idiopathic inflammatory myopathies will be discussed:

- *First-line treatment*:
  - Corticosteroids, either oral prednisone 1–1.5 mg/kg/day or IV methylprednisolone 500–1, 000 mg/day for 3–5 days
  - High-dose oral steroid therapy should be continued for at least 4–6 weeks or until clinical improvement has plateaued
  - A slow taper of no faster than 10 mg/month
- *Second-line treatment*:
  - Required in all but the mildest cases
  - Oral azathioprine 2–2.5 mg/kg/day, oral or IM methotrexate 20–25 mg/week, and mycophenolate mofetil up to 3 g/day in divided doses
- *Third-line treatment*:
  - More refractory cases
  - IV immunoglobulin (IVIg) is an option
- *Fourth-line treatments*:
  - Rituximab
  - Calcineurin inhibitors: Cyclosporine and tacrolimus
  - Cyclophosphamide

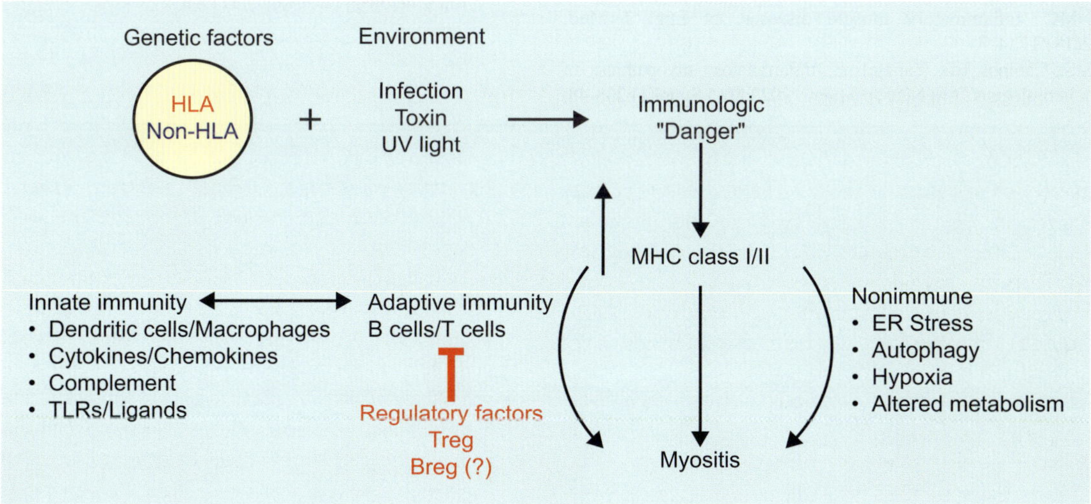


**FIG. 1:** The pathogenesis of polymyositis and dermatomyositis.

*Source*: Ascherman DP. Pathogenesis of Myositis. In: Aggarwal R, Oddis C, (eds). Managing Myositis. Springer: Cham; 2020. https://doi.org/10.1007/978-3-030-15820-0_28

## Points to Ponder

- History and neurological examination to be done to identify the neuroaxis involved and with the focus of pattern recognition of the weakness. The different types of myopathies like inflammatory myopathies, muscular dystrophies, congenital myopathies, metabolic myopathies can be clinically suspected and investigation should be targeted accordingly.
- Inflammatory myopathies are a group of autoimmune diseases with a broad spectrum of clinical presentation, mainly characterized by immune-mediated muscle injury and extra muscular organ involvement.
- The landscape of inflammatory myopathies is evolving-with the advancements of diagnostic tools—improved serology (discovery of MSAs, MAAs), staining marker, muscle pathology led to a better understanding of the disease pathogenesis.
- Needle-EMG, muscle MRI plays an important role in a case of myopathies as they help in pattern recognition of the weakness.
- Individualized treatment regimens using various immunosuppressants such as IVIG, rituximab, cyclophosphamide based on the precise diagnosis, improves prognosis.

## MULTIPLE CHOICE QUESTIONS

1. **MDA5 Ab positivity associated with:**
   A. Amyopathic presentation
   B. Thrombotic complication
   C. Severe ILD
   D. All the above
2. **Anti NXP2 Ab associated with:**
   A. Bimodal presentation
   B. Strong association with malignancy
   C. Calcinosis cutis
   D. All the above
3. **Typical-heliotrope rash, gottron papule, prominent nail fold pathology seen in:**
   A. Anti-Mi-2 Ab
   B. Anti-SAE Ab
   C. Both above
   D. None of the above
4. **Anti-HMGCR-IgG Ab is associated with:**
   A. One-third patients-statin naïve
   B. May be associated with malignancy
   C. IVIG is the first line treatment
   D. All the above
5. **Myositis associated Ab are:**
   A. Anti-Ro52
   B. Anti-U1-RNP antibodies
   C. Anti-PM-SCL-75 and anti-PM-SCL-100
   D. All the above

### Answers

1. (D); 2. (D); 3. (C); 4. (D); 5. (D)

## SUGGESTED READINGS

1. Hochberg MC, Feldman D, Stevens MB. Adult-onset polymyositis/dermatomyositis: an analysis of clinical and laboratory features and survival in 76 patients with a review of the literature. Semin Arthritis Rheum. 1986;15(3):168-78.
2. Dalakas MC. Inflammatory muscle diseases. N Engl J Med. 2015;372(18):1734-7.
3. Silva AMS, Campos ED, Zanoteli E. Inflammatory myopathies: an update for neurologists. Arq Neuropsiquiatr. 2022;80(5 Suppl 1):238-48.
4. Dalakas MC. Inflammatory myopathies: update on diagnosis, pathogenesis and therapies, and COVID-19-related implications. Acta Myol. 2020;39(4):289-301.
5. Connolly CM, Gupta L, Fujimoto M, et al. Idiopathic inflammatory myopathies: current insights and future frontiers. The Lancet Rheumatology. 2024;6(2):e115-e127.

CHAPTER

70

# An Approach to a Case of Recurrent Stroke in Young

*Kaushik Biswas, Tapas Bandyopadhyay, Anirban Paul, Anismita Basu*

## CASE VIGNETTE

Mrs X, a 37-year-old female with no known comorbidities developed sudden onset loss of vision and gait instability 4 months back. She got admitted at a local hospital where MRI revealed left PCA infarct. She was started on single oral antiplatelet and she got better with medical management and physiotherapy. She was discharged after hospital stay of 27 days. Ten days ago, she developed low grade fever. She was taken to a local physician who prescribed her antibiotics but her fever did not subside. 1 week back her husband noticed, on waking up in the morning, that her wife was acting in a strange manner. She was pulling her hair using her left hand and was not following command. She was again taken to a local hospital where MRI revealed a new onset left MCA infarct.

She was then referred to our hospital. Here, examination revealed power in right upper and lower limbs to be 2/5 and 3/5 respectively. Sensation was impaired in the face and upper limb, spared in the lower limb and brisk reflexes on the right side of the body. Blood investigations showed ANA positive in high titer along with anti-dsDNA and anti-cardiolipin antibody. Echocardiography revealed small, localized and sessile echo-densities with well-defined borders adjacent to aortic and mitral valve leaflets, intact IAS and no RV dysfunction. Blood cultures repeated on consecutive days came negative for any growth.

## PROVISIONAL DIAGNOSIS

Recurrent ischemic stroke in a patient of systemic lupus erythematosus with libman–sacks endocarditis.

## DIFFERENTIAL DIAGNOSIS

Refer to **Table 1**.

**TABLE 1: Differential diagnosis for ischemic stroke in a patient with systemic lupus erythematosus.**

| | |
|---|---|
| *Autoimmune*:<br>• Systemic lupus erythematosus (SLE) with secondary APS<br>• Primary APS<br>• Takayasu's disease | *Infective*:<br>• Infective endocarditis<br>• HIV/AIDS<br>• Varicella zoster virus vasculopathy<br>• Tuberculous vasculitis<br>• Neurosyphilis |
| *Cardiac*:<br>• Cerebral embolism (RHD, PFO, pulmonary AV malformation)<br>• Cardioembolic stroke in atrial fibrillation | *Procoagulant states*:<br>• Thrombotic thrombocytopenic purpura (TTP)<br>• Factor V Leiden mutation<br>• Prothrombin gene deficiency<br>• Protein C/S deficiency<br>• Antithrombin deficiency<br>• Hyperhomocysteinemia |
| *Anatomical defect*:<br>• Fibromuscular dysplasia<br>• Craniocervical dissection<br>• CADASIL | *Malignancy*:<br>• Intracranial neoplasm<br>• Paraneoplastic syndromes |
| *Accelerated atherosclerosis*—due to smoking, low physical activity, metabolic syndrome, chronic inflammatory conditions | *Miscellaneous*:<br>• Hyper-viscous condition like polycythemia<br>• Prolonged use of oral contraceptives<br>• Illicit drugs like cocaine, amphetamine |

## CLINICAL APPROACH

### History

- Similar episode in the past
- Duration of altered mental status/limb weakness (TIA, Todd's palsy)
- Recurrent miscarriage (APS)
- Fever with rash in sun exposed areas, oral ulcers, accelerated hair fall and weight loss (SLE)
- Fatigue with limb claudication, hypertension and angina (Takayasu's arteritis)
- Fever with headache, neck rigidity and vomiting (CNS infection)
- Significant weight loss, anemia and anorexia (malignancy, tuberculosis)
- Easy bruising, hematuria, fever and anemia (TTP)
- Use of oral contraceptives/illicit drug

### Physical Examination

- Pulse regular/irregular, palpable or not in the peripheries, equality in bilateral upper limbs
- BP equality in bilateral upper limbs
- Higher functions including speech
- Neck rigidity, Kernig's sign, Brudziński sign

### Cranial Nerve Examination

- Presence of wasting
- Assess the pattern and distribution of weakness
- Presence or absence of sensory deficit
- Plantar response
- Cerebellar, autonomic functions
- Presence of carotid, renal bruit

## ROUTINE INVESTIGATIONS

- CBC with ESR, CRP
- Culture (2 sites)
- Na, K, Ca; urea, creatinine; lipid profile
- HIV serology; VDRL
- Urine R/E, ACR
- ECG

## SPECIAL INVESTIGATIONS

- Autoimmune markers (ANA, anti-dsDNA, anti-phospholipid, anti-cardiolipin, anti-β2GP I)
- Thrombophilia screening
- Lipoprotein(a)
- USG carotid, renal artery Doppler to look for hemodynamically significant stenosis
- Transthoracic/transesophageal echocardiography to look for vegetations, congenital defects
- CT/MRI brain to look for spatial distribution of infarcts
- FDG-PET to look for malignancy

## PATHOPHYSIOLOGY

In systemic lupus erythematosus (SLE), the occurrence a stroke involves a multifactorial pathogenesis:

- *Autoimmune-driven vascular inflammation*:
  - *Endothelial dysfunction*: Damage to the endothelium promotes the adhesion of leukocytes and platelets, setting the stage for thrombosis.
  - *Immune complex deposition*: In cerebral blood vessels, leading to vasculitis.
- *Prothrombotic state*:
  - *Antiphospholipid syndrome (APS)*: Autoantibodies increase the risk of thrombosis by promoting platelet aggregation, impairing fibrinolysis, and interacting with the endothelium and clotting factors.

## INCREASED PLATELET ACTIVATION

- *Accelerated atherosclerosis*—due to chronic inflammation, dyslipidemia, oxidative stress and immune-mediated vascular damage.
- *Complement activation*—direct endothelial damage, increased vascular permeability, and promote a prothrombotic state.
- *Hypertension and cardiovascular complications*: SLE is associated with secondary hypertension due to renal involvement (lupus nephritis) or due to chronic corticosteroid use. Hypertension increases the risk of hemorrhagic stroke and accelerates the progression of atherosclerosis.
- Valvular heart disease (Libman–Sacks endocarditis) and cardiomyopathy in SLE can lead to cardioembolic stroke if thrombi formed in cardiac chambers or on abnormal valves embolize to the cerebral circulation.
- *Role of cytokines and oxidative stress*:
  - *Proinflammatory cytokines*: TNF-α, IL-6, and type I interferons play a critical role in inflammation and cytokine dysregulation. This can affect the blood–brain barrier (BBB), leading to further neuronal and glial injury, contributing to neurological deficits.
  - *Oxidative stress*: Leads to lipid peroxidation and vascular damage, promoting atherosclerosis.
- *Genetic and epigenetic factors*: Its possible genetic predispositions to autoimmune-related thrombosis.

## TREATMENT AND PREVENTION

- *Initial acute management*: In case of recurrent stroke, IV thrombolysis and mechanical thrombectomy is avoided due to increased risk of hemorrhagic transformation of old infarct.

  NIHSS is calculated. If score >5, start dual antiplatelet, else start aspirin alone.
- Prevention of complication secondary to raised intracranial pressure
  - Blood pressure control to keep < 220/120 and < 185/110 if TPA candidate.
  - Head end elevation
  - Isotonic fluid resuscitation
  - IV mannitol (if GCS ≤8 and reversible causes of AMS absent)
- *Prevention of systemic complications*:
  - 2 hourly position change—to prevent pressure sore
  - Eye care—to prevent exposure keratitis
  - Nutrition—monitored feeding with Ryles tube
  - Avoid catheter associated UTI
- *Long-term secondary prevention*:
  - *Anticoagulation*: Routine use of anticoagulants for ischemic stroke in not advised due to increased risk of intracranial bleed. However, given that cardioembolic stroke in SLE often has a high risk of recurrence, the following is recommended:

- Warfarin or direct oral anticoagulants (DOACs) like apixaban or rivaroxaban are recommended for long-term anticoagulation. In cases of APS or high-risk patients, warfarin is often preferred with a target INR between 3 and 3.5.
- *Antiplatelet therapy*: Low-dose aspirin may be considered if anticoagulation is contraindicated.

o *Avoidance of triggers*: SLE patients should avoid factors that can exacerbate disease activity including infections, stress and UV exposure.

- *Management of SLE with DMARDs and immunosuppressants*: Treatment of APS—if APS is diagnosed, anticoagulation is usually lifelong, and strict INR monitoring is crucial to prevent recurrence.
- *Rehabilitation*: Physical therapy, occupational therapy, and speech therapy if needed, to address any residual neurological deficits. In case of vision impairment, a fulltime attendant must be ensured.

## Points to Ponder

- Recurrent stroke in young individuals (ages 18–50 years) accounts for approximately 10–15% of all strokes and the numbers are increasing.
- Early identification and treatment of the etiology is important to reduce the risk for further thrombotic events.
- Common causes of recurrent stroke include cardiac conditions (e.g., atrial fibrillation, patent foramen ovale), vasculitis, infections, arterial dissection and coagulopathies.
- SLE alone can cause stroke. Not all strokes need to be associated with secondary antiphospholipid syndrome.
- Strokes in patients with SLE present unique challenges due to the complex interplay of autoimmune processes, vascular risk factors and rate of recurrence.
- Prevention of stroke and early rehabilitation after stroke are essential for the long term well-being of the patients.

## MULTIPLE CHOICE QUESTIONS

**1. According to EULAR classification criteria of SLE, what titer of ANA serves as the entry criteria?**

A. ≥ 1:320
B. ≥ 1:160
C. ≥ 1: 80
D. ≥ 1:64

**2. Which is true about Libman–Sacks endocarditis?**

A. Right side valves are more affected
B. Bacterial endocarditis that results in arterial emboli
C. Malignancy is one of its causes
D. Vegetations are typically large in size

**3. Which of the following chart is used for predicting pressure sore risk?**

A. Luke
B. Braden
C. Fleming
D. Bracken

**4. At what NIHSS dual antiplatelet therapy is indicated in acute ischemic stroke?**

A. ≥2
B. ≥3
C. ≥4
D. ≥5

**5. Which of the following is correct for diagnosis of APLA?**

A. Any of LA, aCL and aβ2GP I present at an interval of ≥12 weeks
B. Any of LA, aCL and aβ2GP I present at an interval of ≤12 weeks
C. Intracranial venous + arterial thrombosis in the absence of antibodies
D. Arterial thrombosis in ≥2 limbs in the absence of antibodies

### Answers

1. (B); 2. (A); 3. (B); 4. (C); 5. (A)

## SUGGESTED READINGS


1. Kleindorfer D, Kissela B, Schneider A, et al. Eligibility for rtPA in acute ischemic stroke: a population-based study. Stroke. 2004;35(2):e27-9.
2. Schoenfeld SR, Kasturi S, Costenbader KH. The epidemiology of atherosclerotic cardiovascular disease among patients with SLE: a systematic review. Semin Arthritis Rheum. 2013;43(1):77-95.
3. Mikdashi J, Handwerger B, Langenberg P, et al. Baseline disease activity, hyperlipidemia, and hypertension are predictive factors for ischemic stroke and stroke severity in systemic lupus erythematosus. Stroke. 2007;38(2):281-5.
4. Nojima J, Kuratsune H, Suehisa E, et al. Strong correlation between the prevalence of cerebral infarction and the presence of anti-cardiolipin/beta2-glycoprotein I and anti-phosphatidylserine/prothrombin antibodies--Co-existence of these antibodies enhances ADP-induced platelet activation in vitro. Thromb Haemost. 2004;91(5):967-76.
5. Si-Yuan W, Fei-Fei C, Xiang-Ting C, et al. Repeated intravenous thrombolysis in recurrent ischemic stroke within 3 months: a systematic review. BMC Neurol. 2023;23(1):422.
6. Husseini NE, Katzan IL, Rost NS, et al. Cognitive Impairment After Ischemic and Hemorrhagic Stroke: A Scientific Statement From the American Heart Association/American Stroke Association. Stroke. 2023;54(6):e272-91.
7. Ferrone SR, Boltyenkov AT Lodato Z, et al. Clinical Outcomes and Costs of Recurrent Ischemic Stroke: A Systematic Review. J Stroke Cerebrovasc Dis. 2022;31(6):106438.
8. Xiong Y, Wakhloo AK, Fisher M, et al. Advances in Acute Ischemic Stroke Therapy. Circ Res. 2022;130(8):1230-51.

CHAPTER
71

# An Approach to a Case of Paraneoplastic Glomerulopathy

*Madhuchanda Kar*

## CASE VIGNETTE

A 63 63-year-male presented with 1 month history of neck swelling, muffling of voice and anorexia. He had 12 kg weight loss over last 9 months. On clinical examination he was afebrile, vitals were normal, weight 50 kg, BSA 1.5 $m^2$. Clinical examination of neck nodes revealed bilateral hard and fixed levels 1 and 2 lymph nodes , largest measuring 4.5 cm × 3.5 cm. Fiberoptic laryngoscopy revealed hard indurated mass lesion 2.5 cm × 3 cm on the base of the tongue while larynx and hypopharynx were normal. He had no comorbidities.

### Investigations

*Hematological*: Hb-10.6 g/dL, WBC-6030/$mm^3$, platelets- 1.4 lacs/$mm^3$, ESR-66 mm, high creatinine 2.1 mg/dL, electrolytes were normal ($Na^+$ 132 mEq/L, $K^+$ 3.9 mEq/L), FBS was normal (108 mg/dL), LFT was normal except, albumin: 2.42 g/dL, eGFR-225 mL/min, ANCA nonreactive, urine R/E; plenty of RBCs and pus cells –14/npf, pH–5.5, protein ++++, occult blood present but urine C-/S showed no growth.

Biopsy from cervical lymph node revealed B cell non- Hodgkin's lymphoma — diffuse large B cell variety.

Immunohistochemistry revealed CD 45+, CD20+, BCL 6+, CK–, P40–, CD3–, BCL2–, CD10–, Cyclin-D–, MUM1–, FISH for c-MYC bcl-2, and bcl-6 to rule out double/triple hit lymphoma was not performed in this patient due to limited therapeutic implications and scope in presence of gross nephropathy.

In view of gross renal dysfunction, kidney biopsy was performed that yielded 11 glomeruli. It showed diffuse glomerular mesangial matrix expansion, mild mesangial proliferation in the glomerulus with capsular adhesion, extracapillary proliferative lesion and deposition of C3 in the mesangial lesion. Direct immunofluorescence studies (DIF) revealed IgA deposition along glomerular basement membranes.

### Whole Body Pet Scan

#### Head and Neck

FDG avid large soft tissue density lesion is seen involving the left tonsillar fossa with extension into the left base of tongue and left sublingual space, left vallecula measuring 5.3 × 4.4 × 4.2 cm, ($SUV_{max}$ 27.0).

FDG avid enlarged left parapharyngeal, left cervical levels I–IV and discrete lymph nodal mass (4.3 × 3.6 × 8.0) cm, ($SUV_{max}$ 24.6) and discrete right cervical level II and left supraclavicular lymph nodes were also seen.

#### Thorax

FDG avid prominent thoracic-paraaortic nodes measuring 16 × 12 mm ($SUV_{max}$ 13.2) and left internal mammary nodes were seen.

Multiple FDG avid prominent right paraesophageal, pre-epicardial, middle cardiophrenic lymph nodes were seen, measuring 4.4 × 2.0 cm, ($SUV_{max}$ 13.4).

#### Abdomen and Pelvis

FDG avid hypodense lesions in both lobes of liver, measuring 3.3 × 2.0 cm, ($SUV_{max}$ 8.9), and in the splenic hilum, along the anterior and posterior left pararenal fascia, measuring 16 × 14 mm, ($SUV_{max}$ 4.6).

FDG avid prominent left pelvic and inguinal nodes were seen, measuring 12 × 14 mm, ($SUV_{max}$ 8.5) and moderate ascites noted.

## PROVISIONAL DIAGNOSIS

Non-Hodgkin's lymphoma with IgA nephropathy due to paraneoplastic syndrome.

## DIFFERENTIAL DIAGNOSIS

- Primary glomerulopathy in conjunction with a diagnosis of diffuse large B-cell lymphoma (DLBCL) (two separate entities).
- Paraneoplastic glomerulopathy associated with an underlying diagnosis of diffuse large B-cell lymphoma (DLBCL).

## CLINICAL APPROACH

This is a diagnosis of exclusion:

- Temporal profile of glomerulopathy is either concurrent with primary cancer or precedes the diagnosis of primary cancer. It can also be the first manifestation of relapse or metastasis of primary cancer.
- Monitoring of the primary cancer with tumor markers like CEA, CA125, CA19.9, PSA maybe successful in solid cancers but are unhelpful in hematolymphoid malignancies.
- Symptoms of lymphoma like fever, unexplained weight loss or sweating may be helpful for the diagnosis in lymphoproliferative disorder.
- Nuclear—radiological investigations like PET-CT scan may be helpful to clinch the possible underlying diagnosis of cancer in suspected paraneoplastic glomerulopathy.

Diagnosis of paraneoplastic glomerulopathy relies on 3 criteria:

1. Complete clinical and histological remission after surgical removal or chemotherapy or radiotherapy. However, post-remission histological verification is rarely advised for ethical reasons.
2. Renal relapse on recurrence of cancer most commonly in the form of proteinuria that should correlate with the activity of cancer.
3. Demonstration of subepithelial immune deposits.

## PATHOPHYSIOLOGY

In non-Hodgkin's lymphoma (NHL), malignancy of B-cells leads to abnormal immune responses, which can result in the production of abnormal immunoglobulins. IgA nephropathy develops when IgA deposits accumulate in the glomeruli, triggering immune complex-mediated inflammation. This can lead to glomerular injury, mesangial expansion, and impaired renal function. In paraneoplastic syndrome, lymphoma's systemic effects may provoke renal dysfunction through immune dysregulation and cytokine release, further contributing to the development of IgA nephropathy.

## TREATMENT AND PREVENTION

R-CHOP chemotherapy consisting of rituximab, cyclophosphamide, doxorubicin, vincristine, and prednisolone was given at interval of 3 weeks. Postchemotherapy serum creatinine level improved to 0.78 mg/dL. He completed 2 such cycles.

### Points to Ponder

- Glomerular lesions may be associated by malignant lymphomas.
- Among all lymphomas, Hodgkin's lymphoma is a predominant cause of nephrotic syndrome.
- Non-Hodgkin's lymphoma is linked to several glomerulopathies, including membranoproliferative glomerulonephritis (MPGN), membranous nephropathy (MN), rapidly progressive glomerulonephritis (RPGN) and other varieties.
- Immunoglobulin A nephropathy (IgAN) is the commonest type of cause of glomerulonephritis globally detected in 30–50% of biopsy proven glomerulonephritis.
- Malignant lymphoma is rarely associated with IgA nephropathy, except for Hodgkin's lymphoma, angioimmunoblastic T-cell lymphoma, mucosa-associated lymphoid tissue lymphoma and low-grade B-cell lymphoma.
- This is rare case of IgA nephropathy associated with diffuse large B cell lymphoma presenting as paraneoplastic syndrome.

## MULTIPLE CHOICE QUESTIONS

1. **What is the most likely diagnosis in this patient?**
   A. Laryngeal carcinoma
   B. Diffuse large B-cell lymphoma (DLBCL)
   C. Hodgkin's lymphoma
   D. Thyroid malignancy
2. **Which finding in the biopsy is consistent with diffuse large B-cell lymphoma (DLBCL)?**
   A. CD3+
   B. CD20+
   C. BCL2+
   D. CK+
3. **What does the presence of IgA deposition along glomerular basement membranes in the kidney biopsy suggest?**
   A. Membranous nephropathy
   B. IgA nephropathy
   C. Focal segmental glomerulosclerosis
   D. Minimal change disease
4. **What does the presence of FDG-avid lymph nodes in the PET scan most likely indicate?**
   A. Infection
   B. Metastatic carcinoma
   C. Lymphoma involvement
   D. Autoimmune disease
5. **Which renal feature is most likely to worsen the prognosis in this patient?**
   A. Normal urine pH
   B. Presence of RBCs and pus cells in urine
   C. Normal serum electrolytes
   D. High serum creatinine and albumin < 2.5 g/dL

### Answers

1. (B); 2. (B); 3. (B); 4. (C); 5. (D)

## SUGGESTED READINGS

1. de Oliveira Filgueira PH, Vasconcelos LF, da Silva GB, et al. Paraneoplastic syndromes and the kidney. Saudi J Kidney Dis Transpl. 2010;21(2):222-31.
2. Ronco PM. Paraneoplastic glomerulopathies: new insights into an old entity. Kidney Int. 1999;56(1):355-77.
3. Ng MSY, Francis L, Pillai E, et al. Paraneoplastic immunoglobulin a nephropathy and associated focal segmental glomerulosclerosis in asymptomatic low volume B-cell lymphoma—a case report. BMC Nephro. 2018;(19):224.
4. Kakeshita K, Koike T, Imamura T, et al. IgA Nephropathy with Dominant IgA2 Deposition Accompanied by Mantle Cell Lymphoma. Intern Med. 2021;60(8):1243-50.
5. Bacchetta J, Juillard L, Cochat P, et al. Paraneoplastic glomerular diseases and malignancies. Crit Rev Oncol Hematol. 2009;70(1):39-58.
6. Bergmann J, Buchheidt D, Waldherr R, et al. IgA nephropathy and Hodgkin's disease: a rare coincidence. Case report and literature review. Am J Kidney Dis. 2005;45(1):e16-9.
7. Motoyama O, Kojima Y, Ohara A, et al. IgA nephropathy associated with leukemia and lymphoma: report of two cases. Clin Exp Nephrol. 2008;12(2):140-3.
8. Harada Y, Sakai K, Asaka S, et al. Angioimmunoblastic T-cell lymphoma associated with IgA nephropathy. Intern Med. 2017;56(1):85-9.

CHAPTER

72

# An Approach to a Case of Face and Neck Swelling in a Smoker

*Rohini Rokkam, Prashant G Badole, Pranita Sahay, Mudalsha Ravina*

**CASE VIGNETTE**

Mr XYZ, a 59-year-old gentleman presented to the outpatient department (OPD) with complaints of progressive facial puffiness for 15 days. There is no positional variation in the swelling. Along with this he has been experiencing worsening holocranial headache and progressive dyspnea. His wife reports that he has had a recent change in voice. He had an unremarkable past medical and surgical history. He has a significant past smoking history which compounded to 30 pack-years.

On examination he was alert but visibly distressed. He has a blood pressure (BP) of 130/80 mm Hg, pulse of 96 beats/min, and an oxygen saturation of 92% on room air which improved to 95% on a changing his position from supine to recumbent. His neck veins were distended and non-pulsatile. He also had edema of his bilateral upper limbs. There was no significant lymphadenopathy. The respiratory and cardiovascular examinations were within normal limits.

## PROVISIONAL DIAGNOSIS

Superior vena cava (SVC) obstruction (secondary to lung malignancy).

## DIFFERENTIAL DIAGNOSES

- Cor pulmonale—pulsatile JVP, predominantly lower limb edema
- Cardiac tamponade—pulsatile JVP with prominent x-descent, circulatory shock with muffled heart sounds (*the Beck's triad)*
- Cervical lymphadenopathy—palpable nodes
- Angioedema—acute in onset, will have more edema in the lips and around the eyes

## CLINICAL APPROACH

Superior vena cava obstruction syndrome (henceforth referred to as SVC syndrome) is a clinical condition that arises when the SVC, becomes obstructed. This obstruction can lead to a range of symptoms, primarily due to impaired venous return to the heart, resulting in swelling and congestion in the upper part of the body.

The primary diagnosis of our case is superior vena cava obstruction because of the following key findings:

- Edema over face, neck and upper extremities with preserved vitals
- Relative hypoxia which readily improved with proper positioning of the patient
- Distended *nonpulsatile* neck veins

Later imaging findings did reveal a right lung mass encasing and invading the SVC along with mild compression of trachea.

As in any patient, history is the most important aspect of evaluating the patient. The following are key *clinical features* **(Fig. 1)** a patient with SVC syndrome can present with:

- Edema of face and upper limbs (80%)
- Dyspnea (60%) which worsens on lying down
- Facial plethora (80%)
- Distended nonpulsatile neck veins (60–70%)
- Cough (50–60%)

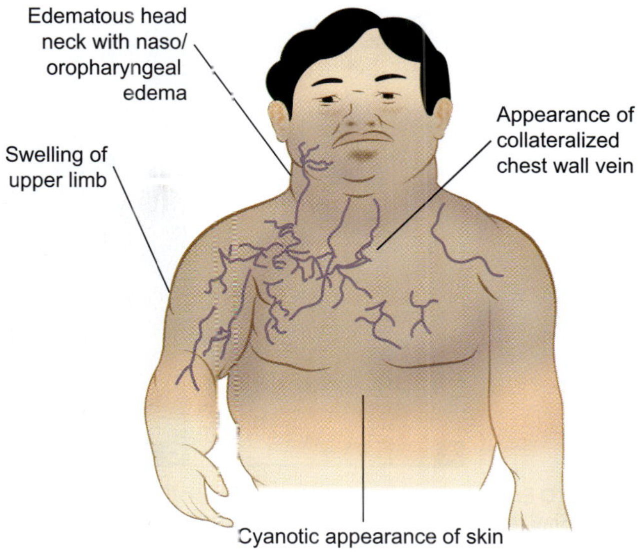


**FIG. 1:** Clinical features of superior vena cava (SVC).

- Distended chest veins (50–60%)
- Hoarseness of voice (10–20%)
- Lymphadenopathy—when present might suggest lymphoma as the cause
- *Stridor (<5%)*: It is an emergency and will require urgent intervention
- *Neurological (<10%)*: Headache, blurred vision, altered mentation may be seen in case of elevated cerebral venous pressure secondary to SVC obstruction. These findings are also emergency and will require prompt action
- *Risk factors*: One should carefully look for risk factors like smoking, pacemaker leads, recent central venous catheterization, history of radiotherapy (may lead to mediastinal fibrosis)

## INVESTIGATIONS

A baseline complete hemogram, liver and renal function test, coagulation profile (especially in cases of SVC thrombosis) and a blood gas analysis should be undertaken to look for any abnormalities.

Targeted investigations include:
- *Chest X-ray*: A chest X-ray is usually the first investigation done. It is cheap, easily available and has minimum radiation exposure. It will usually show any mediastinal widening if present. However, the sensitivity and specificity of the investigation are low.
- *Contrast-enhanced computed tomography* (CECT) is the single most important investigation needed to confirm SVC syndrome. It can show the extent and severity of the obstruction, the etiology and also other complications like laryngeal obstruction and can pick up the extent of collateral circulation. It can pick up thrombus if present. It can also help in characterization of any mediastinal mass and help in a CT guided biopsy. A positron emission tomography (PET) CT further characterizes the lesion. **Figure 2** shows the Contrast CT and PET CT of a female with mediastinal germ cell tumor leading to SVC syndrome. Though there is a risk of contrast nephropathy and radiation exposure, the benefits of the CT far outweigh its benefits.
- *Chest magnetic resonance imaging* (MRI) is not usually required. It can be done in patients who already have renal dysfunction. It also provides details akin to those provided by CT, but is more time consuming and expensive.
- *Other investigations* like upper limb doppler, venography are rarely needed. A 2D echocardiography will rule out any underlying cardiac pathologies.
- *Biopsy:* Biopsy of a mass lesion is required to reach a tissue diagnosis. Bronchoscopy has a sensitivity of 50–70% and CT guided biopsy has a sensitivity of 80% to > 90%. Diagnostic yield is best for a mediastinotomy or a mediastinoscopy directed biopsy.

## PATHOPHYSIOLOGY

The brachiocephalic veins on either side join the form the superior vena cava **(Fig. 3)**. It primarily drains the venous blood of the head and neck and the upper extremities. It also receives the drainage of the azygos vein, which drains the upper lumbar region and the thoracic wall. It ends by draining into the right atrium.

The SVC is a thin muscular structure which is easily amenable to obstruction by both extraluminal or intraluminal pathologies because of its mediastinal location and close relation to the rigid sternum, trachea, pulmonary artery, right main bronchus and numerous lymph nodes. There are various classifications of SVC syndrome.

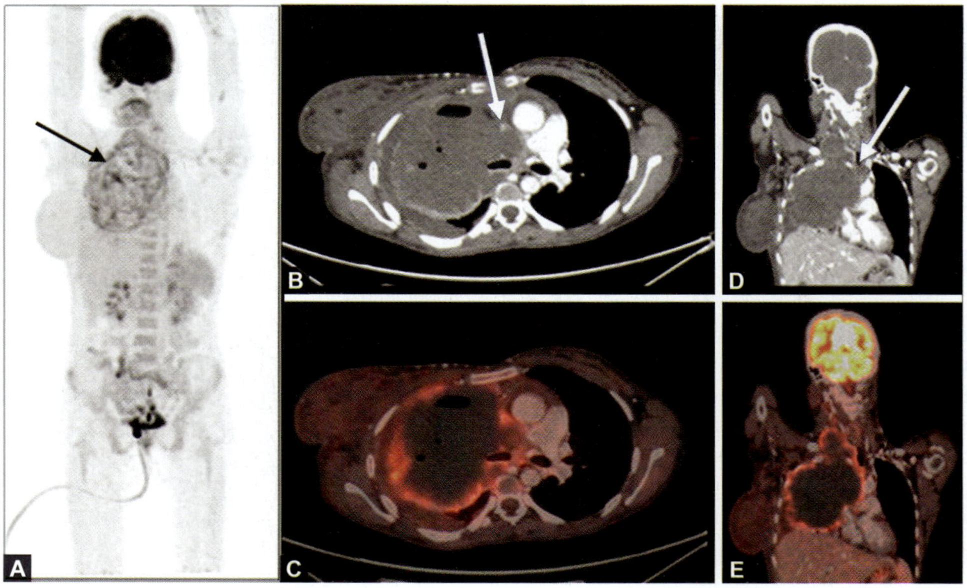


**FIGS. 2A TO E:** The maximum intensity projection (PET). (A) Image revealed inhomogeneous fluorine-18 fluorodeoxyglucose (18F-FDG) uptake in the thorax (black arrow). The axial (B) and coronal (D) contrast-enhanced CT images revealed a peripherally enhancing lesion with large central necrotic area with air foci involving the right hemithorax, superiorly extending to the right supraclavicular and lower cervical regions and medially encasing the trachea, right main bronchus and mediastinal vessels with significant compression (white arrow – compressed superior vena cava). The axial (C) and coronal (E) PET/CT images revealed inhomogeneous 18F-FDG uptake along the periphery of the lesion.

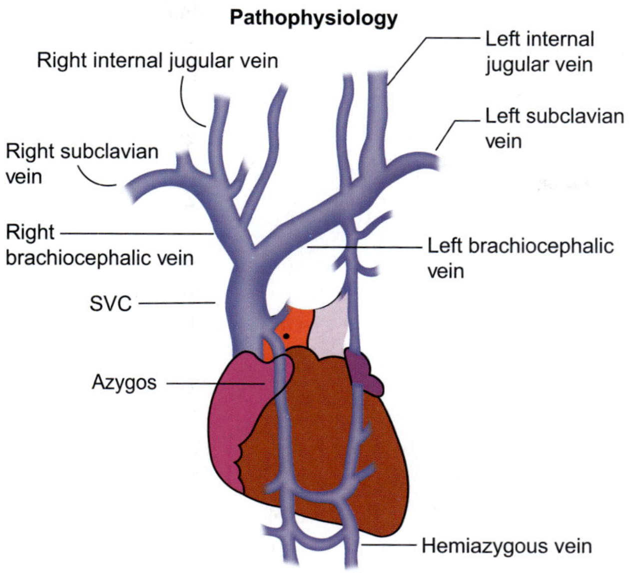


**FIG. 3:** Normal anatomy of SVC.

**TABLE 1: Obstruction classification: Extraluminal versus intraluminal causes.**

| Extraluminal obstruction | Intraluminal obstruction (thrombus) |
|---|---|
| Lung cancer (most common nonsmall lung cancer) | Central venous catheters |
| Lymphomas (diffuse large B cell lymphoma) | Leads of pacemakers, ICDs |
| Thymomas | |
| Germ cell tumors | |
| Metastatic cancers (breast, colon, esophageal, Kaposi's sarcoma) | |
| *Benign causes*: Mediastinal fibrosis, sarcoidosis, aortic arch aneurysm | |

*Classification-based on type of obstruction*: **Table 1** shows the classification.

Malignant extraluminal causes are the most common cause of SVC obstruction. Although small-cell lung cancers are more often associated with SVC obstruction, by numbers nonsmall cell cancer is seen more often in clinical practice. Lately SVC thrombosis is emerging as a common cause of SVC syndrome accounting for almost 30–40% of cases. Most often it is seen following prolonged central venous catheterization. With intracardiac devices the incidence increases with the number of leads used.

*Classification based on location*: **Table 2** highlights the classification based on location of the obstruction.

It is based on severity of obstruction and the collateral flow **(Table 3)**. First introduced by Stanford based on venography findings, it correlates well with the clinical picture **(Fig. 4)**. Most patients with neurological symptoms will have a type III or IV obstruction.

**TABLE 2: Radiological classification: Doty and Stanford classification.**

| Pre-(supra-) azygos | Post-(infra-) azygos |
|---|---|
| Venous congestion and edema of face neck and upper extremities | Venous congestion and edema of face neck and upper extremities along with dilated veins over abdomen |
| Better tolerated | Poorly tolerated |

**TABLE 3: Grading of superior vena cava (SVC) obstruction.**

| Type | Features |
|---|---|
| I | Less than 90% occlusion of the lumen of SVC, with patent azygos vein |
| II | 90–100% occlusion of the lumnen with patent azygos vein |
| III | Complete occlusion of SVC, prominent flow through collaterals, no involvement of mammary and epigastric veins |
| IV | Same as III, with flow through mammary and epigastric veins |

Clinical grading of severity **(Table 4)** is important to decide further management. Grades 3 and 4 require urgent intervention.

## TREATMENT AND PREVENTION

A complete treatment of all the etiologies of SVC syndrome are beyond the scope of this chapter. We will limit to treatment of the SVC syndrome.

As discussed above, clinical stages 3 and 4 are medical emergency. The first step in the management would be to secure the airway by endotracheal intubation or a tracheostomy. It is followed by local radiotherapy with injection dexamethasone 10 mg followed by 4 mg q6h. However, percutaneous endovascular stenting is becoming more commonly used these days, in well-equipped centers. Use of radiotherapy and steroids can alter the tissue architecture and might make the histopathological diagnosis difficult late on.

In case of SVC thrombosis secondary to central venous catheter, first the catheter should be removed followed by local thrombolysis or short course anticoagulation. It should be followed by vitamin K antagonists or direct acting anticoagulants for a duration of 3–6 months. In case of pacemaker or ICD leads leading to SVC obstruction, removal of the leads may carry a high risk of mortality. In this case a percutaneous dilatation or stenting might be a better choice.

Prognosis of SVC syndrome once treated depends on the primary disease. The presence of SVC obstruction, per se, does not worsen the prognosis of the disease.

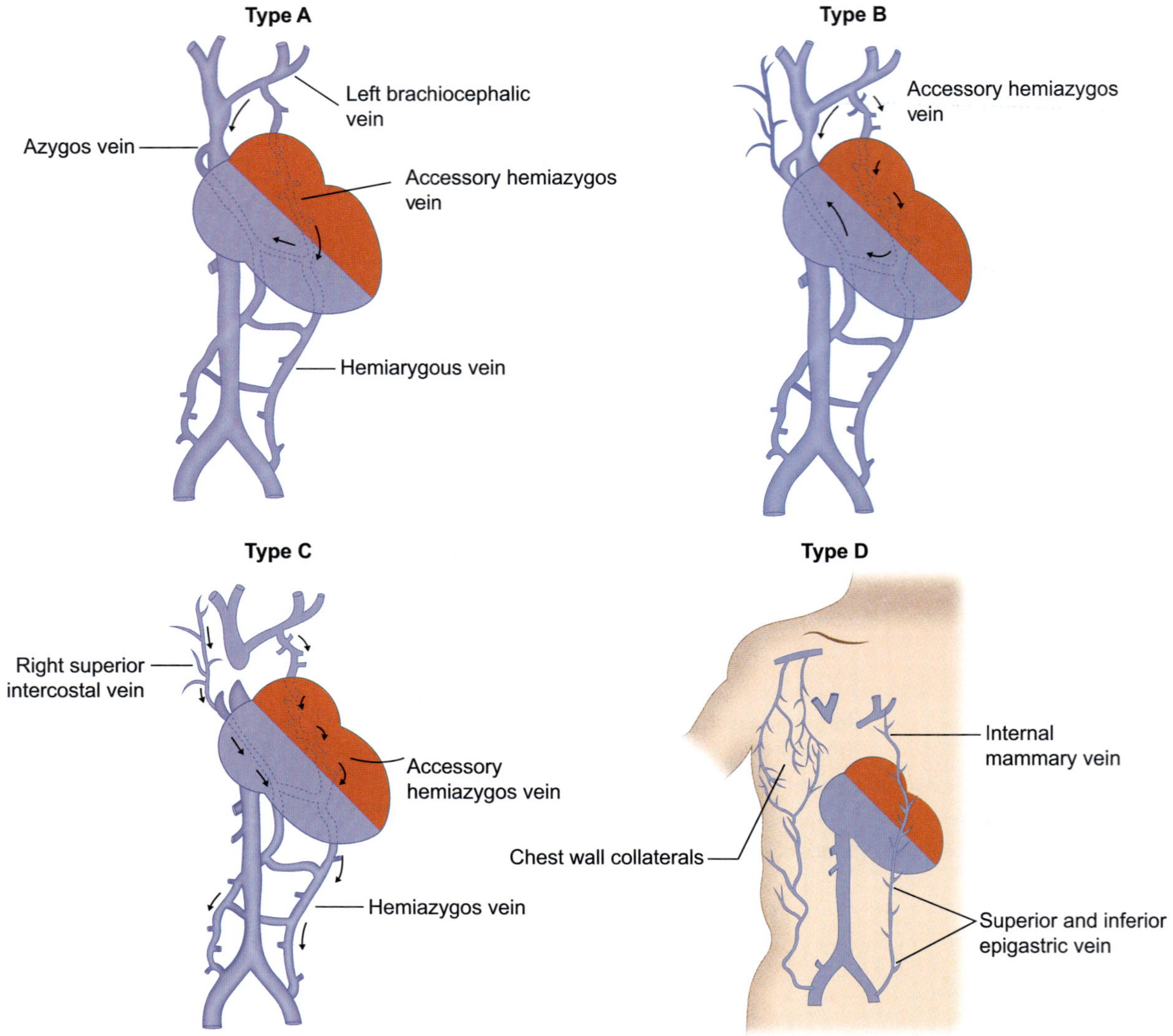


**FIG. 4:** Doty and Stanford classification.

**TABLE 4: Grading severity of clinical features.**

| Grade | Severity | Clinical features |
|---|---|---|
| 0 | Asymptomatic | Only radiological evidence of SVC obstruction |
| 1 | Mild | Head and neck edema, plethora and cyanosis |
| 2 | Moderate | Features of 1 with mild dysphagia, cough, limited neck movement, visual disturbances due to lid edema |
| 3 | Severe | Headache, dizziness due to mild cerebral edema, mild to moderate laryngeal edema, diminished cardiac reserve |
| 4 | Life-threatening | Mental obtundation, stridor, hemodynamic compromise |
| 5 | Fatal | Death due to SVC obstruction |

## Points to Ponder

- SVC obstruction syndrome is a potential clinical emergency, as it can cause significant symptoms due to venous congestion in the upper body.
- Malignancy is the most common cause, particularly lung cancer and lymphoma.
- The approach involves both diagnostic assessment and appropriate treatment of the underlying cause, whether that be a tumor, thrombus, or other pathology.
- Interventional treatments (stenting, chemotherapy, or radiation) are often required to manage this condition effectively.

## MULTIPLE CHOICE QUESTIONS

1. **What is the most likely diagnosis for Mr XYZ based on his presentation?**
   A. Superior vena cava (SVC) syndrome
   B. Congestive heart failure
   C. Chronic obstructive pulmonary disease (COPD) exacerbation
   D. Pulmonary embolism
2. **Which of the following is a likely underlying cause of Mr XYZ's condition, considering his smoking history?**
   A. Tuberculosis
   B. Bronchogenic carcinoma
   C. Sarcoidosis
   D. Pulmonary hypertension
3. **The finding of distended and non-pulsatile neck veins is indicative of which of the following?**
   A. Right-sided heart failure
   B. Venous obstruction
   C. Aortic stenosis
   D. Pericardial effusion
4. **Which investigation would be most useful to confirm the diagnosis in this patient?**
   A. Electrocardiogram (ECG)
   B. Chest X-ray
   C. Contrast-enhanced CT (CECT) of the chest
   D. Arterial blood gas (ABG) analysis
5. **Which of the following is an immediate management strategy for Mr XYZ?**
   A. High-flow oxygen therapy
   B. Administration of corticosteroids and diuretics
   C. Positioning in a semi-recumbent position
   D. Emergency thoracic surgery

### Answers

1. (A); 2. (B); 3. (B); 4. (C): 5. (C)

## SUGGESTED READINGS


1. Lepper PM, Ott SR, Hoppe H, et al. Superior vena cava syndrome in thoracic malignancies. Respir Care. 2011;56(5):653-66.
2. Yu JB, Wilson LD, Detterbeck FC. Superior vena cava syndrome-a proposed classification system and algorithm for management. J Thorac Oncol. 2008;3(8):811-4.
3. Aggarwal K, Chan AK. Superior Vena Cava Syndrome, BMJ Best Practice, 2023.
4. Loscalzo J, Fauci AS, Kasper DL, et al. Harrison's Principles of Internal Medicine, Twenty-First Edition (Vol. 1 & Vol. 2). McGraw Hill Professional; 2022.

# CHAPTER 73 A Case-based Approach to Management of Massive and Submassive Pulmonary Embolism

*Rakhi Sanyal*

## CASE VIGNETTE

A 45-year-old female patient, with a medical history of obesity, recent long-haul flight, and oral contraceptive use, presents with a 2-day history of worsening shortness of breath, pleuritic chest pain, and left calf swelling. She has no prior history of cardiovascular or respiratory disease. On examination, she appears anxious and mildly distressed. Vital signs reveal tachycardia (heart rate 105 bpm), tachypnea (respiratory rate 26 breaths/min), and mild hypoxemia ($PaO_2$ 65 mm Hg). Blood pressure is normal (115/75 mm Hg), and oxygen saturation is 90% on room air. Chest X-ray shows normal lung fields with no signs of consolidation or pneumothorax **(Fig. 1)**. The patient is currently taking ethinylestradiol/levonorgestrel (oral contraceptive).

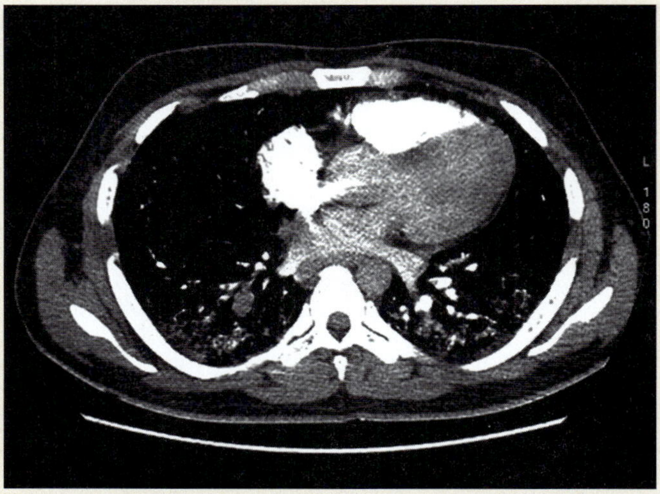


**FIG. 1:** Submassive PE as viewed in CT pulmonary angiography.

## PROVISIONAL DIAGNOSIS

Submassive pulmonary embolism (PE).

## DIFFERENTIAL DIAGNOSIS

Apart from pulmonary embolism, differential diagnosis depends on the following (**Table 1**).

**TABLE 1:** Differential diagnosis of pulmonary embolism.

| Diagnosis | Signs and symptoms |
|---|---|
| Chest pain | Acute myocardial infarction, acute aortic syndromes, pericarditis |
| Dyspnea | Heart failure, pneumothorax, acute exacerbations of chronic lung disease, pneumonia, metabolic, e.g., diabetic ketoacidosis |
| Syncope | Tamponade, malignant arrhythmia, acute aortic syndromes, left ventricular outflow tract obstruction, severe volume loss (e.g., GI bleeding, ruptured ectopic pregnancy) |

## CLINICAL APPROACH

### Clinical Features

Pulmonary embolism (PE) presents with a wide range of features, from no symptoms to shock or sudden death. The most common presenting symptom **(Box 1)** is dyspnea, followed by chest pain, which is classically pleuritic but can also be dull, and cough. However, many patients, including those with large PEs, may havemild or nonspecific symptoms or may be asymptomatic.

## Clinical Likelihood of Pulmonary Embolism

Diagnosing PE is challenging because its clinical features often overlap with other conditions. Therefore, a composite scoring system is used to aid in diagnosis. After taking a comprehensive historyand conducting a clinical examination, determining the pretest probability is the next step. The most widely accepted and validated clinical decision rule is the Wells score **(Table 2)**, which classifies the pretest probability into low, intermediate, and high categories (PE likely or unlikely).

**BOX 1: Presenting signs and symptoms of pulmonary embolism.**

*The most common presenting signs and symptoms include*:
- Dyspnea
- Syncope, presyncope
- Chest pain
- Hemoptysis
- Silent PE
- Sudden cardiac arrest or circulatory collapse
- Hypoxemia
- Tachypnea
- Tachycardia
- DVT

## Investigations

Refer to **Table 3**.

## Risk Stratification

Refer to **Table 4**.

**TABLE 2: Wells score for calculating the likelihood of pulmonary embolism.**

| Criteria | Points |
|---|---|
| Clinical signs/symptoms of DVT | 3 |
| Alternative diagnosis less likely than PE | 3 |
| Tachycardia (>100 bmp) | 1.5 |
| Immobilization/surgery in previous 4 weeks | 1.5 |
| Prior DVT/PE | 1.5 |
| Hemoptysis | 1 |
| Active malignancy (treat within 6 month) | 1 |

| Low-risk | Intermediate-risk | High-risk |
|---|---|---|
| <2 points | 2–6 points | >6 points |
| **PE unlikely** | **PE likely** | |
| ≤4 points | >4 points | |

(PE: pulmonary embolism; DVT: deep vein thrombosis)

**TABLE 3: Primary investigations to diagnose pulmonary embolism.**

**Imaging**

***Echocardiography***

Echocardiography (Echo) is not a primary diagnostic tool for pulmonary embolism (PE), but it is valuable in assessing the hemodynamic impact of a PE, particularly in cases of suspected massive or submassive PE. It can help evaluate right heart function and identify signs of right ventricular strain due to an acute PE

*Echocardiographic findings in pulmonary embolism*:
- *Right ventricular (RV) dilation and dysfunction*:
  - RV dilation: Enlarged right ventricle (RV) compared to the left ventricle (LV) (RV/LV diameter ratio > 1)
  - Hypokinesia or akinesia of the RV free wall: McConnell's sign—right ventricular free wall hypokinesia with apical sparing, is suggestive of acute PE
  - Reduced tricuspid annular plane systolic excursion (TAPSE): Indicates impaired RV function
- *Interventricular septal flattening or paradoxical motion*: Flattening or leftward bowing of the interventricular septum in systole (D-shaped LV), which indicates increased right-sided pressure
- *Pulmonary artery hypertension*: Elevated estimated pulmonary artery systolic pressure (PASP) due to increased resistance from the embolism
- *Tricuspid regurgitation*: Tricuspid regurgitation is often present due to RV dilation and elevated pulmonary artery pressure
- *Dilated inferior vena cava (IVC) with reduced collapsibility*: This indicates elevated right atrial pressure due to RV dysfunction
- *Right atrial enlargement*: Enlargement of the right atrium due to increased pressure from the right ventricle
- *Visualizing clots*: Occasionally, clots may be visualized in the right heart chambers or main pulmonary arteries, though this is rare

*Clinical utility of echocardiography in PE*:
- *Risk stratification*: Identifies patients at high risk of mortality who may benefit from aggressive treatments like thrombolysis
- *Assessment of hemodynamic impact*: Helps determine the extent of right heart strain and failure in acute PE
- *Monitoring*: Useful for monitoring the progression or resolution of right heart strain after treatment

While echocardiography can suggest the presence of PE and help assess its severity, the definitive diagnosis of PE is typically made using CTPA or a V/Q scan

*Continued*

*Continued*

**CT pulmonary angiography (CTPA)**

CT pulmonary angiography (CTPA) is the gold standard for diagnosing pulmonary embolism (PE). The key findings on a CTPA for PE include:

- *Filling defects in pulmonary arteries*: The most characteristic finding is a central or eccentric filling defect within the pulmonary arteries (main, lobar, segmental, or subsegmental branches) where the contrast is absent due to the embolus
- *Partial or complete occlusion*: The clot may cause a partial "railway track" appearance or a complete occlusion with no contrast flow beyond the point of obstruction
- *Peripheral wedge-shaped opacities*: These may indicate areas of infarction or ischemia, often described as "Hampton's hump" on CTPA
- *Enlargement of the pulmonary artery*: An enlarged pulmonary artery may indicate increased pressure due to a significant thrombus burden
- *Right heart strain signs*: This includes right ventricular dilation, interventricular septal flattening or bowing toward the left ventricle, and reflux of contrast into the inferior vena cava (IVC) and hepatic veins
- *Mosaic perfusion pattern*: Due to varying levels of blood flow in different lung regions, showing a patchwork appearance

CTPA is highly sensitive and specific for detecting PE, making it the preferred diagnostic tool in clinical practice

**Ventilation-perfusion (V/Q) scan**

*Indications*:

- Hypersensitivity to iodinated contrast or renal impairment
- *Pregnancy*: If CTPA contraindicated

*Findings*:

- Mismatch defect
- *Normal V/Q scan*: If both the ventilation and perfusion scans are normal, it effectively rules out PE

**X-ray**

- *Chest X-ray*: Most common—Normal
- *Hampton's hump*: A wedge-shaped, pleural-based opacity that indicates lung infarction
- *Westermark sign*: Regional oligemia (loss of vascular markings) in the lung due to obstruction of pulmonary blood flow
- *Elevated hemidiaphragm*: Often seen on the affected side due to atelectasis
- *Atelectasis or pleural effusion*: These are nonspecific findings that may appear in the case of a PE
- *Enlarged pulmonary arteries*: This may suggest pulmonary hypertension secondary to a PE

**Laboratory parameters**

***Troponin***

- Elevated troponin is associated with increased mortality
- The cutoff values might be troponin I >0.1 ng/mL or troponin T >0.03 ng/mL

**D-dimer**

- An elevated D-dimer alone is insufficient to make a diagnosis of PE, but a normal D-dimer can be used to rule out PE in patients with a low or intermediate probability of PE. D-dimer testing should be used in conjunction with clinical probability assessment
- While D-dimer assays are highly sensitive, their specificity is low, usually between 40 and 60%

**Brain natriuretic peptide (BNP) or NT-BNP**

Elevated BNP or NT-proBNP concentrations possess low specificity and positive predictive value (for early mortality) in normotensive patients with PE, but low levels of BNP or NT-proBNP are capable of excluding an unfavorable early clinical outcome, with high sensitivity and a negative predictive value

**Miscellaneous**

***ECG***

ECG signs of (sub) massive PE include RV strain pattern and RV injury pattern:

- *ECG signs of RV strain may include*:
  - Most common ECG finding—Sinus tachycardia
  - T-wave inversions in the right precordial leads (V1–4) ± the inferior leads (II, III, aVF)
  - QR pattern in V1
  - S1Q3T3 pattern
  - Incomplete or complete right bundle branch block

*ECG signs of RV injury pattern may include*:

- ST elevation in inferior (II, III, aVF) and V1–V2 and/or ST depression in I, aVL, V6
- ST elevation in aVR and ST depression in lead I (it has been shown to be associated with a high in-hospital mortality rate)

## PATHOPHYSIOLOGY

Pulmonary embolism occurs when a blood clot, often originating from the deep veins of the legs (deep vein thrombosis), obstructs pulmonary arteries, leading to impaired gas exchange, reduced oxygenation, and strain on the right heart. In submassive PE, the clot causes moderate right ventricular dysfunction and mild to moderate hypoxemia without causing complete circulatory collapse.

## TREATMENT AND PREVENTION (FLOWCHART 1)

In the management of submassive pulmonary embolism (PE) in the ICU, initial resuscitation focuses on hemodynamic support and oxygenation while awaiting definitive clot removal. Hemodynamic support should be achieved by using short-term peripheral lines for vasopressors and adopting a fluid-conservative strategy to avoid right ventricular (RV) over-distention. Intubation should be avoided due to the risk of severe hypotension and cardiac arrest; if necessary, it should be done by an experienced operator with careful management of acidosis and hypercarbia. Anticoagulation should be initiated early to prevent new clots, with the choice of agent based on the patient's clinical factors and risk stratification. Systemic thrombolysis is indicated for high-risk PE and can involve agents like alteplase or tenecteplase, though bleeding risks must be carefully considered. In cases where thrombolysis is contraindicated or ineffective, percutaneous catheter-directed treatments, such as catheter-directed thrombolysis or mechanical thrombectomy, may be considered. Surgical embolectomy is an option for massive PE with absolute contraindications to thrombolysis or failure of other interventions.

TABLE 4: Pulmonary embolism severity index (PESI).

| Parameter | PESI | s-PESI |
|---|---|---|
| Age | Age in years | 1 point (if >80 years) |
| Male sex | +10 points | – |
| Cancer diagnosis | +30 points | 1 point |
| Chronic heart failure | +10 points | 1 point |
| Chronic pulmonary disease | +10 points | |
| Pulse rate ≥ 110 beats pre minute | +20 points | 1 point |
| Systolic blood pressure < 100 mm Hg | +30 points | 1 point |
| Respiratory rate ≥ 30 breaths per minute | +20 points | – |
| Temperature <36° C | +20 points | – |
| Altered mental status | +60 points | – |
| Arterial oxyhemoglobin saturation <90% | +20 points | 1 point |
| **Risk stratification** | | |
| Class I: ≤65 points | Very low 30-day mortality risk (0–1.5%) | |
| Class II: 66–85 points | Low mortality risk (1.7–3.5%) | |
| Class III: 86–105 points | Moderate mortality risk (3.2–7.1%) | |
| Class IV: 106–125 points | High mortality risk (4–11.4%) | |
| Class V: >125 points | Very high mortality risk (10–24.5%) | |
| **Simplified PESI score** | | |
| 0 point = 30-day mortality risk 1% (95% CI 0–2.1%)<br>≥1 point(S) = 30-day mortality risk 10.9% (95% CI 8.5–13.2%) | | |

(PESI: pulmonary embolism severity index; s–PESI: simplified pulmonary embolism severity)

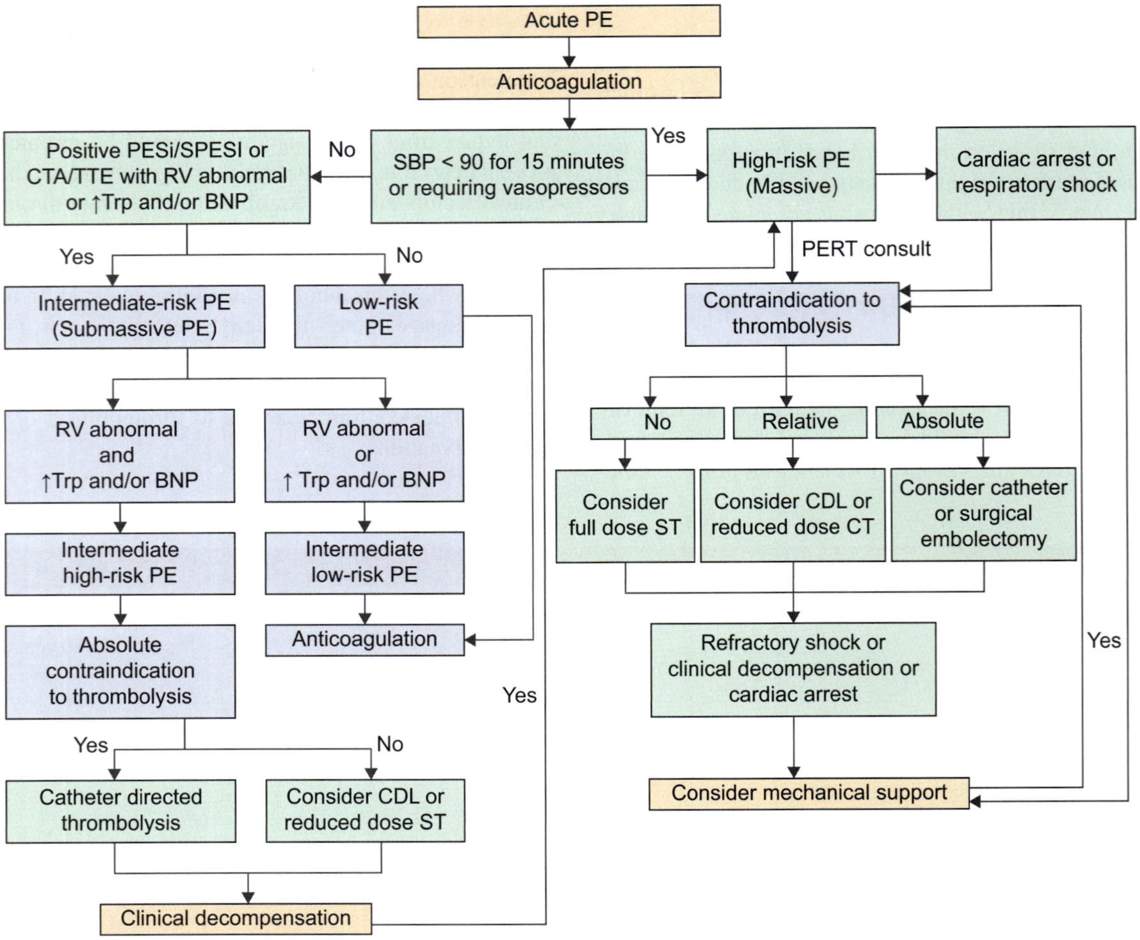


**FLOWCHART 1:** Treatment algorithm of pulmonary embolism.

(PE: pulmonary embolism; CT: computed tomography; RV: right ventricle; SBP: systolic blood pressure; Trp: transient receptor potential; BNP: brain natriuretic peptide; PESI: pulmonary embolism severity index; s–PESI: simplified pulmonary embolism severity index; TTE: transthoracic echocardiogram; CTA: computed tomography angiography; CDL: catheter-directed thrombolysis; ST: streptokinase)

## Points to Ponder

- PE is not uncommon.
- Clinical diagnosis can be very deceptive, and a strong degree of clinical suspicion is required for diagnosis.
- Management depends on clinical severity, pretest probability, risk assessment.
- Pulmonary embolism response team (PERT) should be involved in the immediate management and follow-up of the patients with PE.

## MULTIPLE CHOICE QUESTIONS

**1. What is the most likely cause of the patient's presentation?**

A. Pneumonia
B. Pulmonary embolism
C. Acute asthma exacerbation
D. Myocardial infarction

**2. Which of the following is a risk factor for the patient's condition?**

A. Smoking
B. Obesity
C. History of asthma
D. Family history of heart disease

**3. What is the most concerning finding in this patient's vital signs?**

A. Tachycardia
B. Tachypnea
C. Mild hypoxemia
D. Normal blood pressure

**4. What is the first step in the management of suspected pulmonary embolism?**

A. Administer diuretics
B. Start anticoagulation therapy
C. Perform a chest CT or V/Q scan
D. Start oxygen therapy

**5. Which of the following medications is most likely contributing to the patient's risk of pulmonary embolism?**

A. Statins
B. Oral contraceptives
C. Beta-blockers
D. Antihypertensives

## Answers

1. (B); 2. (B); 3. (A); 4. (C); 5. (D)

## SUGGESTED READINGS


1. Morrone D, Morrone V. Acute Pulmonary Embolism: Focus on the Clinical Picture. Korean Circ J. 2018;48(5):365-81.
2. Rivera-Lebron B, McDaniel M, Ahrar K, et al. PERT Consortium. Diagnosis, Treatment and Follow-up of Acute Pulmonary Embolism: Consensus Practice from the PERT Consortium. Clin Appl Thromb Hemost. 2019;25:1076029619853037.
3. Shonyela FS, Yang S, Liu B,et al. Postoperative Acute Pulmonary Embolism Following Pulmonary Resections. Ann Thorac Cardiovasc Surg. 2015;21(5):409-17.
4. Chopard R, Behr J, Vidoni C, et al. An Update on the Management of Acute High-risk Pulmonary Embolism. J Clin Med. 2022;11(16):4807.
5. Leidi A, Bex S, Righini M, et al. Risk Stratification in Patients with Acute Pulmonary Embolism: Current Evidence and Perspectives. J Clin Med. 2022;11(9):2533.

CHAPTER

74

# An Approach to a Case of Chronic Cough Management

*Sandeep Thareja, Vikas Marwah, Deepu Peter*

**CASE VIGNETTE**

A 61-year-old female presented with complaints of cough for the past 3 months. It increased at night and her sleep was disturbed because of the cough. There was no history of expectoration, fever, wheezing, chest pain, hemoptysis or breathlessness. She was obese and complained of frequent retrosternal burning sensation especially after spicy meal. She was also diagnosed to have primary hypertension five years back for which she had been prescribed Tab. ramipril 5 mg once daily. She had been prescribed repeated courses of antibiotics, bronchodilators and inhaled steroids for her cough over the past 3 months and she claims no benefit with these medications. Her vitals were normal, and systemic examination was also essentially normal.

Chest radiograph and electrocardiograph were also within normal limits. Microbiological examination of sputum revealed commensal flora and was negative for acid fast bacilli. ENT consult showed features of laryngopharyngeal reflux and patient was diagnosed as a case of gastroesophageal reflux disease and was commenced on proton pump inhibitors along with prokinetics and was asked to review after 02 weeks. Patient during her review claimed minimal improvement in cough and her medications were continued and patient was kept on follow-up. However, she reported again after 1 month with persistent symptoms with only 20% relief with medications. In view of this, it was decided to stop ACE inhibitor and switch to calcium channel blockers while continuing PPI and prokinetics. During her next visit to OPD after a month, patient claimed near total resolution of cough, and she was labelled as a case of gastroesophageal reflux disease with ACE inhibitor induced cough.

## PROVISIONAL DIAGNOSIS

Gastroesophageal reflux disease (GERD) with ACE inhibitor-induced cough.

## DIFFERENTIAL DIAGNOSIS

The most common causes of chronic cough are chronic obstructive pulmonary disease, bronchial asthma, nonasthmatic eosinophilic bronchitis, gastroesophageal reflux disease (GERD), and upper airway cough syndrome (UACS). Cough can also be a manifestation of disorders of airway like foreign body, neoplasm and bronchiectasis; or parenchymal abnormalities in the form of interstitial lung disease and lung abscess. Underlying heart failure can also cause a cough which is usually aggravated on lying down.

Drugs like ACE inhibitors, glaucoma medications (Latanoprost)(80) and even calcium channel blockers and bisphosphonates can also cause cough by various mechanisms. Viral or other upper respiratory infections can lead to a cough which can persist beyond the acute period. Abnormalities of the external auditory canal, larynx, pharynx, pleura, diaphragm, pericardium, stomach, esophagus, and thyroid can lead to irritation of the vagus nerve and stimulation of the cough reflex arc.

Other causes of chronic cough include chronic aspiration, swallowing dysfunction and foreign body. Somatic cough disorder, also known as tic cough or psychogenic cough is a rare and troublesome cause of cough. The common causes of chronic cough are mentioned in **Table 1**.

## CLINICAL APPROACH

Detailed history should be obtained from all patients being evaluated for chronic cough. It can be quite nonspecific and care should be taken to rule out the common aggravating factors like smoking, viral infection, ACE inhibitor use, airway disease and other treatable traits. History regarding the duration of cough, presence of expectoration and prior history of similar episode should also be sought. In addition to history of dyspnea, heartburn, hemoptysis, and wheeze, patient should also be asked about associated symptoms of rhinorrhea, excessive sneezing, dysphonia, dysphagia, and swelling of feet. Recent history of viral infection should be ruled out. History of environmental air pollution may also be significant. The danger signs that may warrant urgent attention are hemoptysis, associated chest pain, recurrent or persistent chest infection, hoarseness of voice, dysphagia and age more than 40 years in a smoker or ex-smoker or previous history of asbestosis.

Hemoptysis may be suggestive of lung cancer, bronchiectasis, lung abscess, heart failure, immunologic causes and even rheumatologic causes. Any obstruction of the airway or a

# CHAPTER 74

**TABLE 1: Common causes of chronic cough.**

| | |
|---|---|
| Reflux disorders | • GERD<br>• LPR<br>• UACS |
| Airway disease | • COPD<br>• Bronchial asthma<br>• Bronchiectasis<br>• Chronic bronchitis<br>• Nonasthmatic eosinophilic bronchitis |
| Parenchymal disease | • Interstitial lung disease<br>• Lung cancer |
| Drugs | • ACE inhibitors<br>• Calcium channel blockers<br>• Bisphosphonates<br>• Glaucoma medications (Latanoprost, Timolol) |
| Infectious | • Bordetella pertussis<br>• COVID-19<br>• Bacterial infections |
| Other causes | • Aspiration<br>• Swallowing dysfunction<br>• Foreign body<br>• Heart failure<br>• Irritation of vagal nerve |

pulmonary parenchymal disease can lead to dyspnea. History regarding the progression of dyspnea, any triggers, waxing and waning nature of dyspnea, or associated hoarseness of voice will help deciding on the further course of action. History of smoking is significant as it is an irritant and can be a cause of chronic bronchitis and lung cancer. Smoking cessation can often help improve cough due to cigarette smoking.

Patients who are immunosuppressed, if presenting with cough should be worked up for infections like tuberculosis and pneumocystis pneumonia diligently. Patients with infections in the lung parenchyma or the sinuses can present with history of cough with purulent sputum. Cough secondary to pertussis consists of paroxysmal episodes of cough with whoop prior to the cough, absence of fever, and posttussive vomiting.

Chronic infections like tuberculosis, lung abscess or interstitial lung disease secondary to connective tissue disease can have fever, weight loss or night sweats.

The clinician should obtain family or personal history of allergies, including rhinitis and conjunctivitis and also the use of tobacco products or vaping devices by the patient himself or amongst those staying with him.

Cough frequency and quality can be measured with the help of validated tools which are mostly research tools, and their clinical utility is not clear. History about the effect of cough on QoL including mood should be assessed.

Examination of both the upper and lower airway should be performed. Note should be made of nasal congestion, swelling of tonsils, hoarseness, stridor and pharyngeal edema. Careful examination should be performed for correct identification of wheeze, crackles and squawks.

## INVESTIGATIONS

Patients with chronic cough are commonly subjected to pre- and postbronchodilator spirometric study for assessment of airway abnormalities. Restrictive disorder if identified will require further diffusion and lung volume studies.

If an underlying infection is suspected, then sputum culture should also be ordered. T2 high airway disease can be identified with the help of blood eosinophil count and FENO.

Chest radiograph is usually obtained in all patients with chronic cough. Radiation exposure should be minimised, and routine computed tomography of the chest should not be undertaken. Lung cancer diagnosis cannot be excluded in the presence of a normal chest radiograph. If warning signs are present then patient should be further investigated. Chest CT is not routinely recommended in individuals with normal examination and chest radiograph. It should be performed to look for evidence of disease as in cases of chronic productive cough to rule out bronchiectasis; to exclude malignancy in high risk patients, if patient has hemoptysis or if there is a barking cough suggestive of airway collapsibility.

Bronchoscopy can be helpful in identifying tracheal abnormalities like airway collapsibility, tracheopathia osteochondroplastica and tracheobronchomalacia. Bronchoscopy should be considered in patients with productive cough without obvious cause, suspicion of foreign body and in patients with possibility of infection but the sputum culture is negative. If a patient with CC is suspected to have inducible laryngeal obstruction (ILO), or has persistent rhinosinusitis despite treatment or has hoarseness of voice he/she may benefit from flexible nasal endoscopy and laryngoscopy.

There is limited value for bronchial hyperreactivity tests with mannitol/methacholine in the diagnosis or management of chronic cough. RCC patients should also be not subjected to cough challenges like Capsaicin challenge which are to be performed only in research settings.

Consensus panels have advocated an anatomical diagnostic protocol toward the management of chronic cough. The most common causes of chronic cough are chronic obstructive pulmonary disease, bronchial asthma, gastroesophageal reflux disease, upper airway cough syndrome, and nonasthmatic eosinophilic bronchitis. However, in 30–40% patients, no cause can be identified or do not get better with the treatment of underlying comorbidities using the anatomical diagnostic protocol. There is also a tendency to blindly initiate treatment like proton pump inhibitors even in the absence of symptoms like heartburn. So, the protocol despite being valid requires refinement.

A treatable trait approach has been advocated rather than the protocolised investigation. The treatable trait approach describes phenotypes or endotypes which can be identified with the help of a biomarker which can be measured or evaluated objectively. This approach has been effective in airway pathology, and allows multidimensional clinical assessment of the various factors that cause cough. It proposes that the patient may be labelled as having RCC or CC with a particular trait like reflux, ACEI use, cough hypersensitivity, obesity or dysphonia. This will enable the personalised treatment of the patient rather than empiric treatment. Also, CC can also be seen in individuals with cough hypersensitivity which is often overlooked, and which explains why the protocolised approach becomes ineffective in certain categories of patients.

## PATHOPHYSIOLOGY

Gastroesophageal reflux disease (GERD) occurs when stomach contents, including acid, reflux into the esophagus, causing irritation and inflammation. In GERD, acid can also reach the larynx and pharynx (laryngopharyngeal reflux), leading to symptoms like chronic cough, throat clearing, and burning sensations. ACE inhibitors like ramipril, commonly used for hypertension, can cause a persistent dry cough due to bradykinin accumulation. This is because ACE inhibitors prevent the breakdown of bradykinin, which can trigger cough reflex through local irritation in the respiratory tract. In this case, the patient's cough was attributed to both GERD and the ACE inhibitor.

## TREATMENT AND PREVENTION

### Smoking Cessation

Smoking cessation can help reduce the cough caused due to the chronic bronchitis. On quitting smoking, patients may experience increased cough due to the nicotine withdrawal induced cough hypersensitivity. Nicotine replacement can help prevent this and also enhance rates.

### ACE Inhibitors

ACE inhibitors should be stopped in patients with CC irrespective of the cause of the cough as it can cause cough hypersensitivity.

### Gastro-oesophageal Reflux Disease

It is debatable as to whether GERD is an aggravant or a primary cause of cough. Some studies suggest GERD as the third most common cause of cough. Symptoms of heartburn, dysphonia and sour taste in mouth are reported by many patients with chronic cough. However, in 40% of patients with cough attributable to GERD do not demonstrate any of these symptoms. Despite esophageal dysmotility being a common in patients with CC, therapy with proton pump inhibitors have shown no benefit in systematic studies in patients without acid reflux and only modest benefit in those with acid reflux.

There are numerous mechanisms by which GERD causes cough. The reflux contents can stimulate the receptors in the vagal afferent neurons in the upper respiratory tract. The gastric contents can be aspirated into the lower respiratory tract leading to inflammation. The reflux of acid into the distal esophagus can also cause initiation of the esophageal-tracheobronchial cough reflex.

The diagnosis of GERD induced cough is most often made with the presence of symptoms and response to empiric PPI therapy. In patients with persistent symptoms of GERD despite 3 month antireflux therapy trial are subjected to ambulatory esophageal pH monitoring.

The presence of heartburn is the best predictor of treatment response. In patients without typical reflux symptoms of heartburn, abdominal/chest discomfort, and regurgitation should not be prescribed treatment. In addition to treatment, patients should also be advised about lifestyle modifications like weight loss, raising the head end of the bed and dietary modifications (reducing spicy, fatty, and carbonated drinks, and not eating before bedtime) which might help reduce GERD. In patients with reflux symptoms twice daily PPI should be offered for 1 month. PPI should be taken 30–60 minutes prior to meals and dose should be increased only to control heartburn. Treatment should be discontinued if there is no improvement after 1 month of treatment. There is limited evidence for the use of prokinetic drugs and should be limited to specialist services due to potential adverse effects. Alginates may be prescribed in the presence of typical symptoms of heartburn.

Surgical consultation should also be sought for the management of GERD. Laparoscopic fundoplication surgeries are an effective modality for the control of GERD, however, it is usually associated with numerous complications like dysphagia, flatulence, bloating, and reflux recurrence. In the presence of cough with significant persistent reflux symptoms fundoplication surgeries can be advised after careful assessment and patient counseling.

### Cough with Expectoration

Patients with CC and expectoration should be subjected to an early CT chest in addition to sputum culture. History of smoking, immunodeficiency, tracheal disorders like tracheobronchomalacia and environmental dust exposure should be taken. Bronchoscopy and bronchoalveolar lavage can also help in diagnosing various airway diseases and infections.

Primary goal is to treat and optimize the underlying disease condition. Mucolytic therapy and physiotherapy may also be beneficial in a certain group of patients. If CC persists after these interventions, a therapeutic trial of macrolides can be offered to patients with underlying airway disease or those with productive CC. Evaluation as per the BTS guidance should be performed prior to initiation of macrolide therapy.

### Eosinophilic Disease of the Airways

This comprises of bronchial asthma, cough variant asthma and nonasthmatic eosinophilic bronchitis. It is characterized by increased FENO and blood eosinophil levels, and the presence of >3% eosinophils in the sputum.

FENO >25 ppb should prompt a trial of ICS. BEC $\geq 0.3 \times 10^9$/L in a patient with CC suggests eosinophilic airway disease. This however has poor sensitivity and specificity to make a diagnosis and studies have reported poor relation with treatment response.

In patients with CC with elevated T2 biomarkers even in the absence of any other features of airflow obstruction, a trial of inhaled corticosteroids for four weeks may be considered. If the compliance is good and the technique is optimal, consider increasing the dose or adding an leukotriene antagonist to the regimen. If markers are persistently high, a short course of oral corticosteroids may also be administered.

### Upper Airway Disease

Postnasal drip or secretions dripping from the nasal cavity into the nasopharynx arising out of allergy, or vasomotor rhinitis or rhinosinusitis is thought to cause UACS. Patients may present with frequent throat clearing, chronic cough and sensation of something stuck in throat or a liquid flowing into the back of throat. The term laryngopharyngeal reflex is a popular label used to describe these symptoms despite any obvious mechanism and poor response to treatment. Hoarseness of voice and chronic throat symptoms can also be seen in patients with obesity, psychological stress, snoring, upper airway disorders and hormonal changes.

Persistent dysphonia or progressive dysphagia especially in smokers >45 years of age should be considered as a red flag sign and evaluation for malignancy should be performed.

Inducible laryngeal obstruction, previously known as vocal cord dysfunction, is the dynamic airway obstruction arising out of inadequate laryngeal closure at the glottic or subglottic level. Patients will manifest with acute onset breathlessness, inspiratory wheezing and choking sensation triggered usually by an emotional episode. Functional laryngoscopy can confirm the diagnosis of ILO.

Treatment of UACS consists of intranasal steroids. If the patient reports with symptoms suggestive of chronic rhinosinusitis, then in addition to the intranasal steroids, saline irrigation/rinses administered for a minimum 6 weeks may give symptomatic relief. Studies have shown no benefit with PPI in patients with upper airway symptoms.

## Obstructive Sleep Apnea

Studies have shown a very high prevalence of OSA, varying from 39–68% in patients with CC. Patients with OSA tend to have GERD, rhinitis and upper airway inflammation which can cause cough hypersensitivity. If OSA is suspected in a patients with CC, sleep study followed by a trial of CPAP should be given.

## Obesity

Obesity was found to be high among patients with CC. Increase in body mass index is associated with an increased prevalence of CC. Also studies have shown a high incidence of reflux and OSA which can eventually lead to CC. Weight reduction strategies may also be added to the treatment plan in all patients with CC as it might help reduce the GERD and OSA.

## Management of Refractory Chronic Cough

In patients with RCC, the cough hypersensitivity should be targeted with the help of neuromodulating agents. Certain unlicensed pharmacological agents and nonpharmacological interventions have been shown to be efficacious in patients with RCC.

## Nonpharmacological Management of RCC

A complex multimodality approach consisting of techniques that actively suppress coughing. There was a 40% reduction in the cough in addition in the improvement in QoL as demonstrated by the PSALTI study. This can be offered complimentary to the pharmacclogical treatment and is best delivered by physiotherapists and speech and language therapists.

## Pharmacological Treatment

Sustained release sulphate preparation of morphine at a low dose (5–10 mg/day) has been shown to improve the cough related QoL by reducing the cough frequency by nearly 70%. Tolerance was not seen, however, cough tends to recur on stopping therapy, hence, long term treatment is mandated. It has an addiction or abuse potential and careful monitoring of the patient is required. Studies have shown that codeine is not beneficial in patients with URTI induced acute cough and in COPD. Its usage is not recommended.

Gabapentinoids are a class of drugs which act by inhibition of gamma amino butyric acid. Its predominantly used as an antiepileptic, it has been shown to improve cough related QoL. They also help improve the mood and reduce anxiety. Side effects of the drug mostly limit the dose escalation. Pregabalin is started at a dose of 25 mg twice daily, and then gradually uptitrated to full dose of 75 mg twice daily. Doses of gabapentin are gradually increased from 100 mg thrice daily to full dose of 600 mg thrice daily. Careful monitoring of adverse effects and response to treatment is required.

Amitriptyline has also been shown to be beneficial in treating RCC as compared to codeine/guaifenesin and may be tried especially in patients with coexisting depression/low mood.

Novel agents like gefapixant which is a P2X3 antagonist have been proven to be effective in CC. Its use is limited as it causes significant taste disturbance. Newer agents like camlipixant are undergoing clinical trials and might be available for use in the near future. TRPM8 (menthol receptor) agonist and neurokinin one receptor antagonist are also being evaluated.

## Points to Ponder

- Chronic cough can be attributed to multitude of causes, and hence, warrants multidisciplinary team approach.
- Routine healthcare visits can help prevent the progression of acute respiratory diseases into chronic pathology. General practitioners should consistently be on the look for red flag signs suggestive of malignancy and other serious illnesses.
- The health care provider should educate and emphasize the importance of smoking cessation and avoidance of environmental and other pollutants in prevention of chronic cough. They should also be made aware about the various vaccines available against various preventable respiratory infections.
- Combined efforts by the healthcare provider with the patient can help reduce the burden of chronic cough on the patients' health as well as on healthcare expenditure.

## MULTIPLE CHOICE QUESTIONS

**1. What is the most likely cause of chronic cough in a patient with GERD?**

A. Infection
B. Laryngopharyngeal reflux
C. Asthma
D. Pulmonary embolism

**2. Which medication is associated with ACE inhibitor-induced cough?**

A. Metoprolol
B. Ramipril
C. Amlodipine
D. Losartan

**3. Which of the following is the first-line treatment for GERD-induced cough?**

A. Antibiotics
B. Proton pump inhibitors
C. Inhaled steroids
D. Bronchodilators

**4. What is the primary mechanism by which ACE inhibitors cause a cough?**

A. Increased histamine release
B. Bradykinin accumulation
C. Airway inflammation
D. Direct airway irritation

**5. What is the likely outcome after discontinuing ACE inhibitors in a patient with persistent cough?**

A. No improvement in cough
B. Near total resolution of cough
C. Worsening of cough
D. Development of wheezing

### Answers

1. (B); 2. (B); 3. (B); 4. (B); 5. (B)

## SUGGESTED READINGS

1. Hulme K, Dogan S, Parker SM, et al. 'Chronic cough, cause unknown: A qualitative study of patient perspectives of chronic refractory cough. J Health Psychol. 2019;24(6):707-16.
2. Hulme K, Deary V, Dogan S, et al. Psychological profile of individuals presenting with chronic cough. ERJ Open Research. [Internet]. 2017 Jan 1 [cited 2024 Jun 2];3(1). Available from: https://openres.ersjournals.com/content/3/1/00099-2016
3. Koskela HO, Lätti AM, Pekkanen J. The impacts of cough: a cross-sectional study in a Finnish adult employee population. ERJ Open Research [Internet]. 2018 Oct 1 [cited 2024 Jun 2];4(4). Available from: https://openres.ersjournals.com/content/4/4/00113-2018
4. Koskela HO, Lätti AM, Pekkanen J. Risk factors for repetitive doctor's consultations due to cough: a cross-sectional study in a Finnish employed population. BMJ Open. 2019;9(6):e030945.
5. Hull JH, Langerman H, Ul-Haq Z, et al. Burden and impact of chronic cough in UK primary care: a dataset analysis. BMJ Open. 2021;11(12):e054832.
6. McGarvey LPA. Patterns of cough in the clinic. Pulm Pharmacol Therapeutics. 2011;24(3):300-3.
7. Jo EJ, Song WJ. Environmental triggers for chronic cough. Asia Pacific Allergy. 2019;9(2):e16.
8. Vertigan AE, Kapela SL, Birring SS, et al. Feasibility and clinical utility of ambulatory cough monitoring in an outpatient clinical setting: a real-world retrospective evaluation. ERJ Open Research [Internet]. 2021 Oct 1 [cited 2024 Jun 2];7(4). Available from: https://openres.ersjournals.com/content/7/4/00319-2021
9. Hall JI, Lozano M, Estrada-Petrocelli L, et al. The present and future of cough counting tools. J Thorac Dis. [Internet]. 2020 Sep [cited 2024 Jun 2];12(9). Available from: https://jtd.amegroups.org/article/view/44208
10. Cho PSP, Birring SS, Fletcher HV, et al. Methods of Cough Assessment. J Allergy Clin Immunol. In Practice. 2019;7(6):1715-23.

CHAPTER

# 75

# A Case-based Approach to Miliary Shadows in Chest X-ray

*Kausik Bhar*

## CASE VIGNETTE

A 40-year-old male migrant laborer with no prior comorbidities presented with severe fatigue, extreme exhaustion, low-grade irregular fever, dry cough, and postural dizziness **(Figs. 1 and 2)**.

Physical examination revealed mild pallor, a pulse rate of 104 beats/min (regular), and blood pressure of 90/60 mm Hg (sitting) dropping to 68/46 mm Hg (standing). Laboratory investigations showed anemia of chronic disease (Hb 9.5 g%), hyponatremia (Na 125 mmol/L), normal liver and renal function tests, normal thyroid function, and a negative ICTC test. Morning serum cortisol was 8 µg/dL, and ACTH was 120 pg/mL.

CECT of the abdomen revealed bilateral adrenal space-occupying lesions (SOL). Urinary histoplasma antigen, bronchoscopy findings, BAL AFB, and CBNAAT tests were negative, and urinary metanephrine and normetanephrine levels were normal, ruling out pheochromocytoma before adrenal biopsy. Chest X-ray findings suggested **(Fig. 3)** differential diagnoses, including miliary tuberculosis with adrenal involvement, bronchoalveolar lung carcinoma with adrenal metastasis, and lung histoplasmosis with adrenal involvement.

The patient was diagnosed with adrenal histoplasmosis with presumptive pulmonary histoplasmosis and treated with liposomal amphotericin B followed by fluconazole along with steroid replacement therapy. Gradual improvement was observed, with substantial resolution of chest radiographic findings and symptoms. The final diagnosis was adrenal and pulmonary histoplasmosis with primary adrenal insufficiency.

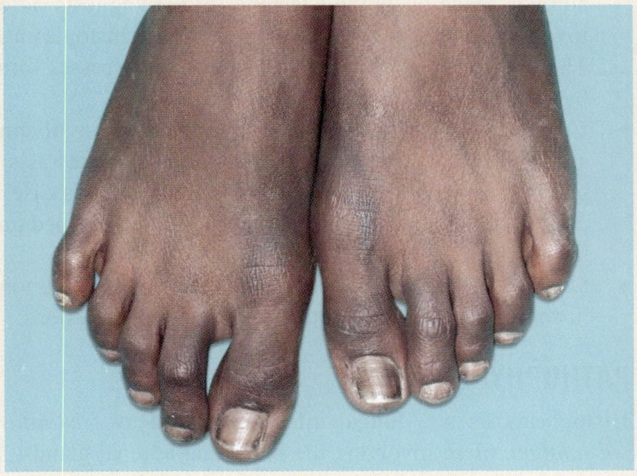

**FIG. 1:** Hyperpigmentation skin more over foot knuckle.

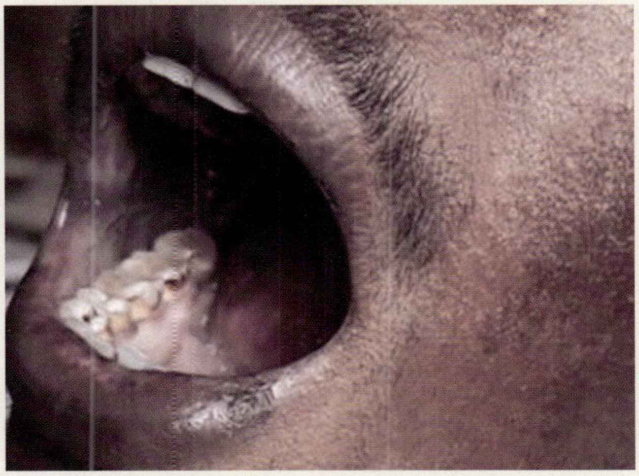

**FIG. 2:** Hyperpigmentation of oral mucosa.

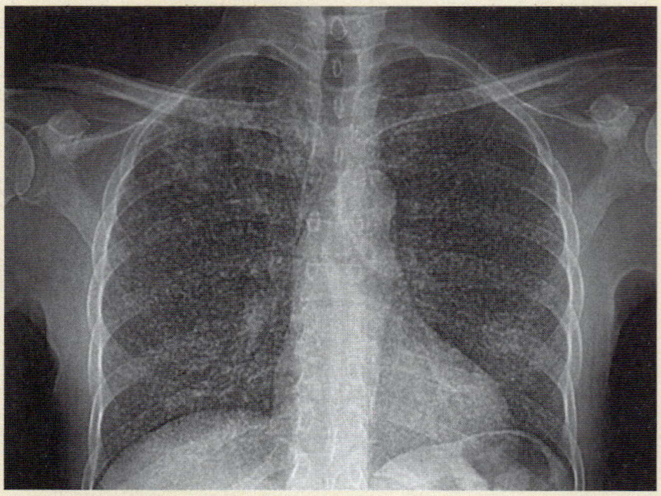

**FIG. 3:** Chest X-ray findings.

## PROVISIONAL DIAGNOSIS

Adrenal histoplasmosis with presumptive pulmonary histoplasmosis and primary adrenal insufficiency.

## DIFFERENTIAL DIAGNOSIS

- Miliary tuberculosis with adrenal involvement.
- Bronchoalveolar carcinoma with adrenal metastasis.
- Lung histoplasmosis with secondary adrenal involvement.

## CLINICAL APPROACH

### History and Symptoms

- *Risk factors*: Obtain a detailed history, including recent exposure to areas endemic for histoplasma capsulatum (e.g., soil or bird droppings in regions like the Mississippi or Ohio River Valleys), occupation (e.g., migrant laborers), and travel history.
- *Presenting symptoms*: The patient may present with fatigue, weight loss, low-grade fever, dry cough, and postural dizziness. In this case, the patient's symptoms of extreme exhaustion, irregular fever, dry cough, and dizziness are suggestive of systemic involvement, which may point to a fungal infection like histoplasmosis affecting multiple organs, including the lungs and adrenal glands.
- *Physical examination*: *Signs of adrenal insufficiency*: Look for clinical signs of adrenal insufficiency, including hypotension, tachycardia, and hyperpigmentation (in chronic cases). The patient's low blood pressure with a postural drop (sitting BP: 90/60 mm Hg, standing BP: 68/46 mm Hg) is suggestive of hypovolemia or adrenal insufficiency.
- *Pulmonary findings*: Perform a thorough lung examination for any signs of respiratory distress, abnormal breath sounds, or crackles that might suggest pulmonary involvement (e.g., pneumonia or pulmonary histoplasmosis).
- *General examination*: Mild pallor may be observed due to anemia, and signs of systemic infection or granulomatous disease may be present.
- *Laboratory investigations: Serum cortisol and ACTH*: The patient's morning serum cortisol is low (8 μg/dL), and ACTH is elevated (120 pg/mL), which confirms primary adrenal insufficiency.
- *Electrolytes*: Hyponatremia (Na 125 mmol/L) is often seen in adrenal insufficiency due to impaired aldosterone secretion, which can lead to water retention and sodium loss.
- *Complete blood count (CBC)*: Anemia of chronic disease may be present, which is common in systemic fungal infections.
- *Adrenal function tests*: The lab results support adrenal insufficiency, necessitating further investigation into the etiology, which in this case is histoplasmosis.
- *Imaging*: *Abdominal CECT*: The presence of bilateral adrenal space-occupying lesions (SOL) suggests adrenal involvement by an infectious process like histoplasmosis. These lesions could be granulomatous or abscesses formed by the infection.
- *Chest X-ray*: Look for signs of pulmonary involvement such as miliary tuberculosis, pulmonary metastasis, or granulomatous diseases like histoplasmosis. In this case, the chest X-ray findings and negative sputum tests helped guide the diagnosis of pulmonary histoplasmosis.
- *CT scan of the chest*: If needed, can help confirm pulmonary histoplasmosis or other potential causes of lung lesions.

## PATHOPHYSIOLOGY

Histoplasmosis is a fungal infection caused by *Histoplasma capsulatum*, often involving the lungs and adrenal glands. The adrenal involvement can lead to adrenal insufficiency, as seen with low cortisol levels. Histoplasmosis typically presents with nonspecific symptoms like fatigue, cough, and fever. In this case, bilateral adrenal lesions and low cortisol, combined with a negative ICTC test and adrenal biopsy, pointed to adrenal histoplasmosis. The infection leads to granulomatous inflammation and can impair adrenal function, resulting in primary adrenal insufficiency.

## TREATMENT AND PREVENTION

Treatment includes antifungal therapy with liposomal amphotericin B, followed by fluconazole for long-term management. Steroid replacement therapy is crucial for addressing adrenal insufficiency. Early detection and treatment of histoplasmosis can prevent severe complications. Preventive measures include avoiding exposure to fungal spores in endemic areas and using appropriate personal protective equipment for individuals at risk. Regular follow-up is necessary to monitor response to treatment and adrenal function recovery.

### Points to Ponder

- Miliary tuberculosis typically does not lead to pleural effusion.
- The coexistence of pleural effusion and miliary shadows should prompt consideration of alternative diagnoses, such as malignancy.
- While adenocarcinoma of the lung rarely presents with a miliary pattern due to intrapulmonary metastases, it can be overlooked in TB-endemic regions where empirical treatment for miliary TB is often initiated without a tissue biopsy.
- Miliary shadows on chest imaging may result from conditions such as miliary TB, fungal infections, sarcoidosis, occupational lung diseases, or hematogenous metastases from cancers like thyroid, renal, and sarcomas.

## MULTIPLE CHOICE QUESTIONS

1. **Which of the following is most likely responsible for the patient's primary adrenal insufficiency?**
   A. Tuberculosis
   B. Adrenal histoplasmosis
   C. Autoimmune adrenalitis
   D. Pheochromocytoma
2. **What finding on the patient's abdominal CECT is most consistent with adrenal histoplasmosis?**
   A. Bilateral adrenal hemorrhage
   B. Adrenal calcifications
   C. Bilateral adrenal space-occupying lesions
   D. Adrenal nodules
3. **The patient's hyponatremia (Na 125 mmol/L) is most likely a result of:**
   A. Excessive fluid intake
   B. Adrenal insufficiency leading to impaired aldosterone secretion
   C. Renal tubular acidosis
   D. Liver failure
4. **What is the first-line treatment for this patient's adrenal histoplasmosis with primary adrenal insufficiency?**
   A. Antifungal therapy with amphotericin B followed by fluconazole and glucocorticoid replacement therapy
   B. Antiviral therapy
   C. Surgical resection of adrenal lesions
   D. Antibiotic therapy with ceftriaxone
5. **Which of the following diagnostic tests helped rule out pheochromocytoma in this patient?**
   A. CT scan of the abdomen
   B. Urinary metanephrine and normetanephrine levels
   C. ACTH and cortisol levels
   D. Bronchoscopy with biopsy

### Answers

1. (B); 2. (C); 3. (B); 4. (A); 5. (B)

## SUGGESTED READINGS

1. Umeoka S, Koyama T, Miki Y, et al. Pictorial review of tuberous sclerosis in various organs. Radiographics. 2008;28(7):e32.
2. Khan D, Danjuma M, Saddique MU, et al. Yassin; Adenocarcinoma of the Lung Mimicking Miliary Tuberculosis. Case Rep Oncol. 2020;13(1):139-44.
3. Kauffman CA, Dismukes WE. Histoplasmosis: A review of the pathophysiology, clinical features, and management of systemic histoplasmosis with special reference to adrenal involvement. J Clin Microbiol. 2004;42(5):1894-1904.
4. Baddour LM, McCarthy MW. Adrenal histoplasmosis: Diagnosis and management. Infect Dis Clin North Am. 2017;31(3):511-27.
5. Shadduck FP, Hoag JB. Pulmonary and adrenal histoplasmosis: A comprehensive overview of clinical presentation, diagnosis, and therapeutic approaches. Mycoses. 2016;59(5):271-81.

# CHAPTER 76

# An Approach to a Case of COPD with Acute Exacerbation

*Satyendra Khichar, Rakesh Kumar*

**CASE VIGNETTE**

A 47-year-old chronic smoker male patient who is a known case of chronic obstructive pulmonary disease (COPD) since last 5 years presented in emergency with chief complaints of fever with sore throat and generalized body ache for 5 days, cough with mucoid sputum production for 5 days, shortness of breath for 2 days which was initially on exertion but now at rest also.

### Physical Examination

On examination respiratory rate was 32 breaths/min, blood pressure was 134/90, JVP was raised, pulse rate was 112 beats/min, regular in rhythm and normal in volume.

Onc auscultation—B/L diffuse wheezing and loud P2 was present. Patient was well oriented, GCS was E4V5M6 and flapping tremors were absent.

## PROVISIONAL DIAGNOSIS

Based on clinical presentation, physical examination and in hospital work up a provisional diagnosis of COPD acute exacerbation **(Fig. 1)** precipitated by acute viral infection was made.

## DIFFERENTIAL DIAGNOSIS

- COPD acute exacerbation.
- Community acquired pneumonia.
- Pulmonary thromboembolism
- CURB 65 – Score 2

After primary stabilization, patient was shifted toward for further management, where he was managed with: Noninvasive ventilation, oxygen therapy, nebulization with bronchodilators, glucocorticoids, empirical antibiotics and other supportive care.

He was discharged after 5 days of hospital stay with advice of smoking cessation, proper education regarding use of metered dose inhalers at home, sign and symptoms of acute exacerbation explained.

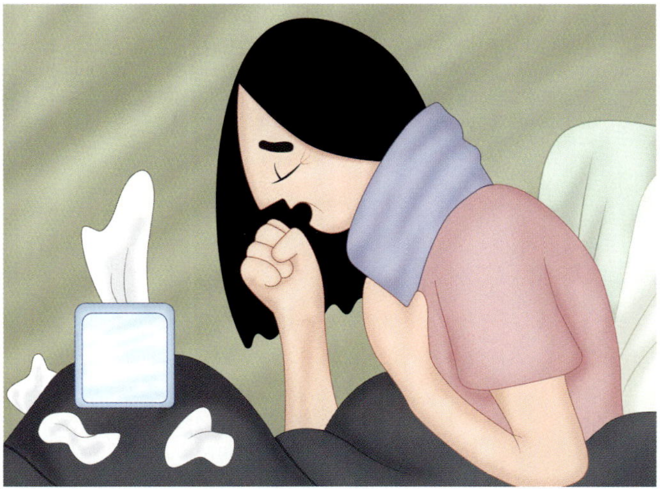

**FIG. 1:** A chronic obstructive pulmonary disorder (COPD) exacerbation.

## CLINICAL APPROACH

### Laboratory Investigations (Table 1)

ABG shows type 2 respiratory failure with $pCO_2$ 62, pH 7.28, $PaO_2$ 52, $SpO_2$ 86% on room air. CXR shows hyperinflated lung

**TABLE 1: Lab investigations of the 47-year-old chronic smoker male patient.**

| Parameter | Value | Parameter | Value |
|---|---|---|---|
| ABG | Respiratory acidosis | Serum creatinine | 1.4 mg/dL |
| ECG | Sinus tachycardia | Blood urea | 52 mg/dL |
| CBC | Hb/TLC/PLT 14/3.9k/1.2L | $Na^+/K^+$ | 134/5.1 (mEq/L) |
| ESR | 54 | RBS | 96 mg/dL |
| SGOT/SGPT | 76/60 | Serum procalcitonin | 0.05 ng/dL |
| Total bilirubin | 0.9 mg/dL | H1N1, COVID-19 | Negative |
| Blood cultures | Sterile | Sputum cultures | Sterile |

fields, right upper zone fibrotic bands and calcified nodules, right para hilar calcified lymph nodes.

*HRCT thorax* was s/o bilateral diffuse ground glass opacities suggestive of acute infective etiology. Changes of old tuberculosis in right upper zone and right parahilar calcified lymph nodes were present. CT pulmonary angiography was normal.

*2D echo*: No RWMA, normal LV systolic function, LVEF 55%. Mild MR, mild TR, RVSP (40 + RAP).

## PATHOPHYSIOLOGY OF COPD WITH ACUTE EXACERBATION

Acute exacerbations of COPD exhibit significant heterogeneity in their pathophysiology, with the inciting agents varying widely in nature and impact. A defining characteristic of COPD is expiratory flow limitation (EFL) resulting from airway inflammation. During exacerbations, airway resistance abruptly rises, triggered by mechanisms such as bronchospasm, mucosal oedema, and thickened sputum.

In individuals with flow limitation, the time available for lung emptying (expiratory time) is often insufficient, preventing the end-expiratory lung volume (EELV) from reaching its natural relaxation volume and leading to lung overinflation. The acute, variable increase in EELV above its baseline is known as dynamic hyperinflation (DH). This phenomenon occurs during exertion when inspiratory tidal volume rises and expiratory time is shortened, which imposes severe restrictive mechanical constraints on ventilation and is associated with respiratory discomfort.

Exacerbations often trigger a rapid, shallow breathing pattern that further restricts the time available for lung emptying, fostering DH in a vicious cycle. Evidence suggests that acute DH may be life-threatening during severe exacerbations in both asthma and COPD.

## ACUTE RESPIRATORY FAILURE IN COPD EXACERBATIONS

COPD exacerbations leading to acute respiratory failure are marked by worsening hypoxemia, often accompanied by elevated carbon dioxide retention and acidemia. Hypoxemia typically results from increased ventilation-perfusion (V/Q) mismatch, though modest increases in shunt fraction may also contribute.

Decompensated hypercapnia during exacerbations is a significant prognostic factor, associated with both short- and long-term mortality risks. Some patients may experience worsened $CO_2$ retention with high supplemental oxygen, likely due to increased V/Q mismatch (from loss of hypoxic vasoconstriction) or a reduced central drive to breathe (from loss of hypoxemic ventilatory drive). Increased hypercarbia risk is also influenced by elevated dead space, leading to alveolar hypoventilation despite increased respiratory drive. Advanced COPD often presents with increased physiological dead space due to underlying V/Q mismatch.

## TREATMENT AND PREVENTION

### Treatment and Management of COPD with Acute Exacerbation

An essential part of initial management is determining the need for hospitalization. Over 80% of COPD exacerbations are managed on an outpatient basis, occasionally after initial treatment in a clinic or emergency department.

### Criteria for Hospitalization

The CURB-65 score:

- Confusion (based upon a specific mental test or new disorientation to person, place, or time)
- Urea (blood urea nitrogen in the United States) >7 mmol/L (20 mg/dL)
- Respiratory rate ≥30 breaths/min
- Blood pressure (BP; systolic <90 mm Hg or diastolic ≤60 mm Hg)
- Age ≥65 years

*Note*: 1 point is assigned for each criterion.

- Score 1 or 2—hospitalization except a score of 1 due to being ≥65 years of age who do not have major comorbidities.
- Score 3 or more—assess for admission in ICU.

### Home or Office Management

- *Bronchodilator therapy:* All COPD exacerbation patients should receive inhaled short-acting bronchodilator therapy. Short-acting beta-agonists (SABA), like albuterol, are the primary treatment for rapid and effective bronchodilation. Muscarinic antagonists like ipratropium are also administered, typically combined with SABA.
- *Oral glucocorticoids:* Systemic glucocorticoids help relieve breathlessness, particularly for patients with elevated eosinophil counts. A common dose is prednisone 40 mg daily for 5–14 days, with caution regarding side effects like hyperglycemia, fluid retention, and hypertension.
- *Inhaled glucocorticoids:* High-dose budesonide has been studied as a systemic glucocorticoid alternative in non-ICU hospitalized patients. Further research is required to confirm its efficacy.
- *Antibiotics:* Empiric antibiotics are recommended for patients with increased sputum purulence, volume, or dyspnea, or those requiring ventilatory assistance, with choice depending on individual factors and resistance trends.
- *Antiviral agents:* Influenza screening is advised during flu season. Molecular assays are preferred over rapid antigen tests, with antiviral therapy beginning immediately if influenza is suspected.
- *Supportive care:* Smoking cessation support, medication adherence advice, nutritional support, and care goals review are important for home-managed patients. Those needing new supplemental oxygen typically begin in hospital care.

### In Hospital Management of COPD with Acute Exacerbation

For hospitalized patients, severity of the acute exacerbation is classified based on clinical signs:

- *No respiratory failure:* Breathing rate ≤24 breaths/min; heart rate (HR) <95 beats/min; no use of accessory respiratory muscles; normal sensorium; pulse oxygen saturation ($SpO_2$) 88–92% with venturi mask 24–35% inspired oxygen (or equivalent); no carbon dioxide retention.
- *Acute nonlife-threatening respiratory failure:* Breathing rate >24 breaths/min; use of accessory muscles of respiration;

normal sensorium; $SpO_2$ 88–92% with venturi mask 24–35% (or equivalent); arterial tension of carbon dioxide ($PaCO_2$) 50–60 mm Hg or increased above baseline.

- *Acute life-threatening respiratory failure*: Breathing rate >24 breaths/min; use of accessory muscles of respiration; acute change in mental status; requiring fraction of inspired oxygen (FiO2) ≥40% to maintain $SpO_2$ 88–92%; $PaCO_2$ increased compared with baseline or >60 mm Hg or associated with acidosis (pH ≤7.25).

## Hospital-based Bronchodilator Therapies

- Inhalation short-acting beta (adrenergic) agonist—(SABAs, e.g., salbutamol, levosalbutamol) due to their rapid onset of action and high efficacy for bronchodilation in COPD patients.
- Combination therapy—combination of a short-acting muscarinic antagonist (SAMA, e.g., ipratropium) and SABA for exacerbations that require emergency department or hospital-based treatment.
- Glucocorticoids—tablet Prednisolone 40 mg daily or equivalent, for 5–14 days. Oral glucocorticoids absorbed rapidly (peak serum levels achieved within one hour of ingestion) with almost complete bioavailability and appear similar in efficacy to intravenous glucocorticoids for treating COPD acute exacerbations.
- Magnesium sulfate—indicated in patients who present with a severe exacerbation that is not responding promptly to short-acting inhaled bronchodilators. It has bronchodilator action.
- Antiviral and antimicrobial agents—most clinical practice guidelines recommend antibiotics for patients having a moderate-to-severe COPD exacerbation that requires hospitalization.
- Antiviral therapy is recommended only for those patients who have clinical and laboratory evidence of influenza infection.
- Oxygen therapy—supplemental oxygen is one of the important components of COPD exacerbation. Oxygen supplementation should target an $SpO_2$ of 88–92% or an arterial oxygen tension ($PaO_2$) of approximately 60–70 mm Hg, to minimize the risk of worsening carbon dioxide retention.
- Noninvasive ventilation—patients with respiratory acidosis [as characterized frequently by $PaCO_2$ >45 mm Hg (6 kPa) and pH <7.35] are most likely to benefit from an initial trial of NIV. Bilevel positive airway pressure is typically used. Timely use of NIV may decrease intubation and mortality rate significantly and is the preferred method of ventilatory support in many COPD patients if no contraindications.
- Invasive ventilation—invasive mechanical ventilation should be administered when patients fail NIV, do not tolerate NIV, or have contraindications to NIV.

## Planning Discharge

Criteria for dischargeitt depends on sufficient improvement in patient's condition including general well-being and decreased need for frequent nebulization.

Before planning discharge, the patient's ability to manage his daily activities at home should be determined along with the need for assistive devices such as a walker, elevated toilet seat, bedside commode, or shower chair.

# PREVENTION

General measures—following measures can reduce the frequency of COPD exacerbation:

- Smoking cessation.
- Proper and regular use of medications (including inhaler technique).
- Vaccination to prevent against seasonal influenza.
- Pneumococcal vaccination.

### Points to Ponder

- Patients should be educated about his disease and proper use of inhalers at home.
- Emphasis should be given on smoking cessation.
- Patients should be educated on the consequences of living with COPD and in how to participate in their own care—detect, react and report changes in symptoms.
- Patients should receive a personalized management plan with regular, proactive reviews.
- Healthcare professionals, patients and the general public should be educated about the numerous risk factors associated with COPD in order to reduce the associated stigma of the condition.

# MULTIPLE CHOICE QUESTIONS

**1. A defining characteristic of COPD is:**

A. Inspiratory flow limitation
B. Expiratory flow limitation
C. Respiratory muscle weakness
D. Increased tidal volume

**2. Criteria for acute life-threatening respiratory failure includes all, except:**

A. Respiratory rate >24 breath/min
B. Use of accessory muscles of respiration
C. Blood pH ≤ 7.25
D. Normal mental status

**3. Hypoxemia during COPD with acute exacerbation occurs mainly due to:**

A. Decreased availability of oxygen
B. Poor inspiratory efforts by patient
C. Ventilation-perfusion (V/Q) mismatch
D. Increased utilization of oxygen by tissues

**4. The CURB-65 score includes all of the following, except:**

A. Confusion
B. Respiratory rate > 32 breath/min
C. Systolic blood pressure < 90 mm Hg
D. Age 65 years or more

**5. Which of the following statement regarding COPD acute exacerbation is not true?**

A. Patients with CURB-65 score more ≥3 should be assessed for ICU admission
B. Short-acting beta-agonists (SABA) are the primary treatment
C. Systemic steroids should be avoided
D. Antiviral therapy should only be considered when influenza is strongly suspected or confirmed with RT-PCR

## Answers

1. (B); 2. (D); 3. (C); 4. (E); 5. (C)

## SUGGESTED READINGS


1. Bhowmik A, Seemungal TAR, Sapsford RJ, et al. Relation of sputum inflammatory markers to symptoms and lung function changes in COPD exacerbations. Thorax. 2000;55:114–20.
2. Vitacca M, Clini E, Porta R, et al. Acute exacerbations in patients with COPD: predictors of need for mechanical ventilation. Eur Respir J. 1996;9:1487-93.
3. Calverley PMA. Respiratory failure in chronic obstructive pulmonary disease. Eur Respir J. 2003;22:26-30s.
4. Seneff MG, Wagner DP, Wagner RP, et al. Hospital and 1-year survival of patients admitted to intensive care units with acute exacerbations of chronic obstructive pulmonary disease. JAMA. 1995;274:1852-7.
5. Connors AFJ, Dawson NV, Thomas C, et al. Outcomes following acute exacerbation of severe chronic obstructive lung disease. The SUPPORT investigators. Am J Respir Crit Care Med. 1996;154:959-67.
6. Global Initiative for Chronic Obstructive Lung Disease (GOLD). Global Strategy for the Diagnosis, Management and Prevention of Chronic Obstructive Pulmonary Disease: 2024 Report. www.goldcopd.org www.goldcopd.org [Accessed on November 16, 2023].
7. Wedzicha JA Ers Co-Chair, Miravitlles M, Hurst JR, et al. Management of COPD exacerbations: a European Respiratory Society/American Thoracic Society guideline. Eur Respir J. 2017;49.
8. McCrory DC, Brown CD. Anti-cholinergic bronchodilators versus beta2-sympathomimetic agents for acute exacerbations of chronic obstructive pulmonary disease. Cochrane Database Syst Rev. 2002;CD003900.

# CHAPTER 77

# An Approach to a Case of Intubated Patient Developing New Lung Opacity

*Saikat Mondal, Nazneen Nahar Begam, Mahesh Ravikumar Jansari, Boudhayan Das Munshi*

**CASE VIGNETTE**

A 56-year-old, known hypertensive male is admitted to the intensive care unit (ICU) with sudden onset left sided hemiparesis since last 2 hours and very poor sensorium (Glasgow Coma Scale – 6). Urgent NCCT head revealed a large hemorrhagic CVA involving right MCA territory. He underwent emergency endotracheal intubation to protect the airway and was put on mechanical ventilation. On 6th day, the patient had developed a low-grade fever with white blood cell (WBC) count of 18,000/μL, and increased purulent tracheal secretions. His oxygenation has also deteriorated, requiring an increase in positive end-expiratory pressure (PEEP) and $FiO_2$ requirement. Upon evaluation, the chest X-ray reveals a new left middle and lower zone opacity as shown in the image **(Fig. 1)**. How do we approach further in this case?

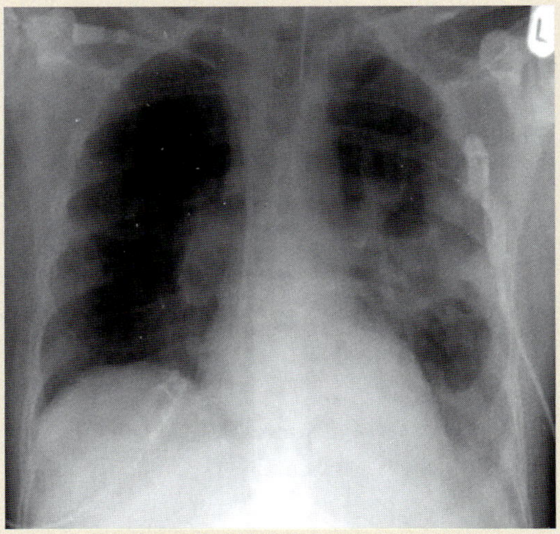


**FIG. 1:** Chest X-ray shows a newly developed opacity in the left middle and lower lung zones.

## PROVISIONAL DIAGNOSIS

The new lung opacity in this intubated patient **(Fig. 2)** is most likely due to ventilator-associated pneumonia (VAP). The clinical presentation, including fever, leukocytosis, worsening oxygenation, and purulent secretions, aligns with this most possible diagnosis.

## DIFFERENTIAL DIAGNOSIS

### Infectious Causes

- *Ventilator-associated pneumonia (VAP)*:
  - Most common cause in intubated patients.
  - Caused by multidrug-resistant pathogens like *Klebsiella* species, *Pseudomonas aeruginosa, Acinetobacter baumannii*, MRSA, etc.
- *Aspiration pneumonia/pneumonitis*:
  - Common in intubated patients due to impaired airway protection.
- *Septic emboli*:
  - Source from infective endocarditis or indwelling catheters (mostly centrallines).

### Noninfectious Causes

- *Atelectasis*: Collapse of alveoli; presents with linear opacities and volume loss.
- *Pulmonary edema*:
  - Cardiogenic: Bat wing appearance on CXR in pulmonary edema
  - Noncardiogenic (e.g., ARDS)

- *Pulmonary embolism (PE)*: Wedge-shaped infarcts or opacity.
- *Lung contusion*: Post-trauma or iatrogenic injury.
- Pulmonary hemorrhage

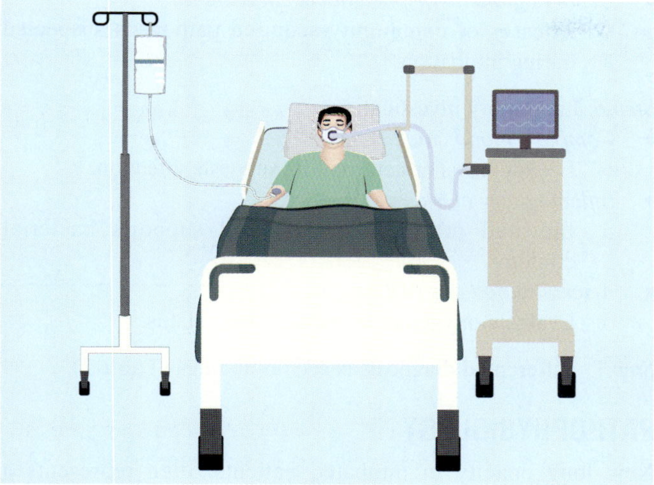

**FIG. 2:** Depicting an intubated patient.

- *Loculated intrathoracic collection*: Air, fluid, blood, chyle, fluid from iatrogenically misplaced catheters (effusion, pneumothorax, pneumomediastinum, subcutaneous emphysema)
- *Fluid overload*: Bilateral pleural effusion, batwing appearance shadow in fluid overload
- *Iatrogenic*:
  - Misplaced catheters: Chest tube, nasogastric tube, central lines, etc.
  - Trauma during intubation: Vocal cord, supraglottic structure
- *Foreign body*: Teeth, other medical parts of medical instrument's accidental migration inside chest
- Progression of ongoing pathological process
- Bony fracture post CPR, post fall from bed
- *Pseudo opacity*: From objects outside the chest wall

## RADIOLOGICAL APPROACH TO LUNG OPACITY IN CRITICAL CARE

Consider the following points before final interpretation of any ICU chest X-ray in **Table 1**.

**TABLE 1: Interpretation of ICU self provided points.**

| | | Interpretation | Comment |
|---|---|---|---|
| Outside chest wall | Opacities outside chest wall | Pseudo opacity | Repeat CXR |
| Soft tissue | • Subcutaneous emphysema<br>• Soft tissue lesion<br>• Postoperative changes (e.g., mastectomy) | Physical examination to reconfirm | |
| Rib cage and bony structure | • Rib fracture<br>• Dislocation of ribs (flail chest)<br>• Other bony structures—sternum, clavicle, scapula<br>• Post surgery complications: Sternotomy wires vertebroplasty kyphoplasty spinal fixation thoracotomy | Trauma | Post CPR |
| Pleura | • Costophrenic angle<br>• Cardiophrenic angle<br>• Fissures (major, minor) | Effusion, pneumothorax, Pus, blood, fluid from misplaced catheter | • USG<br>• Plan aspiration |
| Parenchyma | • Opacity (new, persistent and progression, any characteristic alignment with specific pathological condition)<br>• With air-bronchogram<br>• Interstitial markings or Kerley B lines<br>• Cavitation<br>• Loss of silhouette<br>• Volume loss | Pneumonia, atelectasis interstitial edema | |
| Mediastinum | Cardiomegaly | Cardiac history | 2D echo |
| Vascular marking | Perihilar opacity hilar prominence/cephalization of vessels/ prominent descending pulmonary arteries | Pulmonary edema, pulmonary embolism | Correlate clinically |
| Lines and tubes | Different vascular catheter, intrapleural catheters, any other type of device | Appropriate positioning | Secondary complications |
| Abdomen | • Diaphragm position, pneumoperitoneum/pathological calcifications/bowel gas pattern<br>• Distension of stomach due to esophageal intubation | Diaphragmatic eventration/palsy | Surgical consultation |
| | Serial comparative assessment | Check progression | Clinical correlation |

## CLINICAL APPROACH

### Stepwise Algorithm

*Step 1*: Identify clinical context

- *History and risk assessment*:
  - Duration of mechanical ventilation (>48 hours increases risk of VAP).
  - Presence of fever, leukocytosis, or hypoxemia.
  - Changes in sputum character (increased volume, purulence).
  - Assess recent changes in ventilatory settings (e.g., rising $FiO_2$ or PEEP).

*Step 2:* Perform targeted physical examination

- *Focus on*:
  - *Auscultation*: Localized crackles or diminished breath sounds.
  - Signs of hemodynamic instability, suggesting septic shock.
  - Evidence of extrapulmonary sources of infection.

*Step 3:* Review imaging

- *Initial chest X-ray (CXR)*:
  - Look for new or progressive opacities.
  - Patterns:
    - Consolidation (suggests VAP, aspiration, or pneumonia).
    - Linear atelectasis or volume loss (suggests atelectasis).
    - Wedge-shaped opacity (suggests pulmonary infarction).
    - Bilateral or perihilar distribution (suggests pulmonary edema).
- *Advanced imaging*:
  - If CXR is inconclusive, proceed with CT chest:
    - Detect subtle consolidations, cavitations (lung abscess), or pulmonary embolism.

*Step 4:* Assess ventilator parameters

- Rising plateau pressure or reduced compliance may indicate worsening lung pathology, such as ARDS or atelectasis.

*Step 5*: Microbiological investigations

- *Endotracheal aspirates*:
  - Obtain for culture and Gram staining to guide empirical antibiotics.
- *Bronchoalveolar lavage (BAL)*:
  - Preferred method for distal airway sampling, particularly in unresolved cases.
- *Blood cultures*:
  - Rule out bacteremia or systemic sepsis.
- *Urine Legionella or pneumococcal antigen*:
  - In cases of community-acquired pathogens suspected during intubation.

*Step 6*: Laboratory investigations

- *Complete blood count (CBC)*:
  - Leukocytosis or neutrophilia suggests infection.
- *Inflammatory markers*:
  - Elevated procalcitonin or CRP supports bacterial etiology.
- *Arterial blood gas (ABG)*:
  - Evaluate oxygenation and acid-base status.

*Step 7:* Differential diagnosis based on findings **(Table 2)**.

**TABLE 2: Differential diagnosis.**

| Condition | Key features |
|---|---|
| Ventilator-associated pneumonia (VAP) | Fever, purulent secretions, patchy/diffuse consolidation on imaging |
| Atelectasis | Linear opacities, volume loss, and improvement with recruitment maneuvers |
| Pulmonary edema | Bilateral hazy opacities, "batwing" pattern, rapid improvement with diuresis |
| Aspiration pneumonitis | Opacity in dependent zones, history of aspiration risk |
| Pulmonary embolism (PE) | Wedge-shaped opacity, risk factors like deep vein thrombosis (DVT) |

## PATHOPHYSIOLOGY

New lung opacity in intubated patients often represents a pathological response to inflammation, infection, or mechanical injury.

- *Ventilator-associated pneumonia (VAP):*
  - *Colonization of airway and biofilm formation:* Pathogens bypass host defences, colonizing the oropharynx and upper respiratory tract.
  - *Micro-aspiration*: Subglottic secretions enter the lower airway due to cuff leak or reflux.
  - *Impaired mucociliary clearance*: Prolonged intubation disables normal defences, allowing bacterial growth.
  - *Ventilation-induced lung injury*: High pressures and volumes exacerbate damage.
- *Atelectasis*:
  - Collapse of alveoli due to mucus plugging or impaired surfactant leads to hypoventilation and regional lung opacities.
- *Pulmonary edema:*
  - Fluid shifts due to capillary leak (noncardiogenic, ARDS) or volume overload (cardiogenic).
- *Aspiration pneumonitis:*
  - Chemical injury from acidic gastric contents causes alveolar inflammation and consolidation.
- *Pulmonary embolism:*
  - Vascular obstruction results in ischemic damage and hemorrhagic infarcts, manifesting as opacities on imaging.

## TREATMENT

- *Ventilator-associated pneumonia (VAP)*:
  - *Empiric antibiotics*: Initiate broad-spectrum coverage (e.g., piperacillin- tazobactam or carbapenems) while awaiting culture results. De-escalate based on sensitivities.
  - *Mechanical ventilation strategies:*
    - Minimize sedation and assess readiness for extubation daily.
    - Elevate the head of the bed to reduce aspiration risk.
  - *Pulmonary hygiene*: Regular suctioning and secretion management.

- *Atelectasis*:
  - *Lung recruitment maneuvers*: Adjust PEEP or use intermittent deep breaths.
  - *Chest physiotherapy*: Promote clearance of mucus.
- *Pulmonary edema:*
  - Treat the underlying cause (e.g., diuretics for fluid overload, low tidal volume ventilation for ARDS).
- *Pulmonary embolism:*
  - Initiate anticoagulation if PE is confirmed.
- *Aspiration pneumonitis:*
  - Supportive care, including oxygen therapy, and antibiotics if infection develops.

## PREVENTION

- *Ventilator bundle care*:
  - Elevate head of bed to 30–45°.
  - Minimize sedation, daily extubation trials.
  - Perform oral care with chlorhexidine.
- *Infection control measures:*
  - Hand hygiene and sterile techniques for suctioning.
  - Use subglottic secretion drainage endotracheal tubes.
- *Optimize noninfectious risk factors:*
  - Avoid fluid overload.
  - Provide adequate thromboprophylaxis.

### Points to Ponder

- ❑ Ventilator-associated pneumonia (VAP) is the most likely cause of new lung opacity in intubated patients after 48 hours, presenting with fever, leukocytosis, purulent secretions, and worsening oxygenation.
- ❑ Differential diagnoses include infectious causes (VAP, aspiration pneumonia, septic emboli) and noninfectious causes (atelectasis, pulmonary edema, pulmonary embolism, or lung contusion).
- ❑ A stepwise clinical approach involves evaluating symptoms, imaging, microbiology, starting targeted treatment, and continuously reassessing the patient's progress.
- ❑ Systematic chest X-ray interpretation follows an "outside-to-inside" approach, evaluating external artifacts, soft tissues, bones, pleura, lung parenchyma, mediastinum, and device placement.
- ❑ Key radiological patterns to differentiate conditions include consolidation for VAP, linear opacities for atelectasis, "batwing" opacities for pulmonary edema, and wedge-shaped opacities for pulmonary embolism.
- ❑ Advanced imaging, such as a CT chest, is essential when chest X-ray findings are inconclusive or when subtle pathologies need detailed evaluation.
- ❑ Key microbiological investigations include endotracheal aspirates, bronchoalveolar lavage (BAL), and blood cultures, supported by laboratory tests like CRP, procalcitonin, and ABG.
- ❑ Treatment for VAP includes empiric broad-spectrum antibiotics, de-escalated based on culture results, along with ventilatory adjustments and pulmonary hygiene.
- ❑ Preventive measures include ventilator care bundles such as head elevation, sedation minimization, daily extubation trials, and oral care with chlorhexidine.

## MULTIPLE CHOICE QUESTIONS

1. **Which diagnostic method provides the highest specificity for identifying the causative pathogen in VAP?**
   A. Blood cultures
   B. Tracheal aspirate culture
   C. Bronchoalveolar lavage (BAL)
   D. Sputum smear
2. **What is the first-line empiric antibiotic for suspected VAP?**
   A. Piperacillin-tazobactam
   B. Azithromycin
   C. Linezolid
   D. Doxycycline
3. **What is the recommended elevation angle of the head of the bed to reduce the risk of aspiration in ventilated patients?**
   A. 15°
   B. 30°
   C. 45°
   D. 60°
4. **Which of the following is least likely to cause new lung opacity in an intubated patient?**
   A. Aspiration pneumonitis
   B. Malignancy
   C. Ventilator-associated pneumonia
   D. Atelectasis
5. **Which preventive measure is NOT recommended to reduce VAP incidence?**
   A. Elevation of the head of the bed
   B. Routine changing of ventilator circuits
   C. Daily sedation breaks
   D. Subglottic secretion drainage

### Answers

1. (C); 2. (A); 3. (C); 4. (B); 5. (B)

## SUGGESTED READINGS


1. Kalil AC, Metersky ML, Klompas M et al. Management of Adults with Hospital- acquired and Ventilator-associated Pneumonia: 2016 Clinical Practice Guidelines by the Infectious Diseases Society of America and the American Thoracic Society. Clin Infect Dis. 2016;63(5):e61-111.
2. Torres A, Niederman MS, Chastre J et al. International ERS/ESICM/ ESCMID/ALAT Guidelines for Management of Hospital-acquired Pneumonia and Ventilator- associated Pneumonia: Guidelines for the management of hospital-acquired pneumonia (HAP)/ventilator-associated pneumonia (VAP) of the European Respiratory Society (ERS), European Society of Intensive Care Medicine (ESICM), European Society of Clinical Microbiology and Infectious Diseases (ESCMID) and Asociación Latinoamericana del Tórax (ALAT).Eur Respir J. 2017;50(3):1700582.
3. Kollef MH, Chastre J, et al. Prevention of Ventilator-Associated Pneumonia. Crit Care Med. 2021.
4. Papazian L, Klompas M, Luyt CE et al. Ventilator-Associated Pneumonia in Adults: Diagnosis, Treatment, and Prevention. Lancet. 2020.
5. Chastre J, Fagon JY. Ventilator-Associated Pneumonia. Am J Respir Crit Care Med. 2002;165(7):867-903.Muscedere J, Dodek P, Keena S et al. Comprehensive Evidence-Based Clinical Guidelines for Ventilator-Associated Pneumonia Prevention. J Crit Care. 2008;23(1):126-37.
6. Safdar N, Dezfulian C, Collard HR et al. Clinical and Economic Consequences of Ventilator-Associated Pneumonia : a systematic review. Crit Care Med. 2005;33(10):2184-93.
7. Klompas M, Kleinman K, et al. Culture-Negative Ventilator-Associated Pneumonia. Crit Care Med. 2016.
8. Melsen WG, Rovers MM, et al. Hospital-Acquired Pneumonia and Mortality: A Systematic Review and Meta-Analysis. Crit Care. 2013.

CHAPTER 78

# An Approach to a Case of Massive Hemoptysis

*Abhishek Singhai, Akash Pawar*

**CASE VIGNETTE**

A 55-year-old chronic smoker male presented to the emergency department with complaint of fever, productive cough associated with blood in sputum for one month, followed by three episodes of coughing up a large amount of blood mixed sputum for three days. Other symptoms included exertional dyspnea, weight loss, and decreased appetite. He had a history of pulmonary tuberculosis six years ago for which he did not receive proper treatment. Physical examination reveals that the patient is febrile with hemodynamic instability, including tachycardia, hypotension, low oxygen saturation, pallor, bilateral pedal edema, bilateral rhonchi, crackles predominantly in the right upper lobe on respiratory examination, and a loud P2 and systolic murmur at the tricuspid area on cardiovascular examination.

*Definition*: Hemoptysis is the blood expectorant from the respiratory tract. Massive or life-threatening hemoptysis is defined by volume and frequency of expectorated blood, i.e., >400 mL in 24 hours or >150 mL at one time or 100 mL/h and hemodynamic instability, which requires emergent intervention.

## PROVISIONAL DIAGNOSIS

A case of massive hemoptysis secondary to post-TB sequelae with cardiopulmonary failure and associated with hypovolemic/cardiogenic shock.

## DIFFERENTIAL DIAGNOSIS (FIG. 1)

- Post-tuberculosis lung diseases (PTLDs) spectrum with pulmonary hypertension
- Reactivation of tuberculosis
- Post-tuberculosis sequelae with secondary bacterial or fungal infection
- Bronchogenic carcinoma or lung neuroendocrine tumor
- *Immunological*: Vasculitis, SLE, Goodpasture syndrome
- Pulmonary arteriovenous malformations

## CLINICAL APPROACH

The evaluation of hemoptysis involves history, general physical and systemic examination followed by management which includes diagnostic investigations, supportive, lifesaving immediate measure sand treatment of underlying etiology. Once pseudohemoptysis (arise from epistaxis or hematemesis) is excluded, a targeted clinical history should include questions about the duration of symptoms, frequency of hemoptysis, associated dyspnea, quantity of blood coughed by the patient during 24 hours, history of past illnesses and risk factors like tuberculosis, smoking, etc., immunocompromised status, immobilization, and any recent injury to the airway, such as diagnostic procedures, chest injury, or foreign body. The following is the general approach algorithm to a scenario of hemoptysis presented in **Flowchart 1**.

Physical examination can be valuable for determining the source and severity of bleeding, but they can be normal in the many hemoptysis cases. Careful examination of the thorax can be really helpful in the event of trauma since symptoms of local damage are likely to provide information regarding the location of bleeding. Stridor, crackles, wheezing, or reduced breathing sounds may indicate the existence of a focal obstruction caused by a foreign body, bronchiectasis, or pneumonia. Cardiac auscultation can detect murmurs indicative of mitral stenosis or regurgitation. Skin examination for bruising may indicate coagulopathy, telangiectasia of inherited hemorrhagic telangiectasia, or purpura caused by cutaneous vasculitis **(Fig. 2)**.

## PATHOPHYSIOLOGY

Hemoptysis can occur anywhere along the respiratory tract, from the glottis to the alveolus. The bronchi or medium-sized airways are the most common sites of bleeding, although the entire respiratory system should be evaluated. The lungs contain both pulmonary and bronchial circulations. The pulmonary circulation is a low-pressure system that is required for gas exchange; in contrast, the bronchial circulation originates from the aorta and is thus a higher-pressure system. The bronchial arteries supply the airways and have the ability to neovascularize tumors, bronchitis-induced dilated airways, and cavitary lesions. The majority of hemoptysis is caused by bronchial circulation,

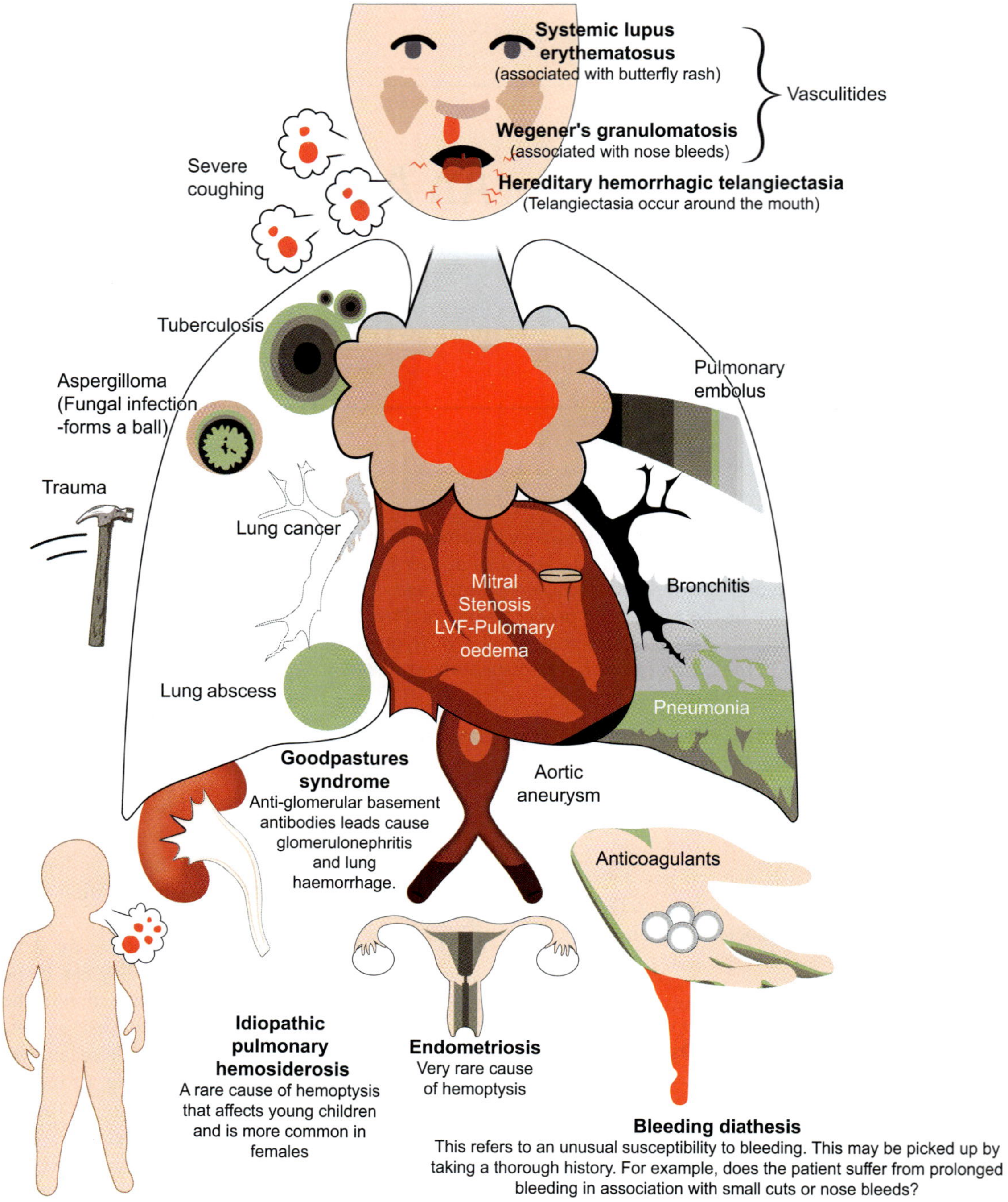


**FIG. 1:** The causes of hemoptysis.

which is more difficult to stop because of the higher pressure in the system.

## TREATMENT AND PREVENTION

Routine laboratory investigations like complete blood count, cross-matching, prothrombin time, liver function test, renal function test, ABG, chest X-ray, sputum gram stain, sputum culture (including *Mycobacterium tuberculosis*, fungi, and bacteria), and cytology should be ordered in patients with massive hemoptysis.

Initial treatment includes securing airway, crystalloid IV fluids, supplemental oxygen (target $SPO_2$ 88–96%). In special situation reversal of bleeding disorders required like fresh frozen plasma to reverse warfarin, platelet transfusion for thrombocytopenia or for platelet defects due to uremia or antiplatelet agents (e.g., aspirin, clopidogrel).

### Endoscopic Approach

Bronchoscopy apart for localization, also provide therapeutic advantage of controlling the bleeding source and prevent asphyxiation by removal of clots and minimizes spilling of blood into unaffected portions of the lung. Flexible bronchoscopy can be performed bedside to an unstable patient. Bronchoscopy being an diagnostic aid and can be combined with local therapies to

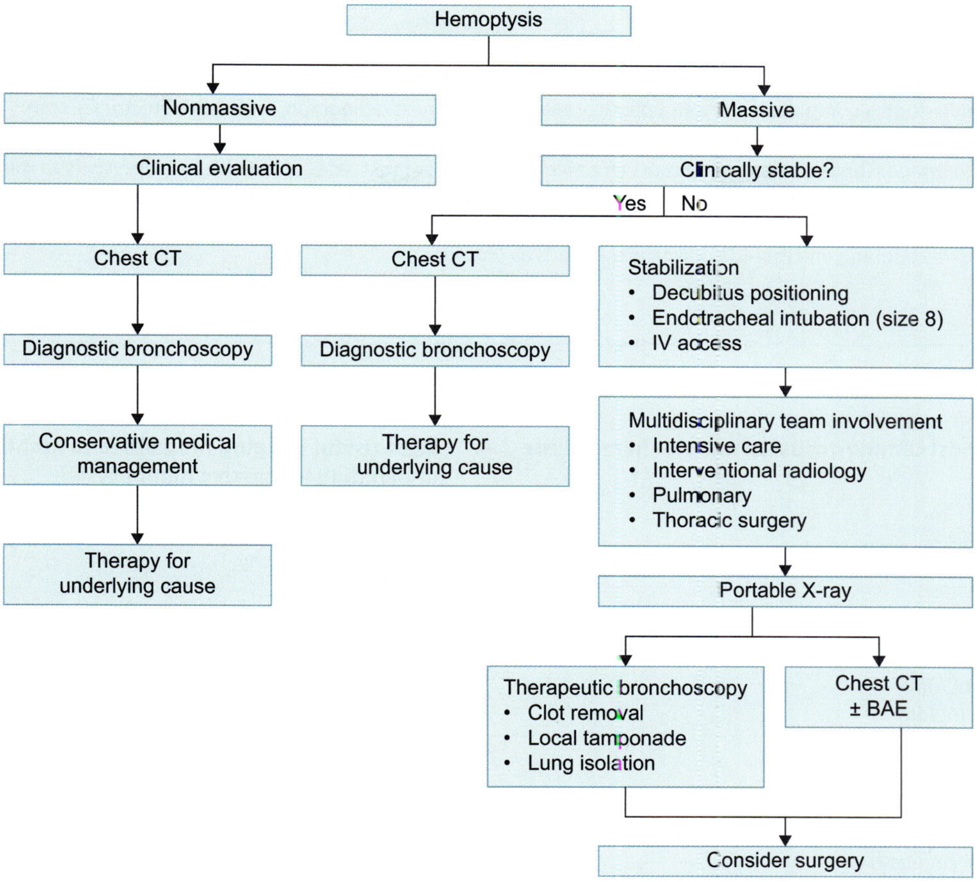


**FLOWCHART 1:** Approach algorithm for the management of the patient with hemoptysis.
(BAE: bronchial arterial embolization; CT: computed tomography; IV: intravenous)

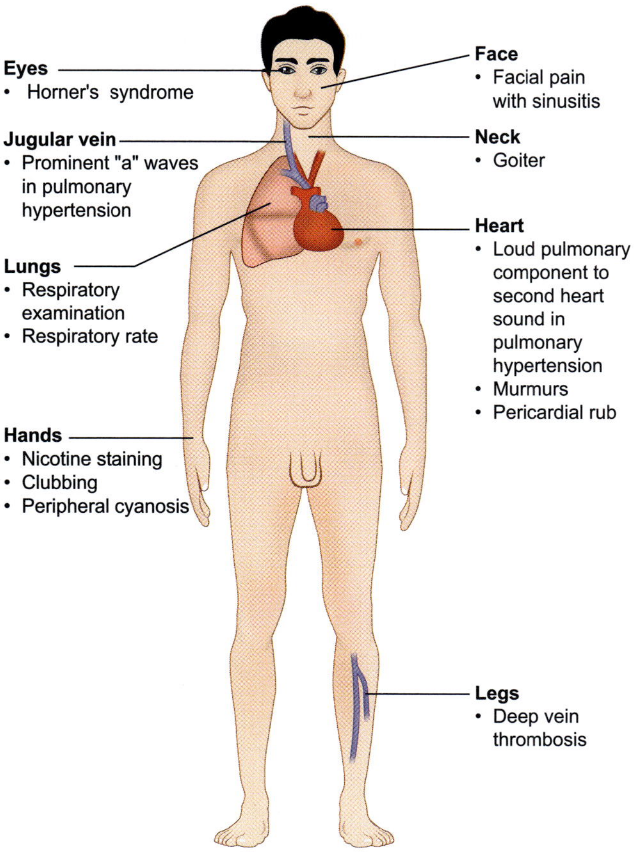


**FIG. 2:** Examining the patient with cough and hemoptysis.

temporize the bleeding (e.g., iced saline, local vasoconstrictors, bronchial blocker/balloon).

## Endovascular Approach

Bronchial artery embolization (BAE) can both localize bleeding vessels and embolize them. As bronchial arteries frequently involves in hemoptysis and the ability of BAE to perform minimally invasive bronchial arteriography in critically patients makes BAE an desirable approach.

## Surgical Approach

Surgical resection may be definitive in the prevention of bleeding recurrence; however, this is typically reserved for cases refractory to all nonsurgical approaches.

## Supportive Therapies

- *Antibiotics*: Antibiotic therapy for patients with acute bronchitis, pneumonia, or exacerbations of bronchiectasis.
- *Bronchodilators*: Inhaled bronchodilator therapy for patients with COPD or asthma
- *Vasopressors*: Vasopressors for hypotension that is refractory to volume resuscitation.
- *Experimental therapy*: Inhaled recombinant factor VIIa (off-label tranexamic acid is generally, only used if other initial therapies have failed).
- Transfusion of packed red cells

### Points to Ponder

- *Airway control*: Immediately secure the patient's airway and isolate the bleeding airway.
- *Early investigation*: Perform a complete history and physical examination, chest radiograph, and multidetector CT scan.
- *Bronchoscopy*: Perform a flexible or rigid bronchoscopy to locate and control bleeding.
- *Endovascular embolization*: This is the safest and most effective treatment for most cases of massive hemoptysis. It's a minimally invasive procedure that involves guiding a catheter to the pathological artery and using embolization agents to control bleeding.
- *Nursing interventions*: Place the patient on bedrest with their head slightly elevated and turned away from the bleeding side. Discourage excessive coughing and provide oral care and fluids as ordered.

## MULTIPLE CHOICE QUESTIONS

**1. What is the most common cause of massive hemoptysis in India?**
A. Lung cancer
B. Tuberculosis
C. Pulmonary embolism
D. Bronchiectasis

**2. Which of the following is considered the threshold volume for defining massive hemoptysis?**
A. 50–100 mL/day
B. 100–200 mL/day
C. 200–600 mL/day
D. >1,000 mL/day

**3. Massive hemoptysis arises most commonly from:**
A. Pulmonary circulation
B. Bronchial circulation
C. Pulmonary circulation more than bronchial circulation
D. None

**4. Most useful imaging modalities to identify the source of bleeding in massive hemoptysis?**
A. Chest X-ray
B. MRI
C. CT angiography
D. PET scan

**5. What is the primary treatment goal in managing a patient with massive hemoptysis?**
A. Treating the underlying disease
B. Replacing blood loss
C. Securing the airway and stop bleeding
D. Immediate lung resection

### Answers

1. (B); 2. (C); 3. (B); 4. (C); 5. (C)

## SUGGESTED READINGS

1. Grippi, MA. Fishman's Pulmonary Diseases and Disorders. McGraw-Hill Education / Medical. 2023.
2. Mason RJ, Slutsky A, Murray JF, et al. Murray & Nadel's Textbook of Respiratory Medicine E-Book. Elsevier Health Sciences. 2015.
3. Loscalzo J, Fauci AS, Kasper DL, et al. Harrison's Principles of Internal Medicine, 21st Edition (Vol. 1 & Vol. 2). McGraw Hill Professional. 2022.

CHAPTER 79

# An Approach to a Case of Management of CTD Related ILD

*Rajesh Kumar, Kanchan Kiran Kujur, Ruthra Kumaran*

**CASE VIGNETTE**

A 44-year-old female presented with a 2 years history of progressive skin binding over the upper limb, face and trunk, Raynaud's phenomenon, progressive shortness of breath, dry cough, pain and swelling in multiple small joints of hand with early morning stiffness of more than 30 minutes and swallowing difficulty since last year. On examination end inspiratory infrascapular crepts were audible.

## DIFFERENTIAL DIAGNOSIS

Interstitial lung disease (ILD) related to connective tissue disease (CTD). The CTD may be systemic sclerosis (SSc), rheumatoid arthritis (RA), mixed connective tissue disease (MCTD), idiopathic inflammatory myopathy (IIM), systemic lupus erythematosus (SLE).

While all CTDs carry a risk of ILD, it is more commonly seen in SSc, RA and IIM.

## CLINICAL APPROACH (FLOWCHART 1)

Approach incorporates the following steps:

1. History taking
2. Meticulous clinical examination.
3. *Relevant investigations*: Autoimmune antibodies, chest HRCT, PFT. Pulmonary function test (PFT). If required diffusing capacity of the lungs for carbon monoxide (DLCO), exercise desaturation test, 6-minute walk test, lung biopsy.
4. Apt treatment as per protocol with proper follow-up.

## PATHOPHYSIOLOGY

Cytokines and growth factors from B cells (TGF-β, IL-6, IL-13), T cells (antitopoisomerase,1, IL-4, -13, -17) JAK/STAT pathways, stimulate fibroblasts and endothelial damage particularly in the skin and lungs. Myofibroblasts formed, leads to excessive collagen and extracellular matrix deposition. Genetics (mutations in TERT, DKC1) and epigenetics has role to play.

Evaluation of patient with CTD:

- *Lab studies*: Routine blood investigation, erythrocyte sedimentation rate (ESR), C-reactive protein (CRP) and autoantibodies **(Tables 1 and 2)**.
- *Echocardiogram*: Screening for pulmonary arterial hypertension (PAH).
- *Pulmonary function tests (PFTs)*: Restrictive pattern [normal/high $FEV_1$/forced vital capacity (FVC)] with reduced FVC and DLCO serial PFTs. (FVC and DLCO) important for follow-up.
- *Chest HRCT* ***(Tables 3 and 4)***: Various patterns of ILD related to CTD as mentioned below. Out of these, NSIP and UIP are mainly found. Others include LIP, OP, DAD, overlap patterns. Extensive disease is present when > 20% lung involvement. Severity is determined by extent of ground-glass opacity (GGOs), reticulation, honeycombing, traction bronchiectasis. CALIPER and pulmonary vascular resistance score (PVRS) are newer modalities of quantitative assessment of fibrosis in chest HRCT.
- Screening tests recommended against include the 6-minute walk test distance and ambulatory desaturation test. Monitoring tests generally not recommended include chest radiography, the 6-minute walk test distance except in certain cases.

*Approach to treatment*: It includes:

1. First line therapy
2. ILD progression despite fiest line therapy.
3. Rapidly progressive ILD

1. *First line therapy*: The first-line therapy for connective tissue disease (CTD)-related interstitial lung disease (ILD) typically involves immunosuppressive agents such as mycophenolate mofetil or corticosteroids, depending on the severity and underlying CTD.
2. *ILD progression despite first line therapy*: If there is worsening of symptoms clinically or changes on serial PFTs (FVC decline of 5%)/chest HRCT on follow over 24 months, then add or switch immunosuppressants **(Tables 5 and 6)** CNI is recommended only for IIM, while tocilizumab is recommended for SSc and MCTD.

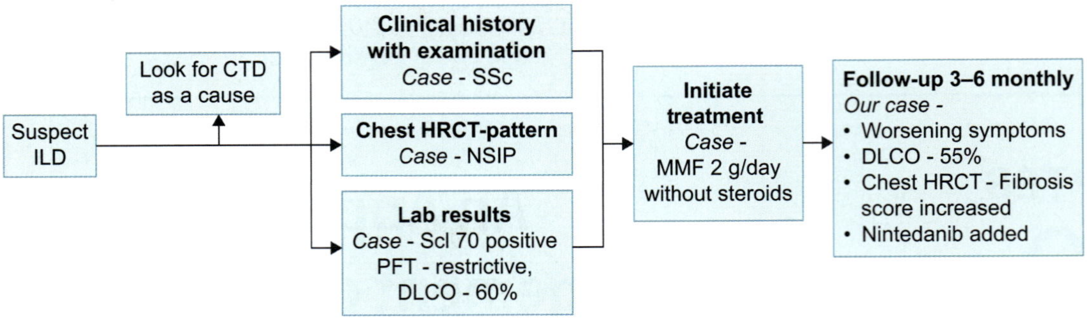


**FLOWCHART 1:** Algorithmic approach of CTD-ILD in consideration of the case.

**TABLE 1: Distinguishing features: RA, SSc and IIM.**

| | RA | SSc | IIM |
|---|---|---|---|
| Clinical features and examination | • Multiple joint pain and swelling primarily affecting the small joints of upper and lower limb with early morning stiffness of > 30 minutes<br>• O/E– tender and swollen joints are present with/without several deformities | • Binding of skin<br>• Raynaud's<br>• Microstomia<br>• Esophageal dysmotility<br>• Mauskopf facies<br>• Digital pitting<br>• Peripheral gangrene<br>• Abnormal nail fold capillaroscopy | Clinical features of proximal muscle weakness of both limbs:<br>• With cutaneous manifestations as in dermatomyositis (DM)<br>○ Heliotrope rash<br>○ Gottron's papules<br>○ Gottron's sign<br>○ Shawl sign<br>○ V-sign<br>• Amyopathic DM<br>• Without cutaneous manifestations PM<br>• Anti-synthetase syndrome ILD, myositis, Raynaud's, fevers, mechanic's hands, and arthritis. Anti-Jo-1 |
| Antibodies | RA factor, Anti-CCP | Anti-Scl-70 | • Myositis specific antibodies<br>• Particularly MDA5, antiJo-1,<br>• Myositis associated antibodies- Anti-Ro, Ku, PM/Scl |
| HRCT chest | Usual interstitial pneumonia (UIP) > nonspecific interstitial pneumonia (NSIP) = organizing pneumonia (OP) > lymphoid interstitial pneumonia (LIP) | NSIP (80%) > UIP (20%) | NSIP/ NSIP with OP > UIP |
| Prevalence of ILD | 19–67% | Up to 90% | Up to 75% |

**TABLE 2: Distinguishing features: MCTD, Sjögren's syndrome and SLE.**

| | MCTD | Sjögren's syndrome | SLE |
|---|---|---|---|
| Clinical features | Overlap of SLE, SSc, and IIM features with high titres of anti-U1 ribonucleoprotein (RNP) | • Glandular features:<br>○ Dry mouth, dry eye xtra glandular features: Distal renal tubular acidosis (RTA), polyneuropathies | Inflammatory arthritis with typical cutaneous features with other systemic symptoms as per ACR-EULAR 2019 criteria |
| Antibodies | Anti-U1RNP | Anti-Ro52, anti-Ro60 anti-La | • Antinuclear antibody (ANA)—IFA homogeneous pattern<br>• Anti-dsDNA, anti-smith and other |
| Chest HRCT | NSIP > OP = UIP | NSIP > UIP > LIP, OP | NSIP > UIP = LIP = OP |

TABLE 3: Common chest HRCT patterns: It's determination helps in identification of CTD.

| UIP | NSIP (most common pattern of ILD) |
|---|---|
| • Subpleural involvement<br>• Honeycombing (clustering of cysts in single or multiple layers)<br>• Traction bronchiectasis<br>• Lower lobe and basal predominant | • Subpleural sparing<br>• Diffuse<br>• Ground glass opacities (GGOs)<br>• Cysts may be present<br>• Good prognosis compared to UIP pattern |
| 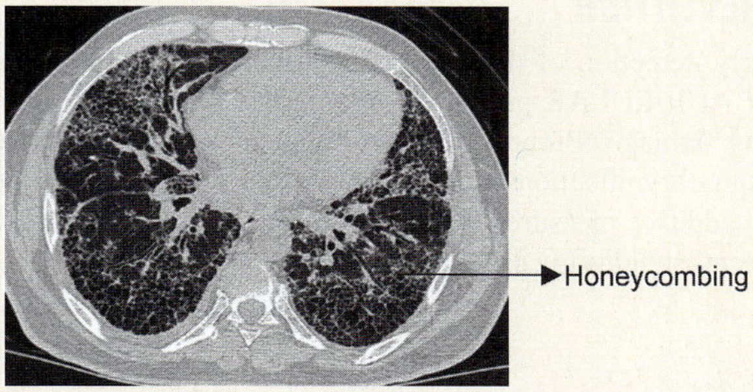  | 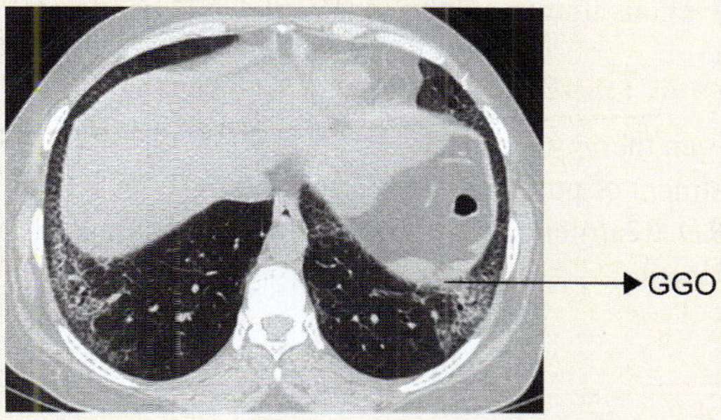  |

TABLE 4: Following specific CT radiographic findings suggest ILD secondary to CTD.

| Anterior upper lobe sign (RA) | Exuberant honeycombing (SSc) | Straight edge sign | Four corners sign (SSc) and island like fibrosis | Esophageal dilatation (SSc) |
|---|---|---|---|---|
| Fibrosis in the anterior upper lobes with sparing of the rest of the upper lobe | Extensive honeycombing covering >70% | Lesions isolated to the lung bases without lateral lung involvement | Lesions in bilateral anterolateral upper and posterosuperior lower lobes | |
| 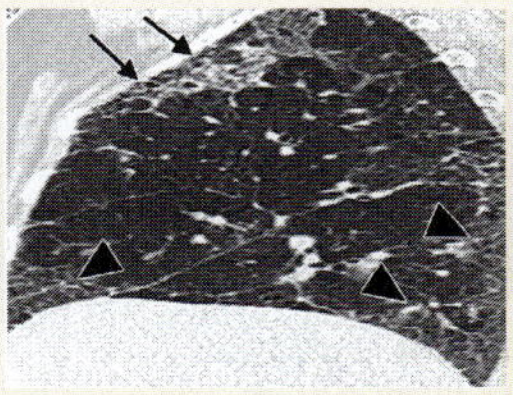 | 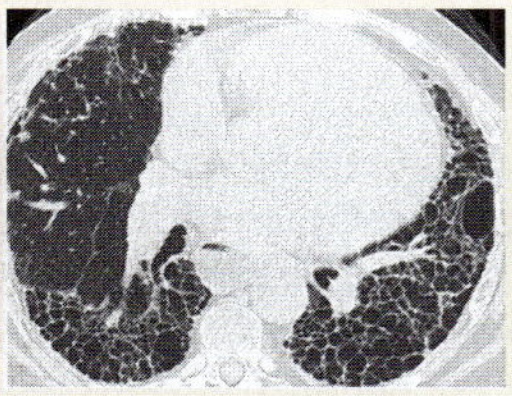 | 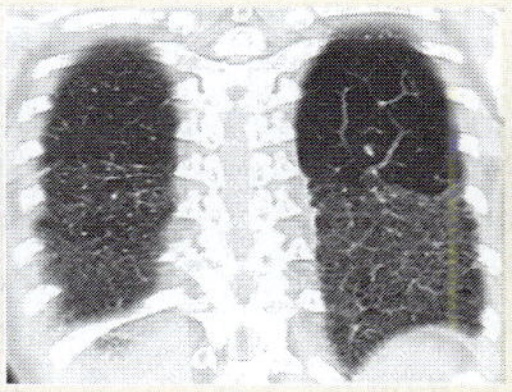 | 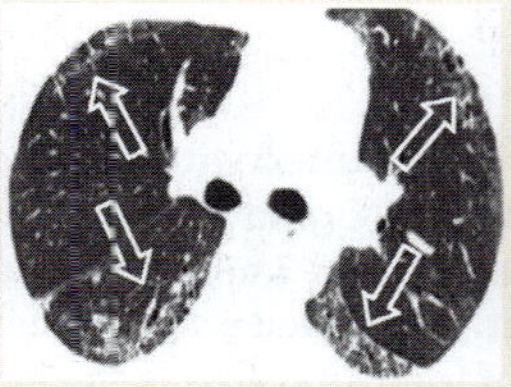 | 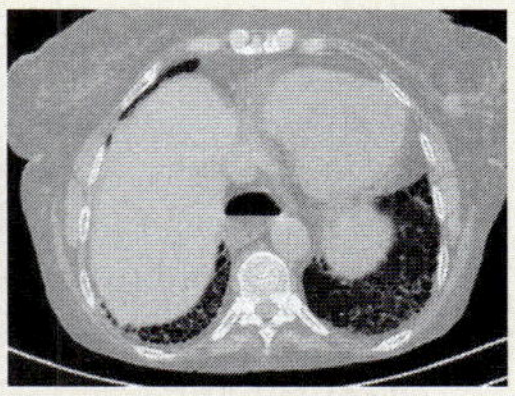 |

TABLE 5: ACR 2023 guidelines of CTD-ILD treatment.

| | SSC–ILD | IIM | MCTD | RA | SJS |
|---|---|---|---|---|---|
| First line therapy preferred (conditional recommendation) | • Mycophenolate<br>• Tocilizumab<br>• [FaSScinate study FocuSSced trial], rituximab<br>• DESIRES multicenter RCT | • Mycophenolate,<br>• Azathioprine, rituximab<br>• CNI<br>• Short-term glucocorticoids (GCs) | • Mycophenolate<br>• Azathioprineand Rituximab<br>• Short term GCs | • Mycophenolate,<br>• Azathioprine Rituximab<br>+<br>• Short term GCs | • Mycophenolate,<br>• Azathioprine and Rituximab<br>+<br>• Short term GCs |
| First line therapy additional options | • Cyclophosphamide nintedanib<br>• Azathioprine | • Janus kinase inhibitors (JAKi)<br>• Cyclophosphamide | • Tocilizumab<br>• Cyclophosphamide | Cyclophosphamide | Cyclophosphamide |

TABLE 6: Recommendations of steroids and antifibrotic therapy in CTD-ILD.

| | Conditionally recommended | Conditionally not recommended |
|---|---|---|
| Steroids (Long-term) | Other CTDs | SSc |
| Nintedanib | SSc | Other CTDs |
| Pirfenidone | RA | Other CTDs |

3. *Rapidly progressive ILD (RP-ILD)*: RP-ILD is a severe form of ILD characterized by rapid deterioration of respiratory function often over 3 months (FVC decrease by > 10% or FVC decrease by 9% with DLCO decrease by 15%. It is commonly seen in melanoma differentiation-associated protein 5 (MDA5) associated antibody IIM and SSc treatment includes parenteral GCs + two additional therapies [Mycophenolate, Rituximab, Cyclophosphamide, intravenous immunoglobulin (IVIg), CNI, JAKI]

## Adjunctive Therapies for ILD

- Oxygen therapy
- Treatment of pulmonary hypertension in ILD
- GERD treatment: High doses of proton pump inhibitors, prokinetic
- Pulmonary rehabilitation
- *Vaccines*: Influenza and pneumococcal vaccines. Additionally, herpes zoster vaccine.
- Supportive/palliative care
- *Lung transplant*: Conditional recommendation is given for early referral for stem cell and/or lung transplantation in progressive lung disease

# PREVENTION

Early detection of the CTD and initiation of apt treatment as per ACR/EULAR protocol is the cornerstone of prevention of lung damage. Stoppage of smoking, prevention of recurrent respiratory infections by vaccines along environmental exposure are additive measures. Regular follow every 3–6 monthly with specialist helps to curb the disease progression.

## Points to Ponder

- In ILD, CTD as a cause should always be ascertained as it has better prognosis than idiopathic form.
- Recognition of definite chest HRCT patterns suggests CTD type.
- Mycophenolate is indicated as first line therapy in all CTDs. Shifting or additional therapy is required if there is worsening.
- There is no role of long-term steroids. Short time steroids are indicated in CTDs except SSc-ILD.
- Regular follow-up is essential. Rapidly progression occurs in ILD related to amyopathic IIM particularly related to MDA5.

# MULTIPLE CHOICE QUESTIONS

**1. A 30-year-old female presented with rapidly progressive shortness of breath (mMRC grade 2 to 4) and dry cough that developed over the past 3 months. O/E: Velcro crepitations present. She tested positive for anti-MDA5 antibodies. Which of following CTD is she likely to have?**

A. IIM
B. RA
C. SS
D. SLE

**2. A 52-year-old male presented with chronic symmetrical inflammatory polyarthritis primarily affecting the small joints of the hands, sparing the DIP joints, for the past 4 years, along with progressive shortness of breath and dry cough for the past 2 years. O/E: Fine end inspiratory crackles were noted. Serology revealed RF and ACPA positivity with high titres. Which of the following ILD pattern is most likely?**

A. NSIP
B. UIP
C. NSIP with OP
D. LIP

**3. A 47-year-old female presented to the OPD with skin tightening over her entire body, Raynaud's phenomenon, and dysphagia for 3 years, along with progressive shortness of breath (mMRC grade 2) and dry cough for 1 year. O/E: Velcro-like crackles were heard PFT revealed a restrictive pattern, and Anti-Scl-70 antibodies. Was positive. Chest HRCT thorax showed a cellular NSIP pattern. What should be the preferred first-line treatment?**

A. Mycophenolate mofetil (MMF)+ Pirfenidone
B. MMF + Nintedanib
C. MMF
D. MMF + tocilizumab

**4. The HRCT thorax radiographic findings of CTD-ILD include all of the following except?**

A. Exuberant honeycombing
B. Straight edge sign
C. Four corner sign
D. Tree in bud

**5. The chest HRCT findings of a patient revealed diffuse GGO, reticular opacities, subpleural sparing, and traction bronchiectasis. Which of the following CTDs is least likely?**

A. MCTD
B. SLE
C. Systemic sclerosis
D. Sjögren's syndrome

## Answers

1. (A); 2. (B); 3. (C); 4. (D); 5. (B)

## SUGGESTED READINGS


1. Tashkin DP, Roth MD, Clements PJ, et al. Mycophenolate mofetil versus oral cyclophosphamide in scleroderma-related interstitial lung disease (SLS II): a randomised controlled, double-blind, parallel group trial. Lancet Respir Med. 2016;4(9):708-19.
2. Khanna D, Denton CP, Jahreis A, et al. Safety and efficacy of subcutaneous tocilizumab in adults with systemic sclerosis (faSScinate): a phase 2, randomised, controlled trial. The Lancet. 2016;387(10038):2630-40.
3. Ebata S, Yoshizaki A, Oba K, et al. Safety and efficacy of rituximab in systemic sclerosis (DESIRES): a double-blind, investigator-initiated, randomised, placebo-controlled trial. Lancet Rheumatol. 2021;3(7):e489-97.
4. Maher TM, Tudor VA, Saunders P, et al. Rituximab versus intravenous cyclophosphamide in patients with connective tissue disease-associated interstitial lung disease in the UK (RECITAL): a double-blind, double-dummy, randomised, controlled, phase 2b trial. Lancet Respir Med. 2023;11(1):45-54.
5. Johnson SR, Bernstein EJ, Bolster MB, et al. 2023 American College of Rheumatology (ACR)/American College of Chest Physicians (CHEST) Guideline for the Treatment of Interstitial Lung Disease in People with Systemic Autoimmune Rheumatic Diseases. Arthritis Rheumatol. 2024;76(8):1182-200.
6. Wells AU, Flaherty KR, Brown KK, et al. Nintedanib in patients with progressive fibrosing interstitial lung diseases—subgroup analyses by interstitial lung disease diagnosis in the INBUILD trial: a randomised, double-blind, placebo-controlled, parallel-group trial. Lancet Respir Med. 2020;8(5):453-60.

CHAPTER 80

# An Approach to a Case of Uveitis and HLA-B27 Positivity

*Sreemanta Madhab Baruah, Nongmaithem Bikash Singh*

**CASE VIGNETTE**

A 25-year-old male presented with an acute onset of pain, foreign body sensation, redness, and photophobia in his left eye, accompanied by blurred vision for 3 days. He also gave similar episodes occurring in either eye monthly for the past 4 months. The patient has no known ocular history and denies any recent infections or systemic illnesses. For the past 5 years, he also reported a significant medical history of episodic low back pain and stiffness, especially during morning time, that improves with physical activity and as the day progresses. No significant family history. Considering recurrent episodes of uveitis and inflammatory back pain, rheumatologic workup was carried out.

## PROVISIONAL DIAGNOSIS

Acute anterior uveitis (most likely recurrent) with a strong suspicion of HLA-B27-associated uveitis, given the association with inflammatory back pain.

## DIFFERENTIAL DIAGNOSIS

- Infectious uveitis could be viral, bacterial, or fungal, but less likely due to the recurrent nature and absence of systemic infection signs.
- Traumatic uveitis no history of trauma or injury to the eye.
- Autoimmune uveitis conditions like Behçet's disease or sarcoidosis, though less likely due to lack of other systemic signs.
- Herpetic uveitis could be considered if there were any history of herpes simplex or varicella-zoster infections, but no specific signs were noted.
- Systemic diseases such as juvenile idiopathic arthritis, but the patient's age and lack of systemic symptoms make this less likely.

## CLINICAL APPROACH

- *Detailed ocular examination*: To confirm the presence of anterior uveitis, check for cells and flare in the anterior chamber, and assess for any keratic precipitates or hypopyon.
- *Systemic evaluation*: Given the history of episodic low back pain and stiffness, further assessment for ankylosing spondylitis (AS) should be done, especially with HLA-B27 testing.
- *Laboratory tests*: HLA-B27 antigen test, ESR, CRP, and CBC to assess for inflammation. If necessary, imaging studies (e.g., X-ray or MRI of the sacroiliac joints) may help in diagnosing ankylosing spondylitis.
- *Referral to rheumatology*: For further management of suspected inflammatory back pain and potential autoimmune conditions like ankylosing spondylitis or other spondyloarthropathies.
- *Treatment plan*: Initial management may include corticosteroid eye drops for the uveitis, and if HLA-B27-associated uveitis is confirmed, consider systemic anti-inflammatory therapy for the underlying rheumatologic condition.

## PATHOPHYSIOLOGY (FIG. 1)

- *Immune system dysfunction*: Due to an autoimmune response which leads to immune dysregulation resulting in an abnormal immune response where the body's immune system mistakenly targets the uvea (the middle layer of the eye, including the iris, ciliary body, and choroid).
- *Inflammatory response*: This leads to activation of immune cells, such as lymphocytes and macrophages, and the release of proinflammatory cytokines (e.g., TNF-α, IL-1, IL-6) which further leads to inflammation of the uveal tissues.
- *Infiltration and cellular damage*: Inflammation results in the infiltration of immune cells, damaging the uveal tissues and disrupting the normal function of the eye. This release enzymes and reactive oxygen species, which can further damage ocular structures.
- *Increased vascular permeability*: Inflammation increases the permeability of the blood-retinal barrier, leading to leakage of proteins and fluid into the uveal tissues causing edema and inflammatory exudates. This can further proceed to complications such as retinal damage, cataracts, glaucoma, or even vision loss.

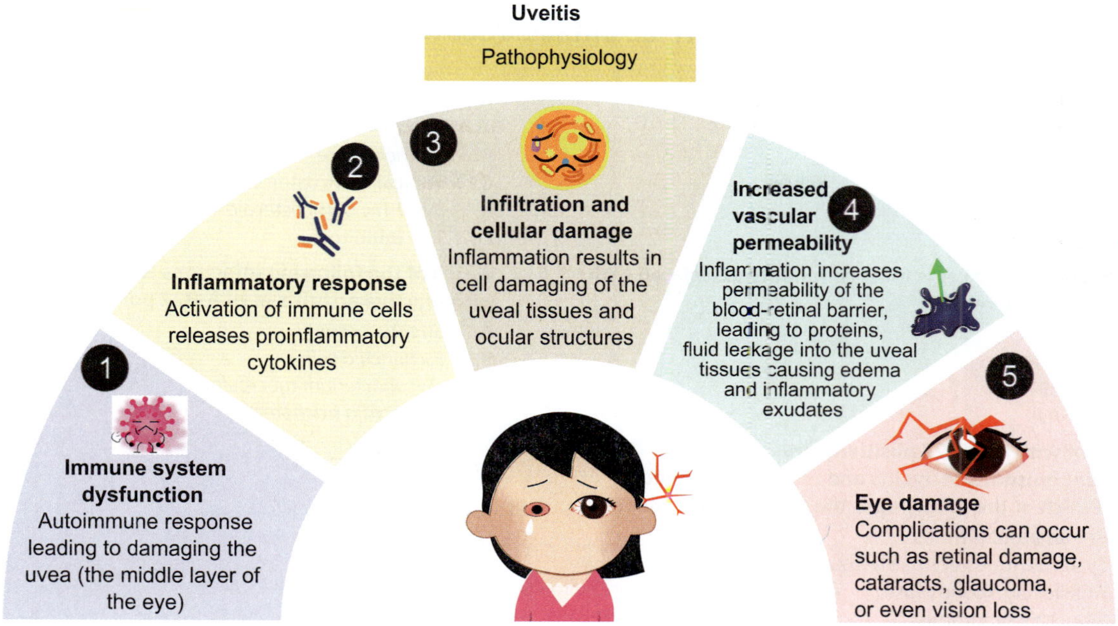


**FIG. 1:** Pathophysiology of uveitis.

## TREATMENT

For acute uveitis:

- *Topical corticosteroids (e.g., prednisolone acetate 1%)*: To reduce inflammation in the anterior chamber.
- *Mydriatic agents (e.g., tropicamide or homatropine)*: To dilate the pupil, prevent synechiae formation, and relieve pain.
- *Systemic nonsteroidal anti-inflammatory drugs (NSAIDs)*: For pain management and to reduce inflammation.

If HLA-B27-associated uveitis is confirmed:

- *Systemic NSAIDs (e.g., ibuprofen or indomethacin)*: For pain relief and management of underlying inflammation.
- *Disease-modifying antirheumatic drugs (DMARDs)*: Such as sulfasalazine or biologics (TNF inhibitors like etanercept or adalimumab) if ankylosing spondylitis is diagnosed and systemic treatment is needed.
- *Steroid-sparing agents*: For long-term control and to minimize steroid use.

Follow-up and monitoring:

- Frequent follow-up to monitor intraocular pressure (to avoid steroid-induced glaucoma) and check for resolution of inflammation.

## PREVENTION

- *Regular monitoring*: Routine eye exams for patients with recurrent uveitis to detect flare-ups early.
- *Manage underlying systemic condition*: Effective management of ankylosing spondylitis or other HLA-B27-associated diseases through appropriate rheumatologic treatment to prevent future uveitis episodes.
- *Patient education*: Advise the patient on recognizing early symptoms of uveitis (pain, redness, photophobia) to seek timely medical attention.
- *Vaccination and infection control*: If there is a risk of infectious uveitis, ensure vaccination against preventable infections (e.g., herpes simplex virus) and good hygiene practices.

### Points to Ponder

- *Recurrent uveitis*: HLA-B27 positivity is strongly associated with recurrent anterior uveitis, often seen in patients with spondyloarthropathies like ankylosing spondylitis.
- *Systemic inflammatory link*: Uveitis in HLA-B27-positive individuals may indicate underlying systemic inflammatory conditions, such as ankylosing spondylitis or psoriatic arthritis.
- *Acute onset*: Uveitis in HLA-B27-positive patients often presents with sudden eye pain, redness, and photophobia, sometimes with blurred vision.
- *Management*: Treatment typically involves corticosteroid eye drops, NSAIDs, and managing the underlying spondyloarthropathy with DMARDs or biologics.
- *Regular monitoring*: Patients with HLA-B27-associated uveitis require close follow-up to monitor for flare-ups and to manage associated systemic conditions.

## MULTIPLE CHOICE QUESTIONS

**1. Which of the following is the most common extra-articular manifestation of spondyloarthritis?**
A. Posterior uveitis
B. Anterior uveitis
C. Psoriasis
D. Enthesitis

**2. Which genetic marker is most commonly associated with acute anterior uveitis?**
A. HLA-B15
B. HLA-DR4
C. HLA-B27
D. HLA-A29

**3. A patient with HLA-B27 positivity presents with recurrent episodes of uveitis and inflammatory back pain. Which of the following is the most likely diagnosis?**
A. Rheumatoid arthritis
B. Systemic lupus erythematosus
C. Ankylosing spondylitis
D. Sjögren's syndrome

**4. What is the first-line treatment for acute anterior uveitis in a patient with HLA-B27 associated spondyloarthritis?**
A. Methotrexate
B. Topical corticosteroids
C. Systemic corticosteroids
D. TNF inhibitors

**5. Which of the following infections is commonly associated with reactive arthritis in HLA-B27 positive patients?**
A. *Streptococcus*
B. *Escherichia coli*
C. *Mycobacterium tuberculosis*
D. *Chlamydia trachomatis*

### Answers

1. (B); 2. (C); 3. (C); 4. (B); 5. (D)

## SUGGESTED READINGS

1. Taurog JD, Gensler LS, Haroon N. Spondyloarthritis. In: Loscalzo J, Fauci A, Kasper D, Hauser S, Longo D, Jameson J. eds. Harrison's Principles of Internal Medicine, 21e. McGraw-Hill Education; 2022. Accessed January 09, 2025. https://accessmedicine.mhmedical.com/content.aspx?bookid=3095&sectionid=264534154
2. Li Z, Khan MK, van der Linden SM, et al. HLA-B27, axial spondyloarthritis and survival. Ann Rheum Dis. 2023;82(12):1558-67.
3. Wakefield D, Clarke D, McCluskey P. Recent developments in HLA B27 anterior uveitis. Frontiers in Immunology. 2021;11.
4. Gopalaswamy R, Dusthackeer VNA, Kannayan S, et al. Extra-pulmonary Tuberculosis—An update on the diagnosis, treatment and drug resistance. Journal of Respiration. 2021;1(2):141-64.
5. Sharma B, Borde P, Priyanka N, et al. Pattern of uveitis in a tertiary eye care center of central India: Results of a prospective patient database over a period of two years. Indian J Ophthalmol. 2020 Mar;68(3):476-81.
6. Jayaprakash T, Muthamilan OL, Leela KV, et al. Association of Genetic Marker HLA-B27 with Spondyloarthritis In A Tertiary Care Centre In South India. Journal of Pure and Applied Microbiology. 2022;16(2):901-8.
7. Vinutha BV, Shetu R, Sundeep, et al. Clinical profile of anterior uveitis in Tertiary Eye Care Center. Journal of Medical Sciences and Health. 2023;9(2):224-8.
8. Rao N. Uveitis in developing countries. Indian Journal of Ophthalmology. 2013;61(6):253.
9. Tay-Kearney ML, Schwam BL, Lowder C, et al. Clinical features and associated systemic diseases of HLA-B27 uveitis. American Journal of Ophthalmology. 1996;121(1):47-56.
10. Agrawal R, Testi I, Bodaghi B, et al. Collaborative Ocular Tuberculosis Study Consensus Guidelines on the Management of Tubercular Uveitis—Report 2. Ophthalmology. 2020;128(2):277-87.

CHAPTER

81

# An Approach to a Case of Dactylitis in Clinical Practice

*Kripasindhu Gantait*

## CASE VIGNETTE

A 40-year-old man presented with painful swelling of his right index and ring fingers, along with right fourth toe for the past 5 days. Severe pain hampered his daily activities. His medical history was unremarkable except that his paternal uncle had psoriatic arthritis (PsA). Physical examination revealed tender, fusiform, swollen soft tissues in the affected fingertips, the fourth toe, and swollen palms. Nails were normal in appearance. Hand radiography revealed mild edema of the soft tissue of the index and ring fingers, but no joint abnormalities. Dactylitis was diagnosed clinically. Then we examined hidden areas and a psoriatic patch was detected on his scalp. Enthesitis was not present. Relevant laboratory tests were unremarkable. PsA was diagnosed based on CASPAR criteria. We put him on methotrexate (MTX) 15 mg once a week, folic acid tablets 5 mg twice a week, and indomethacin 75 mg daily for 10 days then 25 mg daily. At the 2-month follow-ups, the patient had substantial relief from pain and swelling and was able to continue his daily activities.

## CLOSING POINTS

- Dactylitis, a diffuse swelling of a finger or toe, is considered a hallmark clinical feature of PsA
- Dactylitis occurs in 16–49% of patients with PsA, often early in the disease as the inaugural symptom. Recurrent dactylitis, frequently in the same digit, may be the only manifestation of PsA for months to years
- Different treatment modalities have been laid down by various guidelines for the treatment of psoriasis underlying dactylitis ranging from nonsteroidal anti-inflammatory drugs (NSAIDs) to disease modifying antirheumatic drugs (DMARDs). Some physicians recommend injecting corticosteroids in the tenosynovial sheath, joints or soft tissues where dactylitis does not respond to NSAIDs. The Group for Research and Assessment of Psoriasis and Psoriatic Arthritis (GRAPPA) recommends DMARDs including methotrexate, while the European League Against Rheumatism (EULAR) PsA guidelines recommend starting biologic therapy immediately. Biologic medicines have so far been the preferred treatment for PsA and dactylitis. They treat psoriasis as well as synovitis, enthesitis, and noninfectious inflammatory osteitis, which are all common in PsA.
- Because dactylitis is a good indicator of PsA severity, its response to therapy may predict PsA prognosis.

## PROVISIONAL DIAGNOSIS

Psoriatic arthritis presenting with dactylitis.

## DIFFERENTIAL DIAGNOSIS

- Rheumatoid arthritis (RA)
- Gout
- Reactive arthritis
- Septic arthritis
- Sarcoidosis

## CLINICAL APPROACH

Refer to **Table 1**.

## PATHOPHYSIOLOGY

Psoriatic arthritis is an immune-mediated inflammatory disease characterized by aberrant activation of the innate and adaptive immune systems. Genetic predisposition (e.g., HLA-Cw6 and family history) and environmental triggers lead to activation of dendritic cells and T-cells, resulting in cytokine release (e.g., IL-17, IL-23, TNF-α). This drives inflammation, synovitis, enthesitis, and dactylitis, as seen in this patient. Dactylitis **(Fig. 1)**, or "sausage digits," results from inflammation of the tendon sheath, entheses, and soft tissues.

**TABLE 1: Clinical approach of dactylitis.**

| History | Clinical assessment | Investigation |
|---|---|---|
| • Pain → Acute dactylitis<br>• Painless → Chronic dactylitis<br>• LBP and uveitis → SpA<br>• Arthritis → Oligo (ReA) and Poly (PsA)<br>• Skin rash with balanitis → ReA and Skin rash with nail and scalp involment → PsA<br>• Podagra → Gout<br>• Pulmonary involvement → Sarcoidosis<br>• Fever and weight loss → TB<br>• Trauma → TB and blistering distal dactylitis | • Dactylitis is swelling of the whole digit and tenderness being assessed by a simple squeeze at the level of proximal phalanx [C = Tenderness score: 0 = no tenderness, 1 = tenderness]<br>• The dactylitis score is calculated by formula<br>$= [A/B - 1] \times 100 \times C$<br>where,<br>A = the circumference of the affected digit<br>B = the circumference of the digit on the opposite hand or foot<br>• A minimum difference of 10% is used to define a dactylitic digit<br>• If ipsilateral and contralateral digits are thought to be involved, a table of normative values is used to provide the comparison<br>• The Leeds dactylitis index measures the severity and activity of dactylitis. It incorporates a measurement instrument called Leed's dactylometer<br>• The Dactylitis Severity Score for each digit of 0–3 (no dactylitis, mild, moderate and severe) and sums of the score for each digit for a final score ranging from 0–60 | • Diagnosis of dactylitis is usually clinical. Investigations need to find out the underlying etiology<br>• Elevated CRP → Inflammatory<br>• Hb—electrophoresis → to rule out SCD<br>• Hyperuricemia → Gout and PsA<br>• Hypercalcemia → Sarcoids<br>• Hilar lymphadenopathy or pulmonary lesion in chest X-ray → Sarcoids and TB<br>• VDRL → Syphilis Imaging can detect the particular anatomical structures involved, can help to find out the etiology, and can also help to monitor the treatment efficacy. Amongst the imaging MSK-USG and MRI are the most helpful |

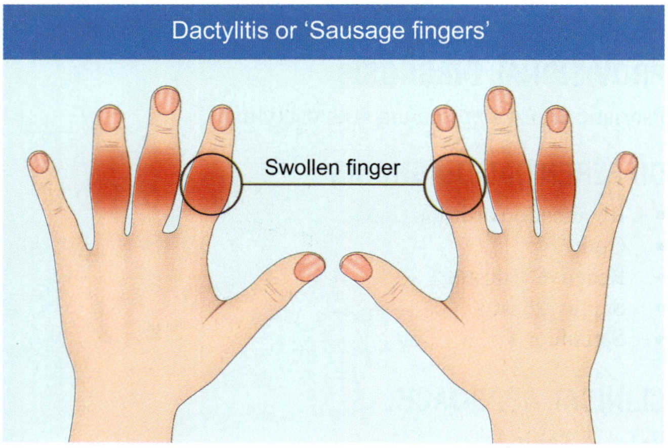


**FIG. 1:** Dactylitis.

## TREATMENT AND PREVENTION

Management of dactylitis usually comprises symptomatic relief as well as the management of underlying etiology:

- For pain control—use NSAID
- For SpA related dactylitis—USG-guided local steroid injection therapy and use cs-DMARDS followed by biological DMARD if needed (Ustekinumab for PsA dactylitis).
- For gouty dactylitis—short course of steroid along with urate lowering therapy
- Sarcoid dactylitis—Steroid + MTX
- TB dactylitis—ATD
- Syphilitic and sickle cell dactylitis—treat underlying cause

### Points to Ponder

- Dactylitis is the uniform diffuse swelling of the digits.
- Acute dactylitis is always painfull but chronic is usually painless.
- PsA is the most common cause of dactylitis among SpA group of diseases, whereas TB is the most common among the infective groups.
- History and clinical examination are helpful for detection of underlying etiology of dactylitis.
- MSK-USG can be helpful in assessment of dactylitis.

## MULTIPLE CHOICE QUESTIONS

1. **What is the most likely diagnosis in a 40-year-old man with painful swelling of his fingers and toe, dactylitis, and a psoriatic patch on the scalp?**
   A. Rheumatoid arthritis
   B. Psoriatic arthritis
   C. Gout
   D. Reactive arthritis
2. **Which diagnostic criteria were used to confirm psoriatic arthritis in the patient?**
   A. ACR/EULAR criteria
   B. CASPAR criteria
   C. Modified Duke criteria
   D. New York criteria
3. **What is the most common site for dactylitis in psoriatic arthritis?**
   A. Fingers and toes
   B. Wrist
   C. Knees
   D. Elbows
4. **What is the first-line disease-modifying therapy (DMARD) used in this patient?**
   A. Methotrexate (MTX)
   B. Leflunomide
   C. Sulfasalazine
   D. Hydroxychloroquine
5. **Which of the following findings is NOT typically associated with Psoriatic Arthritis?**
   A. Dactylitis
   B. Enthesitis
   C. Fusiform swelling
   D. Symmetrical joint involvement in all cases

### Answers

1. (B); 2. (B); 3. (A); 4. (A); 5. (D)

## SUGGESTED READINGS


1. Kaeley GS, Eder L, Aydin SZ, et al. Dactylitis: a hallmark of psoriatic arthritis. Semin Arthritis Rheum. 2018;48:263-73.
2. Rothschild BM, Pingitore C, Eaton M. Dactylitis: implications for clinical practice. Semin Arthritis Rheum. 1998;28:41-7.
3. Fendler C, Baraliakos X, Braun J. Glucocorticoid treatment in spondyloarthritis. Clin Exp Rheumatol. 2011;29:S139-42.
4. Gossec L, Baraliakos X, Kerschbaumer A, et al. EULAR recommendations for the management of psoriatic arthritis with pharmacological therapies: 2019 update. Ann Rheum Dis. 2020;79:700-12.
5. Balakrishnan C, Madnani N. Diagnosis and management of psoriatic arthritis. Indian J Dermatol Venereol Leprol. 2013;79:S18-24.
6. Subasi M, Bukte Y, Kapukaya A, Gurkan F. Tuberculosis of the metacarpals and phalanges of the hand. Ann Plast Surg. 2004;53(5):469-72.
7. Karanas YL, Yim KK. *Mycobacterium tuberculosis* infection of the hand: a case report and review of the literature. Ann Plast Surg. 1998;40:65-7.
8. Ali N, Bhat A, Fatima A, et al. Tuberculous dactylitis: a case series and review of literature. J Pioneer Med Sci. 2014;4(4):184-90.
9. Kotwal PP, Khan SA. Tuberculosis of the hand: clinical presentation and functional outcome in 32 patients. J Bone Joint Surg Br. 2009;91(8):1054-7.

CHAPTER
82

# An Approach to a Case of Nonhealing Ulcers

*Arghya Chattopadhyay*

## CASE VIGNETTE

A 40-year-old lady, presented with a history of inflammatory polyarthritis affecting large and small joints symmetrically for the past 10 years and developing progressive joint deformity for the past 2 years. She also gave a history of a large nonhealing ulcer over lateral aspect of her left leg for the past 2 months. There was no preceding history of trauma, and she did not have any significant systemic symptoms like fever or weight loss. She was advised to take painkillers for her joint disease initially, but later she shifted to ayurvedic treatment for her joint disease. Examination revealed, multiple tender and swollen joints, swan neck deformity affecting her middle finger and index finger on the right side and ring finger on the left side and ulnar deviation of fingers in both hands. There was a large ulcer over her left leg with a violaceous border, a well-defined undermined edge with a necrotic slough at the base and surrounding granulation tissue **(Fig. 1)**. All peripheral pulses were equally palpable and systemic examination findings were unremarkable. The possibility of inflammatory arthritis like rheumatoid arthritis was considered as a primary disease and skin ulcer was suspected as pyoderma gangrenosum. Routine blood investigations were unremarkable except for elevated inflammatory markers (ESR, CRP). Immunological workup showed positive rheumatoid factor (RF) and anti-CCP antibody in high titer. Biopsy was done from the ulcer edge which showed features suggestive of pyoderma gangrenosum **(Fig. 2)**. She was started on a high dose of steroid, weekly methotrexate and anti-TNF (infliximab).

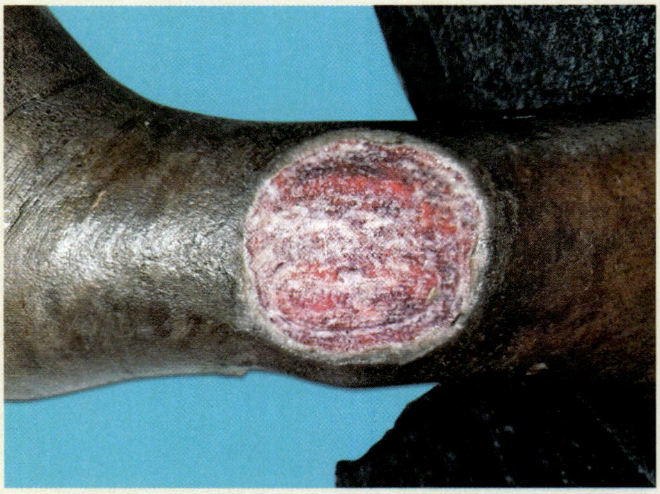

**FIG. 1:** Large nonhealing ulcer over the left leg with a violaceous border, and surrounding granulation tissue.

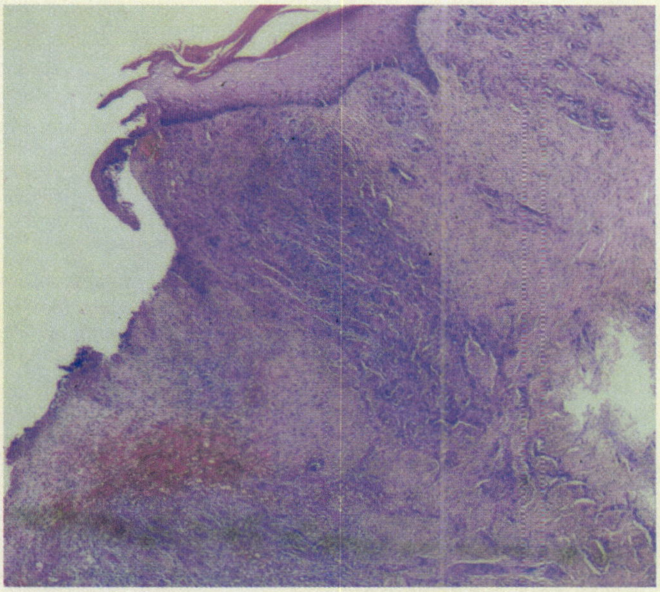

**FIG. 2:** Ulcerated epidermis with intradermal neutrophilic inflammation and dense perivascular inflammatory infiltrate of polymorphs and lymphocytes [H & E(4×)].
*Courtesy:* Dr Rakesh Gupta and Dr Ankita, Department of Pathology, AIIMS Raipur.

## PROVISIONAL DIAGNOSIS

Rheumatoid arthritis with pyoderma gangrenosum.

## DIFFERENTIAL DIAGNOSIS

- Systemic lupus erythematosus (SLE) with cutaneous manifestations.
- Vasculitis-associated ulcer (e.g., polyarteritis nodosa).
- Seronegative spondyloarthritis (e.g., psoriatic arthritis).
- Chronic venous stasis ulcer or arterial insufficiency ulcer.

## PATHOPHYSIOLOGY

The nonhealing ulcer in this case, likely pyoderma gangrenosum, results from dysregulated immune responses associated with rheumatoid arthritis. Overactivation of neutrophils and proinflammatory cytokines (e.g., TNF-α, IL-1, IL-6) leads to tissue inflammation, necrosis, and poor wound healing. The violaceous border and undermined edge are hallmark features caused by immune-mediated vascular damage and impaired reparative processes, compounded by chronic systemic inflammation.

### Causes of Nonhealing Ulcer

Nonhealing ulcers persist despite adequate treatment and often result from impaired blood supply, such as poor venous drainage in venous insufficiency or reduced arterial flow in peripheral arterial disease (PAD). Systemic diseases, including vasculopathy and neuropathy, can cause nonhealing ulcers. These ulcers may also result from bacterial and fungal infections, skin cancer, rheumatological conditions, or recurrent trauma. Multiple causes of nonhealing ulcers are listed in **Table 1**.

## CLINICAL APPROACH

The clinical approach to a nonhealing ulcer includes a thorough history, clinical examination, and focused investigations.

**TABLE 1: Causes of nonhealing ulcers.**

| Pathological condition | Diseases |
|---|---|
| Venous insufficiency | • Varicose vein<br>• Obesity<br>• Past DVT |
| Arterial insufficiency | *Peripheral arterial disease*:<br>• Atherosclerotic<br>• Smoking |
| Systemic diseases | • Diabetes mellitus<br>• Sickle cell disease |
| Cancer | *Skin cancer*:<br>• Primary<br>• Metastatic |
| Neurological disorder | *Neuropathy*:<br>• Diabetes mellitus<br>• Alcoholism<br>• Leprosy<br>• B12 deficiency<br>• Syringomyelia |
| Infection | *Bacterial*:<br>• Tuberculosis<br>• Nontubercular mycobacterial (NTM) infection<br>• Leprosy<br>• Melioidosis<br>• Nocardia<br>*Fungal*:<br>• Sporotrichosis<br>• Actinomycosis<br>• Chromoblastomycosis |

*Continued*

*Continued*

| Pathological condition | Diseases |
|---|---|
| Rheumatological diseases | • Systemic vasculitis (polyarteritis nodosa, ANCA vasculitis, Behçet's diseases, etc.)<br>• SLE<br>• Rheumatoid arthritis<br>• Antiphospholipid syndrome |
| Others | • Pyoderma gangrenosum<br>• Marjolin's ulcer<br>• Recurrent trauma |

The history should cover the ulcer's duration, onset, previous treatments, and any triggering events. Factors hindering proper healing, such as repeated trauma, uncontrolled diabetes, obesity, PAD, and poor wound care, should be considered. In diabetic patients, glycemic control should be assessed, and inquiries about smoking, atherosclerotic cardiovascular disease, or dyslipidemia should be made to rule out PAD. A history of varicosities or deep vein thrombosis (DVT) may indicate venous ulcers, while neuropathic symptoms suggest neuropathic ulcers. Multisystemic symptoms, like joint pain or photosensitivity, may point to underlying rheumatological causes. Bacterial or fungal infections may also be involved, so systemic infection symptoms should be sought.

A detailed local examination is essential, focusing on the ulcer's size, shape, location, and presence of granulation tissue or necrotic material. Specific ulcer types have characteristic features, such as venous ulcers being painful, shallow, and irregular, often located around the medial malleolus. Vasculitic ulcers are sharp and punched-out, while pyoderma gangrenosum presents as large, painful ulcers with violaceous borders. A systemic examination, including testing for venous incompetence, peripheral pulses, ankle-brachial pressure index, and neurological assessment, is critical to rule out venous or arterial insufficiency and neuropathic causes.

Investigations are guided by history and physical examination findings and may include routine blood tests, inflammatory markers (ESR, CRP), and blood glucose levels. Specialized tests like autoimmune serology, cancer markers, or Hb-electrophoresis may be needed based on symptoms. Imaging techniques such as Doppler ultrasound, CT, MRI, or PET-CT can be useful. Microbiological tests are recommended for suspected infective ulcers. Histopathological examination of tissue from the ulcer edge is essential for diagnosing vasculitic ulcers or undiagnosed cases. Key historical points, physical findings, and investigations for different ulcers are summarized in **Table 2**.

## TREATMENT AND PREVENTION

Treatment of nonhealing ulcers is usually a two-pronged strategy, one directed toward treating the ulcer and another directed toward treating the underlying cause. Treatment of the ulcer includes various strategies like debridement of the ulcer, institution of the appropriate antibiotic therapy in case of secondary infection, etc. Techniques like negative pressure therapy, more commonly known as vacuum-assisted wound closure, and growth factor

**TABLE 2: Historical points, clinical findings and required investigation in different types of nonhealing ulcers.**

| Underlying disease/ condition responsible | History and clinical findings | Investigations needed |
|---|---|---|
| Venous ulcer | History of varicose vein, DVT, prolonged standing, obesity<br>*Examination*: Shallow, irregular ulcer with fibrinous material at base, usually medial aspect of the leg, around medial malleolus | Color-flow duplex ultrasound |
| Arterial ulcer | History of atherosclerotic vascular disease like coronary artery diseases, dyslipidemia, smoking<br>*Examination*: Deep, dry ulcer, usually over the distal part of the legs, diminished/absent peripheral pulsation, reduced ankle-brachial pressure index | Color-flow duplex ultrasound, CT angiography |
| Neuropathic ulcer | History of neuropathic symptoms-sensory, or motor, or both; predisposing conditions like history of alcoholism, systemic diseases like diabetes mellitus (DM)<br>*Examination*: Usually on pressure areas like soles, may be coexistent neuropathic/charcot joint | Nerve conduction study |
| Rheumato-logical diseases | History suggestive of multisystem involvement, symptoms like joint pain, photosensitivity, hair fall, young hypertension, unexplained renal dysfunction, and other system involvement in various combinations<br>*Examination*: Sharp punched out ulcer, can happen in both upper and lower limbs, cutaneous infarcts in case of antiphospholipid syndrome, other evidence of rheumatological diseases like presence of arthritis, skin rash | Autoimmune work-up like ANA, rheumatoid factor (RF), anti-CCP, ANCA, antiphospholipid antibodies (APLA), biopsy of the ulcer |
| Infection | History of systemic symptoms like fever, weight loss, evidence of infection in other organ systems<br>*Examination*: Painful ulcer with overlying necrotic material, foul smelling | Gram stain, AFB stain and fungal stain; culture sensitivity, wound swab, tissue, blood; radiological tests like CT/MRI |

*Continued*

*Continued*

| | | |
|---|---|---|
| Systemic diseases | History of uncontrolled/poorly controlled diabetes, history of diabetic complications like retinopathy, neuropathy; history of sickle cell disease (SCD) requiring multiple blood transfusions, history of sickle cell crisis<br>*Examination*: Evidence of neuropathy, retinopathy in case of diabetes, anemia or rarely avascular necrosis of joints in case of SCD | Fasting and post-prandial blood sugar, HbA1c, evaluation of neuropathy/retinopathy in case of DM; sickling test, Hb-electrophoresis in case of sickling cell disease |
| Cancer | History of any previous malignancy, painful ulcer<br>*Examination*: Painful, foul-smelling ulcer, often with bleeding; evidence of any other malignancy elsewhere | Biopsy of the ulcer, imaging like CT/MRI/PET-CT |

therapy have also shown success in some scenarios. In the case of refractory ulcers, skin grafting is also another option.

For treatment of the underlying disease, treatment is directed toward the particular disease. In the case of diabetes mellitus, sugar control needs to be optimized. Transfusion and hydroxyurea are helpful in the treatment of sickle cell disease. Compression stocking and if required sclerotherapy, or stripping can help in venous ulcers. Antiplatelet, vasodilator therapy and revascularization in selected cases can help in arterial ulcers. Appropriate immunosuppressive therapy helps in managing ulcers due to rheumatological diseases. Surgery, radiation and sometimes chemotherapy can help with skin cancers.

To conclude, non-healing ulcers can occur in several underlying systemic diseases. If not addressed, it can be a major cause of morbidity. A detailed history dedicated systemic and local examinations and focused investigation can help in the diagnosis of the exact cause. Treatment depends on the proper diagnosis as treating the underlying cause is the mainstay of treatment.

## Points to Ponder

- An ulcer which does not heal after 3 to 4 weeks of appropriate treatment is usually considered a nonhealing ulcer.
- If not addressed, it can be a major cause of morbidity.
- A detailed history dedicated systemic and local examinations and focused investigation can help in the diagnosis of the exact cause.
- Treatment depends on the proper diagnosis as treating the underlying cause is of paramount importance.

## MULTIPLE CHOICE QUESTIONS

1. **What is the most likely underlying cause of the nonhealing ulcer in the case described?**
   A. Venous insufficiency
   B. Pyoderma gangrenosum
   C. Diabetic foot ulcer
   D. Infectious ulcer
2. **Which serological markers are most specific for diagnosing rheumatoid arthritis in this patient?**
   A. Antinuclear antibody (ANA)
   B. Rheumatoid factor (RF)
   C. Anticyclic citrullinated peptide (anti-CCP) antibody
   D. Erythrocyte sedimentation rate (ESR)
3. **What is the most appropriate first-line treatment for pyoderma gangrenosum in this patient?**
   A. Antibiotics
   B. Surgical debridement
   C. High-dose steroids and immunosuppressants
   D. Local wound care only
4. **Which deformity described in the patient's hands is characteristic of long-standing rheumatoid arthritis?**
   A. Swan neck deformity
   B. Heberden's nodes
   C. Mallet finger
   D. Boutonnière deformity
5. **What is the role of infliximab in the management of this patient?**
   A. It is an antibiotic used to treat secondary infections
   B. It is an anti-TNF agent that reduces systemic inflammation
   C. It is a local steroid injected into joints to relieve pain
   D. It promotes wound healing in chronic ulcers

### Answers

1. (B); 2. (C); 3. (C); 4. (A); 5. (B)

## SUGGESTED READINGS

1. Smolen JS, Aletaha D, McInnes, IB. Rheumatoid arthritis. The Lancet. 2016;388(10055):2023-38.
2. Mishra S, Kancharla H. Pyoderma gangrenosum: A review. Indian Dermatol Online J. 2019;10(6):707-21.
3. Firestein GS, McInnes IB. Immunopathogenesis of rheumatoid arthritis. Immunity. 2017;46(2):183-96.
4. Goodman SM, et al.. Management of rheumatoid arthritis: Clinical guidance. BMJ. 2020;368, m82.
5. Brooklyn T, Dunnill G, Probert C. Diagnosis and treatment of pyoderma gangrenosum. BMJ. 2006;333(7560):181-4.

# CHAPTER 83

# An Approach to a Case of Reactive Arthritis and Management

*Chiranjita Phukan*

**CASE VIGNETTE**

A 42-year-old male presents with a 3-month history of joint pain and swelling, which began 3 weeks after an episode of acute gastroenteritis. He reports intermittent fever, fatigue, and significant pain in his knees, ankles, and lower back. Despite over-the-counter nonsteroidal anti-inflammatory drugs (NSAIDs), his symptoms have progressively worsened, affecting his daily activities and mobility. He has a history of occasional uveitis and recent episodes of eye redness and discomfort. He denies any significant past medical history apart from recent diarrhea and abdominal cramps.

*Physical examination*: Bilateral knee and right ankle swelling with decreased range of motion and tenderness over the sacroiliac joints were noted. The patient was afebrile.

### Laboratory Tests Revealed

- Elevated ESR (45 mm/h) and CRP (30 mg/L)
- Negative rheumatoid factor (RA) and anti-CCP antibodies
- HLA-B27 positive
- Synovial fluid analysis: Sterile with elevated WBC count
- X-rays of the knee: No erosive changes, but signs of joint effusion

### Treatment

The patient was prescribed NSAIDs (naproxen 500 mg twice daily), leading to symptomatic improvement within a week. Physical therapy was initiated to preserve joint function. At a 6-week follow-up, the patient reported significant relief, with no recurrence of gastrointestinal or ocular symptoms.

## PROVISIONAL DIAGNOSIS

Based on clinical presentation, laboratory findings (elevated inflammatory markers and HLA-B27 positive status), and the temporal relationship with a gastrointestinal infection, a diagnosis of reactive arthritis (ReA) **(Fig. 1)** was made.

## DIFFERENTIAL DIAGNOSES

- *Rheumatoid arthritis (RA)*: Rheumatoid arthritis typically presents with symmetric, small joint involvement (e.g., hands and feet). Prolonged morning stiffness lasting over an hour is a key feature, whereas in ReA, stiffness tends to be shorter in duration. Positive RF and anti-CCP antibodies are commonly seen in RA but are negative in ReA.
- *Psoriatic arthritis (PsA)*: It may involve asymmetric oligoarthritis or axial symptoms similar to ankylosing spondylitis. A personal or family history of psoriasis, skin, and nail changes (e.g., nail pitting, onycholysis, or dystrophy) distinguishes PsA from ReA. PsA can present as oligoarthritis, polyarthritis, or axial disease similar to ankylosing spondylitis. Elevated inflammatory markers and Pencil-in-cup deformity of the joints in PsA (especially in

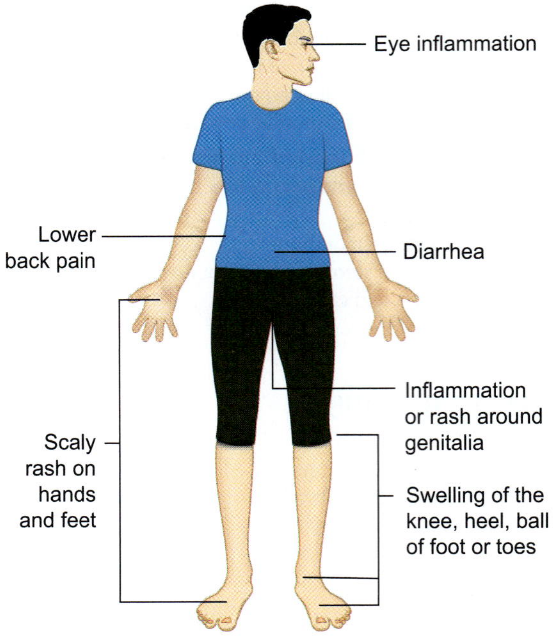


**FIG. 1:** Symptoms of reactive arthritis.

advanced disease) is a classic radiologic feature. Enthesitis and periostitis can also be seen in PsA, as in ReA.

- *Ankylosing spondylitis (AS)*: Both ReA and AS can involve the sacroiliac joints, especially in HLA-B27-positive individuals. However, AS presents with chronic low back pain that improves with exercise and worsens with rest. The onset is typically insidious in young males, and axial symptoms are more pronounced.
- *Septic arthritis*: Septic arthritis often presents with acute monoarthritis and more severe systemic symptoms. In ReA, arthritis develops gradually following an infection. Negative joint fluid cultures and the absence of high WBC count (>50,000/mm$^3$) help differentiate it from septic arthritis.
- *Gout and pseudogout*: Both conditions cause acute monoarthritis, with gout commonly affecting the first metatarsophalangeal joint and pseudogout affecting larger joints like the knee. Patients with gout often have a history of similar episodes. Dietary triggers (high purine intake) or alcohol may precipitate flares. Synovial fluid analysis identifying uric acid crystals in gout or calcium pyrophosphate crystals in pseudogout confirms these diagnoses.
- *Systemic lupus erythematosus (SLE)*: SLE features polyarthritis with systemic involvement (e.g., skin, kidneys) and positive ANA and anti-dsDNA antibodies. Joint involvement is typically symmetric and nonerosive, unlike ReA.
- *IBD-associated arthritis*: Arthritis associated with inflammatory bowel disease (IBD) can mimic ReA but is typically linked to active bowel disease. Peripheral joint involvement is often indistinguishable from ReA, though sacroiliitis and axial involvement are common in both.

## Pathophysiology of Reactive Arthritis

Reactive arthritis is an inflammatory arthritis that develops after an infection in another part of the body, typically involving the gastrointestinal or urogenital systems. It is often triggered by bacterial infections, such as chlamydia, salmonella, shigella, yersinia, or campylobacter. The pathogenesis of ReA involves the activation of the immune system, where molecular mimicry between bacterial antigens and host tissues leads to the inflammation of joints, particularly in the lower limbs. HLA-B27 positivity is commonly associated with ReA, suggesting a genetic predisposition to the disease. The inflammation typically affects peripheral joints (knees, ankles), the sacroiliac joints, and may involve extra-articular manifestations such as uveitis and skin lesions.

# CLINICAL APPROACH

## Comprehensive History Taking

A detailed history is critical for diagnosing ReA. Key points include:

- *Triggering infection history*: Ask about recent diarrhea or dysentery (e.g., *Salmonella*, *Shigella*) or urogenital infections (e.g., *Chlamydia*). Symptom onset typically occurs 1–4 weeks after infection.
- *Joint symptoms*: Large joints (knees, ankles) are often asymmetrically affected, with swelling, pain, and morning stiffness.
- *Axial symptoms*: Low back pain with sacroiliac involvement may be present.
- *Extra-articular symptoms*: Look for uveitis, conjunctivitis, skin lesions (e.g., keratoderma blennorrhagicum), or genitourinary symptoms.
- *Family history*: A history of spondyloarthropathies or psoriasis increases the likelihood of ReA.

## Physical Examination

- *Joint examination*: Look for asymmetric oligoarthritis affecting large joints dactylitis sacroiliitis enthesitis. Assess range of motion, tenderness, and swelling.
- *Axial skeleton examination*: Check for sacroiliac tenderness and use Schober's test for spinal flexibility.
- *Skin and nail*: Circinate balanitis, keratoderma blennorrhagica, psoriatic onychodystrophy, painless ulcers in the mouth.
- *Eye*: Conjunctivitis, corneal ulceration, episcleritis, keratitis, uveitis.
- *Genitourinary*: Cervicitis/salpingitis/vulvovaginitis in women urethritis and prostatitis in men.
- *Gastrointestinal*: Acute diarrhea resembling inflammatory bowel disease.
- *Heart* (rare): Ascending aortitis conduction abnormalities.

## Diagnostic Testing

- *Blood tests:* Elevated ESR and CRP suggest inflammation. CRP helps in assessing the severity and monitoring response to treatment. HLA-B27 is positive in 60–80% of ReA cases. RF and anti-CCP are negative.
- *Microbiological tests:* Stool cultures and urine PCR may identify the triggering pathogens (e.g., *Chlamydia*, *Salmonella*).
- *Joint aspiration:* Synovial fluid analysis shows sterile, inflammatory fluid with elevated WBC count (5,000–50,000/mm$^3$).
- *Imaging:*
  - X-rays are particularly useful in patients with persistent or chronic symptoms to assess structural joint damage. In chronic cases, sacroiliitis may be evident.
  - Ultrasound is particularly useful in detecting enthesitis, a common feature of reactive arthritis may be helpful for detecting soft tissue inflammation and confirming joint effusions or tenosynovitis.
  - MRI is highly sensitive for detecting early inflammation, bone marrow edema, and soft tissue involvement before X-ray changes become evident. MRI is especially useful when sacroiliitis or spondylitis is suspected, or when there is uncertainty in the diagnosis after other imaging modalities have been used.

# TREATMENT AND PREVENTION

## Acute Phase Management

*NSAIDs*: First-line treatment for acute arthritis symptoms. Drugs like ibuprofen, naproxen, diclofenac, or indomethacin can be used for several weeks to months, depending on symptom severity and response. However, they should be tapered off as soon as the acute phase resolves to avoid side effects. Regular monitoring for GI and renal side effects is essential.

## Corticosteroids

- *Systemic corticosteroids*: Short-term use of systemic corticosteroids (e.g., prednisone) for 2–4 weeks can be considered if NSAIDs fail to control inflammation or in cases of severe multijoint involvement or extra-articular manifestations. Short-term use with a gradual taper is preferred to minimize side effects.
- *Intra-articular corticosteroid injections*: Intra-articular steroid injections are effective for managing persistent monoarthritic or oligoarthritic when a specific joint remains inflamed.
- *Antibiotics:* These are only used to treat underlying infections that triggered reactive arthritis, such as urogenital (Chlamydia trachomatis) or gastrointestinal infections (e.g., Campylobacter, salmonella). Antibiotics do not treat the arthritis directly, and there is no benefit from prolonged antibiotic use for the arthritis itself.

### Chronic or Recurrent Reactive Arthritis

#### Disease-modifying antirheumatic drugs (DMARDs)

DMARDs like sulfasalazine, methotrexate are indicated for patients with:

- Chronic reactive arthritis lasting more than 6 months
- Recurrent flares despite NSAID or corticosteroid therapy
- Severe disease with axial involvement or persistent joint damage

Sulfasalazine (Dose 2–3 g/day) is often the first-choice DMARD in reactive arthritis. Methotrexate is particularly useful for peripheral joint involvement and can be used when sulfasalazine is ineffective or poorly tolerated. Both drugs require regular monitoring of liver and kidney function, as well as blood counts, due to potential side effects.

### Biologic Therapy (TNF Inhibitors)

Biologics are used for patients with severe or refractory reactive arthritis that does not respond to DMARDs or those with significant axial involvement (e.g., sacroiliitis). Etanercept, infliximab, or adalimumab are TNF-α inhibitors that have been shown to reduce inflammation, improve function, and prevent structural joint damage in refractory cases of reactive arthritis. Once inflammation is well-controlled and remission is sustained for 6–12 months, tapering or stopping biologic therapy may be considered. However, patients must be closely monitored for relapse.

### Management of Extra-articular Manifestations

- *Eye involvement*: Mild uveitis can be managed with topical corticosteroids, while severe cases may require systemic therapy.
- *Skin lesions*: Topical corticosteroids or calcipotriene may be used for keratoderma blennorrhagicum or balanitis. Severe cases may require systemic therapy.

### Rehabilitation and Physical Therapy

*Physical therapy*: Maintaining joint mobility, flexibility, and muscle strength is essential. Low-impact exercises (e.g., swimming) are encouraged, particularly for axial disease.

### Preventing Flares and Long-term Follow-up

- *Infection prevention*: Safe sexual practices and good hygiene are crucial for preventing recurrent infections.
- *Stress management*: Stress can exacerbate inflammation, so techniques such as mindfulness or counselling may be beneficial.
- *Monitoring*: Regular follow-up with physical exams, inflammatory markers, and imaging helps manage chronic disease.

### Points to Ponder

- ❑ Reactive arthritis can become chronic in 15–20% of cases.
- ❑ Timely diagnosis and treatment of infections can prevent complications.
- ❑ Extra-articular manifestations, including eye and skin involvement, should be monitored closely.
- ❑ Long-term follow-up is essential for patients with recurrent or persistent symptoms.

## MULTIPLE CHOICE QUESTIONS

**1. Which of the following is most commonly associated with the development of reactive arthritis (ReA)?**
   A. Recent viral infection
   B. Recent gastrointestinal infection
   C. Recent dental surgery
   D. Family history of autoimmune diseases

**2. The presence of which genetic marker is most strongly associated with reactive arthritis?**
   A. HLA-DR4
   B. HLA-B27
   C. HLA-A2
   D. HLA-CCP

**3. Which of the following is typically not seen in the laboratory findings of a patient with reactive arthritis?**
   A. Elevated ESR and CRP
   B. Negative rheumatoid factor
   C. Positive anti-CCP antibodies
   D. Synovial fluid with elevated white blood cells

**4. Which of the following is an extra-articular manifestation commonly seen in reactive arthritis?**
   A. Psoriasis
   B. Uveitis
   C. Systemic lupus erythematosus
   D. Rheumatoid nodules

**5. What is the first-line treatment for managing symptoms of reactive arthritis?**
   A. Methotrexate
   B. NSAIDs
   C. Glucocorticoids
   D. Biologic agents

### Answers

1. (B); 2. (B); 3. (C); 4. (B); 5. (B)

## SUGGESTED READINGS


1. Singh JA, Saag KG, Bridges SL Jr, et al. 2015 American College of Rheumatology Guideline for the Treatment of Rheumatoid Arthritis. Arthritis Rheumatol. 2016;68(1):1-26.
2. Guidelines British Society for Rheumatology. Available from: https://www.rheumatology.org.uk/guidelines.
3. Gossec L, Smolen JS, Gaujoux-Viala C, et al. EULAR recommendations for the management of psoriatic arthritis with pharmacological therapies. Ann Rheum Dis. 2012;71(1):4-12.
4. Firestein GS, Budd RC, Gabriel SE, McInnes IB, O'Dell JR. Kelley's Textbook of Rheumatology, 10th edition. Philadelphia: Elsevier; 2016.
5. NICE. Overview Spondyloarthritis in over 16s: diagnosis and management Guidance NICE [Internet]. 2017. Available from: https://www.nice.org.uk/guidance/ng65.

CHAPTER 84

# An Approach to a Case of Hand Joint Deformities

*Kaushik Basu*

**CASE VIGNETTE**

A 50-year-old female presents with progressively worsening deformities of the fingers and difficulty performing daily activities for the past 2 years. She reports morning stiffness lasting over an hour and occasional pain and swelling in the small joints of the hands. Physical examination reveals ulnar deviation, boutonnière deformities of the fingers, and swan neck deformities. The metacarpophalangeal and proximal interphalangeal joints are tender and swollen.

Laboratory investigations show elevated rheumatoid factor (RF) and anticyclic citrullinated peptide (anti-CCP) antibodies, with mildly elevated inflammatory markers (ESR and CRP). X-rays of the hands reveal periarticular osteopenia, joint space narrowing, and erosions at the metacarpophalangeal joints. The clinical findings and investigations are consistent with rheumatoid arthritis.

## PROVISIONAL DIAGNOSIS

Rheumatoid arthritis presenting with progressive hand joint deformities.

## DIFFERENTIAL DIAGNOSIS

- *Rheumatoid arthritis*: Symmetric joint involvement, ulnar deviation, swan neck, and boutonnière deformities.
- *Osteoarthritis*: Heberden's and Bouchard's nodes, with noninflammatory changes.
- *Psoriatic arthritis*: Dactylitis, nail pitting, and asymmetric joint involvement.
- *Systemic lupus erythematosus (SLE)*: Jaccoud's arthropathy with nonerosive deformities.
- *Gout*: Acute episodic joint pain with tophi formation in chronic cases.

## CLINICAL APPROACH

- *History*: Chronicity, joint pain/swelling, stiffness, deformities, systemic symptoms (e.g., fever, rash).
- *Examination*: Assess joint swelling, tenderness, deformities, range of motion, and systemic findings.
- *Investigations*: RF, anti-CCP, ESR/CRP, ANA (if lupus suspected), X-rays (erosions, osteopenia, deformities).
- *Diagnosis confirmation*: Correlation of clinical and serological findings with imaging.

## PATHOPHYSIOLOGY

Rheumatoid arthritis is an autoimmune condition where chronic synovial inflammation leads to pannus formation, cartilage destruction, and bone erosion. Over time, joint deformities develop due to ligament laxity and imbalance between flexor and extensor forces.

## TREATMENT AND PREVENTION

Treatment focuses on controlling inflammation, preventing deformities, and improving quality of life. Disease-modifying antirheumatic drugs (DMARDs) like methotrexate are the cornerstone, supported by NSAIDs or glucocorticoids for symptomatic relief. Advanced cases may require biologics such as TNF inhibitors. Rehabilitation with physical therapy and joint splinting helps maintain joint function. Preventive measures include early diagnosis, timely initiation of DMARDs, and lifestyle modifications like avoiding smoking and maintaining a healthy weight.

**Points to Ponder**

- *Early diagnosis*: Early identification and treatment of rheumatoid arthritis are critical to prevent irreversible joint damage and deformities.
- *Role of anti-CCP*: Anti-CCP is highly specific and helps in early diagnosis, even before radiological changes.
- *Systemic involvement*: Always consider extra-articular manifestations like lung involvement or vasculitis in rheumatoid arthritis.
- *Imaging importance*: X-rays and ultrasonography of hands can detect early erosive changes even before clinical deformities develop.
- *Multidisciplinary management*: Rheumatologists, physiotherapists, and orthopedic surgeons play a collaborative role in the long-term care of patients with joint deformities.

## MULTIPLE CHOICE QUESTIONS

1. **What is the most characteristic deformity in the hand joints of a patient with advanced rheumatoid arthritis?**
   A. Heberden's nodes
   B. Ulnar deviation
   C. Bouchard's nodes
   D. Swan neck deformity
2. **Which laboratory test is most specific for the diagnosis of rheumatoid arthritis?**
   A. Rheumatoid factor (RF)
   B. Antinuclear antibody (ANA)
   C. Anticyclic citrullinated peptide (Anti-CCP)
   D. Erythrocyte sedimentation rate (ESR)
3. **What is the primary mechanism underlying joint deformities in rheumatoid arthritis?**
   A. Crystal deposition in synovium
   B. Chronic synovitis with pannus formation
   C. Ligamentous calcification
   D. Increased osteoblastic activity
4. **What is the first-line treatment for managing joint deformities in rheumatoid arthritis?**
   A. Physical therapy
   B. Methotrexate
   C. NSAIDs
   D. Joint replacement surgery
5. **Which hand joint is most commonly involved in rheumatoid arthritis?**
   A. Distal interphalangeal (DIP) joints
   B. Proximal interphalangeal (PIP) joints
   C. First carpometacarpal joint
   D. Metacarpophalangeal (MCP) joints

### Answers

1. (B); 2. (C); 3. (B); 4. (B); 5. (D)

## SUGGESTED READINGS


1. Firestein GS, Budd RC, Gabriel SE, et al. Kelley and Firestein's Textbook of Rheumatology. 11th edition. Elsevier; 2020.
2. Smolen JS, Aletaha D, McInnes IB. Rheumatoid arthritis. Lancet. 2016;388(10055):2023-38.
3. Scott DL, Wolfe F, Huizinga TW. Rheumatoid arthritis. Lancet. 2010;376(9746):1094-108.
4. van der Heijde D, Ramiro S, Landewé R, et al. 2019 update of the EULAR recommendations for the management of rheumatoid arthritis with synthetic and biological disease-modifying antirheumatic drugs. Ann Rheum Dis. 2020;79(6):685-99.
5. Klareskog L, Catrina AI, Paget S. Rheumatoid arthritis. Lancet. 2009;373(9664):659-72.
6. Furst DE, Keystone EC, So AK, et al. Updated consensus statement on biological agents for the treatment of rheumatic diseases. Ann Rheum Dis. 2010;69(Suppl 1):i2-29.

CHAPTER

# 85

# An Approach to a Case of Raynaud's Phenomenon

*Ritu, Manuj Kumar Sarkar, Surbhi Dogra, Kirandeep Kour, Taranpreet Kour*

**CASE VIGNETTE**

A female of 25 years old complains of recurring episodes of discoloration of fingers over the past two winter seasons which turns pale especially after exposure to cold weather or cold water and during emotional or psychological stress **(Fig. 1)**. The fingers initially turn white, followed by a bluish tinge, and then turn red and warm as the episode resolves. This is associated with numbness and tingling but no significant pain or persistent discoloration. There was no history of any chronic medical illness, any significant drug or medication intake, no history of any joint pains, skin thickening, rashes or dysphagia. She does not smoke and denies a family history of similar symptoms. The patient has no significant past medical history. On examination, her hands appear normal at room temperature with no evident discoloration, ulceration, or cyanosis. The skin of the hands and fingers is soft and intact, with no evidence of sclerodactyly, joint deformities, telangiectasias, or skin thickening **(Fig. 1)**. Capillary refill time is normal. Peripheral pulses are palpable in all extremities and are symmetrical. There are no visible nail fold capillary abnormalities, such as tortuosity or enlargement. Additionally, joint examination shows no deformities, swelling, or tenderness. Systemic examination was normal.

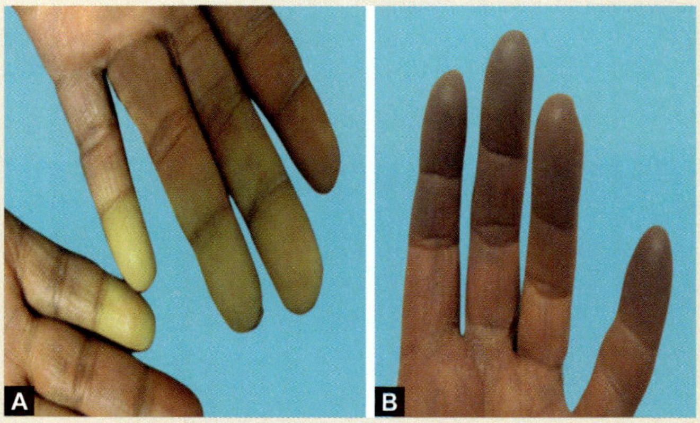


**FIGS. 1A AND B:** Clinical presentation of Raynaud syndrome. (A) Sharply demarcated pallor in several fingers. (B) Cyanosis of the fingertips.

## PROVISIONAL DIAGNOSIS

A typical characteristic triphasic color changes—white (pallor), blue (cyanosis), and red (hyperemia)—in response to cold exposure or emotional stress, are hallmark symptoms of *Raynaud phenomena* (RP). Since Raynaud's phenomenon can be *primary (idiopathic)* or *secondary* to underlying diseases (like systemic sclerosis or systemic lupus erythematosus). In the absence of symptoms such as joint pain, skin thickening, or other systemic complaints, normal physical examination, like no ulcerations, digital pitting, or skin changes supports a provisional diagnosis of *primary Raynaud's syndrome*, which is also called *Raynaud's disease*.

## DIFFERENTIAL DIAGNOSIS

Peripheral vascular disease, excessive cold sensitivity, peripheral neuropathy, complex regional pain syndrome, thromboangiitis obliterans, vasculitis, mixed connective tissue disease, systemic sclerosis, lupus, dermatomyositis, polymyositis, thromboembolic disease, livedo reticularis, acrocyanosis, history of drug intake such as betablocker, cocaine, caffeine, ergotamine, nicotine, chemotherapeutic drugs like bleomycin, vinblastine and chilblains, etc.

## CLINICAL APPROACH

The presenting common complaints with Raynaud phenomenon attacks are usually pin and needles sensation, numbness or finger aches or pain **(Box 1)**.

History of patient with suspected Raynaud phenomenon, should address following points:

- Age of onset
- Location of affected areas
- Presence of symmetry
- Presence of digital ulceration
- Severity of attacks

Provoking factors should be identified like exposure to cold temperatures or sympathetic nervous system stimulation from emotional stress or being startled. The factors which increase frequency or severity of attacks like the presence of stress, female gender, low temperature, and the presence of a concurrent connective tissue disease should be addressed.

The physical examination is necessary to identify areas of tissue loss (e.g., ulceration, gangrene) typically affecting the fingers or toes. Other sites that may be affected by cutaneous vasospasm should also be examined closely, including the skin of the ears, nose, face, knees, and nipples. A complete physical exam should also include a thorough musculoskeletal and cardiopulmonary evaluation, as possible clues of any underlying systemic rheumatic disease may be present. Peripheral pulses should be assessed for evidence of proximal (large) vessel disease.

Clinical features associated with primary RP include the following:

- Vasospastic attack precipitated by cold or emotional stress
- Bilateral symmetric attacks
- No tissue necrosis or gangrene
- No history or physical findings suggestive of secondary cause of RP
- Normal nailfold capillaries
- Normal erythrocyte sedimentation rate (ESR)
- Absence of autoantibodies

If the clinical evaluation defines features consistent with primary RP, then additional diagnostic testing specific for RP is generally not necessary. However, we monitor the patient annually for the development of signs and symptoms of diseases associated with secondary RP.

Laboratory tests in most patients with newly diagnosed secondary RP:

- Complete blood count and differential
- Complete metabolic panel

**BOX 1: Evaluation of Raynaud phenomenon is initiated by asking patient, the following questions.**

- Are your fingers unusually sensitive to cold?
- Do your fingers change color when exposed to cold?
- If the fingers change color, do they turn white, blue/purple, or both

- Urinalysis with urine sediment
- ANA (ideally by indirect immunofluorescence testing)
- Thyroid-stimulating hormone (TSH)
- ESR and/or C-reactive protein (CRP) levels

Additional laboratory tests may be warranted depending on the presence of other clinical symptoms. As examples:

- For patients with sclerodactyly and digital ulcers, antibodies specific for SSc such as antitopoisomerase I (anti-Scl-70), anticentromere, and anti-RNA polymerase III should be done.
- For patents with suspected inflammatory myopathy, creatinine kinase and possibly other myositis-specific autoantibodies (e.g., anti-Jo-1) should be done.
- For patients with suspected SLE or cryoglobulinemia, serum C3 and C4 complement levels should be done.
- For patients with a suspected paraproteinemia, serum protein electrophoresis (SPEP) should be done.

Raynaud phenomena typically affect fingers (distal areas). It is usually sudden in onset with the development of cold digits and the demarcation of "white" areas also known as skin pallor or white attack. Sometimes, there may be cyanotic skin changes, otherwise known as a blue attack. The white or blue attack typically remains for approximately 20 minutes. After the Raynaud phenomenon flare, vascular reperfusion with subsequent rewarming turns it erythematous is known as reactive hyperemia. The episodic attack usually starts out with a single digit and then spreads to other digits symmetrically on both hands.

The criteria for diagnosing primary Raynaud phenomenon include episodic attacks of acral pallor or cyanosis, strong and symmetrical peripheral pulses, absence of digital pitting, ulceration or gangrene, normal nailfold capillaries, negative results on the antinuclear antibody (ANA) test and normal erythrocyte sedimentation rate (ESR).

Patients not fulfilling these criteria require further evaluation. Presences of systemic symptoms like joint pain or skin tightening, which may suggest an underlying autoimmune disorder. The thumb is less commonly affected than other digits in both patients with primary Raynaud phenomenon and those with secondary disease, its involvement raises suspicion of an underlying connective tissue disease.

## INVESTIGATIONS

The basic set of investigations for all patients presenting with Raynaud's phenomena include blood count, ESR, ANA and nailfold capillaroscopy. Usually in patients with primary Raynaud's phenomena all these investigations will be normal. Thyroid function tests, and a thoracic outlet radiograph, to check for a cervical rib may also be done in some cases. If the history or examination indicate the presence of some underlying connective tissue disorder, disease specific autoantibody testing should also be done.

Systemic sclerosis (SSc) is most commonly associated with the most severe RP. SSc specific autoantibodies (including anti-centromere and anti-topoisomerase (anti-Scl-70) should be investigated.

Nailfold capillaroscopy **(Fig. 2)** shows dilated loops, areas of avascularity, distortion of the normal capillary architecture and multiple hemorrhages indicate an underlying SSc-spectrum disorder. Cutolo et al. described a method of scoring the "scleroderma pattern" ("early", "active" and "late"). The capillaries may be visualized using a dermatoscope or with an ophthalmoscope. The newer methods include laser Doppler flowmetry, laser Doppler imaging can also be done.

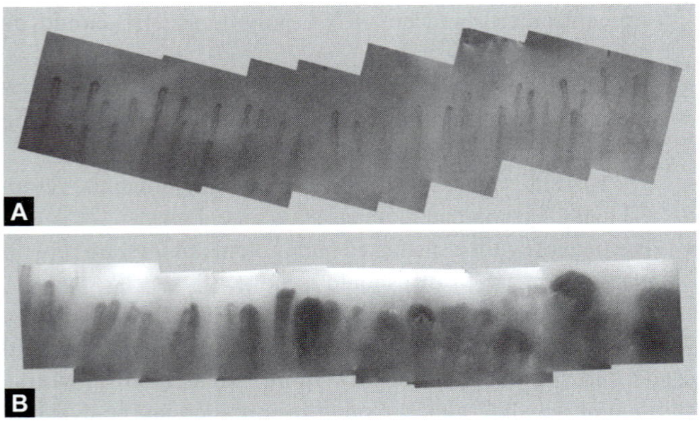

**FIGS. 2A AND B:** (A) Normal capillaroscopy. The capillaries are regular ("hairpin" like) in appearance. (B) Abnormal nailfold capillaroscopy in a patient with SSc. Several capillaries are enlarged, with areas of avascularity.

## PATHOPHYSIOLOGY

Raynaud's phenomenon is marked by vascular abnormalities, with differences in primary versus secondary forms. Secondary RP, commonly seen in systemic sclerosis (SSc), involves structural vascular changes like intimal fibrosis, which restricts blood flow and damages endothelial cells, worsening vasoconstriction Inflammatory mediators such as cytokine growth factors and activated pericytes further disrupt vascular integrity. Functional abnormalities include impaired endothelial regulation of vasodilators like nitric oxide (NO) and prostacyclin, with inconsistent NO levels and reduced prostacyclin contributing to disease progression. Potent vasoconstrictors like endothelin-1 and angiotensin II drive vasospasm and fibrosis, and endothelin-1 receptor antagonists have shown therapeutic benefit in RP. Neural factors also play a role; enhanced sympathetic responsiveness and reduced levels of vasodilatory neuropeptides such as CGRP contribute to dysregulated vascular tone. Additionally, intravascular factors like increased platelet activity and oxidative stress further impair blood flow, particularly in secondary RP, while primary RP typically lacks these structural changes and is largely functional.

## TREATMENT AND PREVENTION

Treatment and prevention is outline in the **Figure 3** below.

**Lifestyle modifications:**
- Avoid exposure to cold; wear warm gloves and socks
- Manage stress levels
- Avoid smoking and caffeine

**Medications**
- *Calcium channel blockers (e.g., nifedipine, amlodipine):* Vasodilators—topical nitroglycerin ointment or oral agents like sildenafil
- *Endothelin-1 receptor antagonists (e.g., bosentan):* Especially beneficial in secondary RP
- *ACE Inhibitors or angiotensin II receptor blockers:* May help by reducing vascular tone
- *Prostaglandin analogs (e.g., iloprost):* Used intravenously for severe cases, especially with ulceration

Treatment and prevention

**Advanced therapies:**
- *Sympathectomy:* Surgical or chemical sympathectomy for severe, unresponsive cases
- *Botulinum toxin injections:* May reduce vasospasm and pain in selected patients
- *Laser therapy:* Multiwave locked system (MLS) laser therapy has been used to improve microvascular health

**Monitoring and prevention:**
- Regular follow-up to monitor progression from primary to secondary RP
- Educate patients on signs of complications (e.g., ulceration) and when to seek medical help

**FIG. 3:** Diagrammatic representation of treatment and prevention for a case of Raynaud's phenomenon.

### Points to Ponder

- The more common variety of RP is primary Raynaud's syndrome, also called Raynaud's disease, which is idiopathic, commonly seen in young females of under 30 years old. This variety does not require any specific treatment, only reassurance and lifestyle changes are sufficient.
- Nine out of 10 systemic sclerosis (SSc) patients develops secondary RP. In majority of these patients RP can be a presenting complaint, so any case of secondary RP must be evaluated for SSc.
- Treatment of primary cause of secondary RP will help majority of individuals.
- Individuals who use hand tools which vibrates (hammers, chain saws, pianist and keyboard operators) are more prone for development of RP.
- Avoidance of precipitant of an attack of RP is very crucial in prevention of symptoms.

## MULTIPLE CHOICE QUESTIONS

1. **In Raynaud's phenomenon, which color change sequence is most typical in the affected digits?**
   A. Red → White → Blue
   B. Blue → White → Red
   C. White → Blue → Red
   D. Red → Blue → White
2. **Which medication is most commonly used as a first-line treatment for Raynaud's phenomenon?**
   A. Aspirin
   B. Calcium channel blockers
   C. ACE inhibitors
   D. Beta-blockers
3. **What differentiates primary Raynaud's phenomenon from secondary Raynaud's phenomenon?**
   A. Primary is associated with underlying diseases like systemic sclerosis
   B. Secondary is less severe and lacks structural vascular changes
   C. Primary has no underlying systemic disease and lacks vascular structural changes
   D. Secondary occurs only in warm environments
4. **Which of the following complications is most associated with secondary Raynaud's phenomenon?**
   A. Digital ulcers
   B. Hyperpigmentation
   C. Hair loss
   D. Muscle weakness
5. **Which neurotransmitter is involved in the exaggerated vasoconstriction seen in Raynaud's phenomenon?**
   A. Dopamine
   B. Serotonin
   C. Norepinephrine
   D. Acetylcholine

### Answers

1. (C); 2. (B); 3. (C); 4. (A); 5. (C)

## SUGGESTED READINGS


1. LeRoy EC, Medsger TA. Raynaud's phenomenon: a proposal for classification. Clin Exp Rheumatol. 1992;10:485-8.
2. Herrick AL. The pathogenesis, diagnosis and treatment of Raynaud phenomenon. Nat Rev Rheumatol. 2012;8(8):469-79.
3. Chikura B, Moore T, Manning J, et al. Thumb involvement in Raynaud's phenomenon as an indicator of underlying connective tissue disease. J Rheumatol. 2010;37:783-6.
4. Koenig M, Joyal F, Fritzler MJ, et al. Autoantibodies and microvascular damage are independent predictive factors for the progression of Raynaud's phenomenon to systemic sclerosis: a twenty-year prospective study of 586 patients, with validation of proposed criteria for early systemic sclerosis. Arthritis Rheum. 2008;58(12):3902e12.
5. Maricq HR, LeRoy EC. Patterns of finger capillary abnormalities in connective tissue disease by 'wide-field' microscopy. Arthritis Rheum. 1973;16(5):619e28.
6. Cutolo M, SullI A, Smith V. Assessing microvascular changes in systemic sclerosis diagnosis and management. Nat Rev Rheumatol. 2010;6(10):578e87.
7. Murray AK, Herrick AL, King TA. Laser Doppler imaging: a developing technique for application in the rheumatic diseases. Rheumatology (Oxford). 2004;43:1210-8.
8. Herrick AL, Clark S. Quantifying digital vascular disease in patients with primary Raynaud's phenomenon and systemic sclerosis. Ann Rheum Dis. 1998;57(2):70-8.
9. Hughes M, Herrick AL. Raynaud's Phenomenon, Best Practice & Research Clinical Rheumatology. 2016, http://dx.doi.org/10.1016/j.berh.2016.04.001
10. Freemont AJ, Hoyland J, Fielding P, et al. Studies of the microvascular endothelium in uninvolved skin of patients with systemic sclerosis: direct evidence for a generalized microangiopathy. Br J Dermatol. 1992;126(6):561-8.

CHAPTER

86

# An Approach to a Case of Vesicular Rashes

*Md Jamil*

**CASE VIGNETTE**

A young female with a diagnosis of systemic lupus erythematosus under treatment with mycophenolate mofetil presented with a history of pain and vesicular eruption over the right scapular region, arm, and forearm. The lesions were preceded by severe pain for 2 days.

## PROVISIONAL DIAGNOSIS

### Herpes Zoster

Vesicular lesions are small, clear fluid-filled lesions < 5 mm in diameter. They are raised above the plane of the surrounding skin and are translucent. They often develop over an erythematous base and are preceded by maculopapular rashes. Though many diseases can present as vesicular lesions, proper history taking, including recent exposure, and thorough clinical examination that includes distribution and pattern (discrete, grouped, irregularly distributed, or linear) of the vesicular lesions can give you a diagnostic clue.

### Etiology

The causes of the vesicular lesion are varied. The common causes of vesicular lesions are viral infections that include infections from varicella zoster virus (VZV) and herpes simplex virus (HSV). Other less common causes of vesicular rashes are bacterial infections like erysipelas, contact dermatitis, coxsackievirus, echovirus, atypical measles, rickettsial pox, COVID-19 and monkeypox (Mpox).

## DIFFERENTIAL DIAGNOSIS

Common differential of vesicular rashes is:

- Herpes simplex viral (HSV-1 and HSV-2) infection
- Varicella-zoster infection
- Contact dermatitis/allergic contact dermatitis
- Mpox
- Rickettsial pox

### Herpes Simplex Viral

Both HSV-1 and HSV-2 can cause genital and orofacial infection, and clinical manifestations caused by two subtypes (HSV-1 and HSV-2) are clinically indistinguishable. Recurrent herpes labialis is more common with the HSV-1 and reactivation of genital herpes is more common with HSV-2 than HSV-1. Clinical diagnosis of herpes lesions can be made accurately if the typical vesicular lesions on the erythematous base are present. Staining scraping from the base of the lesions with Wright's or Giemsa's stain to demonstrate giant cells or intranuclear inclusions of herpesvirus infection, but these methods do not differentiate between HSV and varicella-zoster virus infection. Confirmation of the specific virus is done by detecting the virus, viral antigen, or viral DNA in scraping from lesions. Detection of viral DNA by PCR is the most sensitive test used for laboratory diagnosis confirmation. Sensitively of all the tests depends upon the stage of the lesions, whether lesions are from the first or recurrent episode of the disease, and whether the patient is immunosuppressed or immunocompetent. The test's sensitivity is higher in the vesicular lesion, the first episode of the disease, and the immunosuppressed state.

### Varicella-zoster Virus

Varicella (chickenpox) and herpes zoster (shingles) are the two distinct clinical syndromes caused by VZV. VZV belongs to the family Herpesviridae. Chickenpox occurs because of primary infection with VZV and herpes zoster, resulting from the reactivation of a virus that remains latent in the dorsal root ganglia and is infected during chickenpox. The incubation period is usually 14–17 days (but may vary from 10–20 days), and the disease is characterized by fever, rash, and malaise. Characteristics of skin lesions are diagnostic of the varicella infection and include maculopapular rashes, vesicles, and scabs in various stages. Rashes started over the trunk and face that rapidly speared to the limbs; they started as maculopapular lesions that evolved into vesicles. Rashes are polymorphic and of different ages as they appear in crops over 2–4 days. Immunocompromised individuals have a greater number of lesions and take longer duration to heal.

### Herpes Zoster

Herpes zoster results from reactivation of latent virus from the dorsal root ganglia. It is more common among elderly people over 60 years of age than among young people. It is characterized by unilateral dermatomal vesicular eruption. Vesicular eruptions are often associated with severe pain that may precede the lesion by 2–3 days. Though T3 to L3 dermatomes are commonly involved, they may also involve the other dermatomes and the cranial nerve. The involvement of the ophthalmic division of the trigeminal nerve causes herpes zoster ophthalmicus, and the involvement of the geniculate ganglion of the facial nerve causes Ramsay–Hunt syndrome. Though the vesicular rashes healed within a short time, many, especially the elderly, developed post-herpetic neuralgia in the involved dermatome. More server disease with longer duration of lesion and involvements of multiple dermatomes are common in immunocompromised host.

### Allergic Contact Dermatitis (Poison Ivy)

Allergic contact dermatitis is an inflammatory skin disease caused by a type-4 hypersensitivity reaction. The severity of the lesion depends on the sensitizing ability and concentration of the sensitizer. The pattern and location of the lesion indicate the offending agent. For example, vesicular lesions in poison ivy contact are grouped and in a linear streak, signifying the contact line.

## TREATMENT AND PREVENTION

### Herpes Simplex Viral

Oro-labial herpes—antiviral acyclovir, famciclovir, and valacyclovir are the mainstay of treatment; the duration of therapy is 5–10 days. Tropical acyclovir therapy can also be used and shown to fasten the healing. Acyclovir is the agent most frequently used and is available in IV, oral, and topical formulations. One day high dose famciclovir or valacyclovir can be used at the onset of the prodrome, and it has been shown to reduce pain and fasten healing.

Genital herpes—antiviral acyclovir, famciclovir or valacyclovir are effective and duration of treatment vary from 7 to 14 days.

### Varicella

Good hygiene and meticulous skin care prevent the secondary infection of the skin lesion. Pruritus can be reduced by topical dressing and applying antipruritic drugs. Antiviral acyclovir (800 mg five times a day), famciclovir (250 mg thrice daily), and valacyclovir (1 g thrice daily) for 5–7 days are used for chickenpox of 24 hours duration or less.

### Herpes Zoster

Acyclovir (800 mg five times a day for 7–10 days), famciclovir (500 mg thrice daily for 7 days), and valacyclovir (1 g thrice daily for 5–7 days). Along with antiviral therapy, oral steroid prednisolone 60 mg daily for 1 week followed by 30 mg for 1 week, then 15 mg for 1 week has been shown to improve pain and quality of life in cases of localized herpes zoster.

### Allergic Contact Dermatitis

Avoidance is essential in cases of allergic contact dermatitis. Topical steroids reduce the local inflammation, and anti-histaminics reduce the pruritus.

**Vesicular rashes**
*Detail history taking:* Duration, onset, whether first episodes or recurrent, pain, itching, history of travel, contact, sexual exposure, immune status of the patient

↓

**Detail clinical examination**
*Local examination:* Localized or generalized, grouped or discrete, vesicular or vesiculobullous, condition of the surrounding skin, base of the vesicle
*Systemic examination:*

| Generalized: • Chickenpox, Mpox, • Disseminated HSV | Localized with dermatomal involvement: Herpes zoster | Localized with dermatitis: Allergic contact dermatitis example—Poison ivy | Localized: Grouped without dermatomal involvement—Herpes simplex |
|---|---|---|---|

↓

*Investigations:*
- VZV: Detection of VZV DNA by PCR from lesions, blood or saliva; Tzanck smear; Serological test—FAMA, IAH, ELISA
- HSV: Tzanck smear preparation, detection of HSV DNA by PCR from scraping of lesion;
- *Serological* test—ELISA, radioimmunoassay, indirect immunofluorescence, passive hemagglutination
- Poison ivy: Mostly clinical diagnosis
- Mpox-detection of viral DNA by PCR

↓

*Treatment:*
- *Chickenpox:* Acyclovir, famciclovir or valacyclovir, care for skin rashes—proper hygiene to prevent secondary skin infection
- *Herpes zoster:* Acyclovir, famciclovir or valacyclovir; steroid in selected case
- *Herpes simplex virus:* Acyclovir, famciclovir or valacyclovir, topical antiviral
- *Poison ivy:* Avoidance to irritant. Topical steroid and antihistaminic to reduce pain and pruritus
- *Mpox:* Currently no specific treatment is approved for Mpox. Mostly supportive care and pain control

**FLOWCHART 1:** Clinical approach to a patient with vesicular rashes.

## Monkeypox

Currently, no specific treatment is approved for Mpox. Treatment is primarily supportive care and pain control.

## Vaccination

Vaccination against chickenpox is used for a long duration to prevent the primary varicella infection. Varicella-zoster vaccine is a live attenuated vaccine, and it is administered in two doses. Vaccines to prevent herpes zoster are also available. It is a recombinant vaccine indicated for adults aged 50 years or older and adults (18 years or above) if they are immunosuppressed. It is administered in two intramuscular doses 2–6 months apart. There is currently no licensed vaccine available for HSV-1 or HSV-2. Vaccination against monkeypox is recommended for the particular population at high risk of infection. The two FDA approved vaccines for Mpox are JYNNEOS [Modified Vaccinia Ankara-Bavarian Nordic (MVA-BN)] and ACAM2000.

# CLINICAL APPROACH

Based on the history and clinical examination, we can classify vesicular rashes. Proper detailed history taking helps us in early diagnosis, judicial use of investigation to confirm the diagnosis, and early initiation of specific treatment. The general approach to patients with vesicular rashes is shown in **Flowchart 1**.

### Points to Ponder

- *Onset and distribution of the vesicular rashes*: It gives us clue about the likely pathogen.
- *Detail history taking*: High risk behavior, high risk sexual exposure, travel history, history of contact many time put a patient on risk of acquiring particular disease.
- Many diseases present in a similar pattern of vesicular lesions, so laboratory confirmation is very important.
- Presence or absence of associated condition like atopic dermatitis, herald spot in rickettsialpox help in early diagnosis and judicial use of laboratory test.

# MULTIPLE CHOICE QUESTIONS

1. **The dose of valacyclovir in varicella is:**
   A. 1,000 mg thrice daily for 5–7 days
   B. 500 mg thrice daily for 5–7 days
   C. 250 mg thrice daily for 5–7 days
   D. 250 mg five times daily for 5–7 days
2. **Vesicular lesions in poison ivy are:**
   A. Discrete
   B. In linear group
   C. Respond to antiviral
   D. Nonpruritic
3. **Duration of oral prednisolone in localized herpes zoster is:**
   A. One week
   B. Two weeks
   C. Three weeks
   D. Four weeks
4. **Sensitivity of Tzanck smear to demonstrate multinucleated giant cells is:**
   A. 10%
   B. 20%
   C. 40%
   D. 60%
5. **The secondary attack rate in chickenpox among susceptible household is:**
   A. 10–20%
   B. 30–50%
   C. 50–70%
   D. 70–90%

## Answers

1. (A); 2. (B); 3. (C); 4. (D); 5. (D)

# SUGGESTED READINGS


1. Fernandez-Nieto D, Ortega-Quijano D, Jimenez-Cauhe J, et al. Clinical and histological characterization of vesicular COVID-19 rashes: a prospective study in a tertiary care hospital. Clin Exp Dermatol. 2020;45(7):872-75.
2. Arvin AM. Varicella-zoster virus. Clin Microbiol Rev. 1996;9(3): 361-81.
3. Miller GG, Dummer JS. Herpes simplex and varicella zoster viruses: forgotten but not gone. Am J Transplant. 2007;7(4):741-7.
4. Moore MJ, Rathish B, Zahra F. Mpox (Monkeypox) [Updated 2023 May 3]. In: StatPearls [Internet]. Treasure Island (FL): StatPearls Publishing; 2024. Available from: https://www.ncbi.nlm.nih.gov/books/NBK574519/
5. Emmert DH. Treatment of common cutaneous herpes simplex virus infections. Am Fam Physician. 2000;61(6):1697-706, 1708.
6. Andrei G, Snoeck R. Advances and Perspectives in the Management of Varicella-Zoster Virus Infections. Molecules. 2021;26(4):1132
7. World Health organization [Internet] WHO prequalifies the first vaccine against mpox. [cited 2024 Nov 15]; Available from: https://www.who.int/news/item/13-09-2024-who-prequalifies-the-first-vaccine-against-mpox#:~:text=Available%20data%20shows%20that%20a,effective%20than%20pre%2Dexposure%20vaccination.

CHAPTER

# 87

# An Approach to a Case of Maculopapular Rash

*Yasmee Khan, Manish Khandare*

**CASE VIGNETTE**

A 24-year-old male, hailing from Madhya Pradesh, unmarried, with no known comorbidities presented with history of fever of 5 days duration, of low grade with 1 day history of cephalocaudal progression of rash and history of similar illness among individual from the same office where he was working.

## PROVISIONAL DIAGNOSIS

Viral exanthem (rubella, infectious mononucleosis, measles).

## DIFFERENTIAL DIAGNOSIS

To analyse the differential diagnosis in a case of maculopapular rash, considering centrally and peripherally distribution of rash separately is helpful.

### Central Distribution of Maculopapular Rash (Figs. 1 and 2)

Centrally distributed maculopapular eruptions are more frequently observed than peripheral ones. These eruptions typically begin on the head and neck, spreading outward from there.

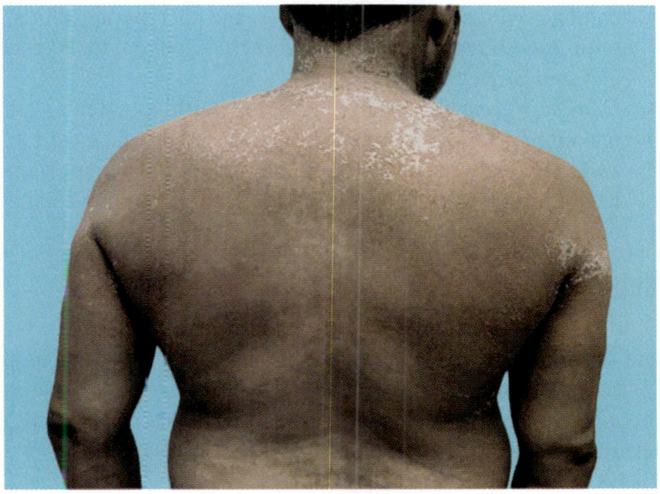

**FIG. 1:** Diffuse maculopapular rash of viral exanthem.

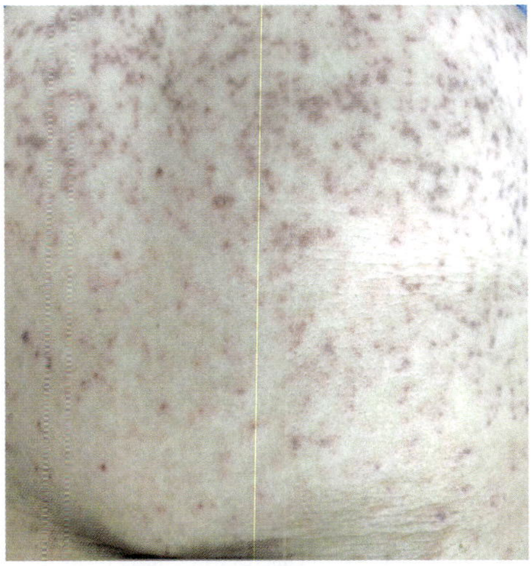

**FIG. 2:** Maculopapular rash due to drug with evidence of target.

### Viral Exanthems

Viral causes of rashes includes rubeola, rubella, erythema infectiosum, and roseola.

- *Rubeola*: The exanthem often appears around the fourth day of fever, starting with distinct lesions that merge as they spread downward from the hairline, while sparing the palms and soles. This rash usually persists for 4–6 days before fading in the order it appeared, often leaving behind a light yellow-brown discoloration or slight peeling. A unique sign of rubeola is Koplik's spots on the oral mucosa.
- *Rubella*: It resembles rubeola but tends to cause milder symptoms and has a shorter rash duration, generally lasting 2–3 days. Rubella presents with a mild fever, tender and swollen glands.
- *Erythema infectiosum or fifth disease*: It is caused by human parvovirus B19. While most commonly affecting children aged 3–12, it can also manifest as a rheumatic condition in adults. The initial symptoms may include fever, sore throat, anorexia, and abdominal pain. Following the resolution of fever, a characteristic bright red "slapped cheek" facial rash

appears, followed within days by a widespread, lacy rash that can persist intermittently for 6–8 weeks.

- *Roseola or exanthema subitum*: It is caused by human herpesvirus 6 and typically affects children under 3 years old. The rash is a pinkish-red, discrete maculopapular rash. The rash begins on the chest and trunk, then spreads to the face and limbs. It is nonconfluent and typically lasts around 2 days.
- *Infectious mononucleosis* **(*Fig. 3*)**: Infectious mononucleosis, caused by the Epstein–Barr virus, commonly presents with fever, tonsillitis, swollen lymph nodes, and hepatosplenomegaly. Upto 20% of children with mononucleosis may develop a pink maculopapular rash on chest and abdomen, often triggered by the use of beta-lactam antibiotics.
- *Enteroviruses*: Enterovirus infections generally present with fever and a pink rash that begins on the face and spreads to the trunk and limbs. The rash features small maculopapules and may include petechiae. These infections are more common in summer and can sometimes lead to aseptic meningitis.
- *Adenoviruses*: Adenovirus infections can lead to various reddish, maculopapular rashes, often accompanied by high fever. These infections may also cause tonsillitis, conjunctivitis, swollen lymph nodes, and pharyngotonsillitis, with blood tests sometimes showing leukocytosis and elevated C-reactive protein levels.
- *Dengue fever*: It usually presents with a macular or maculopapular rash that can appear on the face, chest, abdomen, and limbs, accompanied by itching. Patients often have a history of fever and recent travel to areas experiencing outbreaks of the disease.

## Scarlet Fever

Scarlet fever is characterized by fever, sore throat, vomiting, and tonsillitis, along with swollen cervical lymph nodes and a "strawberry" tongue. The red, rough-textured rash, which spares the area around the mouth, begins in skin folds and spreads, forming a confluent, red appearance. The rash lasts for about 2 days.

## Lyme Disease and Erythema Migrans

Lyme disease, is a vector-borne illness is caused by the spirochete *Borrelia burgdorferi*, transmitted through the bite of an *Ixodes* tick. In approximately 80% of Lyme disease cases, erythema migrans appears as a characteristic rash. This growing, red macular rash begins as a macule or papule at the site of the bite.

The rash commonly appears on the proximal extremities, within body folds, and on the chest. It expands gradually over days to weeks. In early Lyme disease, a painless bluish-red nodule or plaque called Borrelial lymphocytoma may form, typically appearing on the earlobe, nipple, or scrotum. Additional symptoms of Lyme disease can include fever, arthritis, headache, myalgias, neck stiffness, and regional lymphadenopathy.

## Drug-related Eruptions

Drug reactions can present in a variety of dermatologic patterns and occur regardless of age, gender, or race. Exanthematous eruptions are most often associated with penicillins or cephalosporins, NSAIDs, antimalarials and antiepileptic medications. The rash generally appears within the first week of starting the drug and resolves within a few days of discontinuing it. Although drug-related eruptions may be challenging to distinguish from viral exanthems, they tend to be more intensely erythematous and pruritic.

## Peripheral Distribution of Maculopapular Rash

### *Erythema Multiforme*

It is the most common maculopapular rash with a peripheral distribution. Erythema multiforme **(Fig. 4)** initially presents as a macular rash, with dull-red lesions that progress from macules to papules and often display the distinctive target-shaped appearance. Vesicles and bullae may form at the center of these papules, and in numerous cases, the oral mucous membranes are also affected.

The severity of erythema multiforme determines its classification as either minor or major. In erythema multiforme minor, systemic symptoms are absent, and the rash typically appears on the extensor surfaces of the limbs, rarely involving the mucous membranes.

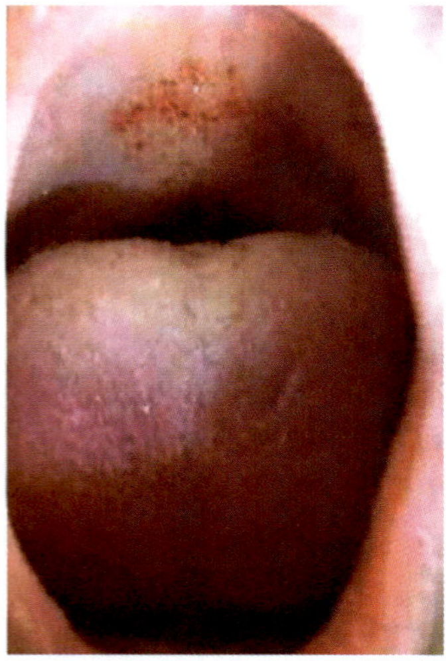

**FIG. 3:** Forchheimer spots in a case of infectious mononucleosis.

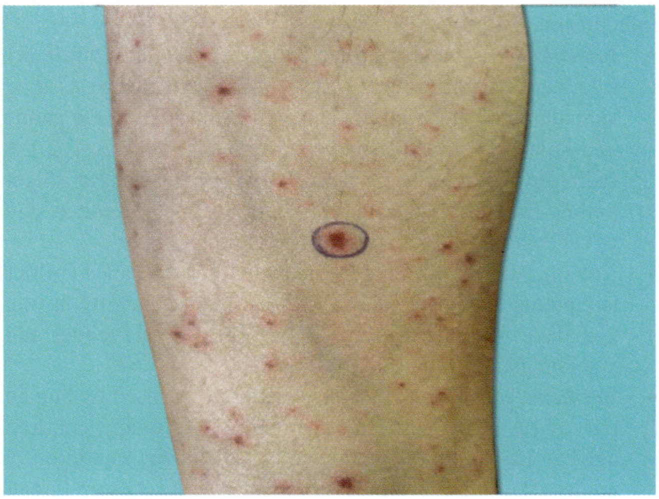

**FIG. 4:** Target lesion in a case of erythema multiforme.

Erythema multiforme major is commonly triggered by a drug reaction, always involving the mucous membranes and frequently presenting with target/targetoid lesions and systemic symptoms such as fever and prostration. Oral intake may be challenging due to cheilitis and stomatitis, and urination may be painful due to balanitis or vulvitis. Severe conjunctivitis can lead to keratitis and ulceration, and lesions may be present in the pharynx, larynx, and trachea.

### Secondary Syphilis

In secondary syphilis, the rash may be widespread, commonly appearing on the head, neck, palms, and soles. These lesions are usually brownish-red or pink macules and papules, but they may also be papulosquamous, pustular, or acneiform. The rash generally appears between 2 and 6 months after the primary infection and 2–10 weeks after the initial chancre.

Individuals present with general symptoms, and symptomless flat-topped macules and papules (mucous patches) are frequently found on the oral and genital mucosa. Typical condyloma lata lesions may be observed in the perineal area.

### Other Conditions

Serious infections such as meningococcemia, Rocky Mountain spotted fever, and dengue fever can initially manifest with erythematous maculopapular lesions that may progress to a petechial exanthem.

## CLINICAL APPROACH

- *History*: As we know history plays a pivotal role in reaching the diagnosis. The relevant history which needs to be consider in a patient with maculopapular rash:
  - Day of onset of rash: Timing of onset of rash. Relation of onset with other symptoms such as fever.
  - Distribution of rash: Has it been spreading or evolving? Is it cephalocaudal spread or centripetal spread or centrifugal in distribution.
  - Associated symptoms: Fever, cough, sore throat, joint pain, malaise, pruritus, or other systemic symptoms.
  - Medications: Drug rash is one of the most common cause of maculopapular rash. History of recent introduction of any drugs (e.g., antibiotics, anticonvulsants, or NSAIDs) is must.
  - Exposure history: Travel history, contact with sick individuals, vaccination status, insect bites, new medications, or known allergies.
  - Past medical history: Any underlying conditions (e.g., immunocompromised states, autoimmune diseases), history similar skin lesions in the past
- *Physical examination*:
  - The approach in examining the case of maculopapular disorder is first and foremost, general examination followed by systemic examination and then dermatological examination that includes examination of the skin, mucous membranes which include oral, ocular, nasal mucosa, and genital mucosa.
  - Pattern and distribution of rash: Is the rash generalized or localized? Is it predominantly on the trunk, face, or extremities? Does it spare certain areas like palms, soles, or mucosal surfaces?
    - Characteristics of rash: Is the rash blanchable or nonblanchable? Does it involve mucous membranes (e.g., oral cavity, conjunctiva).
    - Presence of systemic signs: Fever, lymphadenopathy, or other constitutional symptoms.
    - Examine for any other findings: Enlarged lymph nodes, signs of systemic infection, or joint involvement.

## TREATMENT AND PREVENTION

### Investigations

- *Complete blood count (CBC)*: For signs of infection (e.g., leukocytosis, lymphopenia).
- *Liver function tests (LFTs) and renal function tests (RFTs)*: To assess for systemic involvement (e.g., SLE, DRESS).
- *Erythrocyte sedimentation rate (ESR) and C-reactive protein (CRP)*: Indicators of inflammation.
- *Serologic tests*: For suspected viral causes (e.g., measles, rubella, parvovirus B19, enterovirus).
- *Culture and PCR*: For specific pathogens (e.g., Group A *Streptococcus*, HHV-6).
- *Skin biopsy*: In cases where the etiology is unclear or there is a concern for systemic disease.

### Management

- *Supportive care*: Hydration, antipyretics (acetaminophen or ibuprofen), and symptom management (e.g., antihistamines for itching).
- *Specific treatment*:
  - Antiviral therapy: For specific viral infections (e.g., acyclovir for varicella, HHV-6).
  - Antibiotics: If bacterial infection (e.g., penicillin for scarlet fever).
  - Corticosteroids: In autoimmune conditions or severe drug reactions.
- *Avoidance of causative agents*: If a drug reaction is suspected, the offending drug should be discontinued, and alternative treatments should be considered.

## PATHOPHYSIOLOGY

The pathophysiology of a maculopapulapupular rash depend on the specific etiologies of the rash. For example in case of drug reaction, drugs or their metabolites will act as haptens and become antigenic. Haptenated proteins bind to major histocompatibility complex (MHC) molecules. The hapten-peptide-MHC molecule complexes are then presented to T cells which together with other costimulatory factors may activate and expand drug-reactive T cells (both CD4 and CD8) leading to type IV hypersensitivity reaction.

## Points to Ponder

- Detailed patient history to assess the onset of rash, associated symptoms, recent infections, medications, travel and vaccination history.
- Rash characteristics in form of morphology, distribution, symmetry plays a crucial role to narrow down the differential diagnosis.
- Viral exanthems and drug rash are the most common causes of maculopapular rash.
- Look for systemic signs such as fever, joint pain, or organ-specific symptoms, which may suggest a systemic infection or autoimmune condition.

## MULTIPLE CHOICE QUESTIONS

1. **Which of the following is a common cause of erythema infectiosum?**
   A. Human parvovirus B19
   B. Epstein–Barr virus
   C. Human herpesvirus 6
   D. Cytomegalovirus
2. **Which distinguishing feature is characteristic of erythema multiforme?**
   A. "Slapped cheek" appearance
   B. Target-shaped lesions
   C. Diffuse scaling
   D. Vesicles on the palms and soles
3. **Which of the following conditions is most commonly associated with a maculopapular rash that spares the face and appears after high fever resolves?**
   A. Roseola
   B. Rubeola
   C. Rubella
   D. Erythema infectiosum
4. **Which feature best distinguishes a viral exanthem from a drug-induced rash in many cases?**
   A. Erythema on the face
   B. Itching
   C. Rash onset relative to fever
   D. Rash confined to the trunk
5. **What is the recommended management step for a maculopapular rash suspected to be drug-related?**
   A. Start high-dose corticosteroids
   B. Discontinue the suspected medication
   C. Prescribe antiviral medication
   D. Wait for symptoms to subside on their own

### Answers

1. (A); 2. (B); 3. (A); 4. (C); 5. (B)

## SUGGESTED READINGS

1. Kaye ET, Kaye KM. Fever and rash. In: Fauci AS, et al., eds. Harrison's Principles of internal medicine. 14th ed. New York: McGraw-Hill, Health Professions Division, 1998.
2. Weber DI, Cohen MS, Fine JD. The acutely ill patient with fever and rash. In: Mandell GL, Bennett JE, Dolin R, eds. Mandell, Douglas, and Bennett's Principles and practice of infectious diseases. 5th ed. Philadelphia: Churchill Livingstone, 1999:633-50.
3. Fitzpatrick TB. Color atlas and synopsis of clinical dermatology: common and serious diseases. 3d ed. New York: McGraw-Hill, Health Professions Division, 1997.
4. American Pharmaceutical Association. Infectious diseases handbook: including antimicrobial therapy & diagnostic tests/procedures. 2d ed. Hudson, Ohio: Lexi-Comp; 1996.
5. Nelson WE, Behrman RE, Kliegman RM, Arvin AM, eds. Nelson Textbook of pediatrics. 15th ed. Philadelphia: Saunders, 1996.
6. Edlow JA. Lyme disease and related tick-borne illnesses. Ann Emerg Med. 1999;33:680-93.
7. Schlossberg D. Fever and rash. Infect Dis Clin North Am. 1996;10:101-10.

CHAPTER

# 88

# An Approach to a Case of Purpura

*Taranpreet Kour, Ritu, Kirandeep Kour*

**CASE VIGNETTE**

A 21-year-old male came to OPD with the complaints of rash on his arms and legs for last 15 days. Rash was associated with itching over the lesions. There was no history of preceding trauma, fever, pain abdomen, loose stools, vomiting, oral ulcers, bleeding from any site, joint pains, loss of appetite or loss of weight. There was no history of similar complaints in the past. Patient was a college student with no history of addictions. The family history was not significant.

On examination, he was a thin lean man with BMI of 16 kg/m$^2$. The patient was found to have palpable purpura on his arms and legs. Patient was admitted for further evaluation.

His investigations revealed Hb of 13.4 g%, TLC: 6,500 cells/mm$^3$ with 65% polymorphs, 30% lymphocytes, 3% monocytes and 2% eosinophils, platelet count: 2.5 lakh/mm$^3$. ESR was raised 55 mm. His kidney and liver function tests were normal. His HbA1c was 5.4%, FBS of 98 mg/dL. Viral markers were negative, and his ANA also came out to be negative. Punch skin biopsy was taken which revealed leucocytoclastic vasculitis.

## PROVISIONAL DIAGNOSIS

- Viral exanthem
- Thrombocytopenic purpura
- Drug induced
- Sepsis/DIC
- Henoch–Schönlein purpura
- Connective tissue disorder
- Cryoglobulinemia
- Cutaneous small vessel vasculitis

Let's take a look at the possibilities of the above-mentioned provisional diagnosis:

- *Viral exanthem*: Skin lesions (petechiae, purpura) are mostly generalized all over the body and sometimes, e.g., parvovirus infection can be acral in location. Absence of history of fever, arthralgias or myalgias rules out viral exanthem as cause of purpura.
- *Thrombocytopenic purpura*: Petechiae and purpura are mostly macular and non-blanching in thrombocytopenia and are either widespread in distribution or can be seen only in the dependent location like legs and buttocks. Normal platelet count on CBC rules out this option.
- *Drug induced*: Patients with Stevens-Johnson syndrome can have widespread purpuric lesions, but the absence of history of any drug taken in past rules out this.
- *Sepsis/disseminated intravascular coagulation (DIC)*: Patients will generally present with retiform purpura along with multiorgan dysfunction and coagulopathy.
- *Henoch–Schönlein purpura*: Also called as IgA vasculitis. It is more common among children than adults and is associated with extracutaneous features like abdominal pain, gastrointestinal bleeding, arthralgias and hematuria.
- *Connective tissue disorder*: Absence of history of constitutional symptoms, musculoskeletal manifestations like arthralgias, arthritis rules out this
- *Cryoglobulinemia*: In cryoglobulinemia, the lesions are usually involving ears, nose as well as hands and feet and are typically triggered by cold exposure.
- *Cutaneous small vessel vasculitis*: Typically, the rash involves dependent areas and the area of tight clothing.

## DIFFERENTIAL DIAGNOSIS

After the report of biopsy came out, the diagnosis of cutaneous small vessel vasculitis was made. Cutaneous small vessel vasculitis is idiopathic in 50% of cases and is typically limited to the skin with no systemic involvement. It can also be secondary to infections, autoimmune, or malignancies.

## CLINICAL APPROACH

Purpura is the red discoloration of skin due to hemorrhage into skin or mucus membranes. Purpuric lesions constitute an important examination finding which should never be missed as they can be present in a variety of infectious and noninfectious causes as well.

Purpuric lesions are mostly nonblanchable.

It can be categorized on the basis of size and morphology as: Macular purpura, palpable purpura, and retiform purpura.

Macular purpura—superficial, flat, cutaneous lesions and are further classified on basis of size as:
- Petechiae: < 5 mm in size **(Fig. 1A)**
- Macular purpura: 5–9 mm in size **(Fig. 1A)**
- Macular ecchymoses: ≥1 cm in size **(Fig. 1B)**

Palpable purpura are raised, round, erythematous or purplish lesions that are partially blanchable.

Retiform lesions usually denotes microvascular occlusion of relatively large vessels in dermis and subcutis and typically have a lace-like pattern. They are further classified as:
- Noninflammatory retiform purpura **(Fig. 1D)** and inflammatory retiform purpura.

**Flowchart 1** depicts the algorithm to approach a case of purpura.

## ETIOLOGY OF PURPURA

The underlying mechanisms which can result in purpura can be:
- Increased fragility of blood vessels that can be due to infections, vasculitis, collagen disorders.
- Platelet deficiency or dysfunction
- Derangement in clotting mechanism

The size and location of vessels involved, the extent of hemorrhage and the coagulation status of the patient determine the clinical appearance of the purpuric lesions. So, it becomes pertinent to delineate the morphology of purpura to determine the etiology of purpura.

*Petechiae or macular nonpalpable purpura (< 1 cm)*:
- Thrombocytopenia, abnormal platelet function, increased intravascular pressure, pigmented purpuric dermatosis (also known as Schamberg's disease), and cutaneous small vessel vasculitis.

*Ecchymosis*:
- Coagulation defect like hemophilia, liver disease, anticoagulants or vitamin K deficiency.
- Decreased support of dermal vessels like in actinic (solar) damage, amyloidosis, vitamin C deficiency or due to prolonged use of steroids.
- Collagen vascular disorders like Ehlers–Danlos syndrome.

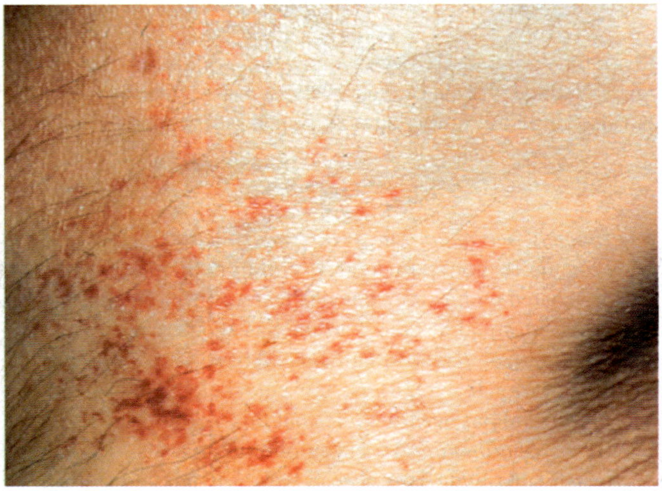

**FIG. 1A:** Macular petechiae and purpura.

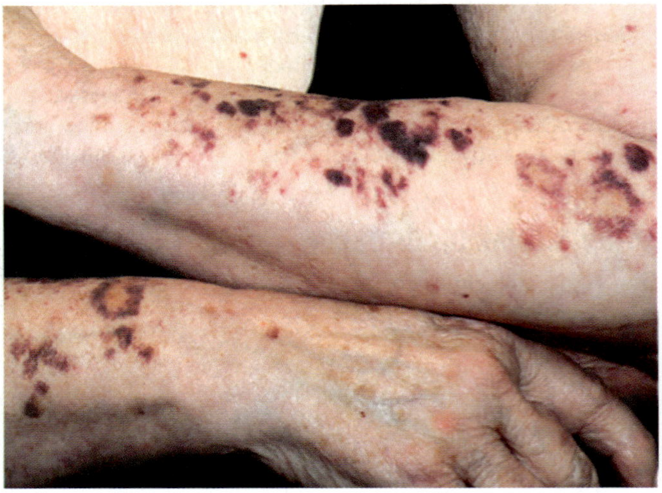

**FIG. 1B.** Macular ecchymoses.

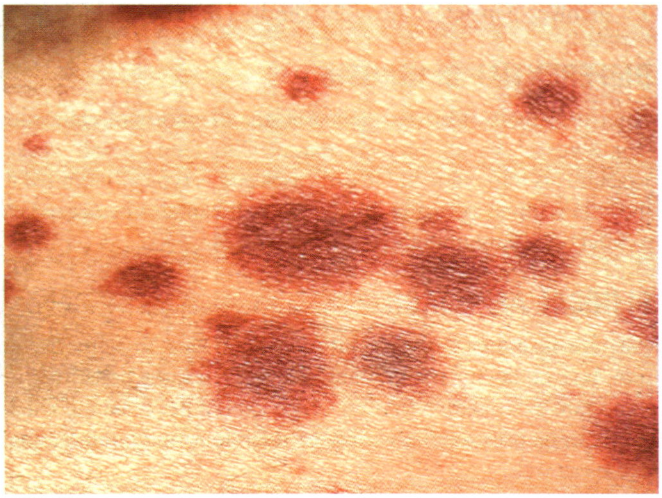

**FIG. 1C:** Palpable retiform purpura.

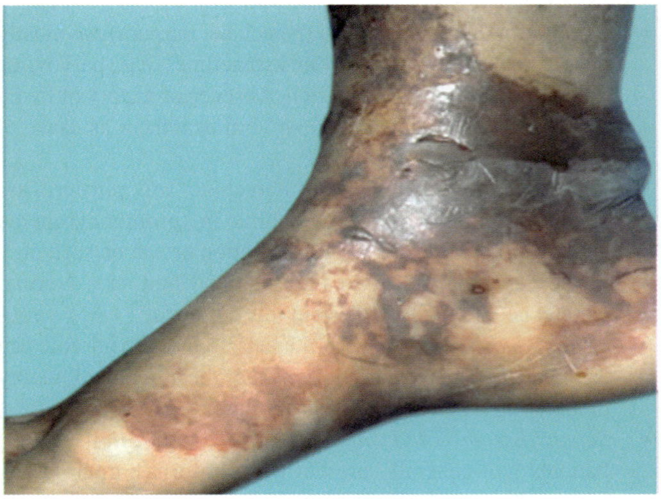

**FIG. 1D:** Noninflammatory retiform purpura.

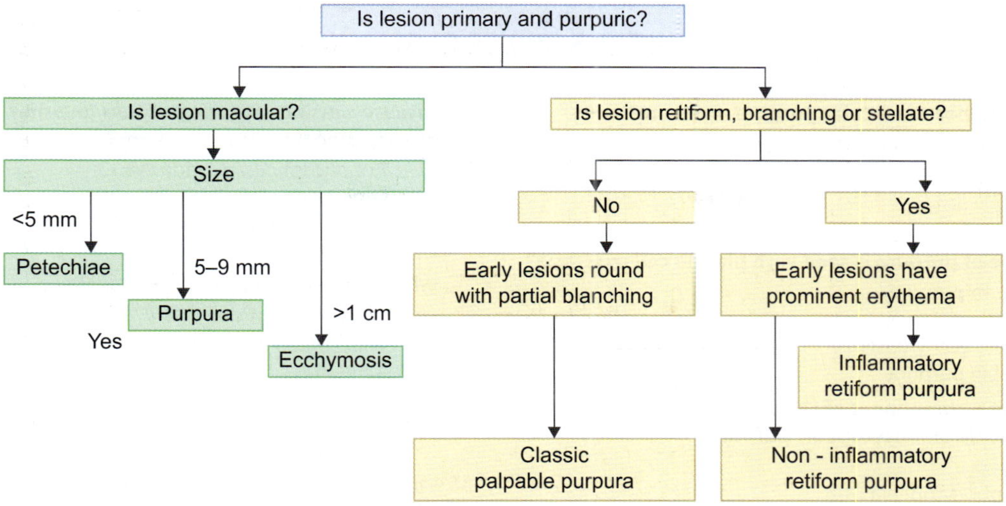


**FLOWCHART 1:** Algorithm to approach a case of purpura.

*Palpable purpura*:
- *Vasculitis (small vessel)*: Hypersensitivity vasculitis, IgA vasculitis, cryoglobulinemia, ANCA associated vasculitis, connective tissue disease associated or erythema multiforme

*Retiform purpura* ***(Fig. 1C)***:
- *Inflammatory:* IgA vasculitis, ANCA associated vasculitis, and connective tissue disease associated
- *Noninflammatory (microvascular occlusion)*: Cryoglobulinemia, antiphospholipid antibody syndrome, calciphylaxis, warfarin necrosis, DIC, hypercoagulable state, embolic condition, angioinvasive infection, and cocaine abuse.

## PATHOPHYSIOLOGY

Purpura results from hemorrhage into the skin as a result of trauma to blood vessel.

Depending on the lesion's age, all purpuric lesions undergo comparable color variations. They start off deep crimson or bright red, turn purple as the heme pigments degrade, then turn green and yellow-brown before fading. The quantity of extravasated blood determines how long it will take to fade. Simple blood extravasation into the skin with minimal inflammation causes petechiae, macular purpura, and ecchymoses, which are categorized as macular or flat purpura. Immune complexes that are deposited on the vessel lumen typically cause vasculitis because they draw neutrophils, which break down the complexes and damage the vessel wall. Occlusion of bigger, slow-flowing arteries causes retiform purpura, while vasculitis causes inflammatory retiform purpura.

## TREATMENT AND PREVENTION

Treatment of purpura consists of treating the underlying cause of purpura. If the purpura is due to infectious cause, then treatment of underlying condition can heal the purpura.

In case of purpura resulting from immune mediated thrombocytopenia, treatment includes corticosteroids, IV immunoglobulins, immunosuppressants, thrombopoietin receptor agonist, and splenectomy. In case of purpura resulting from vasculitis, treatment includes corticosteroids, and immunosuppressants.

### Prevention

It is not possible to prevent the purpura because there are underlying health conditions responsible for it. Preventive measures are helpful in certain types of purpura like actinic purpura that result from sun exposure. In such conditions, using sunscreens in the sun exposed areas can help protect against the purpura development.

### Points to Ponder

- Purpura is reddish discoloration of skin due to hemorrhage into skin.
- Purpuric lesions on skin can be petechiae, macular purpura, ecchymoses, palpable purpura, inflammatory and noninflammatory retiform purpura.
- Purpura can result from infectious, drug induced, inflammatory, malignancies or hematological causes.
- It is important to look for systemic involvement whenever encountering a patient of purpura.
- Punch biopsy of the purpuric lesions is seldom required and only indicated when there is no systemic symptoms and signs suggestive of the underlying disease.

## MULTIPLE CHOICE QUESTIONS

1. **How many types of macular purpura are there?**
   A. 2
   B. 4
   C. 3
   D. 6
2. **Which type of purpura is seen with plasma cell dyscrasia?**
   A. Retiform purpura
   B. Petechiae
   C. Macular ecchymosis
   D. Palpable purpura
3. **What is not a component of the pentad seen in thrombotic thrombocytopenic purpura?**
   A. Fever
   B. Thrombocytopenia
   C. Purpura
   D. Renal dysfunction
4. **Disease causing retiform purpura favoring acral sites and precipitated by cold?**
   A. Antiphospholipid syndrome
   B. Type 1 cryoglobulinemia
   C. Waldenstrom macroglobulinemia
   D. Livedoid vasculopathy
5. **What is the distribution of skin lesions in cutaneous small vessel vasculitis?**
   A. Widespread distribution
   B. Acral sites
   C. Dependent region
   D. Pauci random distribution

### Answers

1. (C); 2. (A); 3. (C); 4. (B); 5. (C)

## SUGGESTED READINGS

1. Arakaki R, Fox L. Updates in the Approach to the Patient with Purpura. Curr Dermatol Rep. 2017;6:55-62.
2. Charrot SC, Sellar RS, Manson JJ. Purpura. Br J Hosp Med. 2017;78(10):C147-51.
3. Chatterjee M, Hemdani R. Approach to purpura. In Dermatological Emergencies. CRC Press. 2019. pp. 315-25.
4. Georgesen C, Fox LP, Harp J. Retiform purpura: a diagnostic approach. J Am Acad Dermatol. 2020;82(4):783-96.
5. Alexandrescu DT, Levi M. The Vascular Purpuras. In: Kaushansky K, Lichtman MA, Prchal JT, Levi MM, Press OW, Burns LJ, Caligiuri M. eds. Williams Hematology, 9th edition. McGraw-Hill Education; 2015.
6. Alpsoy E. Cutaneous vasculitis; An algorithmic approach to diagnosis. Front Med. 2022;9:1012554.
7. Stevens GL, Adelman HM. Palpable purpura: An algorithmic approach. Am Fam Physician. 1995;52(5).
8. Charrot SC, Sellar RS, Manson JJ. Purpura. Br J Hosp Med. 2017;78(10):C147-51.

CHAPTER 89

# An Approach to a Case of Livedo Reticularis

*Ritasman Baisya, Sukdev Manna*

## CASE VIGNETTE

A 25-year-old female presented to the rheumatology outpatient department with a new purple reticular rash on both legs **(Fig. 1)** extending from the mid-leg to the foot. She had a history of recurrent oral ulcers, arthritis, and malar rash. She also experienced two spontaneous second-trimester abortions. On examination, she had a violaceous mottling net-like rash over both legs. A few areas were like broken circles. Investigation showed anemia, leukopenia, a positive antinuclear antibody (ANA) by indirect immunofluorescence, low complement levels, and strongly positive anti-cardiolipin antibodies (IgG).

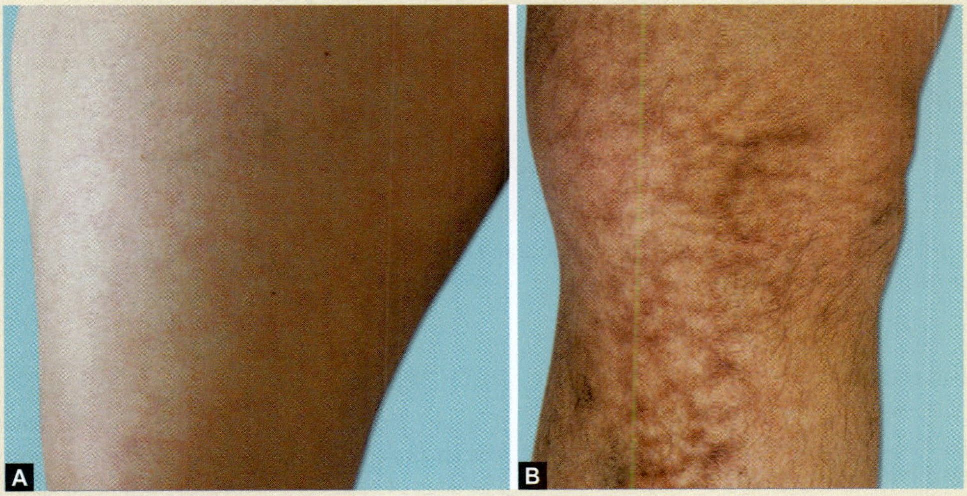


**FIGS. 1A AND B:** (A) Livedo reticularis and (B) livedo racemosa.

*Source*: Adapted from Larché MJ, Lee WH, et al. Livedo Reticularis. McMaster Textbook of Internal Medicine.

## PROVISIONAL DIAGNOSIS

She was diagnosed with systemic lupus erythematosus (SLE) with secondary anti-phospholipid syndrome (APS) with livedo reticularis and livedo racemosa type of skin rash.

## DIFFERENTIAL DIAGNOSIS

The differential diagnosis of the rash includes:

- Livedo reticularis
- Livedo racemosa
- Livedoid vasculopathy
- Erythema ab igne
- Erythema nodosum

The differential diagnosis for the etiology of LR rash is listed in **Table 1**.

## CLINICAL APPROACH

Hebra introduced the term livedo reticularis (LR) to describe a violaceous net-like rash linked to local circulation abnormalities. LR is characterized by a blotchy, reddish-blue to violaceous net-like pattern that encircles a pallor central core. It can occur as a congenital anomaly called cutis marmorata telangiectasia congenital, marked by general LR rash, telangiectasia, and superficial ulceration. LR can also have acquired causes, either idiopathic or associated with diseases. Diagnosis requires

**TABLE 1: Acquired causes of LR.**

| Idiopathic | Isolated, cold-induced arteriolar spasm |
|---|---|
| Disease associated | • *Vessel wall inflammation*:<br>○ Primary systemic vasculitis (PAN, EGPA, and GPA)<br>○ CTD-associated vasculitis (SLE, RA, and dermatomyositis)<br>○ Infectious vasculitis (Lucio phenomenon)<br>• *Intravascular obstruction without inflammation*:<br>○ Thrombosis: APS, Sneddon syndrome, DIC, procoagulant state, cryoglobulinemia<br>○ Embolism: Atrial myxoma, cholesterol emboli<br>○ Vessel wall disease: Calciphylaxis, hyperoxaluria<br>○ Livedoid vasculopathy: LR with painful purpuric lesion seen in malignancy, occasionally SLE/scleroderma<br>• *Pharmacological*: Ergotamine, amantadine, intra-arterial bismuth, quinidine<br>• *Infection*: Tuberculosis, infective endocarditis, meningococcemia, typhus fever, Lucio phenomenon<br>• *Endocrine*: Hypothyroid, pseudohypoparathyroidism, Cushing syndrome<br>• *Miscellaneous*: Cardiac failure, lymphoma, acute pancreatitis |

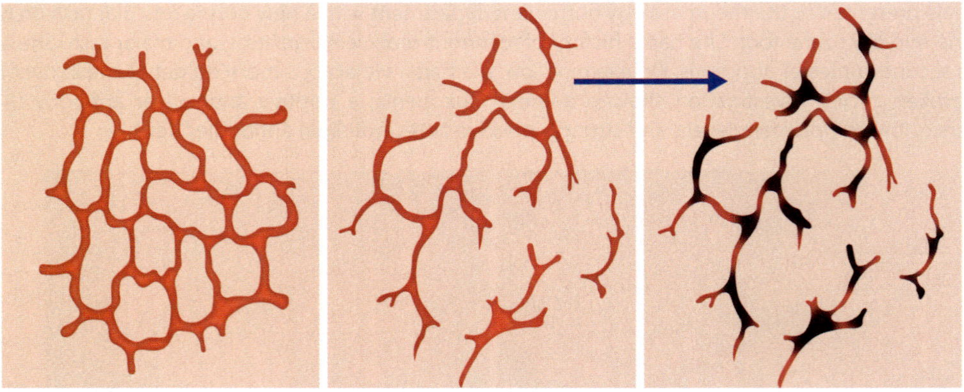

**FIG. 2:** Shows the spectrum of LR, livedo racemosa and retiform purpura.
*Source*: Adapted from Herrero C et al. (2008).

looking for subcutaneous nodules, retiform purpura, necrosis, and ulceration. Some authors differentiate between LR, with complete regular rings, and livedo racemosa **(Fig. 2)**, with incomplete irregular rings. Livedoid vasculopathy is characterized by LR with painful purpuric, necrotic lesions having stellate margins mainly in the malleolar region, healed with atrophic scar (atrophic blanche), has been found in association with carcinomas, lymphoma, myeloma, and occasionally autoimmune diseases like SLE or scleroderma.

A thorough medical history is essential, including information on medications, associated diseases (like renal failure, atherosclerosis, systemic autoimmune disorders), recent surgeries (catheterization, angioplasty), and the history of spontaneous abortion (APS). It's also essential to assess the disease course (chronic, acute, or fulminant), associated symptoms (like fever, shortness of breath, joint pain, rash). Fever may indicate an infection or a severe inflammatory process, such as an exacerbation of SLE **(Flowchart 1)**. A brief laboratory investigation is listed in the flow diagram. For cases of LR with purpura, necrosis, or nodules, a skin biopsy should be performed from affected areas, ensuring it captures the full thickness of the skin down to the hypodermis—a detailed overview of the approach in the flow diagram.

## PATHOPHYSIOLOGY

Renault, Unna, and Spalteholz proposed that the cutaneous vasculature consists of a series of cones measuring 1–3 cm in size. The apex of each cone is located deep in the dermis at the site of an ascending arteriole. According to their model, the density of the arterial bed decreases at the margins of each cone while the superficial venous plexus becomes more prominent. Therefore, any physiological or pathological condition that impedes blood flow to the skin could lead to increased deoxygenated hemoglobin, resulting in a prominent livid coloration, particularly in the predominantly venous areas at the edges of the cones **(Fig. 3)**. Additionally, vessel wall inflammation or intravascular obstruction can reduce blood flow and lead to LR.

A reduction in blood flow through the arterioles can lead to localized responses, while a complete blockage of blood flow can result in hemorrhagic infarcts. Initially, infarcted areas may appear as reticular purpuric lesions or retiform purpura **(Fig. 2)**. Over time, these lesions can become more ecchymotic and may develop into extensive necrosis and secondary ulceration areas

## TREATMENT AND PREVENTION

Systemic vasculitis is treated with corticosteroids and immunosuppressants, with specific doses depending on the

Violaceous retiform mottling rash, suspected livedo reticularis

↓

History:
- Onset and progression, distribution of rash, associated skin changes (nodules, purpura, necrosis)
- Associated symptoms (fever, dyspnea, rash, arthritis, neurological symptoms), recent surgeries (catheterization, angioplasty), pregnancy history
- Medication, comorbidity (CKD, dialysis, diabetes, hypothyroid), addiction (smoking, alcoholism)

↓

Examination:
- Detailed skin examination: Livedo reticularis, livedo racemosa, retiform purpura, livedoid vasculopathy, subcutaneous nodule, cutaneous necrosis, heart murmurs, neck stiffness, vascular bruit, blood pressure, tender or swollen joint, neurological and other systemic examination

↓

Investigation:
- Complete blood count, lipid profile, coagulation studies, kidney function, urinary examination, antinuclear antibodies (ANA), complement levels, ANCAs, cryoglobulin, cryo fibrinogen, antiphospholipid antibodies, and hepatitis B and C serology
- Coagulation factor analysis: Protein C, S levels, factor V Leiden mutations, prothrombin gene mutations, homocysteine levels
- Skin biopsy, nerve biopsy

**FLOWCHART 1:** Depicting clinical approach to livedo reticularis (LR).

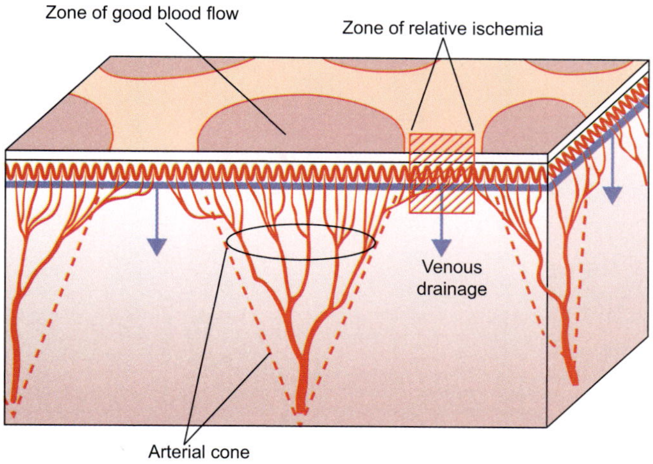


**FIG. 3:** Cone model of LR.

*Source*: Adapted from Copeman BWM. British J Dermatology, 1975.

patient's condition and organ involvement. There are no effective treatments for generalized LR in antiphospholipid or Sneddon syndrome. Skin lesions from thrombosis can be managed with low-dose aspirin or antiplatelet therapy, and some cases may need vitamin K antagonists. Hydroxychloroquine is used for LR in APS. Danazol or stanozolol is prescribed for cryofibrinogenemia. Coumarins or low molecular weight heparin may be necessary for specific hypercoagulable states. Patients with methylenetetrahydrofolate reductase mutations should take folic acid. Patients with plasminogen activator inhibitor abnormalities may benefit from intravenous tissue plasminogen activator.

It's essential to educate patients with livedoid vasculitis or thrombophilia about the importance of quitting smoking or using nicotine substitutes as preventive measures. This aspect of patient care is crucial in managing their condition and preventing further complications.

## Points to Ponder

- LR, a violaceous net-like blotch rash, is usually a common dermatological manifestation of many systemic diseases.
- The presence of LR mandates detailed workup in the line of connective tissue disorders, especially SLE, vasculopathy like APS, and systemic vasculitis like PAN.
- Do not forget to take medication history.
- Treatment depends on the underlying diagnosis and extent of internal organ involvement.

## MULTIPLE CHOICE QUESTIONS

**1. Which of the following is not commonly associated with LR?**

A. APS
B. PAN
C. Cholesterol embolism
D. Ankylosing spondylitis

**2. Which feature(s) characterize(s) LR rash?**

A. Blotchy
B. Purple-blue
C. Network pattern
D. All of the above

3. **Livedoid vasculopathy is mainly caused by which of the following:**
   A. Vessel wall inflammation
   B. Vessel occlusion by thrombosis
   C. Vessel spasm
   D. Infection

4. **Which of the following drugs is a cause of LR?**
   A. Ergotamine
   B. Amantadine
   C. Quinidine
   D. All of the above

5. **Match the following**

| | |
|---|---|
| I. Livedo reticularis | A. Network pattern with incomplete, irregular rings) |
| II. Livedo racemosa | B. Painful purpuric necrotic lesion at malleolus healed with arophic scar |
| III. Retiform purpura | C. Network pattern with complete, regular rings |
| IV. Livedoid vasculopathy | D. Hemorrhagic infarction |

## Answers

1. (D); 2. (D); 3. (B); 4. (D); 5. (I – C, II – A, III – D, IV – B)

## SUGGESTED READINGS

1. Herrero C, Guilabert A, Mascaró-Galy JM. Livedo reticularis de las piernas: metodología de diagnóstico y tratamiento [Diagnosis and treatment of livedo reticularis on the legs]. Actas Dermosifiliogr. 2008;99(8):598-607.
2. Sajjan VV, Lunge S, Swamy MB, et al. Livedo reticularis: A review of the literature. Indian Dermatol Online J. 2015;6(5):315-21.
3. Fleischer AB Jr, Resnick SD. Livedo reticularis. Dermatol Clin. 1990;8(2):347-54.

CHAPTER
90

# An Approach to a Case of Asymptomatic Transaminitis

*Subhendu Jana*

**CASE VIGNETTE**

A 38-year-old male presents for a routine health check-up. He is asymptomatic and has no significant medical history. Laboratory investigations reveal elevated alanine transaminase (ALT) and aspartate transaminase (AST) levels (ALT: 85 U/L, AST: 72 U/L), with a normal bilirubin and alkaline phosphatase. His BMI is 32 kg/m$^2$, and he reports occasional alcohol consumption. Further history reveals no use of hepatotoxic medications, herbal supplements, or intravenous drug use. Viral hepatitis serologies (HBsAg, anti-HCV) are negative, and ultrasound abdomen shows mild hepatic steatosis without hepatomegaly or structural abnormalities.

### Key Considerations Include

- Excluding common causes such as nonalcoholic fatty liver disease (NAFLD), alcohol-related liver disease, and chronic viral hepatitis.
- Investigating less common etiologies like autoimmune hepatitis, hemochromatosis, or Wilson's disease based on clinical and biochemical clues.
- Lifestyle modification as the cornerstone of management in NAFLD with follow-up liver function tests to monitor trends in transaminase levels.

## PROVISIONAL DIAGNOSIS

Asymptomatic transaminitis, likely secondary to nonalcoholic fatty liver disease (NAFLD).

## DIFFERENTIAL DIAGNOSIS

- *Nonalcoholic fatty liver disease (NAFLD)*: Associated with obesity, diabetes, or metabolic syndrome.
- *Alcohol-related liver disease*: History of excessive alcohol consumption.
- *Viral hepatitis*: Chronic HBV or HCV infection.
- *Autoimmune hepatitis*: Unexplained transaminitis, positive ANA, or anti-SMA.
- *Hemochromatosis*: Genetic predisposition with iron overload.
- *Wilson's disease*: Copper accumulation, especially in young patients.
- *Medication-induced liver injury*: Recent drug or herbal supplement use.

## CLINICAL APPROACH

- *History and examination*:
  - Assess alcohol intake, medications, family history, metabolic risk factors.
  - Look for systemic signs like jaundice, hepatomegaly, or stigmata of chronic liver disease.
- *Laboratory workup*:
  - Liver function tests (LFTs), viral hepatitis serology, autoimmune markers (ANA, SMA).
  - Ferritin, transferrin saturation, ceruloplasmin levels if hereditary causes suspected.
- *Imaging studies*: Ultrasound abdomen to evaluate steatosis or structural abnormalities.
- *Liver biopsy (if indicated)*: Consider in unclear cases or if fibrosis is suspected.

## PATHOPHYSIOLOGY

Transaminitis reflects hepatocellular injury due to various insults. In NAFLD, it arises from fat accumulation in hepatocytes leading to oxidative stress, inflammation, and hepatocyte apoptosis. Over time, this may progress to fibrosis or cirrhosis if untreated.

## TREATMENT AND PREVENTION

### Treatment

- *Lifestyle modifications*: Weight loss through diet and exercise (5–10% of body weight).

- *Medical management*: Optimize control of diabetes, dyslipidemia, and hypertension. Consider vitamin E or pioglitazone in selected NAFLD cases.
- *Avoid hepatotoxins*: Stop alcohol and hepatotoxic drugs.

## Prevention

- Maintain a healthy weight and balanced diet.
- Regular exercise and avoidance of excess alcohol.
- Monitor high-risk individuals (e.g., obese or diabetic) with periodic liver function tests.

### Points to Ponder

- Always rule out common and reversible causes of transaminitis, such as alcohol use or viral hepatitis, before pursuing invasive diagnostics.
- Nonalcoholic fatty liver disease (NAFLD) is often associated with metabolic syndrome, emphasizing the importance of managing diabetes, obesity, and dyslipidemia.
- Medication-induced liver injury should be considered, especially in patients on long-term therapies such as methotrexate or amiodarone.
- Liver biopsy is reserved for cases where the diagnosis remains uncertain or when advanced fibrosis or cirrhosis is suspected.
- Early lifestyle modifications, including weight loss and exercise, can prevent progression of asymptomatic transaminitis to chronic liver disease.

## MULTIPLE CHOICE QUESTIONS

1. **What is the most common cause of asymptomatic transaminitis in the general population?**
   A. Autoimmune hepatitis
   B. Viral hepatitis
   C. Nonalcoholic fatty liver disease (NAFLD)
   D. Hemochromatosis
2. **Which test is most specific for diagnosing autoimmune hepatitis in a patient with transaminitis?**
   A. Antismooth muscle antibody (SMA)
   B. Ceruloplasmin
   C. Hepatitis B surface antigen (HBsAg)
   D. Transferrin saturation
3. **What is the first-line imaging modality for evaluating asymptomatic transaminitis?**
   A. MRI abdomen
   B. CT scan abdomen
   C. Liver biopsy
   D. Ultrasound abdomen
4. **Which of the following medications is least likely to cause transaminitis?**
   A. Acetaminophen (high dose)
   B. Amiodarone
   C. Metformin
   D. Methotrexate
5. **What lifestyle intervention has the greatest impact on improving transaminase levels in NAFLD?**
   A. Low-sodium diet
   B. Weight loss through diet and exercise
   C. Vitamin supplementation
   D. Increasing alcohol intake

### Answers

1. (C); 2. (A); 3. (D); 4. (C); 5. (B)

## SUGGESTED READINGS

1. Chalasani N, Younossi Z, Lavine JE, et al. The diagnosis and management of nonalcoholic fatty liver disease: Practice guidance from the American Association for the Study of Liver Diseases. Hepatology. 2018;67(1):328-57.
2. European Association for the Study of the Liver (EASL). EASL Clinical Practice Guidelines: Management of non-alcoholic fatty liver disease. J Hepatol. 2016;64(6):1388-402.
3. Kim WR, Flamm SL, Di Bisceglie AM, et al. Serum activity of alanine aminotransferase (ALT) as an indicator of health and disease. Hepatology. 2008;47(4):1363-70.
4. Hoofnagle JH, Björnsson ES. Drug-induced Liver Injury—Types and Phenotypes. N Engl J Med. 2019;381(3):264-73.
5. Dyson JK, Anstee QM, McPherson S. Non-alcoholic fatty liver disease: A practical approach to diagnosis and staging. Frontline Gastroenterol. 2014;5(3):211-8.
6. Friedman SL, Neuschwander-Tetri BA, Rinella M, et al. Mechanisms of NAFLD development and therapeutic strategies. Nat Med. 2018;24(7):908-22.
7. Adams LA, Anstee QM, Tilg H, Targher G. Non-alcoholic fatty liver disease and its relationship with cardiovascular disease and other extrahepatic diseases. Gut. 2017;66(6):1138-53.

CHAPTER 91

# A Case-based Approach to Improving Quality of Life in Patients with Advanced Chronic Liver Disease

*Sanjay Bandyopadhyay*

**CASE VIGNETTE**

A 45 years old nondiabetic alcoholic male presented with fatigue and pruritus for three months. Fatigue was progressively increasing without any muscle weakness, and pruritus was marked at night disturbing his sleep. There was no history of ascites, pedal edema, altered sensorium, oliguria, bleeding manifestation, or gastrointestinal bleeding. Patient also complained of insomnia since the cessation of alcohol intake. On examination, patient was icteric with scratch marks and spider angiomas, firm hepatomegaly and mild splenomegaly. Laboratory parameters revealed normocytic normochromic anemia, low albumin, raised bilirubin and liver enzymes (of which alkaline phosphatase and gamma glutamyl transferase were predominantly elevated). Imaging findings were suggestive of advanced chronic liver disease (CLD) with features of portal hypertension.

## PROVISIONAL DIAGNOSIS

In CLD patients, fatigue manifests with both central symptoms, characterised by cognitive impairment, sleep disturbance, apathy, and autonomic dysfunction, and peripheral symptoms, characterised by decreased exercise tolerance and reduced physical activity levels.

## DIFFERENTIAL DIAGNOSIS

The differential diagnosis of fatigue in liver disease could be:

- Psychological—depression, anxiety
- Medication toxicity—BZDs, beta blockers, muscle relaxants
- Associated endocrine/metabolic causes—hypothyroidism, hyponatremia
- Superimposed infection—viral hepatitis, tuberculosis
- Anemia
- Occult hepatocellular carcinoma (HCC)

## CLINICAL APPROACH

A thorough medication history should be taken. Then, endocrine abnormalities or electrolyte disturbances should be ruled out by relevant blood tests. Blood biochemistry and serology may diagnose superimposed viral hepatitis. Occult tuberculosis should be ruled out by Mantoux test, interferon gamma release assay (IGRA), high resolution computed tomography (HRCT) thorax, while occult HCC can be diagnosed by triphasic CT scan or dynamic contrast-enhanced magnetic resonance imaging (MRI) along with tumor marker alpha fetoprotein (AFP).

- *History and examination*:
  - Detailed history of alcohol intake and duration.
  - Evaluate symptoms like fatigue, pruritus, insomnia, and signs of advanced liver disease (e.g., jaundice, spider angiomas).
  - Assess for complications like ascites, variceal bleeding, and hepatic encephalopathy.
- *Laboratory investigations*:
  - Liver function tests: Elevated bilirubin, ALP, and GGT suggest cholestasis.
  - Complete blood count: Normocytic normochromic anemia.
  - Albumin levels and INR: Markers of liver synthetic dysfunction.
  - Viral serologies and autoimmune markers to rule out secondary causes.
- *Imaging and diagnostics*:
  - Abdominal ultrasound or CT scan to assess liver morphology, portal hypertension, and splenomegaly.
  - Fibroscan or biopsy for fibrosis assessment, if needed.
- *Management plan*:
  - Treat symptoms: Antipruritic agents like cholestyramine or rifampin.
  - Monitor and manage complications of chronic liver disease and portal hypertension.
  - Address underlying alcohol-related liver damage.

## PATHOPHYSIOLOGY

Chronic alcohol consumption induces hepatic inflammation, oxidative stress, and fibrosis, leading to alcohol-related liver disease (ARLD). Damage progresses to cirrhosis with features of portal hypertension. Pruritus results from cholestasis with accumulation of bile salts and pruritogens. Insomnia postalcohol cessation reflects a disruption in neurotransmitter regulation.

## TREATMENT AND PREVENTION

- *Treatment*:
  - o Symptomatic management:
    - Pruritus: Cholestyramine (bile acid sequestrant), rifampin or naltrexone.
    - Fatigue and insomnia: Supportive care and sleep hygiene.
  - o Portal hypertension: Nonselective beta-blockers (e.g., propranolol) and endoscopic surveillance for varices.
  - o Liver support: Nutritional supplementation, including vitamins and minerals.
- *Prevention*:
  - o Complete alcohol cessation and counseling to prevent further liver damage.
  - o Lifestyle modifications: Balanced diet, avoiding hepatotoxic drugs.
  - o Vaccination against hepatitis A and B.
  - o Regular follow-up for early detection and management of complications.

### Points to Ponder

- ❑ Presence of fatigue, pruritus, muscle cramps and sleep disturbances adversely affect the quality of life in patients with chronic liver disease.
- ❑ Though common, these symptoms are often not enquired and frequently not addressed in clinical practice.
- ❑ Treatment principle should focus on to reverse what we can, relieve what we cannot and help patients cope with symptoms.

## MULTIPLE CHOICE QUESTIONS

**1. Which enzyme elevation is most characteristic of alcohol-related liver disease with cholestasis?**
   A. Alanine aminotransferase (ALT)
   B. Gamma-glutamyl transferase (GGT)
   C. Aspartate aminotransferase (AST)
   D. Lactate dehydrogenase (LDH)

**2. Which symptom is most commonly associated with cholestasis in chronic liver disease?**
   A. Pedal edema
   B. Pruritus
   C. Bleeding tendencies
   D. Ascites

**3. What is the first-line treatment for pruritus due to cholestasis?**
   A. Rifampin
   B. Naltrexone
   C. Cholestyramine
   D. Ursodeoxycholic acid

**4. What imaging feature is suggestive of portal hypertension?**
   A. Liver calcifications
   B. Splenomegaly
   C. Peritoneal carcinomatosis
   D. Hepatic adenoma

**5. Which complication is not directly related to portal hypertension?**
   A. Ascites
   B. Esophageal varices
   C. Hepatic encephalopathy
   D. Hepatocellular carcinoma

### Answers

1. (B); 2. (B); 3. (C); 4. (B); 5. (D)

## SUGGESTED READINGS

1. Kok B, Whitlock R, Ferguson T, et al. Health-related Quality of Life: A Rapid Predictor of Hospitalization in Patients with Cirrhosis. Am J Gastroenterol. 2020;115(4):575-83.
2. Kosnik A, Wojcicki M. Fatigue in chronic liver disease patients: prevalence, pathophysiology, and management. Gastroenterol Rev. 2022;17(1):21-7.
3. Marenco-Flores A, Sierra L, Goyes D, et al. Managing pruritus in chronic liver disease: An in-depth narrative review. Clin Liver Dis. 2024;23:e0187-7.
4. Mehta SS, Fallon MB. Muscle cramps in liver disease. Clin Gastroenterol Hepatol. 2013;11(11):1385-91.
5. Shah NM, Malhotra AM, Kaltsakas G. Sleep disorder in patients with chronic liver disease: a narrative review. J Thorac Dis. 2020; 12(Suppl. 2):S248-60.

CHAPTER 92

# An Approach to a Case of Fever with Jaundice and Oliguria

*Paramita Bhattacharya*

**CASE VIGNETTE**

A 35-year-old male presents to the emergency department with a 5-day history of fever, jaundice, and reduced urine output. He reports associated symptoms of malaise, dark urine, and pale stools. The patient has a history of recent travel to an endemic area, where he consumed untreated water. On examination, he is febrile, with a yellowish tint to the skin and sclera, and significant abdominal tenderness in the right upper quadrant.

## PROVISIONAL DIAGNOSIS

Acute viral hepatitis, likely due to hepatitis A virus (HAV) given the travel history and symptomatology.

## DIFFERENTIAL DIAGNOSIS

- Acute viral hepatitis (HAV, HBV, and HCV)
- Leptospirosis
- Hemolytic uremic syndrome (HUS)
- Acute kidney injury due to nephrotoxic agents
- Biliary obstruction (cholecystitis or cholangitis)
- Sepsis with multiorgan dysfunction

## CLINICAL APPROACH

- *History taking*:
    - Detailed travel history, exposure to contaminated water, food history, and vaccination status.
    - Medication history including recent antibiotics or nephrotoxic agents.
    - Family history of liver disease or hematological disorders.
- *Physical examination*:
    - Assess vital signs, level of consciousness, and hydration status.
    - Examine for signs of liver dysfunction (ascites, splenomegaly) and kidney failure (edema, electrolyte imbalances).
- *Laboratory investigations*:
    - Complete blood count (CBC) to check for leukocytosis or thrombocytopenia.
    - Liver function tests (LFTs) including bilirubin levels, AST, ALT, and alkaline phosphatase.
    - Renal function tests (creatinine, electrolytes).
    - Serology for HAV, HBV, HCV, and leptospirosis.
    - Urinalysis to assess for hematuria, proteinuria, and casts.
- *Imaging studies*:
    - Abdominal ultrasound to evaluate liver size, biliary tree, and any obstructive processes.
    - Consider CT abdomen if biliary pathology is suspected or if complications arise.

## PATHOPHYSIOLOGY

Jaundice arises from an accumulation of bilirubin due to impaired liver function or hemolysis. Oliguria may result from acute tubular injury secondary to toxic metabolites, reduced renal perfusion from dehydration or sepsis, or obstructive uropathy. In viral hepatitis, the liver's ability to conjugate and excrete bilirubin is compromised, leading to increased serum bilirubin levels and subsequent jaundice.

## TREATMENT AND PREVENTION

- *Supportive care*:
    - Hydration and electrolyte balance correction.
    - Monitoring of liver and renal function.
- *Specific treatment*:
    - Antiviral therapy is not indicated for HAV; supportive measures are sufficient.
    - For suspected leptospirosis, initiate doxycycline or penicillin.
    - Address complications such as coagulopathy or renal failure as necessary.
- *Prevention*:
    - Vaccination against hepatitis A for travelers.
    - Education on safe drinking practices and food hygiene in endemic areas.

## Points to Ponder

- Always consider recent travel history when evaluating jaundice and fever.
- Hepatitis A is highly infectious and preventable through vaccination.
- Oliguria can indicate serious renal involvement; timely intervention is crucial.
- A multidisciplinary approach may be needed for comprehensive management.
- Regular monitoring of liver and kidney function is essential in cases of acute viral infections.

## MULTIPLE CHOICE QUESTIONS

**1. What is the most common cause of jaundice in travelers returning from endemic areas?**
A. Hepatitis A
B. Hepatitis B
C. Leptospirosis
D. Gallstones

**2. Which laboratory finding is most indicative of hepatocellular injury?**
A. Elevated alkaline phosphatase
B. Elevated AST and ALT
C. Elevated bilirubin
D. Thrombocytopenia

**3. What is the first-line treatment for leptospirosis?**
A. Acyclovir
B. Doxycycline
C. Rifampicin
D. Amoxicillin

**4. Oliguria in the context of liver dysfunction may indicate which of the following?**
A. Increased renal perfusion
B. Acute tubular necrosis
C. Chronic kidney disease
D. Biliary obstruction

**5. The most appropriate initial imaging study for a patient with jaundice and right upper quadrant pain is:**
A. MRI abdomen
B. Abdominal ultrasound
C. CT scan of the abdomen
D. X-ray of the abdomen

### Answers

1. (A); 2. (B); 3. (B); 4. (B); 5. (B)

## SUGGESTED READINGS

1. McHugh R, McGowan C, O'Reilly E, et al. Clinical features and outcomes of acute hepatitis A: a case series. J Hepatol. 2021;75:1392-9.
2. Bhattacharya D, Chatterjee S, Patra S, et al. Epidemiology and management of leptospirosis in endemic areas. Trop Med Health. 2022;50:38-45.
3. Liu J, Wang L, Xu W, et al. Acute kidney injury in viral hepatitis: A clinical review. Kidney Dis. 2020;6:126-33.
4. Rafiq S, Beattie A, Virdi S, et al. Jaundice in adults: A practical approach to diagnosis and management. BMJ. 2019;364:k4930.
5. Ahn J, Choi S, Lee J, et al. The role of ultrasound in the diagnosis of acute liver disease. Clin Gastroenterol Hepatol. 2023;21:2005-13.
6. Kumar S, Sharma R, Singh A, et al. Review of complications in patients with leptospirosis: A focus on renal impairment. Infect Dis Clin Pract. 2022;30:312-8.
7. Montano C, Gonzalez L, Arevalo J, et al. Preventing hepatitis A infection in travelers: vaccination strategies and recommendations. Travel Med Infect Dis. 2021;39:101949.
8. Zhao Y, Li Y, Zhang X, et al. Laboratory diagnosis of viral hepatitis: new perspectives. J Clin Virol. 2023;162:105305.

CHAPTER 93

# An Approach to a Case with Liver Nodules/SOL

*Jayeeta Bhowmick, Saikat Mondal, Boudhayan Das Munshi*

**CASE VIGNETTE**

A 55-year-old male, known alcoholic presented in gastroenterology OPD with ascites and pedal swelling. On clinical examination it is found that he has grade 2 ascites with jaundice. It is also associated with spider, bilateral parotid swelling on general survey. Patient underwent USG whole abdomen and it was found that liver is cirrhotic and there is a solid SOL of around 2 × 2 cm at right lobe of liver.

## PROVISIONAL DIAGNOSIS

Alcohol-related liver cirrhosis with suspected hepatocellular carcinoma (HCC).

## DIFFERENTIAL DIAGNOSIS

The differential diagnosis of solid liver lesions is broad, but many can be diagnosed noninvasively. In some cases, predominantly solid liver lesions may have cystic components, as may be seen with hemangiomas or tumors that have areas that are necrotic. Conversely, predominantly cystic liver lesions may have solid areas, particularly in the setting malignancy. There are numerous causes of solid liver lesions, both benign and malignant is important to establish a correct diagnosis, especially when the potential therapy exists. The diagnosis requires consideration of the clinical history, risk factors, laboratory test findings, imaging studies, and in some cases, pathologic examination of the lesion.

In this case differential diagnosis may be:
- Hepatocellular carcinoma (HCC)
- Regenerative nodule (RND)
- Cholangial carcinoma (CC)

Before going to provisional diagnosis, we should know what are the types of liver SOL.

- *Common solid benign liver SOLs are*:
  - Nodular hyperplasia (FNH)
  - Hepatic adenoma
  - Nodular regenerative hepatic hemangioma
  - Focal nodular hyperplasia (FNH)
  - Focal fatty changes
  - Inflammatory pseudotumor
- *Common malignant solid liver SOL*:
  - Hepatocellular carcinoma
  - Cholangiocarcinoma
  - Metastatic disease

Now going back the case. Any solid liver SOL in cirrhotic patient, always we have to rule out HCC.

So differential diagnosis of focal liver SOL in cirrhotic patient:

Now what are the clues for HCC?
- USG showing a lesion >1 cm
- An elevated or rising alpha-fetoprotein (AFP) level even in the absence of liver lesion in USG

  In that case CT/MRI should be performed.

Now here comes the importance of imaging. Most important imaging is triple phase CT scan of abdomen. Livers get most of its blood supply through the portal vein (80%) and 20% from hepatic artery. 100% of liver tumor receives blood supply from hepatic artery. Depending upon the difference in blood supply results in different enhancement patterns between liver tumors and normal liver parenchyma in the various phases of contrast enhancement. There are 3 phases in triple phase CT. Arterial, portal venous and equilibrium phase depending upon time interval between contrast injection and detection of liver SOL.

Classical arterial phase enhancing lesions:
- HCC
- Hemangioma

## CLINICAL APPROACH

### History

- Assess the patient's alcohol consumption history (amount, duration, and pattern).
- Evaluate symptoms of liver dysfunction (e.g., ascites, jaundice, fatigue, pruritus, and loss of appetite).
- Inquire about any signs of portal hypertension (e.g., esophageal varices, spontaneous bacterial peritonitis).
- Check for any recent changes in weight, stool color (melena), or altered mental status.

### Physical Examination

- Jaundice, spider nevi, parotid swelling, and hepatomegaly are classic findings in cirrhosis.
- Ascites should be graded (1+, 2+, 3+).
- Look for signs of hepatic encephalopathy (altered mental status, asterixis).
- Assess for signs of coagulopathy (easy bruising, petechiae).

### Laboratory Investigations

- *Liver function tests*: ALT, AST, bilirubin, albumin, alkaline phosphatase, GGT.
- *Coagulation profile*: INR, PT
- Complete blood count to assess anemia, thrombocytopenia (common in cirrhosis).
- Serum AFP—to evaluate for HCC.
- Hepatitis serology (hepatitis B, C) to rule out viral etiology.

### Imaging

- *Ultrasound of the abdomen*: For liver cirrhosis, ascites, and identification of focal lesions like a solid mass suggestive of HCC.
- *CT/MRI abdomen*: To assess the characteristics of the solid liver lesion and confirm the diagnosis of HCC.

### Diagnosis

- *Cirrhosis* is confirmed through clinical findings, liver function tests, imaging, and biopsy if necessary.
- *HCC* is confirmed if the solid lesion is consistent with the characteristics of malignancy on imaging (e.g., arterial phase hyperenhancement) and elevated AFP levels.

## PATHOPHYSIOLOGY

Alcoholic cirrhosis is a result of chronic liver injury due to prolonged excessive alcohol consumption. The liver undergoes fibrosis and regeneration, leading to cirrhosis. Cirrhosis leads to the development of portal hypertension, which can cause ascites, varices, and splenomegaly. Chronic liver damage increases the risk of HCC due to genetic mutations, inflammation, and hepatocyte regeneration in the setting of cirrhosis. The development of HCC is facilitated by a proinflammatory environment, altered cell signaling, and chronic hepatocellular injury.

## TREATMENT AND PREVENTION

### Management of Cirrhosis

- *Alcohol cessation* is the most important step in preventing further liver damage.
- *Symptomatic treatment*: Diuretics (spironolactone, furosemide) for ascites, beta-blockers for portal hypertension, and lactulose for hepatic encephalopathy.
- *Liver transplantation* is indicated for patients with decompensated cirrhosis or liver failure.

### Management of HCC

- *Surgical resection* or *liver transplantation* for resectable tumors.
- *Ablation therapies* (radiofrequency or microwave ablation) for smaller tumors.
- *Transarterial chemoembolization (TACE)* for unresectable tumors.
- *Targeted therapy (Sorafenib)* for advanced-stage HCC.
- *Screening* for HCC is recommended for cirrhotic patients, especially with elevated AFP levels and liver imaging every 6 months.

### Prevention

- *Avoid alcohol* to prevent further liver damage.
- *Vaccination* against hepatitis B to prevent viral liver diseases.
- *Regular screening* for HCC in cirrhotic patients through AFP levels and ultrasound.
- *Hepatitis C treatment* to prevent further liver damage.

### Points to Ponder

- ❑ The role of alcohol cessation in halting the progression of cirrhosis and reducing the risk of HCC.
- ❑ The need for regular screening for hepatocellular carcinoma in patients with cirrhosis using AFP and ultrasound.
- ❑ The impact of portal hypertension on the development of ascites, varices, and splenomegaly.
- ❑ The role of liver transplantation in patients with decompensated cirrhosis and hepatocellular carcinoma.
- ❑ The implications of managing both cirrhosis and HCC, particularly regarding treatment options like surgery, TACE, and targeted therapy.

## MULTIPLE CHOICE QUESTIONS

**1. Which of the following is the most common cause of cirrhosis in a 55-year-old male with a history of chronic alcohol consumption?**

a. Hepatitis B infection
b. Hepatitis C infection
c. Nonalcoholic fatty liver disease
d. Alcoholic liver disease

**2. What is the first-line imaging modality to evaluate a liver lesion in a patient with cirrhosis?**

a. MRI abdomen
b. CT abdomen
c. Abdominal ultrasound
d. X-ray abdomen

**3. Which of the following is the most important treatment for alcoholic cirrhosis?**

a. Liver transplantation
b. Alcohol cessation
c. Diuretics
d. Antiviral therapy

**4. In a patient with cirrhosis and suspected hepatocellular carcinoma, which of the following is most likely elevated?**

a. Hemoglobin
b. Alpha-fetoprotein (AFP)
c. Prothrombin time
d. Serum calcium

**5. Which of the following is a typical complication of cirrhosis related to portal hypertension?**

a. Ascites
b. Hyperkalemia
c. Diarrhea
d. Hypercalcemia

## Answers

1. (D); 2. (C); 3. (B); 4. (B); 5. (A)

## SUGGESTED READINGS


1. Llovet JM, et al. Hepatocellular carcinoma. Lancet. 2015;378(9790): 1757-69.
2. Schuppan D, Afdhal NH. Liver cirrhosis. Lancet. 2008;371(9615): 838-51.
3. Bruix J, Sherman M. Management of hepatocellular carcinoma: an update. Hepatology. 2011;53(3):1020-2.
4. Osna NA, Donohue Jr TM, Kharbanda KK. Alcoholic Liver Disease: Pathogenesis and Current Management. Alcohol Res. 2017;38(2):147-61.
5. El-Serag HB. Epidemiology of viral hepatitis and hepatocellular carcinoma. Gastroenterology. 2012;142(6):1264-73.e1.
6. Dufour JF, Kullak-Ublick GA. Alcoholic liver disease and hepatocellular carcinoma. Am J Gastroenterol. 2004;99(6):1086-95.
7. Finkelstein J, Torres S. Management of hepatocellular carcinoma. Current Gastroenterology Reports. 2004:6(4);302-8.

CHAPTER 94

# An Approach to a Case of Jaundice with Antitubercular Treatment

*Vishakha Jain, Vahini Golla, Harshita Vaddi*

**CASE VIGNETTE**

A 35-year-old male, nondiabetic, nonhypertensive, alcohol abuser (about 180 mL of whisky 3–4 times/week) and no other comorbidities, had presented 6 weeks back to medicine OPD with complaints of fever since 4 weeks; productive cough with hemoptysis since 2–3 weeks. Patient was diagnosed as sputum positive (3+) tuberculosis with fibrocavitatory lesion, sensitive to both rifampicin (RIF) and isoniazid (INH). Patient was started on antitubercular treatment (ATT)—isoniazid, rifampicin, pyrazinamide and ethambutol (HRZE) as per his weight and was registered under DOTS. He came to us after 3–4 weeks of starting treatment with complaints of vomiting—2–3 episodes, abdominal pain since past 3 days and wife had noticed yellowish discoloration of eyes. We investigated him and he was found to have deranged liver function tests (LFT)—total bilirubin = 3.3 mg/dL with conjugated bilirubin = 2.4 mg/dL, SGOT = 157 IU/mL, SGPT = 186 IU/mL.

## PROVISIONAL DIAGNOSIS

Antitubercular therapy (ATT)-drug induced liver injury (DILI)/TB–DILI/ATT induced hepatitis supported by the temporal association of starting ATT and development of liver injury.

## DIFFERENTIAL DIAGNOSIS

There could be various differential diagnosis.

- *Viral hepatitis*:
  - Acute hepatitis (HAV, HBV, HCV, HEV) should be considered, especially if the patient has risk factors.
  - Chronic hepatitis (HBV, HCV) could also worsen with anti-tubercular therapy.
- *Alcoholic hepatitis*: History of alcohol consumption and typical features (macrovesicular steatosis) help in differentiation. AST > ALT (typically around 2:1 ratio) and elevated GGT are supportive findings.
- *Liver involvement in tuberculosis*: Tubercular hepatitis or miliary tuberculosis can cause liver dysfunction and mimic DILI. A biopsy or specific imaging may be necessary for diagnosis.
- *Drug-induced liver injury (DILI) from other drugs*: Other allopathic medications, herbal supplements, and over-the-counter drugs should be reviewed, as they can also contribute to hepatotoxicity.
- *Underlying liver disease exacerbated by anti-tubercular therapy*: Patients with pre-existing cirrhosis or hepatitis may have exacerbated liver injury on anti-TB drugs. Baseline liver function tests can help determine pre-existing liver conditions.
- *Wilson's disease*: Although rare, Wilson's disease can present with hepatotoxicity in younger patients. Low serum ceruloplasmin, elevated urine copper, and Kayser–Fleischer rings support the diagnosis.
- *Autoimmune hepatitis*: Typically associated with elevated immunoglobulins and positive autoantibodies (ANA, SMA).

## PATHOPHYSIOLOGY

Refer to **Table 1**.

**TABLE 1: Pathophysiological mechanism of hepatic injury by ATT.**

| Drug | Mechanism of action | Pathway of hepatotoxicity |
|---|---|---|
| Isoniazid (INH)<br>*Idiosyncratic DILI* | Isoniazid is a prodrug that, once activated by the bacterial enzyme KatG, inhibits the synthesis of mycolic acids, essential components of the mycobacterial cell wall | Isoniazid is metabolized in the liver, primarily by acetylation (via the enzyme N-acetyltransferase 2, NAT2) and by the cytochrome P450 enzyme system. The metabolism produces acetyl hydrazine, which can form hepatotoxic metabolites leading to liver cell damage. Variations in NAT2 enzyme (slow vs. fast acetylators) affect INH metabolism, with slow acetylators being at higher risk of toxicity |

*Continued*

*Continued*

| Drug | Mechanism of action | Pathway of hepatotoxicity |
|---|---|---|
| Rifampicin (RIF)<br>*Dose dependent DILI* | Rifampicin inhibits bacterial DNA-dependent RNA polymerase, preventing transcription and bacterial replication | Rifampicin is a potent inducer of cytochrome P450 enzymes, which can enhance the metabolism of other drugs, including INH, increasing hepatotoxic metabolite formation. Additionally, RIF and its metabolites can cause oxidative stress in hepatocytes, leading to lipid peroxidation and cellular damage |
| Pyrazinamide (PZA)<br>*Both dose dependent and independent DILI* | Pyrazinamide is converted by mycobacterial pyrazinamidase into pyrazinoic acid, which disrupts the mycobacterial cell membrane's transport function and energy production | The hepatotoxicity of PZA is dose-dependent and involves both direct cytotoxic effects and metabolic activation that forms hepatotoxic intermediates. These intermediates cause oxidative stress, which damages liver cells and results in hepatocyte necrosis |
| Ethambutol (EMB) | Ethambutol inhibits the synthesis of arabinogalactan, an essential component of the mycobacterial cell wall | Ethambutol itself is relatively nonhepatotoxic compared to other anti-tubercular drugs but may contribute to hepatic injury when combined with other hepatotoxic drugs |

## CLINICAL APPROACH

Refer to **Flowchart 1**.

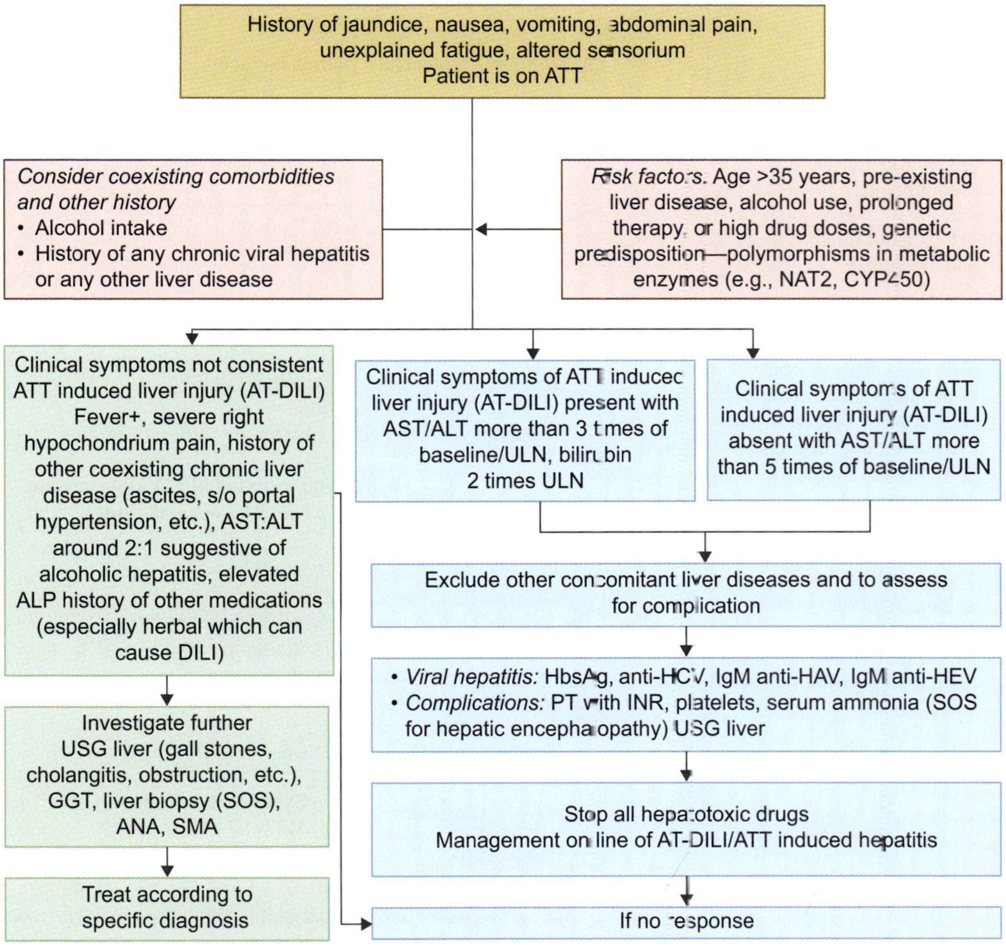


**FLOWCHART 1:** Diagnostic approach to AT-DILI or ATT induced hepatitis.

## TREATMENT AND PREVENTION

### Treatment

Refer to **Figures 1 and 2** and **Flowchart 2**.

### Prevention

- *Screening*: Before initiating ATT, screen for pre-existing liver disease (e.g., hepatitis B and C, cirrhosis of liver, etc.)
- *Dose adjustment*: Use lower doses or monitor liver function closely in patients with pre-existing liver conditions. Liver

| Urgent ATT: Life or organ threatening | No need for urgent ATT |
|---|---|
| • Sputum + pulmonary TB<br>• TB meningitis or CNS TB<br>• Pericardial TB<br>• Any form that is life-threatening, e.g., intestinal TB with intestinal obstruction<br>• Ocular TB<br>• Joint or spinal TB | • Sputum+ve pulmonary TB<br>• TB lymphadenitis<br>• Tubercular pleural effusion<br>• Tubercular ascites<br>• Intestinal TB<br>• Genitourinary TB<br>• Bone TB |

**FIG. 1:** Decision regarding continuing ATT in AT-DILI.

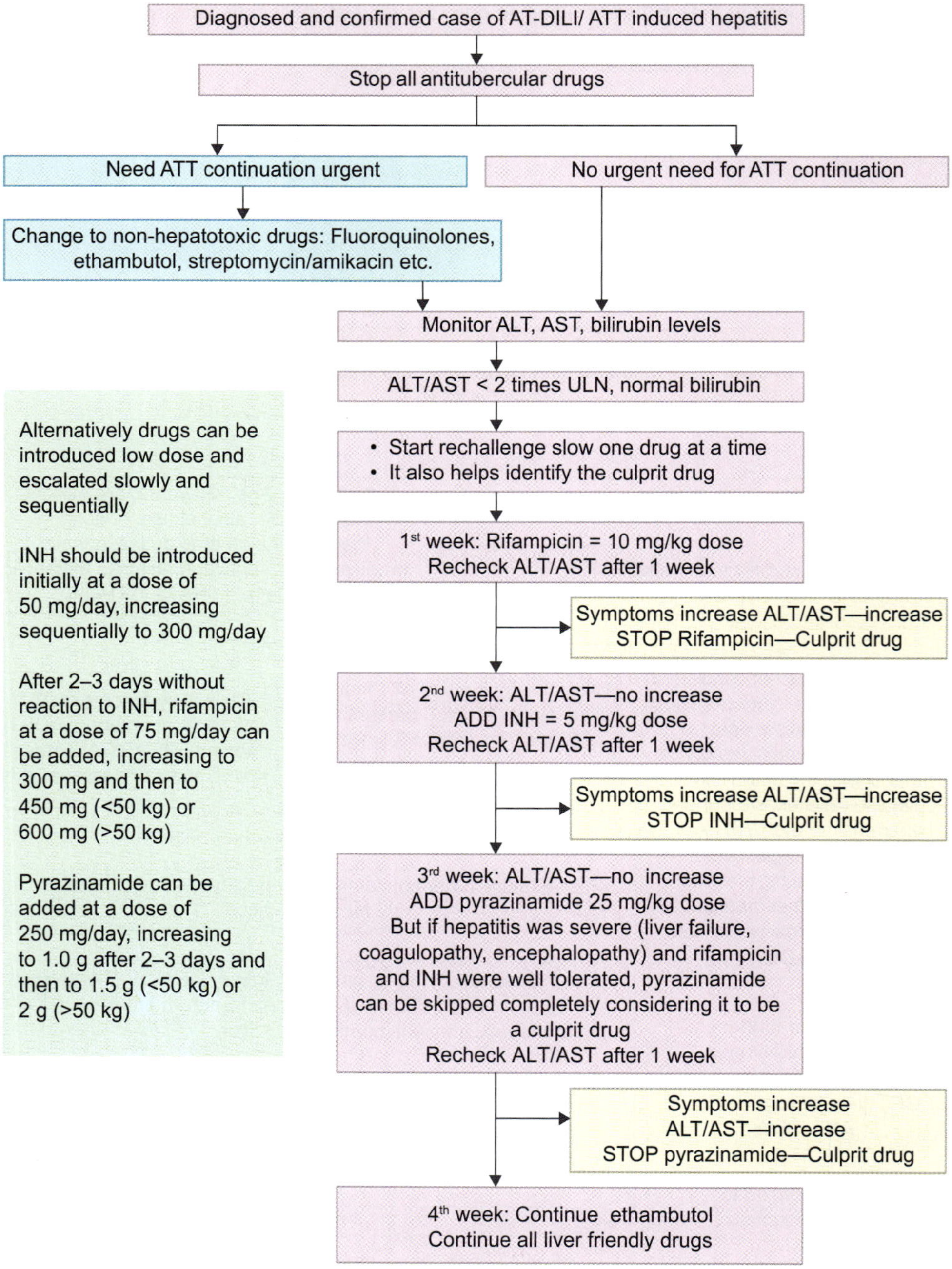


**FLOWCHART 2:** Treatment approach to AT-DILI or ASTT induced hepatitis.

| Child-Turcotte-Pugh (CTP) score | | | |
|---|---|---|---|
| | Score 1 | Score 2 | Score 3 |
| Bilirubin | <2 mg/dL | 2–3 mg/dL | >3 mg/dL |
| Albumin | >3.5 g/dL | 2.8–3.5 g/dL | <2.8 g/dL |
| INR | <1.7 | 1.7–2.2 | >2.2 |
| Ascites | Absent | Slight | Moderate |
| Encephalopathy | Absent | Grade 1–2 | Grade 3–4 |

**Hepatic encephalopathy grade**

- Grade 0: Normal consciousness, personality and neurological examination
- Grade 1: Restless, disturbances in sleep, irritability or agitated, tremors, handwriting affected
- Grade 2: Lethargy, disorientation to time, asterixis, ataxia
- Grade 3: Somnolent and stuporous, disoriented to place, hyperactive reflexes, rigidity
- Grade 4: Unarousable coma, decerebrate

| Child Status | Suggested ATT |
|---|---|
| • Child A cirrhosis (Score 1–6)<br>• Stable liver disease | • 9 months of therapy with HRE OR<br>• 2 months of therapy with HRE followed by 7 months of HR |
| • Child B cirrhosis (Score 7–10)<br>• Advanced liver disease | One hepatotoxic drug regimen can be used: Two months of therapy with INH OR RIF with ETH and aminoglycoside, followed by 10 months of therapy with INH/RIF and ETH |
| • Child C cirrhosis (Score 11–15)<br>• Very advanced liver disease | • No hepatotoxic drug<br>• 18 to 24 months treatment using a combination of ETH, FQL, cycloserine and aminoglycoside/capreomycin |
| In acute hepatitis | • Avoid hepatotoxic drugs<br>• ATT with non-hepatotoxic drugs if urgent ATT required<br>• Wait till improvement in liver function if no urgent need of ATT |

**FIG. 2:** ATT selection for underlying liver disease.

function test should be carried out before initiating ATT, for baseline levels as it has been seen that patients with abnormal baseline transaminases levels are at increased risk of developing hepatic injury eventually. Liver function should be repeated twice weekly for the first 2 weeks followed by weekly monitoring till the end of two months and then monthly investigations till the end of the treatment.

- *Patient education*: Advise on alcohol avoidance, avoidance of other hepatotoxic supplements (herbal, etc.), and regular follow-up visits.
- *Vaccination*: Hepatitis B vaccination for unvaccinated patients.

## Points to Ponder

- Incidence of ATT induced DILI varies from 2 to 28%. It accounts for 46–58% of DILI, 65–71% of drug-induced ALF, and 23% of drug-induced ACLF in India.
- DILI from anti TB drugs occur usually in the first two months of treatment.
- The ATT drugs implicated in AT-DILI: INH + RIF > INH alone >> PZA alone > RIF alone > Ethionamide > PAS
- Early increase in transaminases (usually within first 15 days) has been attributed to rifampicin and isoniazid-induced hepatotoxicity. Late toxicity (usually after one month) has been attributed to pyrazinamide-induced hepatotoxicity.
- Severe unstable liver disease should not be given any hepatotoxic drug. Combination regimen (at least three antitubercular drug) are ethambutol, aminoglycosides, fluoroquinolones, ethionamide, cycloserine and other newer nonhepatotoxic drugs should be considered for a duration of 18–24 months.

## MULTIPLE CHOICE QUESTIONS

**1. What is the most likely cause of jaundice in a patient on ATT?**
   - A. Hepatitis B
   - B. Isoniazid-induced hepatotoxicity
   - C. Hepatitis A
   - D. Gallstone disease

**2. Which is not a risk factor for developing ATT-induced hepatitis?**
   - A. Age above 35 years
   - B. Chronic alcohol use
   - C. HIV infection
   - D. High-protein diet

**3. In cases of ATT-induced hepatitis, the first-line drug often reintroduced after normalization of liver enzymes is:**
   - A. Isoniazid
   - B. Rifampicin
   - C. Ethambutol
   - D. Pyrazinamide

**4. Which of the following is not a recommended action in managing a patient who develops ATT-induced hepatitis?**
   - A. Stop the hepatotoxic drugs immediately
   - B. Reintroduce hepatotoxic drugs gradually once liver enzymes normalize
   - C. Switch to a single-agent therapy immediately
   - D. Provide supportive care to manage symptoms

**5. ATT-induced hepatitis generally develops within what time frame after starting therapy?**
   - A. Within 24 hours
   - B. Within 7 days
   - C. Within 1–2 months
   - D After 6 months

## Answers

1. (B); 2. (D); 3. (B); 4. (C); 5. (C)

## SUGGESTED READINGS

1. European Association for the Study of the Liver. Electronic address: easloffice@easloffice.eu; Clinical Practice Guideline Panel: Chair; Panel members; EASL Governing Board representative. EASL Clinical Practice Guidelines: Drug-induced liver injury. J Hepatol. 2019;70(6):1222-61.
2. World Health Organization (WHO). Treatment of tuberculosis: Guidelines for treatment of drug-susceptible tuberculosis and patient care, 2017. 20th ed. Geneva: World Health Organization; 2017.
3. Lim WS, Avery A, Kon OM, et al. Anti-tuberculosis drug-induced liver injury. BMJ. 2023;383:e074866. [Erratum in: BMJ. 2023;383:p2806].
4. Hosack T, Damry D, Biswas S. Drug-induced liver injury: a comprehensive review. Therap Adv Gastroenterol. 2023;16: 17562848231163410.
5. Standard Treatment Workflow (STW) for the Management of antitubercular therapy related hepatitis 2022. [cited 2024 Nov 15]. Available from: https://www.icmr.gov.in/icmrobject/uploads/stws/1725964686_3_antitubercular_therapy_hepatitis_18032022.pdf
6. British Thoracic Society (BTS). BTS guidelines for the management of tuberculosis. Thorax. 2000;55(Suppl 1).
7. American Thoracic Society (ATS). ATS/CDC/IDSA: Treatment of tuberculosis. Am J Respir Crit Care Med. 2003;167(4):603-62.

CHAPTER
95

# An Approach to a Case of Fever, Jaundice, and Hypoxemia

*Atanu Chandra, Debaditya Chatterjee*

## CASE VIGNETTE

Mr MM, a 32-year-old farmer hailing from a rural area of Southern Bengal, presents to the emergency department with a 7-day history of high-grade fever, jaundice and increasing shortness of breath. He reports that the fever started abruptly, associated with chills and malaise. Over the next few days, he developed yellowish discoloration of the skin and sclera. This was accompanied by shortness of breath and nonproductive cough. He has no known history of liver disease, diabetes or hypertension. On further inquiry, he reveals that he has been in contact with water from flooded fields and has sustained minor cuts on his hands and feet in the past week. He does not report any recent use of medications or history of alcohol abuse.

On examination, the patient appears ill, with a fever of 39.5°C, pulse rate was 110 beats/min, blood pressure was 90/60 mm Hg, respiratory rate was 28 breaths/min and peripheral oxygen saturation was 85% on room air. There was mild conjunctival pallor and jaundice of the sclera. Respiratory system examinations revealed bilateral basal crackles and decreased breath sounds in the lower lobes. Abdominal examination was remarkable for tender hepatomegaly (2 cm below the costal margin) without any splenomegaly or ascites. No rashes or petechiae were present. Other systemic examinations did not reveal anything abnormal.

On admission, laboratory tests showed hemoglobin of 10.5 g/dL, elevated total leukocyte count of 14,800/µL (reference range, 4,500–11,000) and a reduced platelet count of 64,000/µL. The serum creatinine level was significantly raised at 3.0 mg/dL (reference range, 0.6–1.4). Liver function tests indicated hyperbilirubinemia, with a total bilirubin level of 8.9 mg/dL (reference range, 0.0–1.2) and direct bilirubin exceeding 5.0 mg/dL. Alanine aminotransferase (ALT) and aspartate aminotransferase (AST) levels were mildly elevated at 76 IU/L and 68 IU/L, respectively. Seum alkaline phosphatase was not elevated. Chest radiography demonstrated bilateral, predominantly peripheral, patchy opacities.

## PROVISIONAL DIAGNOSIS

Based on the clinical presentation of fever, jaundice and hypoxia in a farmer with recent exposure to contaminated water, the provisional diagnosis is leptospirosis (Weil's Disease). Leptospirosis **(Fig. 1)**, particularly its severe manifestation known as Weil's disease, presents with a combination of fever, jaundice and multiorgan involvement (including liver and kidneys). The patient's history of exposure to floodwaters and minor cuts on his hands and feet makes this a likely diagnosis. Additionally, the presence of hepatomegaly, jaundice and hypoxia (which could indicate pulmonary complications or sepsis) further supports this diagnosis.

An infectious disease screening panel, including tests for malaria parasite, malaria dual antigen, dengue IgM antibody, IgM scrub typhus antibody, and IgM leptospira antibody was sent, and the patient was started on intravenous ceftriaxone and doxycycline. The IgM leptospira antibody returned strongly positive. Tests for antinuclear antibody (ANA), c-myeloperoxidase (c-MPO) and proteinase 3 (PR3) were negative. By 3rd day of hospitalization, the patient became afebrile, with gradual normalization of liver and renal function tests, and he was able to maintain an oxygen saturation above 92%. He was discharged in a stable condition on day 7th, with oral doxycycline continued for a total of 10 days.

## DIFFERENTIAL DIAGNOSIS

- *Plasmodium falciparum* malaria
- Scrub typhus
- *Viral hepatitis (hepatitis A, B and E)*: In fulminant hepatic failure complicated with sepsis or acute respiratory distress syndrome (ARDS), patient may be hypoxemic.
- Gram-negative bacterial sepsis with hepatic dysfunction and hypoxia due to septic shock or ARDS
- *Atypical pneumonia*: Severe pneumonia, particularly from organisms like *Legionella* or *Mycoplasma*
- Drug-induced liver injury (e.g., acetaminophen overdose) or autoimmune hepatitis can cause jaundice and encephalopathy, leading to hypoxia
- *Systemic lupus erythematosus (SLE)*: Lupus pneumonitis or SLE-related hepatitis can cause hypoxia, fever and jaundice.
- Antineutrophil cytoplasmic antibody (ANCA)-associated vasculitis

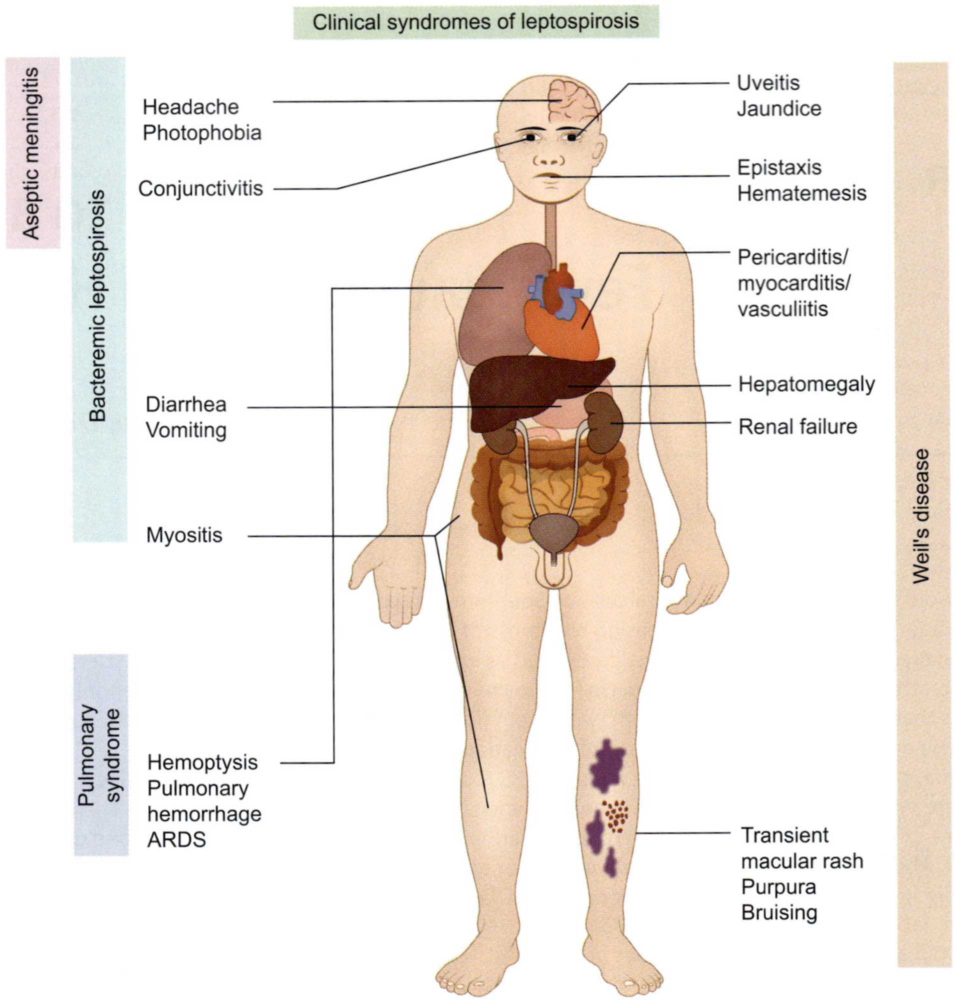


**FIG. 1:** Leptospirosis (Weil's Disease).

## CLINICAL APPROACH

A previously healthy 32-year-old man presented with an acute febrile illness characterized by marked fatigue and myalgia, complicated by hypoxic respiratory failure and jaundice. In developing a clinical approach, I will consider acute febrile illnesses prevalent in our region that can affect immunocompetent patients and rapidly progress to critical illness with multisystem organ failure.

### *Acute Febrile Illness*

Acute febrile illness is a common clinical syndrome with various etiologies. In the Indian setting, acute febrile illness in immunocompetent adults is often attributable to a diverse array of infectious agents. Common bacterial causes include enteric fever and leptospirosis, particularly during the monsoon season. Vector-borne infections, such as dengue, malaria, chikungunya and scrub typhus, are prevalent and can present with overlapping symptoms, posing diagnostic challenges. Viral etiologies like influenza and COVID-19 also contribute significantly.

Malignancies and inflammatory conditions can also present with acute febrile illness and should be included in the differential diagnosis. However, this patient's complete blood count shows no significant abnormalities in the white-cell differential or blasts suggestive of hematologic malignancy. Inflammatory conditions, such as ANCA-associated vasculitis, may cause severe illness with diverse manifestations, potentially involving the lungs, kidneys and skin; thus, a high index of suspicion is essential. While the patient's chest radiograph reveals nonspecific patchy opacities, these findings could be seen in various infectious or inflammatory conditions, including ANCA-associated vasculitis or SLE. Given the acute onset of symptoms, an infectious etiology is more likely, warranting consideration of a broad range of bacterial, viral, parasitic, fungal and tickborne infections.

Tickborne illnesses such as Lyme disease, babesiosis and Rocky Mountain spotted fever can lead to severe febrile illnesses with multisystem involvement; however, these are exceedingly rare in India. Fungal infections caused by typical pathogens, such as *Candida*, are unlikely in this patient given the absence of risk factors like immunosuppression or intravenous substance use. Endemic fungal infections, including coccidioidomycosis, blastomycosis and histoplasmosis, are also very uncommon in India and do not typically produce the liver dysfunction pattern observed in this case. Among viral infections, Epstein–Barr virus and cytomegalovirus can affect multiple organs but rarely cause severe illness without immunosuppression and they generally present with elevated liver enzymes rather than isolated hyperbilirubinemia. Acute HIV infection may manifest as a nonspecific febrile illness; however, hyperbilirubinemia is unusual in acute retroviral syndrome.

### *Conjugated Hyperbilirubinemia*

Acute febrile illness with jaundice in an immunocompetent male often raises suspicion for several infectious etiologies. Leptospirosis, a zoonotic bacterial infection, frequently manifests with fever, jaundice and renal impairment. Malaria, particularly from *Plasmodium falciparum*, can also lead to hemolysis-induced jaundice alongside fever, though it is usually unconjugated hyperbilirubinemia. Anicteric hepatitis is the commonest form of hepatic dysfunction seen in dengue fever.

Viral hepatitis, especially hepatitis A and E, is a primary consideration in febrile jaundice, characterized by a marked rise in liver enzymes and predominantly conjugated hyperbilirubinemia. In uncomplicated viral hepatitis, fever commonly subsides as jaundice appears. This pattern aligns with the typical clinical course of acute viral hepatitis, where the initial prodromal phase presents with nonspecific symptoms such as fever, malaise and fatigue, which tend to diminish or resolve once the icteric phase with jaundice develops. In fulminant hepatic failure complicated with sepsis or ARDS, patient may be hypoxemic. Scrub typhus, another endemic illness, may present with jaundice due to hepatic involvement, often requiring differentiation from other vector-borne infections. To distinguish these infectious causes, targeted diagnostics are essential along with exclusion of noninfectious etiologies such as drug-induced liver injury or autoimmune hepatitis that can mimic these presentations in febrile patients with jaundice. Infectious causes of conjugated hyperbilirubinemia such as cholangitis, hepatic abscess and tuberculosis are generally associated with cholestatic hepatitis. However, our patient did not exhibit signs of cholestatic injury.

### *Acute Febrile Illness with Hypoxemia*

Viral pneumonias, notably influenza and COVID-19, are common and may progress to hypoxemia, especially in those with underlying risk factors. Scrub typhus can cause interstitial pneumonia leading to hypoxia due to alveolar damage. Other vector-borne infections, such as severe dengue, can result in plasma leakage syndrome, pulmonary edema and consequent hypoxia. Leptospirosis, particularly in its severe pulmonary hemorrhagic form, can lead to acute respiratory distress and hypoxia. Additionally, certain bacterial infections like *Streptococcus pneumoniae* and *Mycoplasma pneumoniae* can cause community-acquired pneumonia, presenting with fever and hypoxia. Gram-negative sepsis may lead to jaundice due to hepatic dysfunction and hypoxia due to septic shock or ARDS.

Acute eosinophilic pneumonia, often triggered by environmental exposures or medications, can present with fever, dyspnea, and hypoxemia, along with diffuse lung infiltrates. Autoimmune conditions like ANCA associated vasculitis or SLE can also cause fever and respiratory involvement, resulting in hypoxia and chest radiograph abnormalities.

## PATHOPHYSIOLOGY

Leptospirosis is among the most prevalent zoonotic infections globally, primarily transmitted through contact with environments contaminated by the urine of infected animals, especially rodents. Humans are at higher risk in crowded urban areas with poor sanitation, as well as through occupational exposures in agriculture, veterinary fields and water treatment. Additional risks include contact with stagnant water, freshwater activities and floodwaters, as in this patient's case, likely due to minor skin abrasions. With an incubation period of 3–30 days, symptoms typically emerge within 2 weeks of exposure.

The global incidence of leptospirosis appears to be on the rise, driven by climate change and urbanization. Extreme weather events, particularly flooding, facilitate human exposure to environmental and animal reservoirs, while overcrowding in urban settings increases contact with rodent vectors. Diagnosing leptospirosis is challenging, especially in resource-limited settings, as it often presents with symptoms that overlap with other infections like dengue, malaria and rickettsial diseases. Leptospirosis and dengue frequently co-occur, making clinical differentiation difficult. Given delays in diagnostic testing, empirical treatment is usually initiated when leptospirosis is suspected.

Leptospirosis has diverse clinical manifestations, often self-limited, but icteric cases can present with severe symptoms, including fever, hyperbilirubinemia, acute kidney injury and conjunctival suffusion **(Fig. 1)**. Severe cases may lead to complications like pulmonary hemorrhage, evident in this patient's respiratory failure and diffuse lung opacities, which are associated with a poorer prognosis. Hypotension may result from cardiovascular compromise, potentially due to myocarditis, while other possible complications include aseptic meningitis, uveitis and various neurologic symptoms.

Polymerase chain reaction (PCR) testing is a highly sensitive method that can detect *Leptospira* DNA in blood or urine during the early stages of infection, allowing for timely diagnosis. Serological tests, such as the microscopic agglutination test (MAT), remain the gold standard for confirming leptospirosis, though they are generally more useful later in the disease due to the time needed for antibody production. Enzyme-linked immunosorbent assays (ELISA) provide a rapid and accessible alternative for detecting antibodies, useful in both early and convalescent phases. Newer methods, including point-of-care tests, are under development to facilitate diagnosis in resource-limited settings and help curb disease progression by enabling prompt treatment.

## TREATMENT AND PREVENTION

The cornerstone of managing icteric leptospirosis is supportive care aimed at mitigating end-organ damage. This includes oxygen therapy and ventilatory support for those with ARDS, as well as renal replacement therapy for patients experiencing anuric acute kidney failure. Mild cases of leptospirosis can be effectively managed with doxycycline, azithromycin or amoxicillin. For severe cases, as seen in this patient, intravenous ceftriaxone or doxycycline is recommended. In some severe icteric cases, adjunct therapies such as glucocorticoids and plasmapheresis have been employed, though robust evidence supporting their efficacy is limited. While many patients recover without antimicrobial therapy, the likelihood of leptospirosis in this patient was high enough on presentation that we promptly initiated empirical doxycycline/ceftriaxone therapy while awaiting diagnostic confirmation.

Preventing leptospirosis in Indian scenario involves minimizing exposure to contaminated water sources, particularly during the monsoon season when floodwaters increase the risk. Public health measures, such as improving sanitation and controlling rodent populations in densely populated urban areas, are critical to reducing transmission. Individuals at higher risk, including those in agriculture, veterinary work and water treatment sectors, should wear protective clothing. Public awareness campaigns highlighting the risks associated with contact with stagnant water and promoting hygiene practices can further help curb the incidence of leptospirosis.

## Points to Ponder

- Leptospirosis is primarily transmitted through contact with water contaminated by infected animal urine, especially from rodents.
- It is common in areas with poor sanitation, recent flooding or occupations involving water exposure.
- Weil's disease can present with fever, jaundice, renal failure, respiratory symptoms and multiorgan involvement.
- Leptospirosis symptoms overlap with other infections like dengue and malaria, making early clinical suspicion crucial.
- Start antibiotics like doxycycline or ceftriaxone promptly in severe cases without waiting for diagnostic confirmation.
- Severe cases may require oxygen, renal support, and intensive monitoring for organ dysfunction.

## MULTIPLE CHOICE QUESTIONS

**1. Which of the following laboratory findings is MOST suggestive of icteric leptospirosis in a patient with acute febrile illness, jaundice and renal dysfunction?**

A. Elevated aminotransferases with a pattern of hepatocellular injury.
B. Isolated hyperbilirubinemia with mild elevation in aminotransferases.
C. Markedly elevated alkaline phosphatase.
D. Severe thrombocytopenia with marked transaminitis.

**2. In a patient suspected of leptospirosis, which diagnostic test would most accurately confirm the infection during the early phase of illness?**

A. Microscopic agglutination test (MAT)
B. IgM antibody serology for leptospira
C. Polymerase chain reaction (PCR) for leptospira DNA
D. Blood culture for leptospira

**3. Which of the following organ systems is MOST commonly affected in severe icteric leptospirosis, besides the liver and kidneys?**

A. Cardiovascular
B. Respiratory
C. Gastrointestinal
D. Central nervous system

**4. What is the primary mechanism by which leptospirosis can lead to hypoxemic respiratory failure in severe cases?**

A. Interstitial pneumonia
B. Pulmonary hemorrhage
C. Bronchial obstruction
D. Pleural effusion

**5. In the treatment of severe icteric leptospirosis, which of the following statements is TRUE regarding the use of adjunctive therapies?**

A. Glucocorticoids and plasmapheresis are recommended as standard therapies.
B. Glucocorticoids may be considered in severe cases with pulmonary hemorrhage, although evidence is limited.
C. Plasmapheresis is required in all patients with icteric leptospirosis to reduce bacterial load.
D. Antimicrobial therapy should be withheld until serological confirmation is obtained.

### Answers

1. (B); 2. (C); 3. (B); 4. (B); 5. (B)

## SUGGESTED READING


1. Varyani U, Singhal T, Sheth S, et al. An unusual cause of fever and jaundice. Indian J Med Microbiol. 2021;39:320-2.
2. Hillmann WC, Chung R, Mohareb AM, et al. Case 31-2024: A 37-Year-Old Man with Fever, Myalgia, Jaundice, and Respiratory Failure. N Engl J Med. 2024;391:1343-54.
3. Anand AC, Garg HK. Approach to clinical syndrome of jaundice and encephalopathy in tropics. J Clin Exp Hepatol. 2015;5:S116-30.
4. Haake DA, Levett PN. Leptospirosis in humans. Curr Top Microbiol Immunol. 2015;387:65-97.
5. Rajapakse S. Leptospirosis: clinical aspects. Clin Med (Lond). 2022;22:14-7.
6. Bottieau E, Van Duffel L, El Safi S, et al. Etiological spectrum of persistent fever in the tropics and predictors of ubiquitous infections: a prospective four-country study with pooled analysis. BMC Med. 2022;20:144.
7. Singhi S, Rungta N, Nallasamy K, et al. Tropical Fevers in Indian Intensive Care Units: A Prospective Multicenter Study. Indian J Crit Care Med. 2017;21:811-8.
8. Muthaiah B, Thippeswamy T, Kondareddy S, et al. Study of Aetiology and Outcome in Acute Febrile Illness Patients with Multiple Organ Dysfunction Syndrome. J Clin Diagn Res. 2016;10:OC16-8.

CHAPTER

96

# An Approach to a Case of Fundoscopy in Febrile Illness Diagnosis

*Saikat Datta*

**CASE VIGNETTE**

A 32-year-old male presents to the emergency department with a 5-day history of high-grade fever, chills, and malaise. The fever is persistent, not responding to over-the-counter antipyretics, and is associated with body aches, headache, and a nonproductive cough. He denies any recent travel or significant medical history but mentions being in close contact with a sick family member who had similar symptoms. On examination, his temperature is 39.2°C, pulse 110 bpm, blood pressure 110/70 mm Hg, and respiratory rate 22 breaths/min. The patient appears febrile and slightly confused but is oriented to time and place.

Physical examination reveals mild conjunctival injection, neck stiffness, and a petechial rash over the trunk. Routine laboratory tests show a raised white blood cell count (15,000/μL), thrombocytopenia (platelets 90,000/μL), and a significantly elevated C-reactive protein. A chest X-ray shows no evidence of pneumonia. Given the patient's febrile state and unusual findings, a fundoscopy is performed, revealing retinal hemorrhages with cotton-wool spots, raising suspicion for a systemic infective cause such as dengue fever or meningococcemia.

This case highlights the role of fundoscopy in diagnosing febrile illnesses, as retinal changes can provide critical clues, especially in cases of severe sepsis or viral infections.

## PROVISIONAL DIAGNOSIS

The provisional diagnosis for the case is dengue fever with retinal hemorrhages (also known as dengue-related retinopathy).

## DIFFERENTIAL DIAGNOSIS

- Meningococcemia with retinal involvement
- Malaria with retinal hemorrhages
- Typhoid fever with systemic involvement
- Severe leptospirosis
- Sepsis of unknown origin with retinopathy

## CLINICAL APPROACH

- *History and symptoms*: Thorough history including fever onset, travel history, mosquito exposure, and family contacts. Look for warning signs of severe dengue such as bleeding, organ dysfunction, and shock.
- *Physical examination*: Focus on assessing the extent of fever, rash, and signs of systemic involvement (petechiae, hepatomegaly). Perform a fundoscopy to check for retinal hemorrhages, which suggest more severe dengue or possible meningoencephalitis.
- *Lab tests*: Complete blood count showing thrombocytopenia, elevated liver enzymes, and elevated hematocrit. Dengue IgM/IgG serology or PCR to confirm the diagnosis.
- *Imaging*: Chest X-ray to assess for signs of severe dengue, including pleural effusions.

## PATHOPHYSIOLOGY

Dengue fever is caused by the dengue virus, which is transmitted through the bite of infected Aedes mosquitoes. The virus leads to vascular leakage and capillary fragility, contributing to the development of hemorrhages in multiple organs, including the retina. Retinal hemorrhages, along with other systemic manifestations such as thrombocytopenia, contribute to the severity of the disease. The inflammation and vascular damage during severe dengue may lead to retinal ischemia, leading to cotton-wool spots and hemorrhages visible on fundoscopy.

## TREATMENT AND PREVENTION

Treatment for dengue is primarily supportive, focusing on maintaining hydration, managing fever, and monitoring for complications like shock or bleeding. Platelet transfusions and blood products may be necessary in severe cases. Analgesics like paracetamol should be used cautiously, avoiding NSAIDs due to the risk of bleeding. Prevention relies on controlling mosquito populations and avoiding bites through the use of repellents, nets, and wearing protective clothing. Vaccination may be considered in endemic regions for those previously infected.

## Points to Ponder

- Early detection of retinal hemorrhages can significantly impact the management and prognosis of severe dengue fever.
- Dengue fever should be considered a differential diagnosis when a patient presents with fever, bleeding tendencies, and retinal involvement in endemic areas.
- The fundoscopic examination is crucial for detecting retinal hemorrhages, which is a marker of severe dengue-related vasculopathy.
- Thrombocytopenia in dengue fever can be associated with increased risk of bleeding, which requires careful monitoring and supportive care.
- Dengue prevention strategies, such as reducing mosquito breeding sites and using personal protection, are critical in controlling the spread of the disease.

## MULTIPLE CHOICE QUESTIONS

**1. Which of the following is a key sign in diagnosing dengue fever with retinal hemorrhages?**
- A. Hypertension
- B. Retinal hemorrhages on fundoscopy
- C. Reduced oxygen saturation
- D. High blood sugar levels

**2. Which mosquito is primarily responsible for transmitting the dengue virus?**
- A. Anopheles mosquito
- B. Aedes mosquito
- C. Culex mosquito
- D. Tabanid fly

**3. What is the most appropriate supportive treatment for a patient with dengue fever showing retinal hemorrhages?**
- A. Steroids
- B. Intravenous fluids
- C. Blood transfusion
- D. Antiviral therapy

**4. What is the primary laboratory test used to diagnose dengue fever?**
- A. PCR for dengue virus
- B. Complete blood count
- C. Liver function tests
- D. Dengue serology (IgM and IgG)

**5. Which of the following is a key warning sign of severe dengue fever?**
- A. Mild abdominal pain
- B. Petechiae and bleeding tendency
- C. Weight gain
- D. Decreased liver enzymes

### Answers

1. (B); 2. (B); 3. (B); 4. (D); 5. (B)

## SUGGESTED READINGS

1. World Health Organization. Dengue: Guidelines for Diagnosis, Treatment, Prevention, and Control. Geneva: WHO, 2009.
2. Simmons CP, Farrar JJ, Nguyen VV, et al. Dengue. The Lancet. 2012;379(9816):351-63.
3. Endy TP, Nisalak A. Dengue and Dengue Hemorrhagic Fever. Int J Infect Dis. 2002;6(5):289-97.
4. Thomas SM, Andrews EM. Retinal findings in dengue fever. J Clin Ophthalmol. 2016;10:101-4.
5. Wilder-Smith A, Schwartz E. Dengue in travelers. N Engl J Med. 2005;353:924-32.
6. Kittayapong P, Rattanarithikul R. The epidemiology and vector control of dengue in Thailand. Southeast Asian J Trop Med Public Health. 2006;37(6):24-8.

CHAPTER

97

# An Approach to a Case of Unknown Poisoning

*Amandeep Kaur, Niket Verma, Preeti Singh Dhoat, Rohit Raina*

**CASE VIGNETTE**

A 28-year-old female resident of the Malwa region of Punjab, presented to the emergency of AIIMS Bathinda with a history of ingesting an unknown pesticide following a marital dispute. Within 15 minutes of ingesting the unknown substance, the patient felt dizzy, followed by nausea and painful swallowing. After admission in the hospital, 2 hours after ingestion of the pesticide, the patient scored 13 out of 15 on the Glasgow coma scale, with equal and bilaterally reactive pupils and normal deep tendon reflexes. At presentation, the patient had bradycardia, with a heart rate of 37 beats/min, blood pressure of 114/60 mm Hg and a respiratory rate of 14 breaths/min. Gastric lavage was immediately performed, followed by bolus and maintenance doses of intravenous fluids. The patient's bradycardia persisted for 48 hours, and she remained drowsy for 54 hours. Although she was experiencing nausea, there was no vomiting, and she had not passed stools for the past two days. Respiratory depression, convulsions and hypothermia did not occur and urine output remained normal.

Electrocardiogram (ECG) revealed sinus bradycardia with a normal QT interval, and blood sugar levels were consistently within normal limits. The complete blood counts, liver function tests, renal function tests and serum electrolytes were monitored, and all showed normal results. Urine routine and serum creatinine remained normal and arterial blood gas (ABG) analysis indicated a pH of 7.41, $HCO_3$ of 22 and $PCO_2$ of 38 mm Hg, with no signs of hypoxia.

## PROVISIONAL DIAGNOSIS

Based on the clinical picture and history given by the patient's attendants a provisional diagnosis of poisoning with unknown substance was made.

## DIFFERENTIAL DIAGNOSIS

The following differentials may be kept in mind:

- Drug overdose (sedatives-hypnotics)
- Organophosphate (OPC) poisoning
- Carbamate toxicity

Based on the signs and symptoms of bradycardia and altered sensorium with a high suspicion of poisoning, cholinergic insecticidal poisoning was considered initially. But due to the presence of normal pupils with no cholinergic features, OPC or carbamate poisoning was ruled out.

## CLINICAL APPROACH

**When to suspect poisoning?**

- A history of any one or more of the following should arouse suspicion of poisoning
- Appearance of unexplained symptoms
- Altered sensorium without any obvious cause
- Psychiatric illness
- Recent declaration of exam/assessment results
- Discordant relationships at home/workplace
- Recent change in behavior

Any patient who presents with suspected poisoning should be assessed/managed as per the following protocol:

- Stabilization and maintaining C-A-B (circulation-airway-breathing)
- History taking
- Physical examination
- Laboratory assessment
- Toxidrome recognition
- Decontamination of the gastrointestinal tract, skin, or eyes
- Administration of specific antidote(s)
- Symptomatic and supportive care

A detailed physical examination should include vital signs, neurological examination, pupils, reflexes and posture, mental status, bowel sounds, mucous membranes and skin appearance, characteristic odors, nosebleeds, needle tracks and blistering. Changes in vital signs can help predict the underlying etiology in suspected poisoning cases. A few examples are shared in **Table 1**.

Toxidrome refers to the constellation of symptoms and signs seen in poisoning, which are characteristic to the type of toxic substance. Identifying the group of symptoms that make up a toxidrome, helps in identifying the broad class of the toxic substance and helps to guide treatment in the absence of a definitive etiology. Few important toxidromes and their characteristic clinical features are outlined in **Table 2**.

**TABLE 1: Probable etiology of poisoning based on changes in vital signs.**

| Bradycardia | Tachycardia |
|---|---|
| Beta-blockers, opiates | Cocaine, antipsychotics, amphetamines |
| Anticholinesterase drugs, antiarrhythmics | Anticholinergics, antihistamines, sympathomimetics |
| Clonidine, calcium channel blockers | Alcohol withdrawal |
| Ethanol or other alcohols | Solvent abuse, strychnine |
| Digoxin, digitalis | Thyroid hormones |
| **Hypotension** | **Hypertension** |
| Digoxin, digitalis | Cocaine, nicotine |
| Antidepressants, aminophylline, antihypertensives | Thyroid supplements |
| Rodenticides (containing arsenic, cyanide) | Sympathomimetics |
| Sedative-hypnotics, opiates | Caffeine, anticholinergics, amphetamines |
| **Hypothermia** | **Hyperthermia** |
| Carbon monoxide | Neuroleptic malignant syndrome, nicotine |
| Opioids, alcohol | Antihistamines, alcohol withdrawal |
| Oral hypoglycemics, insulin | Salicylates, sympathomimetics, serotonin syndrome |
| Sedative-hypnotics | Anticholinergics, antidepressants, antipsychotics |
| **Hypoventilation** | **Hyperventilation** |
| Sedative-hypnotics | Paraquat, pneumonitis (chemical), phosgene |
| Alcohols, opioids, marijuana | Salicylates, nerve agents |
| | Noncardiogenic pulmonary edema, toxin-induced metabolic acidosis |
| **Miosis** | **Mydriasis** |
| Cholinergics, clonidine, carbamates, sedative-hypnotics | Sympathomimetics |
| Opiates, organophosphates | Anticholinergics |
| Phenothiazines, pilocarpine, pontine hemorrhage | Withdrawal |

**TABLE 2: Important toxidromes and their characteristic clinical features.**

| Cholinergic toxidrome (OPCs, carbamates, pilocarpine) | Nicotinic side effects (OPCs, carbamates) |
|---|---|
| Diarrhea, diaphoresis | Mydriasis |
| Salivation, emesis, urination, lacrimation | Tachycardia |
| Miosis | Salivation |
| Bradycardia, bronchorrhea | Tremor, fasciculations, seizures |
| Lethargy, paralysis | Weakness, somnolence |
| **Anticholinergic toxidrome (antihistamines, atropine, datura, tricyclic antidepressants, antipsychotics)** | **Sympathomimetic toxidrome (antihistamines, atropine, datura, tricyclic antidepressants, antipsychotics)** |
| Mydriasis | Mydriasis, diaphoresis |
| Tachycardia, flushing, dry skin | Tachycardia, tachypnea |
| Hyperthermia | Hypertension, hyperthermia |
| Decreased gastric motility, urinary retention | Tremors, seizures |
| **Opioid toxidrome** | **Drug withdrawal** |
| Miosis | Lacrimation, diarrhea |
| Hypotension | Mydriasis, goose flesh, cramps |
| Hypoventilation | Tachycardia, hypertension |
| Coma | Yawning, hallucinations, seizures |

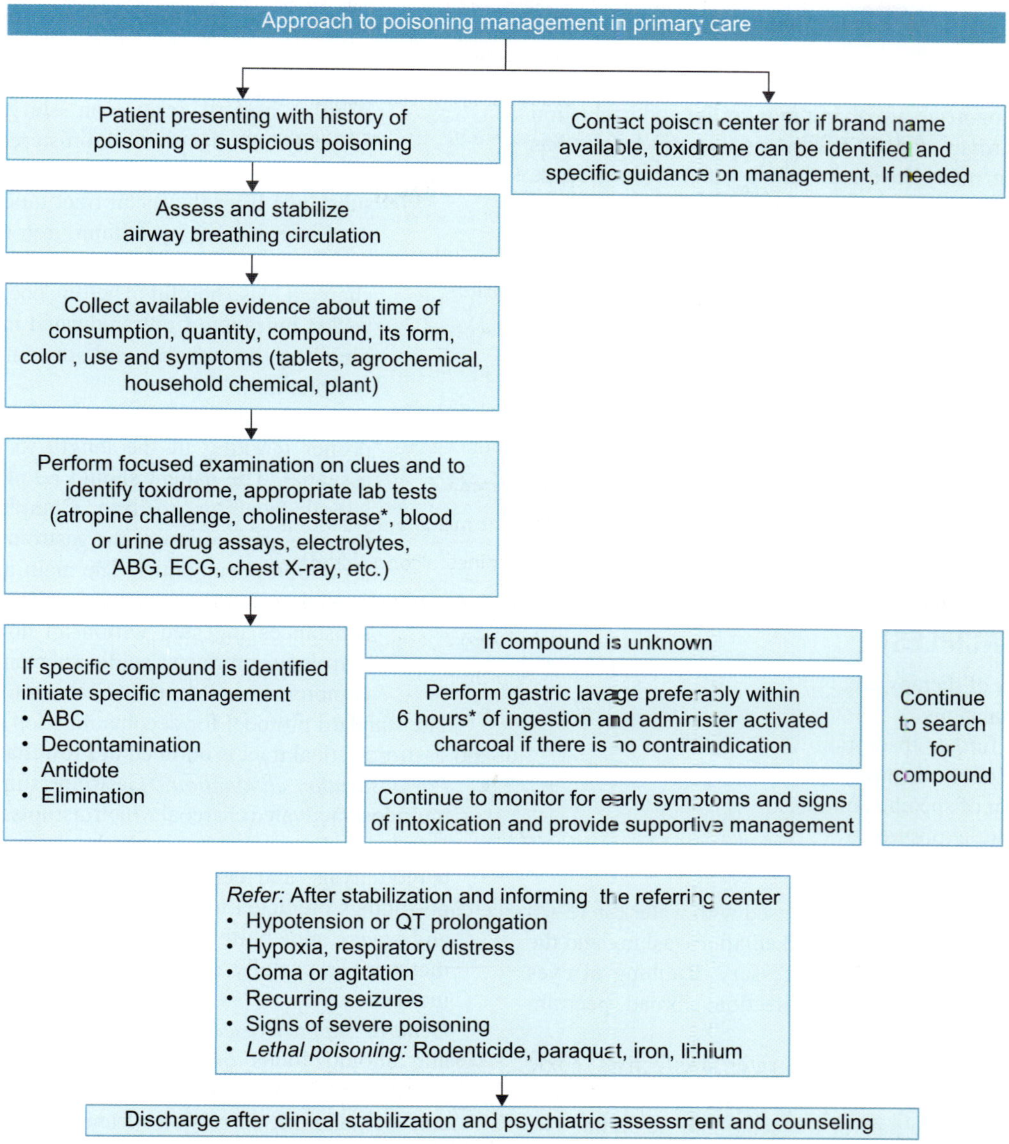


**FLOWCHART 1:** The standard approach to a case of unknown poisoning.

*Source*: Reproduced from Handbook of Poisoning Management Primary Care to Tertiary Care [Internet]. National Health Mission; 2022 [cited 2024 Nov 10]. Available from: chrome-extension://efaidnbmnnnibpcajpcglclefindmkaj/https://www.nhm.tn.gov.in/sites/default/files/2023-02/Hand%20Book%20poisoning%20management.pdf

The standard approach to a case of unknown poisoning is outlined in **Flowchart 1**.

## PATHOPHYSIOLOGY

Poisoning can be unintentional, suicidal, homicidal or of undetermined intent. Poisoning (26%) is the most common method of suicide in India (2019) after hanging (54%). Data from poison information centre of All India Institute of Medical Sciences (AIIMS) has shown that the highest incidence of poisoning is in the 14–40 years age group, with male preponderance. The common mode of poisoning was oral (88%) and the unknown category constituted 2.9% of the total poisonings.

In the above case, a diagnosis of Amitraz poisoning was made. Amitraz acts as an agonist on alpha-2 adrenergic receptors, stimulating these receptors in the central nervous system (CNS) and both alpha-1 and -2 receptors in the periphery, while also inhibiting the activity of monoamine oxidase and prostaglandin E2 synthesis. Its effects resemble those of clonidine and can often be mistaken for organophosphate poisoning or carbamate toxicity. Clinical manifestations include CNS and respiratory depression and cardiovascular effects. Most patients recover within 48 hours, with our patient recovering in 72 hours and being discharged. Action on alpha-1 and -2 receptors can cause bradycardia and hypotension, with some patients requiring atropine and intravenous fluids for resuscitation. Serum electrolyte levels and blood urea nitrogen are typically within normal limits in most cases.

There is no specific antidote for amitraz poisoning, and management is supportive, involving monitoring and evaluation of respiratory, cardiac, and CNS systems. Gastric lavage has been attempted in many cases, including ours, with atropine sulfate used to increase heart rate and prevent amitraz-induced bradycardia. Yohimbine, an alpha-2 antagonist, has been shown to prevent various effects of amitraz poisoning.

Gastric lavage should be performed only if the patient presents within 1 hour of ingestion and if a potentially lethal ingestion has occurred. In our case, due to early presentation and an unclear dose, gastric lavage was performed after excluding contraindications and the patient was then managed symptomatically. Although activated charcoal could have been considered, it was not administered. The case fatality rate of amitraz poisoning is 1.9%, and our patient was discharged asymptomatic on the third day.

## TREATMENT AND PREVENTION (GENERAL PRINCIPLES)

The primary goals of therapy are:
- Support of vital signs
- Prevention of further absorption
- Enhancement of elimination
- Administration of specific antidotes
- Prevention of re-exposure

*Decontamination*:
- *Eyes*: The affected eye should be rinsed with water for 15–20 minutes. The eye should be rechecked after washing and the procedure may be repeated if necessary. Rubbing of eyes should be avoided and in case of infection, a broad spectrum eye ointment should be prescribed.
- *Skin*: Rinsing or showering with water is effective. Toxic particles should be removed from under the nails, behind the ears and from the hair of the scalp and genitalia. The washing may be repeated after every 10 minutes till the toxic particles are completely removed. Contaminated clothing should be removed. In the case of skin burns caused by toxin exposure, the established burns management protocol must be followed.
- *Gastrointestinal tract:*
  - Pre-absorption elimination:
    - Gastric emptying—preferably within 60 minutes of ingesting a poison
    - Activated charcoal—binds different substances, making them less accessible for systemic absorption in the gastrointestinal tract. It is effective if administered within an hour after ingestion. Multiple-dose activated charcoal can eliminate life-threatening toxic doses of substances that undergo enteroenteric or enterohepatic circulation, e.g., salicylates, phenobarbital, dapsone, digitoxin, quinine, theophylline, etc. Not recommended in poisoning due to heavy metals, acids, alkalis or alcohol.
    - Whole bowel irrigation—large amount of polyethylene glycol is administered through either mouth or nasogastric tube to remove the toxic substance from the rectal tract quickly. Commonly used in poisoning by lithium, iron or enteric-coated drugs which are poorly absorbed by activated charcoal. Also helpful in heroin, cocaine, and opioids packet ingestion. Contraindicated in gastrointestinal bleeding or mechanical or functional bowel obstructions.
    - Gastric lavage—correct selection of tube size and proper marking of the length to be inserted are essential. The patient should be placed in the left-lateral decubitus position. Complications include hypoxia, perforation of the gastrointestinal tract and aspiration pneumonitis. The main indication for the procedure is to prevent severe harm caused by the substances ingested within an hour. Ingestion of petroleum products, acidic substances, and airway compromise are contraindications to this procedure.

The standard protocol for decontamination of the skin, eyes and gastrointestinal tract is outlined in **Flowchart 2**.

- *Postabsorption elimination*: "Gastrointestinal dialysis" uses multidose-activated charcoal which disrupts the enterohepatic circulation. Extracorporeal methods, e.g., peritoneal dialysis, hemodialysis, and hemoperfusion, should be utilized for poisonings predicted to result in toxic metabolic activation and severe metabolic acidosis, e.g., ethylene glycol and methanol, especially when other treatment modalities are ineffective.
- *General supportive care*: It should continue side by side and should focus on airway protection, oxygenation/ventilation, hemodynamic support, treatment of seizures and arrhythmias, correction of temperature and metabolic abnormalities derangements.
- *Antidote administration*: In most cases, an initial use of an antidote is recommended for stabilization within the first hour following exposure to a known substance. Some examples of toxins and their specific antidotes are shared in **Table 3**.
- *Monitoring and discharge*: In many cases of poisoning, the specific toxic substance is unknown. It is crucial to closely monitor the patient's oxygen saturation, vital signs, and cardiac rhythm, especially in those with underlying medical conditions. Unstable patients whose airways cannot be protected may need to be transferred to an intensive care unit for continuous monitoring and ventilator support. A comprehensive monitoring strategy must be prepared and a multidisciplinary team approach is highly recommended. The decision to discharge a patient who has intentionally self-poisoned must be made after a thorough psychiatric assessment.

**Poisoning management-decontamination**

Skin should be washed thoroughly with soap and water including genital area and clothes changed, if skin contamination is present

For eyes exposure—cleaned using syringe with clear saline or water for injection for 10–15 minutes

Gastric lavage

*Indications:*

- Life-threatening poisoning and unconscious presentation within 1 hour with precautions to prevent aspiration
- For pesticide poisoning—gastric lavage is useful within 6 hours and can be extended even after 6 hours if clinical condition warrants
- Tablet poisoning with anticholinergic effects presentation within 4 hours
- Sustained release preparation, salicylates, heavy metals within 12 hours
- Iron or lithium poisoning

*Contraindications:*

- Corrosive
- Comatose patients (secure airway before gastric lavage)

*Procedure:*

- Left lateral position.
- Use Ryle's tube
- First aspirate the stomach contents and store the first content for medico legal purpose
- Use normal saline or clean tap water, infuse 200 mL at time and aspirate. Repeat process till the aspirate is clear.

*Complications:*

- Aspiration
- Trauma

*Activated charcoal* 1 g/kg as a single dose for poisoning with significant toxicity, if ingestion less than 1–2 hours

Multiple dose activated charcoal 1 g/kg q4h

*Indication:* Oleander poisoning, carbamazepine, dapsone, phenobarbital, quinine and theophylline

Both can be given orally or through Ryle's tube diluted in 150 mL of water

*Contraindications:* Ileus, vomiting, corrosive poisoning, kerosene poisoning

*Polyethylene glycol (PEG)*

*Indications:* Poisonings where activated charcoal alone is not satisfactory

- Iron and lithium
- Sustained release preparations (e.g., theophylline and verapamil)
- Toxins that form pharmacobezoars (e.g., salicylates)

*Procedure:* PEG given either orally or through nasogastric tube at 2 L/h for 2–6 hours

**FLOWCHART 2:** The standard protocol for decontamination of the skin, eyes and gastrointestinal tract in suspected poisoning.

*Source*: Reproduced from Handbook of Poisoning Management Primary Care to Tertiary Care [Internet]. National Health Mission; 2022 [cited 2024 Nov 10]. Available from: chrome-extension://efaidnbmnnnibpcajpcglclefindmkaj/https://www.nhm.tn.gov.in/sites/default/files/2023-02/Hand%20Book%20poisoning%20management.pdf

**TABLE 3: Examples of toxins and their specific antidotes.**

| Toxin | Antidote |
|---|---|
| Ethylene glycol, methanol | Fomepizole |
| Organophosphates | Atropine, pralidoxime |
| Opioids | Naloxone |
| Benzodiazepines | Flumazenil |
| Methemoglobinemia | Methylene blue |
| Beta-blockers | Glucagon |
| Cyanide | Sodium nitrite |
| Tricyclic antidepressants | Bicarbonate |
| Iron | Deferoxamine |
| Coumadin anticoagulants | Vitamin K |
| Acetaminophen | N-acetylcysteine |
| Anticholinergics | Physostigmine |

**Points to Ponder**

Remember the 10 golden rules regarding the management of a case of unknown poisoning:

1. Correct immediate life-threatening respiratory and circulatory disturbances.
2. Many patients of suspected poisoning may recover with simple supportive measures.
3. Alleviate the anxiety of the patients and the family members.
4. Assess the condition and vital signs of the patient frequently.
5. Encourage attendants to bring the remaining poisonous substance for identifying the agent and the antidote.
6. All cases of poisoning may not necessarily require tertiary care.
7. Never be carried away just because vital signs are stable at the time of presentation, since the toxic manifestations may appear later.
8. It is ideal to observe the poison cases for 24–48 hours before discharge.
9. Every poison case is different from others.
10. Treating the patient is more important than identifying the causative agent.

## MULTIPLE CHOICE QUESTIONS

1. **Which one of the following is an antidote for organophosphate poisoning?**
   A. Atropine
   B. Physostigmine
   C. Magnesium sulphate
   D. Penicillamine
2. **The cholinergic toxidrome include all of the following, except:**
   A. Diarrhea
   B. Diaphoresis
   C. Mydriasis
   D. Bronchospasm
3. **Toxicity of which one of the following may cause hypothermia?**
   A. Antihistamines
   B. Anticholinergics
   C. Salicylates
   D. Oral hypoglycemics
4. **Which one of the following is not a contraindication of gastric lavage?**
   A. Coma
   B. Sulphuric acid poisoning
   C. Convulsions
   D. Organophosphate poisoning
5. **Activated charcoal is effective in poisoning with which one of the following?**
   A. Corrosive agents
   B. Ethylene glycol
   C. Kerosene
   D. Carbamazepine

### Answers

1. (A); 2. (C); 3. (D); 4. (D); 5. (D)

## SUGGESTED READINGS

1. Handbook of Poisoning Management Primary Care to Tertiary Care [Internet]. National Health Mission; 2022 [cited 2024 Nov 10]. Available from: chrome-extension://efaidnbmnnnibpcajpcglclefindmkaj/https://www.nhm.tn.gov.in/sites/default/files/2023-02/Hand%20Book%20poisoning%20management.pdf
2. Prakash J, Singh PK, Kotwal A, et al. Unknown poisoning amongst serving personnel. Med J Armed Forces India [Internet]. 2009;65(1):41-3
3. Kaswa R. An approach to the management of acute poisoning in emergency settings. S Afr Fam Pract. [Internet]. 2024;66(1):e1-5.
4. Raina R, Singh R, Dhoat PS, et al. Amitraz poisoning: a rare case of suicidal poisoning from Malwa region of Punjab and role of early gastric lavage in preventing complications. Int J Community Med Public Health. 2024;11:4064-6.

# Index

Page numbers followed by *b* refer to box, *f* refer to figure, *fc* refer to flowchart, and *t* refer to table.

## A

## B

## C

## D

## E



## F

## G



## H

## I



## J



## K



## L

## M

## P

## Q



## R